FUNCTIONAL
MOVEMENT
DEVELOPMENT
Across the Life Span

FUNCTIONAL MOVEMENT DEVELOPMENT
Across the Life Span

FOURTH EDITION

EDITORS

Donna J. Cech, PT, DHS, Certified Specialist in Pediatric Physical Therapy (PCS)
Professor and Program Director (retired)
Physical Therapy
Midwestern University
Downers Grove, Illinois
United States

Suzanne "Tink" Martin, PT, PhD
Professor Emerita
Physical Therapy
University of Evansville
Evansville, Indiana
United States

ASSOCIATE EDITOR

William H. Staples, PT, DHSc, DPT, Clinical Specialist in Geriatric Physical Therapy (GCS), FAPTA
Professor Emeritus
Krannert School of Physical Therapy
University of Indianapolis
Indianapolis, Indiana
United States

ELSEVIER

Elsevier
3251 Riverport Lane
St. Louis, Missouri 63043

FUNCTIONAL MOVEMENT DEVELOPMENT ACROSS THE LIFE SPAN,
FOURTH EDITION

ISBN: 978-0-323-87799-2

Notice

Practitioners and researchers must always rely on their own experience and knowledge in evaluating and using any information, methods, compounds or experiments described herein. Because of rapid advances in the medical sciences, in particular, independent verification of diagnoses and drug dosages should be made. To the fullest extent of the law, no responsibility is assumed by Elsevier, authors, editors or contributors for any injury and/or damage to persons or property as a matter of products liability, negligence or otherwise, or from any use or operation of any methods, products, instructions, or ideas contained in the material herein.

Senior Content Strategist: Lauren Willis
Content Development Specialist: Ranjana Sharma
Publishing Services Manager: Deepthi Unni
Senior Project Manager: Kamatchi Madhavan
Design Direction: Margaret Reid

Printed in India

Last digit is the print number: 9   8   7   6   5   4   3   2   1

To our families for their support and to all of the therapists we have had the pleasure of meeting as they began their careers. We also want to thank our former patients who have taught us so much about what it means to be a therapist. To the current students utilizing this text, we hope to generate a passion to become the best therapist you can be. Our hope is to impart the knowledge we have gained on our professional journeys to the next generation of therapists.

Many thanks to Tim for his chapter contribution through the past editions and his support in this fourth edition, as he played a key role in the merging of Posture, Balance, and Locomotion into one chapter. His consultation related to current best literature is much appreciated. His contributions to chapters on Motor Learning and Motor Control have also been an important part of this book in several editions.

Many thanks to Susan V Duff, EdD, OTR/l. PT, CHT, DCP, for her contributions to the first three editions of this book, writing and updating the chapter, Prehension. Her framework and content in the first three editions of the book have been maintained in this fourth edition, and we hope that the updates we have included meet with her approval.

CONTRIBUTOR

Timothy Hanke, PT, PhD
Professor
Physical Therapy
Midwestern University
Downers Grove, Illinois
Posture, Balance, and Locomotion

ABOUT THE AUTHORS

Donna Joy Cech, PT, DHS, retired as professor and program director of the physical therapy program at Midwestern University in Downers Grove, IL. She earned a Bachelor of Science and Physical Therapy from the University of Wisconsin, Madison, WI; a Master of Science in Physical Therapy from Rosalind Franklin University, North Chicago; and a Doctor of Health Science degree from the University of Indianapolis. Donna was recognized as a Board Certified Specialist in Pediatric Physical Therapy in 1986, the first year the American Board of Physical Therapy Specialties offered the specialization, and has maintained this certification since that time. She has practiced in pediatric settings of hospitals (in the United States and Switzerland), school systems, early intervention, and home health. Donna has taught in two different entry-level education programs over 33 years, including serving 18 years as a program director. She has been a member of the American Physical Therapy Association for over 50 years; a member of Academies of Pediatrics and Education, APTA; and International Organizations of Physical Therapists in Pediatrics (World Physiotherapy). Currently, Donna continues to serve as a volunteer in physical therapy education and services, primarily in South America.

Suzanne "Tink" Martin, PT, MACT, PhD, is a Professor Emerita of the University of Evansville, Department of Physical Therapy. She earned a Bachelor of Science in Biology from Tulane University; Certificate in Physical Therapy from Duke University; a Masters of Art in College Teaching (Pediatric Physical Therapy) from the University of North Carolina; and a PhD in Rehabilitation Sciences from the University of Kentucky. Tink's pediatric clinical experience includes acute and outpatient care in a children's hospital, early intervention, and rehabilitation. Tink taught in an entry-level program for 37 years with a focus on pediatrics and neurologic rehabilitation. She has coauthored two entry-level textbooks: *Functional Movement Development Across the Lifespan*, fourth edition in press and *Neurologic Interventions in Physical Therapy*, fourth edition. Tink has been an APTA member for 54 years, serving as delegate and chief delegate of the Indiana Chapter, and President of the Academy of Pediatric Physical Therapy. She is an Emerita Fellow of the Academy of Cerebral Palsy and Developmental Medicine. Tink has received the Dean's outstanding teaching award and the Sadelle and Sydney Berger Scholarship award from the University of Evansville. She has also received outstanding service awards: the Bud DeHaven, Section on Pediatrics, APTA; the Fran Ekstam, Indiana Chapter, APTA; and the Lucy Blair Award, APTA.

William "Bill" Staples, PT, DHSc, DPT, FAPTA, is a Board-Certified Specialist in Geriatric Physical Therapy, Certified Exercise Expert for Aging Adults, Advanced Credentialed Exercise Expert for Aging Adults, and is an Associate Professor at the Krannert School of Physical Therapy at the University of Indianapolis. He earned a Certificate in Physical Therapy and Masters from Columbia University. He earned his Doctor of Health Science and Doctorate of Physical Therapy from the University of Indianapolis. Bill was named as a Catherine Worthingham Fellow in 2021. He has been a Geriatric Clinical Specialist (GCS) since 1995 and is a past president of the Academy of Geriatric Physical Therapy. Bill has lectured locally, nationally, and internationally on a variety of geriatric physical therapy issues and is an instructor in the Certification for Exercise Experts for Aging Adults program. His research has investigated exercise and Parkinson disease, fear of falling, use of dementia screening by physical therapists, comparison of mood to physical function in older adults, and attitudes toward working with patients with dementia. He has also authored a textbook entitled *Geriatric Physical Therapy: A Case Study Approach*, which was first published in 2016, and a second edition in 2021. Bill maintains his clinical skills by working part-time at a rehabilitation hospital.

Movement is a key to fully participating in meaningful life activities. It is necessary for safety, survival, mobility, occupation, leisure, health, and fitness. Functional movement plays a role throughout the span of everyone's life and contributes to our complete development. The ability to move changes across the life span—influenced by the development of the body systems that contribute to movement (muscular, skeletal, nervous, cardiopulmonary, endocrine). The motivation to move is innate, but the sociocultural environment and the psychological development influence each person's development and functional movement. Each person's experiences in life are unique and affect development. This perspective reflects how important it is for a health care provider to integrate a thorough understanding of life course perspectives (physical, psychological, and social-emotional development), the role/function of each body system contributing to movement across the life span, and the World Health Organization model, the International Classification of Functioning, Disability, and Health (ICF), into the care provided to individuals across the life span.

The fourth edition of this text continues to be intended primarily for students of physical therapy, occupational therapy, and other professions that address movement dysfunction. This edition continues to emphasize normal development and focuses on the definitions of function and participation, how they are attained, and how participation is optimized across the life span. For therapists to best support optimal participation for patients and clients, they must appreciate not only the physical, social-emotional, and psychological developmental sequences but also a unique understanding of the normal development of the cellular and systems development that contribute to functional movement across the life span. An understanding of these factors contributes to the therapist's clinical decision-making.

In the fourth edition, we welcome associate editor William Staples, PT, DHSc. His expertise in geriatric physical therapy as well as his understanding of exercise principles for older adults have been a valuable addition to this new edition. With Dr. Staples contributions

to each chapter of this book, we are confident that this edition provides an up-to-date, in-depth insight into functional movement for the adult and older adult populations. Another expansion to the fourth edition is the inclusion of the movement system framework, acknowledging the role of muscular, skeletal, cardiopulmonary, nervous, integumentary, and endocrine systems in functional human movement.

This book is organized into three units that will provide the reader with the background and tools necessary to understand the components of functional movement. Unit I reviews the biophysical, psychological, and sociocultural domains of development. This information assists the therapist in effectively communicating and working with patients of any age. Readers are also guided in integrating important theories of development into clinical decision-making models. The most current information about motor development, motor learning, and motor control is provided.

Unit II adds a comprehensive review of how body systems develop and affect functional movement from the prenatal period through older adulthood. All chapters have been updated to include current best evidence related to their development and role in functional movement. Basic information on anatomy, physiology, and histology of the systems has been condensed to identify only those aspects of body system function and structure that change across the life span and influence functional mobility. Clinical Implications sidebars are included to help students apply the information to clinical practice.

Unit III focuses on functional outcomes key to mobility and participation in meaningful life activities. Age-related trends in balance, posture, locomotion, and prehension are presented. Finally, Chapter 13 discusses the issues of health and fitness, heightening awareness of the therapist's role in wellness and prevention issues across the life span. Clinical Implications sidebars again give the reader insights into the relationships between normal development and clinical practice.

The combined content of all three units of this text provides the reader with key information related to life span development, which when considered within clinical decision-making, supports optimal development of function, participation, health, and quality of life of the patients served.

Donna J. Cech, PT, DHS
Board-Certified Clinical Specialist in Pediatric
Physical Therapy
Professor and Program Director (retired)
Physical Therapy Program
Midwestern University
Downers Grove, Illinois

Suzanne "Tink" Martin, PT, PhD
Professor Emerita
Department of Physical Therapy
University of Evansville
Evansville, Indiana

William H. Staples, PT, DHSc, DPT, FAPTA
Board-Certified Clinical Specialist in Geriatric
Physical Therapy (GCS)
Certified Exercise Expert for Aging Adults (CEEAA)
Fellow of the American Physical Therapy
Association
Associate Professor
Krannert School of Physical Therapy
University of Indianapolis
Indianapolis, Indiana

ACKNOWLEDGMENTS

We wish to thank the professional colleagues and many students who have provided feedback on our efforts and have offered encouragement since the inception of this book. We appreciate the contributions of Susan Duff, EdD, OTR/L, PT, CHT, BCP, over more than 20 years and many editions of this book. Many thanks to Jennifer Bottomley, PT, PhD, for helping us better address issues related to older adults in earlier editions of this book and contributions of Ann F. Vansant, PT, PhD, Patricia Wilder, PT, PhD, and Lori Quinn PT, EdD, to the first and second editions of the book, helping set the course for the book as it has developed and matured.

We also want to thank our friends and family for their continued support and encouragement. Terry, Jim, Linda, and Alec, your patience and understanding are so important to us. We acknowledge our parents for instilling in us the confidence that helped us to pursue a project of this scope.

We would also like to thank the many people in the publishing world who have supported and worked with us over the course of this project. We would like to thank our development editor, Ranjana Sharma, for providing access to the resources needed to complete such an immense project and overseeing the final product. We would like to thank Lauren Willis at Elsevier for recognizing the need for a major update of this text. Our special regards go to Margaret Biblis for starting this entire process and for her continued friendship and encouragement.

TINK

Meg Atwater-Singer, the access librarian at the University of Evansville, has been an immense support during the updating of this edition. She and her staff procured voluminous numbers of interlibrary loans. A special thank you to Tim Hanke, PhD, PT, from Midwestern University, who did a magnificent job of reviewing two chapters and guiding the merger of them into a new updated chapter on Posture, Balance, and Locomotion. He has provided expertise and a sense of humor during the process. Our associate editor, Bill Staples, brought his vast geriatric knowledge to the entire project and provided balance to the life span concept so integral to this text. Thank you to Donna, a friend and colleague for the majority of my years in the physical therapy profession. She was the rudder of the project, the quality controller, and the maintainer of the vision of this extraordinary text. She also helped me stay on track and avoid interesting but deadly rabbit holes.

DONNA

This project could not have been completed without the friendship and contributions of Tink over the past three plus decades. Also many thanks to Bill Staples for joining us in this fourth edition and helping us best address issues related to aging and older adulthood, as well as his general editorial improvements. I would also like to thank the University of Evansville library for assisting me in accessing up-to-date evidence supporting the text.

BILL

I would like to thank the co-editors, Tink and Donna, for inviting me to join this edition of the text. As a lifelong learner, this enhanced my understanding of the movement system, especially since childhood is an area outside my normal knowledge base. To the University of Indianapolis library for granting me access to a multitude of materials, many thanks. Lastly, I would like to thank my wife, two daughters—Catherine and Courtney—and three grandsons—Luke, James, and Graham—for the patience they showed while I missed some time together that enabled me to complete this project.

It is such a simple idea to think about looking at movement across a life span but it is a daunting task to make sense of all the information and new discoveries that occur on a daily basis. We have succeeded in raising the level of understanding of how the body systems change over time and how those changes support movement and function for individuals across the life span in this fourth edition.

Thank you
Donna J. Cech, PT, DHS
Board-Certified Clinical Specialist in Pediatric
Physical Therapy (PCS)

Suzanne "Tink" Martin, PT, PhD, MACT

William H. Staples, PT, DHSc, DPT, FAPTA
Board-Certified Clinical Specialist in Geriatric
Physical Therapy (GCS)
Certified Exercise Expert for Aging Adults (CEEAA)
Fellow of the American Physical Therapy Association

CONTENTS

*Contributing author

CONTENTS

1

Functional Independence: A Lifelong Goal

OBJECTIVES

After studying this chapter, the reader will be able to:
1. Define function as it relates to participation in life roles.
2. Appreciate the interrelationship of all domains of function in everyday life.
3. Discuss the relationship of functional abilities to health status.
4. Discuss factors contributing to participation in life roles within the framework of the
International Classification of Functioning, Disability, and Health.
5. Discuss the role of the movement system in optimizing participation in life roles and health status.
6. Appreciate life span issues related to participation and functional ability.
7. Identify the aspects of physical function that relate to quality of performance.

As humans, we strive to fully and actively participate in life roles and learn to exist within our environment. Throughout our life span, we constantly develop or adapt our abilities and skills to live our lives in a satisfying and meaningful manner. The capacity to exist within the environment is influenced by our ability to function, and the quality of our functional ability is related to all aspects of development: physical, social, emotional, and mental. In this book, we approach development as an ongoing, lifelong process and explore its influence on functional movement ability.

Improving our client's ability to fully participate in life roles is frequently our goal as health care professionals. Various health care professionals strive to help their clients optimize different aspects of function to realize the most satisfying and meaningful life possible. To meet this goal most effectively, we must understand the meaning of the word *function* within our respective disciplines. For example, physicians and nurses may focus primarily on the attainment and maintenance of good health as related to function, whereas social workers concentrate on an individual's ability to function within a social system. Occupational therapists work to improve the ability to function in daily life and to perform occupational tasks, whereas physical therapists structure programs to enhance physical function and mobility. All of these aspects of function are, of course, interdependent, and when considered as a conceptual whole, they help to reflect a person's ability to function or participate within our society and environment. The World Health Organization[1] defines the involvement of an individual in life situations as participation within the International Classification of Functioning, Disability, and Health (ICF).

1

FUNCTION

Widely accepted definitions of the word *function* include such phrases as "normal, characteristic actions," "purpose," and "group of related actions." More generally, function is a natural, required, or expected activity. When related to the roles and activities of people, the term *function* can describe the action of an individual body part or the person as a whole. The heart functions to pump blood through the body, delivering nutrients to other organs and tissues. The legs function to support our body weight during standing and to propel us forward during walking. We gain mastery over the environment, functioning to complete roles and tasks important to everyday life.

Function as Related to Health

Function is very closely related to health. As globally defined by the World Health Organization (WHO), *health* is a state of complete physical, mental, and social well-being, not merely the absence of disease and infirmity.[2] This simple definition is difficult to use clinically because well-being is hard to measure and too broad a concept to accurately portray an individual's status. More specifically, health influences our ability to successfully complete the tasks expected by society. Without the necessary functional abilities, it is difficult to complete these tasks or to demonstrate a state of complete physical, mental, and social well-being. Well-being has been defined as the state of being happy and healthy. Within

the field of psychology, well-being is "a state of happiness and contentment, with low levels of distress, overall *good* physical and mental *health* and outlook, or *good* quality of life." From another perspective, well-being and functional ability can be disrupted as a result of poor health. Disease, infirmity, and illness interfere with our capacity to perform socially expected roles. It therefore is not difficult to understand why health professionals endeavor to improve how an individual functions.

International Classification of Functioning, Disability, and Health

The ICF provides a biopsychosocial model to describe the health of people as they function within their environment, highlighting the relationship between function and health. The ICF provides a framework from which to examine the relationships between the biological, personal, and social factors influencing health (Fig. 1.1). How well a person functions and participates in socially expected roles is influenced by a person's health condition, body structure and function, and personal and environmental factors.

The ICF considers the biological construct of function through consideration of the body functions and structures. *Body functions* reflect the physiological processes that support a person's health and ability to participate in important activities. Anatomical support for health and function is reflected by consideration of *body structures*. The brain and all components of the nervous system are part of that support so that mental functions

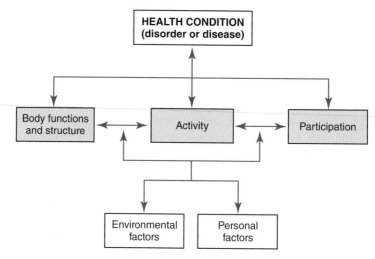

Fig. 1.1 Model of the International Classification of Functioning, Disability, and Health (ICF).

and sensory functions are included along with motor functions in this construct. Physical and psychological functions are both supported by body functions and structures.

Personal factors also contribute to a person's overall health and ability to perform tasks related to participation in life activities. In defining health, obvious personal factors such as sex, race, and age are considered. In addition, a person's lifestyle, level of fitness, social background, culture, and value system are important personal characteristics that contribute to the definition of health. People who believe they have the ability to positively influence their own health and well-being are more likely to value advice from a health care professional and shift from risky behavior to healthy behavior. Promotion of health and wellness involves participation in positive health behaviors such as participation in an active lifestyle and self-management of chronic health conditions.

Similarly, health is certainly influenced by the environment in which one lives. In considering the environmental context of health, not only the physical environment, but also the social and attitudinal environments need to be considered. The *physical environment* includes consideration of basic factors such as climate and geography. Living in urban or rural settings also influences the physical environment in which a person functions. Similarly, where a person lives also helps define the person's social and attitudinal environment. *Social environment* includes a person's support system and social relationships. Family, friends, community, and civic groups are some of the many social relationships a person may have. Health professionals are part of the support system for a person with health issues. The *attitudinal environment* not only reflects the general attitudes of society but also includes the programs provided within a community to support health and well-being, the policies that define these resources, and the systems in place within a community that support health and well-being. For example, availability of public education, parks and recreation facilities, and public transportation are services. Examples of local and national laws and policies include local ordinances banning smoking and national health insurance regulations such as Medicare or Medicaid. Health insurance availability and regulations also contribute to the attitudinal environment. The multiple facets of the environment impact significantly upon a person's health, functional abilities, and participation.

Client Assessment

To identify client needs and to develop interventions, health professionals must be able to measure an individual's health status. Health status can be measured by looking at three primary arenas: (1) physical manifestations, (2) client symptoms, and (3) functional status.[3] *Physical manifestations* are those aspects of body function that can be measured or observed, such as muscle strength, body temperature, blood pressure, and the presence of edema. *Client symptoms* reflect the client's impression of her health. The client may report a painful knee, weakness, fatigue, or generally feeling good. *Functional status* reflects how well the client is able to perform day-to-day activities. Illness and injury, then, influence health status and can reduce one's ability to function. The impact of this reduction varies. Some people lose little ground in keeping up with their day-to-day tasks, whereas others may not be able to do the things they need to do. The reduction in function may also reflect where the person is on the developmental continuum. The amount of physiological reserve or resilience available to come back from an illness or injury lessens with older age. The terms *disability* and *handicap* are frequently used when daily tasks cannot be performed.

In general, *disability* refers to an individual's diminished functional capacity.[3] *Handicap* is a frame of reference defined by society; when individuals are no longer viewed as being able to perform the tasks expected by society, they are considered handicapped. However, the loss of functional ability does not necessarily result in disability or handicap. A person may lose some shoulder range of motion without incurring a problem with function, whereas the loss of a limb would be considered a disability and depending on architectural barriers may be a handicap. *Disability* is the overarching term to connote impairments, activity limitations, or restrictions in participation. Changes in health and functioning can take place at any time of life because of disease, disorder, or injury and take place inevitably as we get older.[4]

In the evaluation of the health status of individuals, health care providers need to understand each client's life roles and optimal levels of participation. Such assessment allows the provider to focus on the issues most important to the individual and to consider whether interventions can minimize an activity limitation or diminish participation restrictions. The ICF directs the provider to identify not only the impairments but also the personal and environmental factors that may be limiting performance of activities and participation in life roles. From this framework, an intervention approach can be designed that will focus on function rather than one solely directed to remediation of impairments. For example, work simplification may be as effective in improving function as a strengthening program for a person with chronic pain. Use of the ICF framework when working with clients helps the health care provider focus on assisting the person in maximizing participation in life situations and roles. Solutions are looked for within the social and attitudinal environments in which the person functions and within the person's physical environment.

In working with people of different ages, it is also important to understand the role of development in the acquisition of functional skills and the ability to perform activities. Is the 3-year-old child who cannot tie a shoe disabled? Of course not. Developmentally, it is normal for a young child to require adult assistance with this task. By 8 years of age, the child usually has developed this skill and no longer needs adult assistance. If older adults with severe arthritis cannot put on their shoes because of limitations in hip flexion or finger mobility, are they disabled? Again, not necessarily. The person may be quite good at completing the task by using a long-handled shoehorn. Similarly, it is not uncommon for adults to use glasses or hearing aids to maximize ability to participate in life roles as they age. Developmental issues, social expectations, family attitudes, and adaptability of the environment are all issues that help determine whether limitations are present.

Functional Activities Leading to Participation

Functional activities are those activities that contribute to an individual's physical, social, and psychological well-being. These activities include self-care, household, vocational, and recreational tasks, allowing an individual to perform as independently as possible in all settings. Functional skills and activities not only support our biophysical and psychological well-being but also allow us to incorporate what we view as important into meaningful, everyday life. From early infancy to late adulthood, we must develop or adapt functional skills to best access the environment in which we live and to meet our own needs as independently as possible. The performance of functional activities not only depends on our physical abilities but also is affected by our emotional

status, cognitive ability, and sociocultural expectations. These factors together define an individual's functional performance.

In general, certain categories of functional activities, such as eating, maintaining personal hygiene, dressing, ambulating, and grasping, are common to everyone. Other tasks related to our job or recreational activities vary from one person to the next. Within the health care model, personal care activities such as ambulating, feeding, bathing, dressing, grooming, maintaining continence, and toileting are referred to as *basic activities of daily living (BADL)*. Other important activities relate to how well we manage within the home setting and in the community. These activities are referred to as *instrumental activities of daily living (IADL)* and include tasks such as cooking, cleaning, handling finances, shopping, working, and using personal or public transportation. The health care provider often assesses BADL and IADL to define client status and to develop appropriate intervention programs. In addition to BADL and IADL, participation in life roles, social activities, and leisure activities is important to consider in defining a person's function and participation. Life roles may include going to school, performing a job, and parenting. Social activities include activities with friends and relatives, membership in a church, and participation in community activities. Leisure activities include hobbies, sports and recreation, and vacations.[5]

Function From a Life Span Perspective

Function defines mastery and competency over the environment. Throughout the life span, from conception until old age, we demonstrate varying abilities and levels of mastery over our environment. Initially, we are concerned with being able to survive and master a level of function concerned with the locus of self-need and control. Next, we learn to function well within the home environment, and finally we learn to function within the community (Fig. 1.2). For example, to ensure survival, the infant learns to cry for food or when experiencing discomfort. The infant can also turn the head to keep the airway clear and can coordinate important tasks, such as breathing and swallowing. The toddler learns to function safely within the home: avoiding electrical outlets, climbing stairs, independently eating, and using the toilet. The school-age child learns to safely cross the street on the way to school. These same levels of mastery are mirrored at all life stages as functional expectations

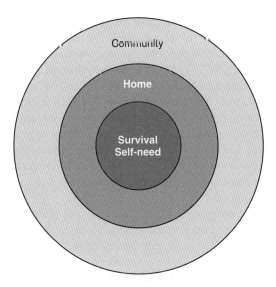

Fig. 1.2 Acquisition of function. The concentric circles illustrate that acquisition of function begins with a focus on self, the locus of self-need and control, which evolves to increased levels of mastery over a broadening environment.

change. The adult masters the self-care tasks of eating by shopping and cooking or dining out and providing a clean and warm shelter. Finally, the adult masters functioning in a larger community, including the workplace.

From these examples, it is obvious that our functional ability is in part defined by age. As children become older, they are expected to gain independence in a wide variety of functional tasks and in an expanding environment. The 5-year-old child must meet the challenges of becoming competent within the new environment of school. Many 16-year-old youths assume the responsibilities of safely driving a car and functioning within their community. The functional expectations of adults expand as they have children and assume job responsibilities. Older adults may appear to be faced with fewer functional expectations as they retire and their children become independent. They may also be faced with challenges related to maintaining functional independence of even basic needs as they adapt to fixed incomes and declining physical abilities. Older adults, when asked to define successful aging, have emphasized the importance of being able to care for themselves and coping with challenges in their later years,[6] emphasizing the importance of functional independence and participation. It is clear that the definitions of function and

functional independence change across the life span as our abilities change and the expectations of society vary.

Physical Growth and Function

In many ways, our functional abilities depend on physical abilities. Physical development not only influences the ability to perform physical activity but also affects our ability to interact with the environment. Movement has been related to cognitive development, social activity, and communication. Across the life span, the physical capacity of the individual changes and helps to define functional capacity. Observation and analysis of movement is a primary skill for therapists to master. Current theories of motor control emphasize that movement comes from the complex interaction between the environment, the specific task, and the individual.[7,8]

During the embryonic development of a human, the first 7–8 weeks after conception are devoted to growth. Functional systems, although being formed, have not yet begun to work at their tasks. In the fetal period (8 weeks after conception until birth), the organ systems begin to function and the developing fetus becomes competent within the protective environment of the womb. After birth, the neonate must accommodate another environment, governed by the force of gravity. Infants attain functional skills in this new environment and systematically continue growing. The 1-year-old toddler may be very proud and excited about the ability to walk. Children who are 2–3 years old add important functional skills such as feeding and dressing themselves. Throughout childhood, physical growth occurs as the child becomes taller and stronger and demonstrates increasing endurance. The child actively explores the community on a bicycle, roller blades, or a skateboard.

The balance between body growth and functional mastery continues until physical maturity is attained in young adulthood. Adults should strive to attain and maintain functionally active lifestyles at home, in the workplace, and during leisure activities. The wear and tear that sometimes results from their functional activities can frequently be balanced by growth and the repair abilities of the body. By the time an adult reaches old age, growth and repair functions may be insufficient to maintain the optimal functional state of the body.

Wide variations in functional ability are seen among older adults. Most adults continue to live an active life, adapting as necessary to physical changes in their body systems. In other older adults, changes in strength, posture, balance, or endurance may make efficient movement and physical function more demanding and difficult. Presence of chronic illnesses such as heart disease, arthritis, and diabetes also impacts an older adult's functional ability. Age-related changes and presence of chronic illness may negatively impact the older adult's ability to participate in activities that are important to them, diminishing their ability to function and maintain a level of mastery over the environment.[9] Limitations in the ability to perform physical activities can be seen in adults over the age of 50 years and increase with age. Over 30% of adults ages 70–79 years demonstrate limitations in 1–3 physical activities, while almost 49% of individuals 80 years of age and above have reported physical activity limitations.[10]

The average life expectancy continues to increase in the United States and across the world. Many older adults will live into their 80s and 90s. In the United States, the number of older adults 65 years of age and older was 52.4 million people (a 35% increase from 2008) and is expected to be almost 95 million people by 2060.[11] The number of older adults in the United States, at least 100 years of age, also increased from approximately 50,000 people in 2010 to almost 94,000 people in 2018.[11] A concomitant compression of the period of morbidity at the end of life has been demonstrated, most notably in older adults who have practiced good health behaviors (e.g., stress reduction, exercise, hydration, nutrition) throughout their life span.[12] Recent studies have shown that older adults who participate in exercise programs can improve levels of physical function, self-efficacy, and quality of life.[13,14,15]

Relationship Between Development and Function

Each individual develops throughout the life span. Development occurs not only as a result of physical changes within the body but also because of environmental influences. As we interact within family, community, social, and cultural contexts, our development is shaped and functional roles or tasks are defined. From this perspective, development and function are intertwined throughout the life span, much like a piece of cloth is woven.

Development is a lifelong process. Through childhood, growth of the body systems occurs, and various new tasks are learned. Through adulthood, the body systems maintain a steady state and the individual continues to learn new skills and develop new interests. Finally, in older adulthood, participation in and development of skills and interests may continue, but biological "aging" may begin to impact physical function. "As people age, it becomes more difficult to adapt to stresses placed on the body, our organ system's capacity decreases, function decreases, and impairments and disabilities increase."[16] *Senescence* is the progressive physiological decline that results in increasing vulnerability to stress and the progressing likelihood of death. Just like other phases of development, senescence is not a single process but rather many processes.

The *development of function* does not refer just to the growth process related to youth or to the decline often associated with senescence and aging. Similarly, it cannot necessarily be reflected linearly. Growth and development imply change, either positive or negative, which can be observed at any point within the life span. If the life span and functional development are considered two separate continuums, pleated onto one another to resemble the bellows of an accordion, their impact on each other is obvious (Fig. 1.3). As adolescents experience growth spurts, attaining new height, they also experience losses in flexibility because muscle growth

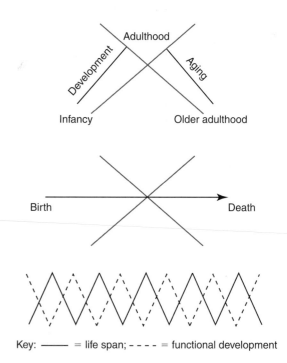

Key: ———— = life span; - - - - = functional development

Fig. 1.3 Interaction of life span and functional development.

does not keep up with bone growth. Adults may achieve new levels of productivity in the workplace but at a cost to family or social interactions. The life span approach to development and function appreciates all of the changes seen in an individual's abilities at any point in the life cycle, whether the changes reflect progression, regression, or reorganization.

Domains of Function

Functional activities with similar outcomes can be grouped together into categories or domains. We consider three domains of function here: biophysical domain, psychological domain, and sociocultural domain (Fig. 1.4). The *biophysical domain* includes the sensorimotor skills needed to perform activities of daily living, such as dressing, ambulating, maintaining hygiene, and cooking. The *psychological domain* is influenced by intellectual activities. Motivation, concentration, emotions, problem solving, and judgment are all factors that contribute to psychological function, as well as affective function, which allows a person to cope with everyday stresses. The psychological domain also influences how we perceive our ability to function. Factors such as anxiety, depression, emotional well-being, social skills, self-awareness, and self-esteem influence affective function. The *sociocultural domain* relates to our ability to interact with other people and to successfully complete social roles and obligations. Cultural norms or expectations help define social function.

These domains of function parallel domains of development discussed in Chapter 2, reinforcing the interrelationship of function and development. No one domain of function stands alone. Similarly, development within each domain is reflected by the progression of activities in each functional domain. For example, within the motor, psychological, and sociocultural domains of function, the young child focuses on learning motor skills such as walking, jumping, and running as they participate in play activities. Over time the child's functional skills expand into learning and being a student, and then assuming job or career roles. Development of relationships with family members and friends begins in childhood and then expands as adults form intimate relationships with friends and life partners. Many sociocultural functions depend on our mobility and ability to physically manipulate objects. Likewise, our physical level of function can be easily influenced by emotional status, intellectual ability, or motivation. Positive psychological functioning contributes to obtaining optimal physical health.[17] All three domains of function are interrelated and interdependent in meeting everyday challenges. Although all three domains of function are important, the primary focus of the rest of this chapter will be the domain of physical function.

PHYSICAL FUNCTION

Physical function can also be thought of as goal-directed movement. Function is the link between the physical actions we call movement and the environmental context in which they take place. For the act of reaching to be meaningful and therefore functional, it must take place when there is an object to reach for. Walking is functional because it is a means of moving from one place to another. People use movement every day as they interact with their environment. Goal-directed movement is important for an individual to survive, adapt, and learn within the environment. When our movement is

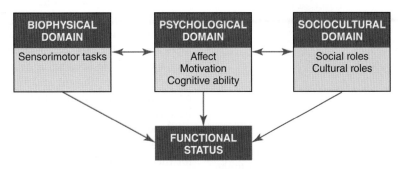

Fig. 1.4 The three domains of function—biophysical, psychological, and sociocultural—must operate independently as well as interdependently for human beings to achieve their best possible functional status.

inhibited, we may be less able to meet day-to-day needs. The young athlete with a broken leg suddenly must depend on crutches, making simple tasks such as walking to the bathroom or opening the door a challenge. As movement becomes less efficient, an individual may be faced with diminished functional independence. The individual with arthritis may not be able to quickly and efficiently button clothes. The person may also have difficulty picking up coins when paying for purchases in a store. As physical function becomes impaired, people frequently turn to health professionals for assistance.

The Movement Systems Role in Physical Function

Physical, occupational, and speech therapy intervention is frequently focused on improving physical function and maximizing an individual's ability to participate in life roles. Improved physical functioning also may be a positive influence on psychological and sociocultural functioning. The therapist has a thorough understanding of the movement system (Fig. 1.5) and utilizes this knowledge to design therapeutic intervention programs that will optimize a person's participation and health status. The movement system includes several body systems (cardiovascular, pulmonary, endocrine, integumentary, nervous, and musculoskeletal systems) that work together to support efficient movement and physical function.[18] After the therapist identifies a client's

basic participation restrictions and activity limitations, additional assessment of sensory, cardiovascular, pulmonary, neurological, endocrine, integumentary, and musculoskeletal systems may then identify impairments that interfere with overall physical function. Such impairments may include anatomical or physiological changes such as limited range of motion, impaired balance, or diminished strength. Therapeutic programs can then be devised to improve function. Therapy may focus on adapting a task or the environment in which the task takes place, or it may address an isolated impairment of body structure or function, which interferes with the patient's level of participation. The success of the therapeutic programs is measured based on the functional change demonstrated by clients and their ability to participate in meaningful activities, not on isolated changes in range of motion or strength impairments.

It is important for therapists to understand how biophysical function changes over time, the relationship of physical function to other domains of function, and the components of physical function that contribute to the quality and efficiency of movement. Knowledge of normal function of all body systems and how movement develops provides a means to detect movement dysfunction. With this knowledge, therapists can effectively create interventions that best meet a patient's individual need to be an active participant in life.

Development

How does physical function develop? What factors influence its development? Age, environment, and social expectations all contribute to a definition of normal biophysical function. Age not only defines size and biological capacity for movement but also reflects expectations about lifestyle.

During infancy and childhood, body size and the maturity of the body systems involved in movement limit and define functional abilities. For example, toddlers are able to walk, but because of their short legs, they have trouble keeping up with their parents. It is frequently more efficient and functional for them to be carried or pushed in a stroller. Young children may have trouble sitting at the table without fidgeting at a meal, perhaps because their feet do not reach the floor, and they cannot easily sit in the large chair provided for them. Functional limitations in these examples are closely related to the immaturity of the child's skeletal system, but the neuromuscular and cardiopulmonary

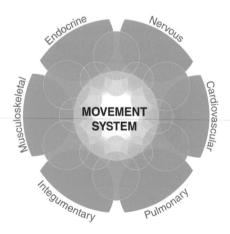

Fig. 1.5 The movement system, American Physical Therapy Association. (From Saladin L, Voight M. Introduction to the movement system as the foundation for physical therapist practice education and research. *Int J Sports Phys Ther.* 2017;12(6):858-861.)

systems are also undergoing rapid development during this time frame and affect the child's physical abilities. Fundamental motor skills such as postural control, locomotion, and prehension develop rapidly during childhood.

Functional expectations of the infant and child also influence their development of functional skills. A young infant's abilities are basically survival oriented. An infant can lift and turn their head; coordinate suck, swallow, and breathing; cry to indicate needs; and socially interact with caregivers. As the infant begins to control their movement, the major job or task is to explore the environment. Through play, an infant learns about the world and develops language; as the toddler and young child associate play with functional activities, such as eating and dressing, caregivers begin to have higher expectations for functional independence.

Through childhood and adolescence, social roles and expectations continue to undergo constant change. Body growth and maturation of the body systems also continue. Once maturity is attained in adolescence or young adulthood, the systems of the body that contribute to motor performance have completed their development. At this point, these body systems are ready to operate at peak efficiency. Practice and motivation to excel contribute to our ability to learn and refine new motor tasks. Skills are refined as we try to improve performance through recreational activities such as baseball, ballet, and gymnastics.

Societal roles and lifestyle changes that accompany adulthood again redefine physical function and may result in decreased physical activity levels. Commuting time, combined with a full day at work, may limit time available for physically active recreational pursuits. As activity levels decrease, so does our level of fitness. Cardiopulmonary functioning and muscle strength may not be supported to full capacity, resulting in decreased endurance and weakness. Refinement of skills associated with job pursuits continues through adulthood. Some job skills may put repetitive stress on the musculoskeletal system, which can lead to injury. As the body systems are continually used in day-to-day activities, wear and tear, as well as ongoing developmental changes related to adulthood, may decrease the efficiency of the body in physical functioning. To optimize physical function across the life span, individuals of all ages are encouraged to maintain an active and healthy lifestyle.

In the older adult, biophysical functional ability may decline because of wear and tear on the body systems, normal development (senescence), and lifestyle changes. Retirement from a physically demanding job may result in a less active lifestyle. A common assumption made about older adults is that they have a diminished ability to perform physical activities. An important fact to remember is that much variation exists in the abilities and activity levels demonstrated by older adults. Each older adult has a unique history, experiences, and changes attributed to aging. When one considers the total population of older adults, the majority do not have significant functional limitations. They live independently and maintain a relatively active and satisfying lifestyle. Functional ability does decrease with age, but it is in the oldest populations (more than 80 years old) that physical disability is the greatest.[9] Numerous functional tasks are required of people who live independently, including BADL (self-care and mobility) and IADL (cooking, shopping, housekeeping, and transportation). Older adults report increasing level of IADL disability with increasing age. Fig. 1.6 reflects the percentage of older adults in the United States indicating limitations in IADL and driving, confirming the percent of the population reporting limitations increases most for individuals 85 years of age and older.[19] Fig. 1.7 demonstrates a similar trend of individuals over 85 years of age reporting the most difficulty with BADL.[19] Older adults who remain physically active maintain higher levels of physical function than their peers who are less active.[20-23]

Components

"Efficient," "effective," "graceful," "fluid," and "smooth" are all adjectives frequently associated with movement. "Clumsy," "awkward," "disjointed," and "wasted" can also describe movement, but these words paint a very different picture. Sports science, physical education, and physical and occupational therapy professionals have tried to define the factors that contribute to efficient, effective movement. Flexibility, balance, coordination, power, and endurance are some dimensions that affect the quality of physical function. Both quality and efficiency of movement are important to optimal physical function.

Flexibility

Flexibility is reflected by a person's ability to move through space without being restricted by the

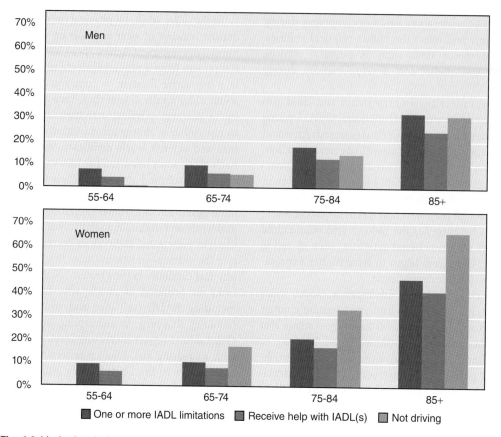

Fig. 1.6 Limitation in instrumental activities of daily living, by age: 2002. (From National Institute on Aging: *Growing older in America: the health and retirement study*, Bethesda, MD: NIH Publication No. 07-5757, March, 2007.)

musculoskeletal system. Most simply, *flexibility* refers to the capacity to bend. Flexibility can be described for a specific joint, a series of joints, or a specific person. Within human movement, flexibility depends on joint integrity, extensibility of the soft tissue (i.e., muscles, connective tissue, and skin), and joint range of motion. The tissues must maintain an appropriate resting length and pliability to allow the joint mobility necessary for the completion of activities of daily living. When a person has good flexibility, movement is more effective and efficient. Flexibility contributes to the ability to easily open the hand just enough to grasp a pencil or a glass, the ability to squat down to pick something up, and the ability to climb stairs.

Two types of flexibility can be assessed. *Static flexibility* refers to the range of motion available at a joint. *Dynamic flexibility* describes the resistance offered to active movement of the joint. As resistance increases, dynamic flexibility decreases. When optimal levels of resistance balance the motion around a joint, efficiency of movement is achieved. As flexibility increases, greater force can be exerted in a movement, and the speed of performance increases.

Developmentally, flexibility is fairly stable in boys from age 5 to 8 years and then decreases slightly until age 12 to 13 years. After that time, it again increases slightly until age 18. In girls, flexibility is stable from age 5 to 11 years and then increases until age 14. After that time, flexibility reaches a plateau. At all ages, females are more flexible than males.[24] In older adults, flexibility may decrease because of cross-linkage of collagen fibers in connective tissue, inactivity, decreased muscle strength, and joint changes. Active older adults maintain greater levels of flexibility than do their more sedentary peers.[25-27]

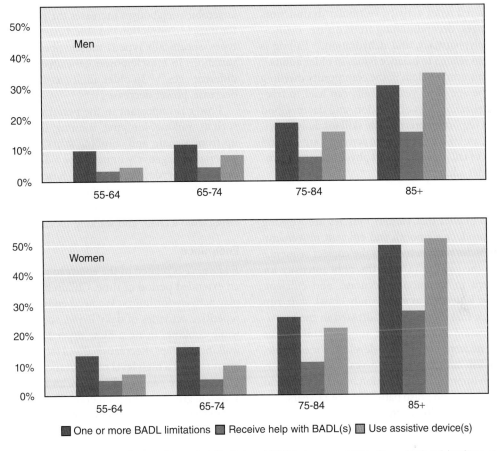

Fig. 1.7 Limitation in basic activities of daily living (BADL), by age: 2002. (From National Institute on Aging: *Growing older in America: the health and retirement study*, Bethesda, MD: NIH Publication No. 07-5757, March, 2007.)

Our flexibility is defined by the types of physical activities we pursue each day at work and engage in during recreational activities. Flexibility also influences health and physical function across the life span. The flexibility of the baseball pitcher's throwing arm is certainly greater than that of a typist's arm. A gymnast is probably more flexible than a football player. Levels of flexibility in adolescence have been shown to relate to decreased risk of neck problems in adulthood.[28] Flexibility exercises are also a component of most fall prevention programs for older adults, reinforcing the importance of flexibility for effective movement.[27,29–31]

Balance

Balance is related to a state of equilibrium and is an important component of skilled movement. Balance is achieved when we can maintain our center of gravity over our base of support, thereby maintaining equilibrium with gravity. Several factors contribute to the ability to balance, including efficient function of the nervous system, musculoskeletal system, and sensory systems. Balance is necessary during static activities such as standing still (*static balance*) and during movement (*dynamic balance*).

Throughout childhood, balance improves.[31,33] Girls appear to perform better than boys in balance activities. In adolescence, both groups reach a plateau in balance skills; boys may perform slightly better than girls in this age group.[21] In older adulthood, poor balance is frequently reported as a problem and may be related to developmental changes or impairments in the body systems that contribute to balance. Some of these changes include impaired reflex activity, vestibular dysfunction, posture changes, deconditioning from disuse, medications and polypharmacy, and dehydration.[34] Falling is also a problem related to balance issues in older adults.[27] Falls are a common problem in the community dwelling adult over the age of 65 years.[35] Falls can lead to fractures, hospitalization, loss of function, and death. Good balance is an important prerequisite skill for daily activities of living, and therefore balance activities are integral components of fall prevention and physical activity programs for older adults.[26,27,36-39]

Coordination

Coordination implies that various muscles are working together to produce a smooth and efficient movement. The right muscles must activate in the correct sequence and work at the right time, with the right intensity for the movement to be smooth, accurate, and efficient. Coordination is needed to successfully crawl, skip, run to catch a bus, make a bed, or get dressed in the morning. Coordination develops over time in children as sensory and neuromotor systems develop. For example, reach and grasp coordination in 6-year-old children is variable, with improved coordination by age 8 years and an adult-like reach and grasp pattern at age 11 years.[40] In older adults, coordination decreases, negatively impacting motor performance.[41,42]

Power

Power refers to the rate at which work is done, the ability to exert force quickly. Related to movement, it is the amount of work a muscle can produce per unit time.[43] Power is then related to both strength and speed. In childhood, power depends on size and maturity of the neurological and musculoskeletal systems. In particular, development of muscle fiber types able to work using anaerobic metabolism increases the power and force of the muscle contraction possible. Changes in muscle fiber types, specifically type II muscle fibers, are reflected in variations in muscle power generated by individuals of different ages.[44,45] In older adults, as strength and speed decrease, power decreases.[44,46,47]

Power is important in the performance of activities such as walking, jumping, running, throwing, standing up from a chair, and climbing stairs. Decreased power generation negatively impacts the older adult's ability to perform everyday motor tasks. Research studies have shown that when older adults participate in power training programs, functional abilities such as stair climbing, rising from a chair, and walking speed improve.[12,13,48,49]

Endurance

Endurance is related to the ability to perform work over an extended period of time. Children, for example, can play actively for hours. We need endurance to perform repetitive activities of daily living, such as stirring food while cooking, using a blow dryer to dry our hair, or walking up steps. Recreational and job-related tasks also often require a high level of endurance.

Endurance can be affected by an individual muscle, a muscle group, or the total body. Total body endurance usually refers to cardiopulmonary endurance, reflecting the ability of the heart to deliver a steady supply of oxygen to working muscle. Muscle endurance reflects the ability to sustain repeated muscle contraction and is related to muscle strength. Developmentally, muscle endurance has been shown to increase linearly in boys between 5 and 13 years of age, after which a spurt is observed. A steady linear increase in muscle endurance is seen in girls.[21] Endurance decreases in older adults, with elite senior marathon runners demonstrating diminished endurance after the age of 50 years.[50,51]

▋ SUMMARY

Human function is an elusive entity. We discuss function from a life span perspective and its relationship to the broader context of health. Optimal function contributes to an individual's well-being and is associated with biological health, but is also influenced by personal and environmental factors. The interactions and interdependence of the biophysical, psychological, and sociocultural domains are what define our ability to function. The domain of biophysical function requires in-depth understanding because this is the area that we, as physical and occupational therapists, hope to improve when working with our clients. The components that make movement efficient, effective, and, most important, functional have been reviewed. Using this knowledge base, we can assess how our clients are functioning and help them successfully meet their goals of improving function and maximizing their ability to participate in life roles.

REFERENCES

1. World Health Organization. *International Classification of Functioning, Disability, and Health*. Geneva: World Health Organization; 2001.
2. World Health Organization. *The First Ten Years of the World Health Organization*. Geneva: World Health Organization; 1958.
3. Jette AM. State of the art in functional status assessment. In: Rothstein J, eds. *Measurement in Physical Therapy*. New York: Churchill Livingstone; 1985:137–168.
4. Nieuwenhuijsen ER, Zemper E, Miner KR, et al. Health behavior change models and theories: contributions to rehabilitation. *Disabil Rehabil*. 2006;28:245–256.
5. Jette AM. Toward a common language for function, disability, and health. *Phys Ther*. 2006;86:726–744.
6. Phelan EA, Anderson LA, LaCroix AZ, et al. Older adults' view of "successful aging"—how do they compare with researchers' definitions? *J Am Geriatr Soc*. 2004;52:211–216.
7. Latasch ML, Levin MF, Scholz JP, et al. Motor control theories and their applications. *Medicina*. 2010;46: 382–392.
8. Latash ML. Biomechanics as a window into neural control of movement. *J Hum Kinet*. 2016;52(1):7–20.
9. Grimmer M, Riener R, Walsh CJ, Seyfarth A Mobility related physical and functional losses due to aging and disease - a motivation for lower limb exoskeletons. *J Neuroeng Rehabil*. 2019;16(2). https://doi.org/10.1186/s12984-018-0458-8.
10. Holmes J, Powell-Griner E, Lethbridge-Cejku M, et al. Aging differently: physical limitations among adults age 50 years and over: United States. *2001-2007. NCHS Data Brief*. 2009;20:1–8.
11. Administration on Aging, US Dept. of Health and Human Services, May 2020. 2019 Profile of Older Americans. https://acl.gov/sites/default/files/Aging%20and%20Disability%20in%20America/2019ProfileOlderAmericans508.pdf, accessed 6/2/2021
12. Blocker WP. Maintaining functional independence by mobilizing the aged. *Geriatrics*. 1992;47:42–56.
13. Henwood TR, Rick S, Taaffe DR. Strength versus muscle power-specific resistance training in community dwelling older adults. *J Gerontol A Biol Sci Med Sci*. 2008;63A(1):83–91.
14. Hazell T, Kenno K, Jakobi J. Functional benefit of power training for older adults. *J Aging Phys Act*. 2007;15: 349–359.
15. Lui C, Shiroy DM, Jones LY, Clark DO. Systematic review of functional training on muscle strength, physical functioning and activities of daily living in older adults. *Euro Rev Aging Phys Act*. 2014;11:95–106. https://doi.org/10.1007/211556-014-0144-1.
16. Staples WH, ed. *Geriatric Physical Therapy: A Case Study Approach*. 2nd ed. New York, NY: McGraw-Hill; 2021.
17. Kubzansky LD, Boehm JK, Segerstrom SC. Positive psychological functioning and the biology of health. *Social and Personality Psychology Compass*. 2015;9(12):645–660. https://doi.org/10.1111/spc3.12224.
18. American Physical Therapy Association. *White Paper - Physical Therapist Practice and the Movement System*. Alexandria VA: American Physical Therapy Association; 2015.
19. National Institute on Aging. *Growing older in America: the health and retirement study*. Bethesda, Md: NIH Publication; 2007.No. 07-5757, March.
20. Brach JS, Simonsick EM, Kritchevsky S, et al. The association between physical function and lifestyle activity and exercise in the health, aging and body composition study. *J Am Geriatr Soc*. 2004;52:502–509.
21. Vaughn L, Leng X, LaMonte MJ, et al. Functional independence in late life: maintaining physical functioning in older adulthood predicts daily function after age 80. *J Gerontol A Biol Sci Med Sci*. 2016;71(Suppl 1):S79–S86.
22. Patterson DH, Warburton DER. Physical activity and functional limitations in older adults: a systematic review related to Canada' Physical Activity Guidelines. *International Journal of Behavioral Nutrition and Physical Activity*. 2010;7:38. https://doi.org/10.1186/1179-5868-7-38.
23. Liao WL, Chang JH. Age trajectories of disability in insturmental activities of daily living and disability-free life expectancy among middle-aged and older aduts in Taiway: an aa-year longitudinal study. *BMC Geriatr*. 2020;20(530). https://doi.org/10.1186/s12877-020-01939-4.
24. Malina RM, Bouchard C, Bar-or O. *Growth, Maturation, and Physical Activity*. Springfield, IL: Human Kinetics Press; 2004. 2nd ed.
25. Kaplan GA, Shawbridge WT, Camachs T, et al. Factors associated with change in physical functioning in the elderly. *J Aging Health*. 1993;5:140–153.
26. Walker JM, Sue D, Miles-Elkousy N. Active mobility of the extremities in older subjects. *Phys Ther*. 1984;64: 919–923.
27. Inami T, Shimizu T. Long-term stretching program in older active adults increase muscle strength. *J Exer Sports Orthop*. 2014;1(2):1–8.
28. Millesson LO, Nupponen H, Kaprio J, et al. Adolescent flexibility, endurance strength, and physical activity as predictors of adult tension neck, low back pain, and knee injury: a 25-year follow up study. *Br J Sports Med*. 2006;40:107–113.
29. Costello E, Edelstein JE. Update on falls prevention for community-dwelling older adults: review of single and multifactorial intervention programs. *J Rehabil Res Dev*. 2008;45(8):1135–1152.

30. Rubenstein LZ, Josephson KR. Falls and their prevention in elderly people: what does the evidence show? *Med Clin North Am.* 2006;90:807–824.

31. Batista LH, Vilar AC, de Almeida-Ferreira JJ, et al. Active stretching improves flexibility, joint torque, and functional mobility in older women. *Am J Phys Med Rehabil.* 2009;88(10):815.

32. Kakebeeke TH, Knairer E, Chaouch A, et al. Neuromotor development in children. *Part 4: New norms from 3-18 years. DMCM.* 2018;60:810–819.

33. Conner BC, Petersen DA, Pigman J, et al. The cross-sectional relationship between age, standing static balance and standing dynamic balance in typically developing children. *Gait Posture.* 2019;73:20–25. https://doi.org/10.1016/j.gaitpost.219.07.128.

34. Lord SR, Clark RD, Webster IW. Physiological factors associated with falls in an elderly population. *J Am Geriatr Soc.* 1991;39:1194–1200.

35. Sturnieks DL, George R, Lord SR. Balance disorders in the elderly. *Clin Neurophysiol.* 2008;38:467–478.

36. Paterson DH, Jones GR, Rice CL. Ageing and physical activity: evidence to develop exercise recommendations for older adults. *Can J Public Health.* 2007;98(Suppl 2): S69S108.

37. Sherrington C, Whitney JC, Lord SR, et al. Effective exercise for prevention of falls: a systematic review and meta-analysis. *J Am Geriatr Soc.* 2008;S2:2234–2243.

38. Jin J. Prevention of falls in older adults. *JAMA.* 2018;319(16):1734. https://doi.org/10.1001/jama.2018.4396.

39. Abraham MK, Cimino-Fiallos N. *Falls in the Elderly: Causes, Injuries, and Management. Medscape.* Medscape; 2021. https://reference.medscape.com/slideshow/falls-in-the-elderly-6012395.

40. Oliver I, Hay L, Bard C, et al. Age-related differences in the reaching and grasping coordination in children: unimanual and bimanual tasks. *Exp Brain Res.* 2007;179(1):17–27.

41. Fujiyama H, Garry MI, Levin O, et al. Age-related differences in inhibitory processes during interlimb coordination. *Brain Res.* 2009;1262:38–47.

42. Paquette C, Paquet N, Fung J. Aging affects coordination of rapid head motions with trunk and pelvis movements during standing and walking. *Gait Posture.* 2006;24(1):62–69.

43. Adams K, Sevene T. *Strength, Power, and the Baby Boomer.* Indianapolis, IN: American College of Sports Medicine 2017.

44. Clemencon M, Hautier CA, Rahmani A, et al. Potential role of optimal velocity as a qualitative factor of physical functional performance in women aged 27 to 96 years. *Arch Phys Med Rehabil.* 2008;89:1594–1599.

45. Hakkinen K, Kraemer WJ, Kallinen M, et al. Bilateral and unilateral neuromuscular function and muscle cross-sectional area in middle-aged and elderly men and women. *J Gerontol A Biol Sci Med Sci.* 1996;51AB21B29.

46. Rogers MA, Evans WJ. Changes in skeletal muscle with aging: effects of exercise training. *Exerc Sport Sci Rev.* 1993;21:65–102.

47. Sayers SP, Gibson K. High-speed power training in older adults: a shift of the external resistance at which peak power is produced. *J Strength Cond Res.* 2014;28(3):616–621. https://doi.org/10.1519/JSC.0b013e3182a361b8.

48. Katula JA, Marsh A, Rejeski WJ. Strength training and quality of life in older adults: the POWER Study. *Health Qual Life Outcomes.* 2008;6:45.

49. Cancela JM, Varela S, Ayan C. Effects of high intensity training on elderly women: a pilot study. *Phys Occup Ther Geriatr.* 2008;27(2):160–169.

50. Tanaka H, Seals DR. Endurance exercise performance in masters athletes: age-associated changes and underlying physiological mechanisms. *J Physiol.* 2008;586(1):55–63.

51. Leyk D, Erley O, Ridder D, et al. Age-related changes in marathon and half-marathon performances. *Int J Sports Med.* 2007;28(6):513–517.

SUGGESTED READING

Liao WL, Chang YH. Age trajectories of disability in instrumental activities of daily living and disability-free life expectancy among middle-aged and older adults in Taiwan: an 11-year longitudinal study. *BMC Geriatr.* 2020;20:530. https://doi.org/10.1186/s12877-020-01939-4.

Purath SW, Buchholz DL. Kark. Physical fitness assessment of older adults in the primary care setting. *J Am Acad Nurse Pract.* 2009;21(2):101–107.

Singh AS, Chin A, Paw MJ, Bosscher RJ, van Mechelen W. Cross-sectional relationship between physical fitness components and functional performance in older persons living in long-term care facilities. *BMC Geriatr.* 2006;6:4.

World Health Organization, 2002. *Toward a common language for functioning, disability, and health:* ICF. Geneva, Switzerland. https://cdn.who.int/media/docs/default-source/classification/icf/icfbeginnersguide.pdf?sfvrsn=eead63d3_4 (accessed 8/30/2021).

Theories of Development

OBJECTIVES

After studying this chapter, the reader will be able to:

1. Define domains, periods, and concepts of development.
2. Discuss concepts of growth, maturation, adaptation, and learning in all developmental domains.
3. Define the concept of life span development.
4. Identify theories of life span development.
5. Define and differentiate life span and health span.
6. Discuss how specific biophysical, psychological, and sociocultural theories are related to function at various ages.

Development is a topic covered in many professional education curricula, including biology, education, psychology, sociology, and health sciences programs. Each discipline focuses on aspects of development unique to its profession, and significant amounts of information exist within these specialized areas. Our collective knowledge substantiates that an individual develops across the broad continuum of the life span, strongly influenced by three interrelated domains. Normal human development is shaped by interaction between the biophysical, psychological, and sociocultural domains.

A general introduction to biophysical, psychological, and sociocultural theories of development describes how the different domains and disciplines are basic to our lives and the study of human behavior. For example, a child in the United States learns to eat with a fork within the first year of life. This social skill cannot develop until physical coordination is sufficiently advanced to allow fine controlled movements of the arm and hand. The child must cognitively understand the relationship between food, the fork, hunger, and the action taken to satisfy that hunger. Social customs shape how the child performs the skill. In fact, an Asian child will be meeting the same functional need at about the same age but will be using chopsticks.

HUMAN DEVELOPMENT

Human development refers to changes that occur in our lives from conception to death. Change can occur on many levels: the cell, tissue, organ, body systems, and in physical, psychological, and social domains. Change can be progressive, reorganizational, or regressive. In muscle, for example, where tissue increases during growth, fiber types differentiate or atrophy because of use, loss of innervation, and nutrition. Form and function change during the process of development, as occurs when a sapling grows into an oak tree or a caterpillar turns into a butterfly. The form a movement takes is shaped by its intended function. Because functional demands vary with age, the movement forms that emerge during development change. Function or the way in which the body and its parts are used can change over time and can result in structural changes. Human behavior is the outward manifestation of development and changes through four processes: growth, maturation, adaptation, and learning. These processes occur simultaneously and concurrently in all domains of human development. Their importance may change relative to the domain or point in developmental time.

Domains of Development

The processes of growth, maturation, adaptation, and learning operate at the same time in three different domains: biophysical, psychological, and sociocultural. Physical growth and development are accompanied by the acquisition of motor skills, intellectual and language development, and socioemotional development. Knowledge is gained about movement and the people and objects within the immediate environment. For example, intellectually, infants may be unable to communicate verbally or understand their own physical actions. Parents supply meaning to the gestures, looks, or early sound production. This assistance shapes infants' actions to parents' expectations for motor performance or communication. Parents may interpret a random swipe as a reach or the sound "ma" as recognition of mother.

We see the interrelationships of development in multiple domains when the infant develops perceptual awareness concurrently with motor control, beginning cognition, and attachment. A social smile is evident in most 2-month-old infants, although it usually takes two additional months before the infant demonstrates sufficient head control to focus attention on caregivers or objects and to be able to direct reaching. The process of human development is interactive, with each domain exerting a positive or negative impact on the other domains. The temperament of a baby can affect the quality of interaction with the caregiver or therapist and thereby affect the attachment process. The biophysical, psychological, and sociocultural selves interact to produce a unique individual. Therefore, no two people are exactly alike.

Each domain contributes to our understanding of motor behavior. We are biological organisms that develop within a psychological and sociocultural environment. This relationship is schematically represented in Fig. 1.4. Our primary therapeutic emphasis has always been on an individual's ability to move. As therapists, we must consider the cognitive, psychosocial, and emotional status of individuals with whom we work. What are their life expectations? Each individuals' motor behavior will reflect their age, ability, experience, and culture.

Periods of Development

The life span is most often divided into age-related segments or periods (Table 2.1). The prenatal period averages 38 weeks in length, beginning with conception and culminating in birth. It is divided into three stages: the *germinal* period, the first 2 weeks of gestation; the *embryonic* period, when all major organ systems form (weeks 2–8); and the *fetal* period, when organ systems differentiate and rapid body growth occurs (weeks 9–38).

The lengthy postnatal period is usually divided into the categories of infancy, childhood, adolescence, and adulthood. *Infancy* spans the first 2 years of life, from birth to the second birthday. *Childhood* begins at 2 years of age for both girls and boys but ends at different ages

TABLE 2.1 Periods of Development	
Period	**Time Span**
Prenatal	Conception to birth
• Germinal	• 1–2 weeks' gestation
• Embryonic	• 2–8 weeks' gestation
• Fetal	• 9–38 weeks' gestation
Infancy	Birth to 2 years
Childhood	2–10 years (female)
	2–12 years (male)
Adolescence	10–18 years (female)
	12–20 years (male)
Young adulthood	18–40 years
Middle adulthood	40–65 years
Older adulthood	65 years to death
• Young-old	• 65–74 years
• Middle-old	• 75–84 years
• Oldest-old	• 85 years to death

because of the time difference in the onset of puberty. Classically, *adolescence* lasts 8 years, beginning at approximately age 10 for girls and age 12 for boys. It is divided into three stages: *prepubescence*, the 2 years before the onset of puberty; *pubescence*, the 4 years in which hormones produce secondary sexual characteristics; and *postpubescence*, the final 2 years of adolescence in which the final maturity of adulthood is reached.

Adulthood is concerned less with age than with role transition. Most of us are considered adult when we reach our 20s. Going to college, getting a job, and being able to vote have all been used as markers of adulthood, but no one task or age clearly defines this period. In fact, Jeffrey Arnett[1] has made a strong case that the transition from adolescence to adulthood is protracted and has introduced a new developmental stage he calls emerging adulthood. His theory of adult development will be discussed further in that section. Adulthood can be divided loosely into young, middle, and older adulthood.

Although transitions have been identified among the various divisions of adulthood, none appear to be as easily defined as the periods of child development.

Geriatrics and gerontology were established as fields of human service and research in the 1950s. Since that time, the field of gerontology has fostered an explosion of information on aging. Demographics document that the population continues to age. In 2006, only 12% of the total population of the United States was age 65 and over. A turning point in population growth will be seen by 2030 when all of the baby boomers will be over 65 years of age and make up 20% of the population.[2] Additionally, population growth is projected to slow and become more racially and ethnically diverse. By 2060, one in four Americans will be an older adult (Fig. 2.1). As research continues to focus on the oldest citizens, older adulthood has been divided into young-old, middle-old, and oldest-old. Many studies are only focusing on centenarians or those over age 100.

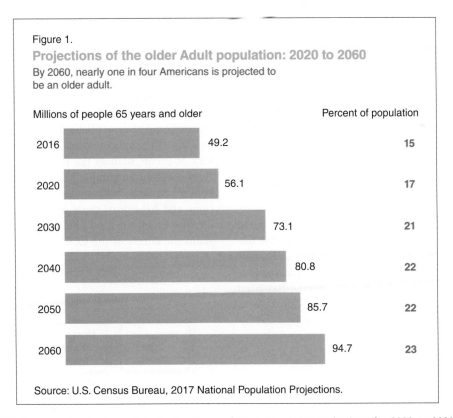

Figure 1.

Projections of the older Adult population: 2020 to 2060

By 2060, nearly one in four Americans is projected to be an older adult.

Millions of people 65 years and older		Percent of population
2016	49.2	15
2020	56.1	17
2030	73.1	21
2040	80.8	22
2050	85.7	22
2060	94.7	23

Source: U.S. Census Bureau, 2017 National Population Projections.

Fig. 2.1 Demographic turning points for the United States: population projections for 2020 to 2060. US Census Bureau. (From https://www.census.gov/content/dam/Census/library/publications/2020/demo/p25-1144.pdf Accessed June 14, 2021.)

Concepts of Development

Maturity

Development from birth to the attainment of biophysical, psychological, and sociocultural maturity constitutes the first part of the life span. *Maturation* is the process whereby an organism continues to grow, differentiate, and change from conception until achieving a mature state. Maturity is usually attained during adulthood between 25 and 30 years of age. Biological maturation is typically attributed to an individual's genetic makeup, whereas psychological and social-emotional maturity results from a combination of maturation and learning. Maturation is not considered the only determinant of development.

Senescence

Development continues throughout adulthood with structural and functional changes seen as a normal part of healthy aging. Therefore, aging can be viewed as a continuation of the developmental process. The term *senescence*, however, is appropriately used to describe later life because aging can refer to any time-related process. *Senescence* is the progressive physiological decline that results in our increasing vulnerability to stress and the progressing likelihood of death. Just like other phases of development, senescence is not a single process but rather many processes. Age-related changes produced in our organ systems and personal identity result from a lifetime of interactions between our internal environment, culture, and society.

Life Span

The concept of life span development is not new. Baltes[3] originally identified five characteristics to use when assessing a theory for its life span perspective. The following list reflects the original four criteria and a new fifth one used to view development from a lifelong perspective. Context, the original fifth criteria, has been replaced by multicausal, meaning that one can arrive at the same destination by different means or by a combination of means.

- Lifelong
- Multidimensional
- Plastic
- Embedded in history
- Multicausal

When Baltes, Lindenberger, and Staudinger[4] revisited the theoretical underpinnings of life span theory, they reinforced the idea that development is *not* complete at maturity. The multidimensional quality of life span theory provides a complete framework for ontogenesis (development). Culture and the knowledge gained from all domains make a significant impact on a person's life course. Biological plasticity is accompanied by cultural competence, so there is a gain/loss dynamic that occurs during development. There are no gains without losses and no losses without gains. In essence, this is the adaptive capacity of the person. Life span development is not constrained to travel a single course or developmental trajectory.

No one period of life can be understood without looking at its relationship to what came before and what lies ahead. History affects development in three ways as seen in Fig. 2.2. Firstly, the normative age-graded influence is seen in those developmental tasks described by Havighurst[5] for each period of development. Age-graded physical, psychological, and social milestones would fall into this category. Walking at 12 months and obtaining a driver's license at 16 years of age are examples of a physical age-graded task. Understanding simple concepts, such as all round objects bounce, and getting along with same-age peers in adolescence are examples from the psychological and social domains. Secondly, normative history-graded influences come from the effect of when a person is born. Each of us is part of a birth cohort or group. Some of us are baby boomers, gen Xers, or millennials. All people in an age cohort share the same history of events such as the terrorist attack of 9/11, the Boston Marathon bombing, and the election of Obama.[6] When you were born makes a difference in expectations and behaviors; these historical events shape the life of the cohort. It will be decades before we understand the effects of the COVID-19 pandemic. The last

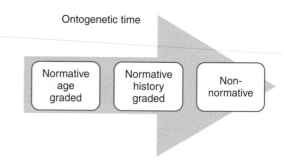

Fig. 2.2 Three major biocultural influences on life span development.

history-related influence comes from things that happen to a person and that have no norms or expectations such as winning the lottery, losing a parent, or having a child with a developmental disability. These experiences are part of your own unique personal history. Life span development provides a holistic framework in which aging is a lifelong process of growing up and growing old. Development within the biophysical, psychological, and sociocultural domains is enriched when viewed through a life span perspective.

Life span is also defined as the maximum survival potential for a particular species. Most gerontologists agree that our life span is species-specific and therefore intrinsically regulated. Theoretically, the maximum length of life biologically possible for a human is 120 years, although documentation exists for one individual who lived to be 122. Numerous social and environmental factors, such as war, famine, pandemics, and toxic chemicals, can negatively affect this figure. Although catastrophic disease is often thought to dramatically shorten our life spans, statistics reveal that if all major causes of death were eradicated, only 15 years would be added to our life expectancy.[7,8]

Individual Differences

The development of human behavior is strongly influenced by both maturation and experience. Genetically, we are provided the physical base of our body that continually changes during our life span. The complete set of genes that are inherited is one's *genotype*. Each of us builds a sense of identity and psychological wholeness within our mind, influenced by experiences within the social environment of our family, culture, and society. The genetic instructions along with these environmental influences produce a *phenotype*, a person's physical, psychological, and behavioral features (Fig. 2.3).

Intelligence and personality can be influenced by the environment and heredity. Intelligence, the ability to learn and solve problems, is highly heritable but can be affected by environmental influences up until adolescence. Recent genetic studies have identified genome sequence differences that explain 20%–50% of heritable intelligence.[9] Children exposed to enriched environments often improve their native intelligence. Conversely, environmental deprivation may contribute to a decrease in intellectual performance. After adolescence, the influence of a shared family environment has little influence on individual differences.[10] Heredity

$$[genotype] + [(diet, lifestyle, and environment)] = [phenotype]$$

Fig. 2.3 Genes do not change but their expression does: [genotype] + [diet, lifestyle, and environment)] = [phenotype]. (From Anton B, Vitetta L, Cortizo F, et al. Can we delay aging? The biology and science of aging. *Ann NY Acad Sci.* 2005;1057:527.)

can also influence the type of experiences an individual seeks, such as finding our niche in the world. Picking a place for one's self in society by seeking social environments that fit with the person's heredity is called niche-picking.[11] Sociability has a genetic component that affects whether a child enjoys social interaction or prefers to observe the world from a distance. Shy children will tend to seek situations that allow peace and quiet, while extroverted children seek social contact. Even with a genetic component, siblings' temperament and social development are different. Researchers have not found out very much about the specific environmental influences that make siblings different within the same family. Despite the same parenting, siblings' personal and social developments differ.[12]

Life Span and Health Span

Longevity is affected by genetics, environment, race, gender, and ethnicity. Heredity accounts for about 25% of our longevity.[13] In other words, one predictor of a longer life is to come from a family of long-lived people. The remaining influences on life span and health span are attributed to environment, physical, social, and lifestyle factors. Lifestyle factors considered to affect longevity include smoking, diet, stress, alcohol consumption, and exercise. Life expectancy has increased for the last three decades but more recent data show that the rate of change is slowing.[14] Average life expectancy has decreased in 2020.[15] Health span, which is the amount of time spent in good health, has also decreased. It is an indicator of population health.[16] As more chronic diseases are controlled by medical interventions, a person may live longer with a disability but have a shorter health span.

Environment and lifestyle account for the remaining influence on life span and health span. Living in a hostile physical or social environment also can be counterproductive to a long life. Within the United States, African Americans have a shorter life expectancy than European Americans by about 5 years.[17] Hispanic Americans' life expectancy exceeds European Americans at all ages, despite access problems to health care for many. This advantage in life expectancy has recently declined due to the pandemic.[18] Women in general live longer than men, with the disparity increasing from 5.1 years (2019) to 5.4 years (2020).[18]

Epigenetics studies the environment's effect on gene expression. Epigenetic changes can be inherited and thus may protect older individuals from developing age-related problems.[13,19] Epigenetic aging estimates have been able to predict longevity[20] and studies of individuals over age 100 years have shown that they differ in their ages of age-related disease onset.[21,22] In supercentenarians (those who are 110–119 years old), health span was found to approximate life span. Extreme longevity (EL) (living over 105+ years) has been found to be associated with genetic variants.[23]

Processes of Development

Growth refers to the changes in physical dimensions of the body. Growth rates vary for specific body systems and tissues. Fig. 2.4 provides a comparison of the general growth curve with that of specific systems and tissues. The general growth curve reflects rapid growth in infancy, slower growth in childhood, and again rapid growth in adolescence. Head circumference, height, and weight are all examples of dimensions that can be used to assess growth and can be ploted on growth charts. Changes in growth can be used to assess development

by comparing the percentile growth achieved in these anthropometrical measures. Growth that falls between the 10th and 90th percentiles is considered normal. Large variations among these measurements, such as when height and weight are at radically different percentiles, may signal a growth problem. Healthy children exhibit stable trends in growth through the developmental stages of life, although different body sections grow at proportionately different rates (Fig. 2.5).

Maturation contributes to development by producing physical changes that cause organs and body systems to reach their adult form and function. Changes that occur on a genetically controlled timetable can usually be attributed to the process of physical maturation. Maturation occurs in all body systems. One example from the skeletal system is the appearance of primary and secondary ossification centers in the bones (see Chapter 5). Reflexes and reactions emerge sequentially in response to maturation of the nervous system; myelination is one hallmark of nervous system maturation. Structures that function first are myelinated first, thus paralleling the development of function of those neuroanatomical structures (see Chapter 8). The integrity of nervous system development can be assessed by evaluating the presence of developmentally appropriate reflexes and reactions. Maturation is also defined within the psychological and social domains of function. The genetic

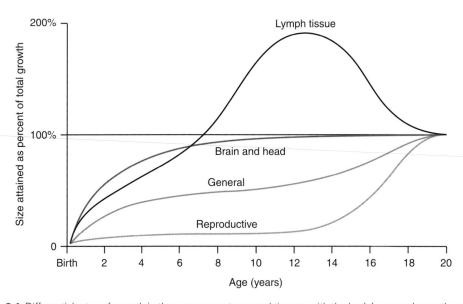

Fig. 2.4 Differential rates of growth in three organ systems and tissues with the body's general growth curve.

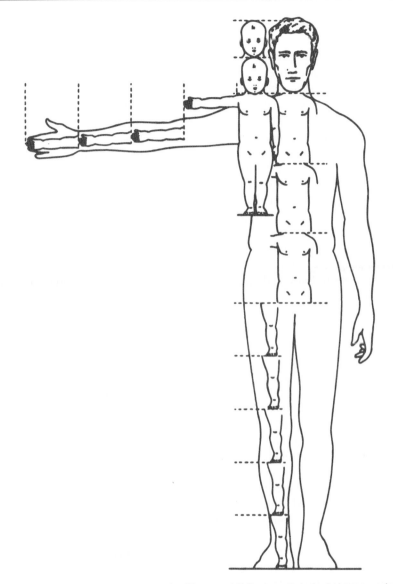

Fig. 2.5 Proportional growth changes across the life span. While the whole body increases in length from birth to maturity, the length of the head increases about two times, the trunk increases about three times, the arms increase about four times, and legs increase about five times. (From Valadian I, Porter D. *Physical growth and development from conception to maturity.* Boston: Little, Brown; 1977.)

substrate of behavior does not simply imprint its code on the environment; rather, the genetic base allows us to adapt to our environment. The environment can also influence maturation through adaptation and learning.

Adaptation and learning are sometimes difficult to separate from maturation. *Adaptation* is the body's accommodation to the immediate environment. Some structures and functions of organ systems are adaptations to exposure to the internal or external environment. Adaptation, such as development, can produce positive or negative change. A positive change is exhibited by the production of antibodies after exposure to chicken pox. An example of negative environmental impact is seen in the delayed development of understimulated infants.[24]

Exposure to some type of stimulus induces change, such as development of joints in the embryo, which requires primitive muscles to pull on bone to produce a joint cavity. If the muscles fail to produce movement, joint deformities occur in utero and result in *arthrogryposis*. Although each of us adapts differently, we all mature at varying rates in a similar manner.

Learning is a relatively permanent change in behavior resulting from practice and, as such, may be considered a form of adaptation. For example, rollerblading, or inline skating, is an adaptation to having wheels on our shoes. To adapt to having wheels on our shoes, we must learn different ways to balance, start moving, and stop. To rollerblade takes practice. Many motor abilities, such as riding a bike, playing soccer, reading, writing, and speaking a foreign language, are learned. We do not know if there is an optimal time for learning these tasks. We do know that experience plays a crucial role in mastering abilities that are not innate.

Factors Affecting Development

The process of development is strongly influenced by four factors: genetics, maturation, environment, and culture. None of these influences alone can account for the many changes that occur throughout our life span. The interaction between maturation and experience within specific biophysical, psychological, and sociocultural domains may account for individual differences. Two children grow up in the same neighborhood but have vastly different lives. What makes the difference? The values and life goals inherited from our family, society, and culture are just as real as our biological heritage.

Genetics and maturation contribute to and control our body's internal environment or milieu. The body's internal chemistry must be balanced to support growth, development, and functional activities such as movement. Hormones play a major role in controlling physical growth and initiating puberty, and they regulate the body's metabolism and ability to use chemical sources of energy for growth, maturation, adaptation, and learning.

Nutrition is part of the internal and external environment and contributes to the production of a healthy body. Adequate nutrition supplies fuel for efficient energy production, tissue development, and tissue repair. For example, adequate nutrition is critical for the development and function of the nervous system,

enabling the execution and control of movement. A lack of folic acid is linked to an increased likelihood of having a child with a neural tube defect. Poor nutrition during pregnancy has been associated with intrauterine growth retardation, a significant cause of developmental disability in low-birth-weight infants. Prenatal malnutrition can cause permanent stunting of brain development. Fat must be present in the diet to produce myelin. Effects of nutritional deprivation on brain development have been so thoroughly established that US manufacturers have added supplements to baby formula to provide sufficient fatty acids for nervous system maturation. Postnatal growth is supported by the secretion of growth hormones (see Chapter 10). Infants who fail to thrive (i.e., do not gain sufficient weight at an appropriate rate) have poorer motor skills than do adequately nourished peers. Inadequate nutrition, especially during periods of rapid growth, can have long-lasting effects on development. Appropriate nutrition supports prenatal and postnatal development.

Our external environment or surroundings and culture contribute to the definition of personal nutrition. There is a vast nutritional difference between having rice and fish as dietary mainstays and having red meat and potatoes. These two different diets have been associated with Asian and Western cultures, respectively, and have been linked to differing incidences of illness. Asian eating habits contribute to lower mortality from heart disease.[25] "In developed countries, almost as many cancer cases are attributable to an unhealthy diet and an inactive lifestyle as to smoking."[26] Studies of the age at onset of puberty highlight the effect of adequate nutrition and health. In countries where health and nutrition are adequate, menarche occurs earlier than in countries with poorer health care and nutrition.[27] Nutrition also affects the aging process. For example, the "Mediterranean diet" is associated with a lower mortality in Europeans[28] and a decreased incidence of cancer.[29] The effects of inadequate nutrition are painfully obvious in areas of the world that experience food shortages.

Culture helps us identify values and determine the task demands and roles that we play. There are similarities between cultural expectations and differences. Cultural expectations affect child-rearing practices and the attainment of adult status especially in selecting activities/actions that represent role transitions. Cultures vary in their focus on an individual or the group. Western cultures tend to focus on the individual, whereas Eastern cultures are collectivistic systems where the group is more important than the individual.

THEORETICAL ASSUMPTIONS

The theoretical approach used to describe human development provides a framework for a discussion of the reasons for change and allows us to test our hypotheses regarding the ability of a theory to predict future development. The major assumptions about development center on the role of maturation and learning and on the nature of developmental change over time. Theories and theorists differ in the way in which the origin of behavior is viewed. Is behavior innate, or is it a product of our experiences? Maturationists argue that our genetic blueprint produces commonalities in our growth and development. Behaviorists take the stand that experience plays a strong role in our personal and social development. While maturation still plays a role, it appears that experience can affect change in an individual's genetic makeup through the process of epigenesis and is the more important influencer of development.[30]

The theorists discussed here have tried to explain the nature of developmental change over time (Table 2.2). All agree that sequential changes occur from simple to complex behavior in all domains of function. They differ on whether these changes occur in a smooth, continuous manner (continuity, or nonstage development) or with abrupt stops and starts (discontinuity, or stage development). *Continuity of development* implies that later development is dependent on what came before. If development is viewed as continuous, earlier skills lead to the development of later skills. Continuity can be observed in psychological development. In Erikson's theory,[31] successful resolution of each psychological dilemma is required to proceed to the next level. Development of cognition can be thought of as a continuous line from start to finish.

Stage theory provides another approach and can be thought of quantitatively: a stair-step arrangement specifies different motor skills, such as head control or sitting on each step. Stage theory also postulates that there are qualitative changes that occur throughout development. At each successively higher level of development, or next step, a new characteristic appears that was not previously present. In stage development, discontinuity is more prevalent than continuity in motor development. For example, sitting and standing are sufficiently different to be considered stages in motor development, not continuous events.

A third viewpoint related to development is that of thinking that a child is a miniature adult. In some parts of the skeletal system, where miniature models of bones are first formed out of cartilage and then replaced by bone, it might appear that the theory is correct. Differential growth, however, occurs in the bones of the face during puberty, so that the adolescent looks much different from the child. Many body systems do not function on an adult level in the child. Because there are more instances in which this theory does not hold true, it is typically not accepted.

It is important to understand that theories provide a starting point from which to understand the complexity of human development. Regardless of the domain considered, theories attempt to explain why changes can and do occur over time. The time span covered by each developmental theory varies greatly. For example, Piaget's theory of intelligence begins at birth and ends in adolescence. Levinson's theory deals exclusively with adult development, a less well-understood phenomenon than either early or later development. Erikson's theory of personality development is the most easily recognized life span approach because his theory accounts for changes that occur from birth to senescence. Therefore, his theory can be used to place the individual in the appropriate stage of psychosocial development relative to what is happening in other domains.

LIFE SPAN THEORIES OF DEVELOPMENT

Biophysical Development
Genetics and Epigenetics

Genes carry the blueprint for how the body systems are put together, how the body changes during growth and development, and how the body operates over a lifetime. Your genetic code coordinates the production of proteins which direct growth, adaptation, and repair.[32] Proteins are constructed from individual amino acids and include structural proteins, hormones, enzymes, and other classes of biomolecules. All cells of the body carry genetic material in chromosomes. The chromosomes in the body cells are called *autosomes*. Because each of us has 22 pairs of autosomes, every cell in the body has 44 chromosomes and two *sex chromosomes*. Reproductive cells contain 23 chromosomes (22 autosomes and either

TABLE 2.2   Theories of Human Development

Domain	Life Span	Child Development	Adolescence	Adulthood	Senescence
Biophysical	Genetics/epigenetics Dynamic systems -Smith and Thelen -Shoots and Yates	Maturation - Gesell Neuronal group selection -Edelman	Sexual maturation Dynamic systems -Fisher and Bidell		Error Programmed Combination
Psychological	Stages of psychosocial development - Erikson	Stages of intelligence - Piaget Perceptual cognitive -Gibson Social cognitive Theory of mind	Self-regulation Self-determination -Deci and Ryan	Career consolidation -Valliant Emerging adulthood -Arnett Established adulthood -Mehta et al. Midlife -Infurna et al. Seasons of Life -Levinson	Processing speed - Salthouse Cognitive reserve - Stern
Sociocultural	Social learning - Bandura Motivation -Maslow Self-determination -Deci and Ryan Environmental - Bronfenbrenner	Behaviorist -Skinner Temperament - Thomas et al. Social cognitive - Vygotsky Play	Gender identity Social role Interpersonal -Cooley -Brown -Neuman and Neuman	Social clock -Neugarten Keeper of meaning -Valliant Culture/well-being -Kitayama et al.	Selective optimization with compensation - Baltes Disengagement Activity Continuity Proactivity -Khana and Khara

an X or Y chromosome). After fertilization of the egg by the sperm, the genetic material is combined during *meiosis*, determining the sex of the child by the pairing of the sex chromosomes. Two X make a female, whereas one X and one Y make a male.

The color of your hair is genetically determined. One hair color, such as brown, is more common than another color such as blond. A trait that is passed on as *dominant* is expressed, whereas a *recessive* trait may be expressed only under certain circumstances. Each gene inherited by a child has a paternal and a maternal contribution. Alleles are alternative forms of a gene, such as H or h. If someone carries identical alleles of a gene, HH or hh, the person is homozygous. If the person carries different alleles of a gene, Hh or hH, the person is heterozygous. Gene expression depends on messenger RNA (mRNA), which is produced by transcription.[33] Transcription involves unzipping and making a photo negative of the DNA. mRNA leaves the cell nucleus and goes to the ribosomes in the endoplasmic reticulum. The ribosomes translate the "photo negative" from the mRNA and assemble three-dimensional proteins called polypeptides.

Epigenetics is the study of how environmental factors can change the expression or repression of genes.[34]

Environmental factors such as exercise, stress, and nutrition change gene expression and make adaptation possible.[32,35,36] Epigenetics literally means above the genome (Fig. 2.6). Metabolism is a key part of how environmental changes impact gene expression.[34] For example, gestational diabetes mellitus (GDM), a common metabolic condition that can occur during pregnancy, can result in complications for the mother and baby. Franzago and colleagues (2019)[36] provided a review of epigenetic modifications during pregnancy and GDM due to nutritional and environmental factors that could result in transgenerational inheritance of metabolic disorders (Fig. 2.6). Early exposure to environmental insults can result in different health outcomes in the offspring (Palma-Gudiel et al., 2019).

Epigenesis is the process whereby gene expression can be modified. Epigenetic changes do not change the DNA. They are not mutations. Epigenetic "tags" are applied to the DNA by methylation or histone acetylation. These modifications are stable and can be inherited via cell division either through *mitosis* or *meiosis*.[32] The transcription/translation process of producing proteins may be highly influenced by epigenetic modifications resulting in a *phenotype* that is reflective of pervasive

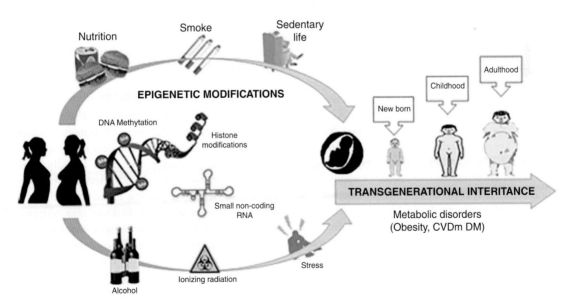

Fig. 2.6 Epigenetic modifications induced by nutrition, hyperglycemia, smoking, radiation, psychological stress, alcohol consumption, etc., can lead to a range of long-term metabolic disorders in offspring. (From Franzago M, Fraticelli F, Stuppia L, et al. Nutrigenetics, epigenetics and gestational diabetes: consequences in mother and child. *Epigenetics.* 2019;14:215-235, Fig. 1.)

environmental influences. An individual or cell's *genotype* or DNA code remains stable unless there is a mutation. *Genomic imprinting* occurs when an inherited trait is expressed differently depending on the gender of the parent who contributes the allele.[33]

Genomic testing involves examination of a person's DNA and goes beyond just identification of a known genetic disorder. Clinical genomics can provide information on a person's susceptibility to some diseases and possible response to both physical and pharmacological interventions.[37] For therapists, research into epigenetic modification is critical for understanding which genes can be modified in response to exercise.[32,38] Because a lack of physical activity increases the risk for metabolic disease, knowledge of epigenetic markers may be able to determine or monitor a person's risk.

Most other theories of biophysical development focus on one age group. The only theoretical approach that remotely approximates a life span perspective is the *dynamic systems theory*. Researchers from developmental psychology and gerontology have applied dynamic systems theory to early development and aging.[39,40] Lockman and Thelen[39] introduced the term *development biodynamics* to explain the organization of motor behavior based on interaction between perception and action. According to this theory, motor behavior emerges from that interaction rather than from nervous system maturation, as previously theorized. The relationship of dynamic systems theory to motor development is discussed in Chapter 3.

Dynamic systems theory grew out of *chaos theory*, which originated in mathematics and physical science to explain change over time in nonlinear systems. As a biological system, the human organism is an open system. Open systems are more complex. The human organism interacts with the internal and external environment. Open systems self-organize. "Dynamic systems theory hypothesizes that internal or external fluctuations of nonequilibrium systems can pass a critical point (transformation point) and create order out of disorder through a process of self-organization."[40] Energy is used in the development of a single cell into interacting organ systems. Living systems exhibit periods of stability or equilibrium and periods of disequilibrium. During the period of disequilibrium, significant change may occur. Energy is also used to keep the body going, make repairs, and preserve capacities in all systems. Living systems fluctuate and behave in complex ways.

Schroots and Yates[40] applied dynamic systems theory to development and aging because they saw development and senescence as having similar features. These common features are (1) change over time, with gradients; (2) tapping of energy resources; and (3) the production of new structures and functions. Each new structure and function adds new dynamic constraints and information to the body through feedback to the genetic blueprint. Differences between early development and senescence are the degree and rate of change that take place. During early development, the system is highly changeable; when maturity is reached, the system is more stable. The rate of change is faster during early development and slower during senescence. The first processes are negentropic or anabolic and initially obscure the ongoing entropic or catabolic process of senescence.

Homeodynamics is the process whereby complex systems maintain stability. The concept goes beyond homeostasis, which implies a static condition. In homeodynamics, the body's systems are working dynamically to cope with an ever-changing internal metabolism. The age-related failure of homeodynamics is caused by the accumulation of molecular damage and is generally accepted as the explanation for biological aging.[41] The more disordered the system, the more vulnerable it is to disease and degradation, and eventual cessation of activity. In fact, aging has been defined as a progressive shrinkage of the homeodynamic space. Think of the space as a buffer zone that is attenuated with advanced age and possible chronic illness.

Psychological Development

Erikson[31] transformed Freud's psychoanalytical theory into a psychosocial view of human development. Erikson's view combined biological needs with cultural expectations, producing the most broadly applicable theory of human psychological development for present-day society by replacing Freud's sexual focus with traits of social interaction. Erikson also addressed the entire life span in his original eight stages of psychosocial development. These stages incorporate more than one domain of function and are identified as necessary for an individual's growth. Each revolves around a psychosocial conflict that must be resolved to advance in the developmental process.

As Erikson aged, his work increasingly dealt with adult stages and aging. He and his colleagues[21] looked at generational differences and the role of expectations

TABLE 2.3 Erikson's Stages of Development

Life Span Period	Stage	Characteristics
Infancy	Trust vs. mistrust	Self-trust, attachment
Late infancy	Autonomy vs. shame or doubt	Independence, self-control
Childhood (preschool)	Initiative vs. guilt	Initiates own activity
School age	Industry vs. inferiority	Works on projects for recognition
Adolescence	Identity vs. role confusion	Sense of self in all domains
Early adulthood	Intimacy vs. isolation	Relationship with significant other
Middle adulthood	Generativity vs. stagnation	Guiding the next generation
Late adulthood	Involvement vs. resignation	Live life despite aging changes
Later adulthood	Integrity vs. despair	Sense of wholeness and wisdom

From Erikson EH. *Identity, Youth, and Crisis.* New York: WW Norton; 1986; Erikson EH, Erikson JM. *The Life Cycle Completed* (extended version). New York: WW Norton; 1997; Erikson EH, Erikson JM, Kivnick HQ. *Vital Involvement in Old Age. The Experience of Old Age in Our Time.* New York: WW Norton; 1986.

in aging. His wife proposed a new eighth stage (involvement vs. resignation) of psychosocial development.[42] The ninth stage is the former stage 8 (integrity vs. despair), which remains the final stage in psychosocial development.[43] The change in placement of this stage occurred because of increased research into aging as a mass phenomenon. Erikson's complete stages are outlined in Table 2.3 and discussed later.

Stage 1

The infant's first psychosocial conflict is whether to trust or mistrust the people within the world. Through physical contact and caregiving, the infant forms positive attachments that are mutually reinforcing. If a positive attachment does not occur, negative attachments or mistrust of others, of the environment, and even of the self may result. The basis of trust is seen in the establishment of positive contact with the environment and the people in it, including touch and the meeting of the infant's needs.

Stage 2

In toddlers, the basic trust learned in infancy is enhanced by resolving the next psychosocial conflict. The toddler expresses newfound independence using both motor and social skills, with the ever-popular statement, "Me do it." It is important during this stage that the toddler be permitted to be as independent as possible to prevent feelings of doubt concerning emerging abilities. Learning to control one's movements and those of

people and objects within the environment is very important in early development. However, with the assertion of this newfound independence can come conflict between the child's wants and parental boundaries, as seen in the so-called terrible twos.

Stage 3

Self-regulation develops slowly in the third stage as the child learns the boundaries of appropriate social behavior. Just as an infant learns the rules of moving by experimenting with movement, the child experiments with learning how to behave socially. A growing sense of identity plus parental guidance allows for the development of self-regulation, whether that means becoming toilet trained, learning to share, or learning to take turns. Between 3 and 5 years, the preschooler has learned to master many tasks and feels free to initiate their own activities. By teaching the child which behaviors are acceptable under what circumstances, the parents encourage the child's confidence in carrying out a plan of action without fear of a negative result or the burden of guilt. During this time, the parents' most important task is to encourage self-regulation of behavior. When children begin to regulate their own behavior, they begin to rely on internalized value and reward systems.

Stage 4

The school-age child deals with the conflict between industry and inferiority. The initiative developed in the previous stage is applied to learning how to work hard on a project and to enjoy the satisfaction of a job done well. A positive self-image grows out of achievement. Without success, the child may learn to be helpless, which in turn can produce a negative self-image. The initial self-image formed between 2 and 3 years of age is expanded during middle childhood in the struggle with success or failure in school. As students' awareness of their values, goals, and strategies increases, they become more sensitive to the needs and expectations of others. It is during this time that tasks are often undertaken to gain the approval of a favorite teacher.

Stage 5

Adolescence produces one of the most trying psychosocial dilemmas: identity versus role confusion. Adolescents' identity is a unique blend of what they were in childhood and what they will become in adulthood. Identity formation is affected by social and sexual experiences, cognitive abilities, and self-knowledge. An adolescent must be capable of the highest level of cognition to ponder the philosophical question of "Who am I?" Anticipation of what an adolescent will do in a variety of situations causes the individual to enact every possible life scenario before it actually transpires. Self-knowledge is gleaned from past life experiences. This knowledge includes physical information gained from the five senses as well as the knowledge of bodily functions. Emotionally, self-knowledge includes self-esteem and self-image.

The self is very important to the adolescent, so much so that self-centeredness or egocentrism engenders a feeling of performing on stage. Although emotions are part of adolescent development, they play only one role in the development of a stable identity: achievement of emotional independence from parents and other adults. Socially, adolescents are expected to develop appropriate behavior toward their own and the opposite sex. Sexual identity is established along with a moral ideology to guide socially responsible behavior. The successful end result is a unique and stable view of self, a life philosophy, and a career path. The pursuit of a career or vocation allows the adolescent to move away from her previous egocentrism.[31]

The term *role confusion* describes the failure to form an identity during adolescence. Role confusion may result if adequate support systems are not available. The inability to form an identity leaves an adolescent confused about their role in society and makes it difficult to formulate a life philosophy, forge a career, or start a family.

Stage 6

Once an identity has been established, the young adult must deal with the conflict of intimacy versus isolation. Forming an intimate relationship with a significant other involves sharing the values, hopes, goals, and fears found during the search for identity. A person learns to share love in many different forms: parental love, spousal love, child love, friend love, and spiritual love. The negative result from losing the battle for intimacy is to become self-absorbed and unable to relate openly with other people. Social and emotional isolation may lead to an overly developed sense of righteousness and outward prejudice toward those with whom we disagree.

Stage 7

Generativity is an unconscious desire to guide and assist the next generation. The traditional way that this assistance is given is through parenting, but it can also be expressed through an occupation such as teaching or an avocation such as Big Brother or Big Sisters. At the age of 80, Erikson[44] wrote that making creative contributions to the world and caring for other people's children could substitute for having our own children. The common denominator in this stage is fostering another's well-being. To help others, we must be productive and creative. Stagnation and cynicism are alternatives to generativity—the "Is that all there is?" attitude toward life.

Stage 8

This stage represents the person's ability to face one's old age in every dimension—mind, body, and society.[42] Involvement is characterized as living life on your own terms and accepting the changes as a result of aging. Involvement is not synonymous with activity. Involvement is being engaged in life in any way that is enjoyable and pleasurable. The opposing dilemma is resignation in which no new activities are undertaken. Old activities may cease and the person may feel as if it is useless to continue any activities. People who embrace this conflict resign from caring about their life. They consciously withdraw. This stage and the final stage are representative of the struggles in older adulthood. For those who choose to be involved, the courage of older people can be meaningful for the world.

Stage 9

The last hurdle of development is the conflict between integrity and despair—not ethical integrity, but ego integrity—a sense of wholeness of self related to the life already lived and life yet to be experienced. There is a sense of vitality, expectation, and wisdom that comes from the life cycle being reflected back on itself.[44] If the older adult does not achieve ego integrity because inner resources from successful handling of previous psychosocial dilemmas have not been built up, despair replaces vitality. Involvement learned from the previous stage can provide strength to carry on and transcend the remaining challenges faced in older adulthood.

Another of the social theories of aging is Robert Peck's stages of psychological development, in which he expanded upon Erikson's middle and late adulthood stages with four specific and detailed areas: mental flexibility versus mental rigidity, emotional flexibility versus emotional impoverishment, socializing versus sexualizing in human relationships, and valuing wisdom versus physical powers. Peck elaborated on Erikson's stages by suggesting that older adults go through three developmental stages to reach full psychosocial development.[45]

Stage 1—Ego differentiation versus work role preoccupation

Stage 2—Body transcendence versus body preoccupation

Stage 3—Ego transcendence versus ego preoccupation

In stage 1, as a person matures, that person moves from work role preoccupation, which is a concept that describes defining oneself through work or an occupation. A person finds new meaning and value in his or her life. This process is called ego differentiation. In stage 2, the theory states that those in old age must redefine themselves in ways that do not relate to their work roles or occupation. A person either accepts the limitations that accompany the aging process called body transcendence or dwells on diminishing abilities called body preoccupation. In stage 3, self-examination occurs. If a person believes their life has worth and has "life contributions" that will live on after death, the person experiences ego transcendence. Otherwise, the person may feel that they have lived a useless life and experience ego preoccupation.[45]

Realistically, we understand that all determinants of late life satisfaction are not under our control. The body ages physically as well as psychologically. The physical self and the life situation, including socioeconomic status (SES), activity level, and availability of transportation, have an impact on successful aging (SA). There is a complex relationship between internal and external factors that shape the end result of a process that includes our past achievements and how we reacted to them. The task of coming to terms with how we led our life, the choices made, and the paths not taken is not easy. The challenge is best met with a strong sense of self-respect and good sense of humor, remembering that "No one gets through this life alive." "A well-lived life is also a well-lived old age."[42]

Sociocultural Development
Social Learning

Bandura's social learning theory explains observational learning.[46] As such, it may be more relevant to understanding the abstract learning that occurs from adolescence through adulthood. However, an essential process in Bandura's cognitive social learning theory is that of *modeling*. Modeling is described as a type of cognitive patterning. Some skills are taught directly by modeling the behavior being taught, such as having a child watch an adult sweep the floor. More complicated behaviors, such as learning values and developing problem-solving approaches, are transmitted more subtly. Adults are always amazed at what behaviors children pick up.

Social theory teaches us that experience is invaluable. We register personal experience with reference to our own level of biological and psychological maturity. A parent's raising their voice to a toddler may stop the child from an unwanted activity, but verbal warnings often go unnoticed by a teenager. Experience by itself is only an occurrence in time; experience paired with memory connotes learning. The pairing is possible because of the interaction between behavior, cognition, and the environment. Each area influences another; cognition can influence the environment, and the environment can influence behavior. For example, teaching children not to play with matches does not preclude them from learning how to safely light a campfire.

Observational learning is used in the socialization process of becoming a professional. Expectations play a large role in structuring or motivating performance. The clinical instructor expects a certain level of performance from a student therapist, and that expectation motivates the student to perform. Therefore the reality that is observed in the clinic is more highly valued than a laboratory simulation. Learning is not the result of a single event but of many events within the context of interpersonal relationships.

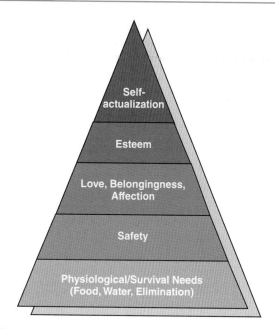

Fig. 2.7 Maslow's hierarchy of needs.

Motivation

Maslow[47] generated a theory to counteract the seemingly nonhumanistic approach of the psychoanalysts and the behaviorists. His theory of motivation is based on his perceived human needs hierarchy (Fig. 2.7), in which each life stage is seen from the perspective of fulfilling a specific need. Maslow identified how those needs change in relation to a person's social and psychological development. He preferred to use a hierarchy rather than stages. We all have an innate drive to survive, grow, and find meaning to life. The sequence of needs progresses from the physiological needs related to survival and safety to the needs for love, self-esteem, and ultimately, self-actualization. The last stage occurs when we have become all that is possible for us to be, and it cannot be achieved unless all other needs have been met. A self-actualized person is self-assured, independent, and autonomous; oriented to solving problems; and not self-absorbed.

Self-determination is another theory of motivation which identifies three basic needs: autonomy, competence, and relatedness.[48] People who are self-determined make their own decisions; those who are competent have the need to master tasks important to them. Human beings need to be connected to other human beings, which includes physical closeness and affection. Adolescents and young adults make healthier life choices if they exhibit autonomous motivation and competence.[49] Intrinsic motivation is also linked to increased attention and learning.[50]

Ecology

Bronfenbrenner's ecological systems approach is the application of the biological concept of studying organisms in their natural habitat or ecosystem to human development.[51] For example, a biologist studies trout in a trout stream, not in a saltwater marsh. The model in Fig. 2.8 represents Bronfenbrenner's perception of the family, community, and culture as interacting systems of society. Each system is named for its relationship to the child and encompasses an ever-widening sphere of influence. The child interacts with the members of the family, community, and culture, and they in turn act on the child. The mesosystem connects the various microsystems as they are likely to influence one another. The exosystem does not affect the child directly but indirectly as it represents social settings. All three of these systems are embedded in the macrosystem. Research has focused on the effects of the varying levels of the system on developmental competence, child-rearing practices and developmental outcome, and parental attitudes within neighborhoods. Family-centered care in early intervention is based on this theory and others.[52]

THEORIES OF CHILD DEVELOPMENT

Biophysical Development
Maturationists

The maturationist's view of motor development correlates all movement acquisition with the onset of changes in the nervous system relative to the onset and integration of reflexes/reactions, hierarchy of control, and a timetable of myelination. As biologists, maturationists might have considered the possibility that the maturation of other tissues, such as the muscle or bone, could contribute to movement production. However, the theory was based on the idea that central nervous system maturation was the primary determinant of motor behavior. Gesell and McGraw are the primary proponents of a biological maturation theory of development. Our discussion will be confined to Gesell's contributions.

The maturationists attributed developmental change to genetics and tended to ignore the role of experience. Gesell and associates[53] studied motor development as

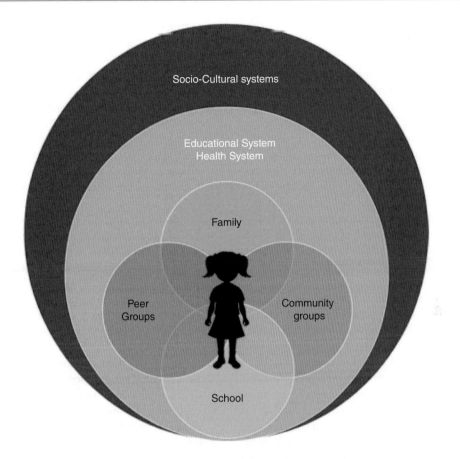

Fig. 2.8 Bronfenbrenner's ecological model is one of the few comprehensive frameworks for understanding the role of the environment in the child's development. (Modified from: Moustafa: Mental Health Effects of COVID-19; Elsevier Inc.)

a means to understand mental development. Gesell became known as the "father of developmental testing." Gesell viewed motor development as the physical entity that allowed functional behavior. A believer in structure, he defined stages of motor development that he thought governed behavior during each age period. Gesell also recognized the role of individual differences in temperament as a variable during the development of stability and change in motor patterns.

Neuronal Group Selection

Edelman's (1987)[54] theory of neuronal group selection supports the dynamic systems theory of motor control and motor development. The brain and nervous system are guided during development by a genetic blueprint and initial activity, which establishes rudimentary neural circuits. Use of certain circuits reinforces synaptic efficacy and strengthens those circuits. Selectivity comes from exploring different ways of moving. Maps are developed that provide the organization of patterns of spontaneous movement in response to mover and task demands. The cornerstone of development is the linking of these early perception-action categories. Other body systems, such as the skeletal, muscular, cardiovascular, and pulmonary systems, develop and interact with the nervous system so the most efficient movement pattern is chosen for the mover. The brain is not hard-wired with movement produced to meet the task and environmental demands. This theory supports the idea that neural plasticity may be a constant feature across the life span. See Chapter 3 for more information on this theory and Chapter 4 for more on neural plasticity.

Psychological Development

Intelligence

Piaget, a well-known developmental psychologist, identified four stages of cognitive development in children: sensorimotor, preoperational, concrete operations, and formal operations.[55] Each stage is characterized by different ways of interacting with the environment, as identified in Table 2.4 and described in detail later. His theory explained how humans acquire and process information about the world. His theory of how children learn to think is predicated on an active construction of cognitive ability. Although research has not completely supported the exact ages to which Piaget attributed these stages, the stages do occur in this order. Even Piaget recognized that children move through the stages at their own rate.

Piaget[55] identified two basic functions of all organisms that make this mastery possible. The first function is the individual's ability to *organize*, which is to make a coherent whole out of the parts. It involves integration at some level. The second basic function is *adaptation*, which is further divided into two processes of *assimilation* and *accommodation*. When a new way of acting becomes completely your own, you have assimilated it, taken it in, and made it a part of your own way of acting. Some objects or actions do not fit into existing structures or actions and require modification. The process of modification of the environment is accommodation. If an infant cannot grasp a block because something is covering it, the obstacle must be removed. The inborn strategies of adaptation—assimilation and accommodation—provide a basis for development of schemas.

Sensorimotor period. Schemas are the basic unit of Piaget's cognitive structure. The infant begins to form these schemas by combining sensory and motor actions. Because the first two years of life are so critical to intellectual development, the sensorimotor period is divided into six stages. Each stage has its own hallmarks.

Stage 1. Stage 1 is *reflexive* and lasts for only the first month of life when the infant's interactions with the world are largely based on reflexes such as rooting, sucking, and kicking. Sucking is not confined to ingesting food. The infant sucks on its fingers, the blanket, and clothes. All kinds of objects are assimilated into the sucking schema. Accommodation begins as the infant makes subtle adjustments of lips and head while feeding.

Stage 2. Stage 2 occurs from 1–4 months and is characterized by *primary circular reactions*. When an infant repeats a volitional act over again, it is considered a circular reaction. The initial action may be purely by chance. The reactions are considered primary because these activities are focused primarily on the infant's body. Examples would include thumb sucking or repetitive grasping of body parts or clothing.

Stage 3. Stage 3 brings about *secondary circular reactions*. Now infants expand their horizons to include events and objects in the external world. Grasping, shaking, and banging objects are all examples of such actions. Even vocalizations become greater as infants recognize

TABLE 2.4 Piaget's Periods of Cognitive Development		
Life Span Period	**Piaget's Period**	**Characteristics**
Infancy	Sensorimotor six stages	Babies pair sensory and motor action schemes, such as sucking, hitting, and grasping, as a means to deal with the immediate surroundings in their world.
Preschool	Preoperations	Children have a one-dimensional awareness of the environment. They use symbols and internal representations to think, but thinking is illogical and unsystematic.
School age	Concrete operations	Children solve problems and think systematically, but only with real objects and activities.
Pubescence	Formal operations	Adolescents solve abstract problems by using induction and deduction. Systematic thinking is applied on a purely abstract level.

that their noise-making prompts those around them to make noises back to them. This stage occurs from 4–8 months.

Stage 4. Stage 4 (8–12 months) brings big changes when there is *coordination of secondary schemas.* Now the infant can put two schemes together to accomplish a goal. Behavior becomes goal-directed, and infants become capable of intentionality. When faced with an obstacle, the infant can figure out how to remove it to get what is wanted. For example, an infant will push one toy out of the way to get to the toy that is partially exposed under it or use a stick to get to another object. *Object permanence* emerges during this stage. The ability to know that an object or person still exists even if not in view is a profound realization. However, the concept is only emerging at this stage and will continue to mature over the next several months as evidenced by the following response to a hidden object. Infants at this stage may still be fooled if a toy is first hidden under one blanket and then another. They will search only the first hiding place. This error is not due to lack of object permanence.[56]

Stage 5. During the second year of life, 12-month-olds begin to seek new, unexpected results by varying their actions. For example, a toddler may experiment with dropping various objects off the highchair tray to see the consequences. Another child might put a hand under the faucet while in the bathtub and observe the different results depending on how close the hand was to the faucet. Trial-and-error experimentation is an obvious primary activity for this stage, which is termed *tertiary circular reactions.* The child deliberately varies actions within schemas to observe the consequences. When playing with toy cars on a ramp, the toddler can comprehend that if the car is let go at the top of the ramp, it should be looked for at the bottom of the ramp. Before this time, the infant would still look for the toy car at the top of the ramp.

Stage 6. The last stage of the sensorimotor period is the *beginning of thought* (18–24 months). The title for stage 6 is quite profound because it connotes the child's ability to exhibit mental representation. Children must be able to mentally represent objects or persons not in plain view in order to think symbolically. Once mental representation is possible, understanding causality becomes more sophisticated. Mentally being able to represent past events or actions allows for the ability to pretend. Deferred imitation is the ability to imitate in the absence of a model.

Preoperations. From 2 to 7 years is the preoperational stage of intelligence. During this time, children are able to represent the world by symbols, such as words and objects. The increased use of language marks the beginning of symbolic thought. Preschoolers exemplify the child in preoperational thought. The child labels all forms of transportation as "ride" or all four-footed animals as "dog" or "cat" depending on the frame of reference. Children in this period demonstrate egocentric behavior in that their reasoning is always in relation to themselves. They are unable to take another's viewpoint. Centration is exhibited when the child centers on only one characteristic of an object to the exclusion of other salient features. In deciding which beaker has more liquid, a typical 4-year-old may focus on the height of the liquid in a beaker and ignore the diameter (Fig. 2.9). The last characteristic of the preoperational period is that of appearance as reality. Scary masks or costumes transform a known person into someone scary. Toward the end of this period, most children begin to have some understanding of time, which eventually allows them to learn how to wait.

Concrete operations. During this stage, the school-age child develops the ability to classify objects according to their characteristics. The child can solve concrete problems, that is, those in which the actual objects are physically present, as in "Which cup is bigger?" or "Which string is longer?" Most of Piaget's famous conservation experiments were carried out to demonstrate a child's ability to transform objects from one set of circumstances to another while preserving the idea that the objects were unchanged. When a child in concrete operations is asked about which beaker has more liquid, as seen in Fig. 2.9, all aspects of the container will be considered. Conservation of liquid is generally achieved by 7 years of age. The school-age child demonstrates symbolic thinking and has acquired the ability to mentally

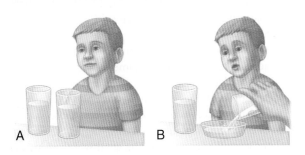

A   B

Fig. 2.9 Conservation of liquids.

reverse thoughts. For example, if they learned that 4 plus 6 equals 10, then 6 plus 4 would also equal 10.

Formal operations. Piaget and Inhelder[57] described the highest level of cognitive development as formal operations. This stage begins in adolescence, which, according to our time periods, begins at 10 years in girls and 12 years in boys. Early adolescents are able to think about and thus deal with hypothetical as well as real situations. Now, instead of engaging in trial-and-error experimentation, the formal operations thinker formulates a hypothesis and plans a way to study a problem. For example, in the problem if Sally is shorter than Terry, and Terry is taller than Steve, the adolescent can figure out who is the tallest without having to line her classmates up and compare their heights. Being able to generate a hypothesis, engage in deductive reasoning, and check solutions are all characteristics of logical decision making. Not all adolescents and adults apply this type of thinking to all aspects of life. They may tend to selectively use the ability only in particular personal or professional situations.

Perceptual Cognitive Theory

Perception has been linked to cognition from the beginning of the field of psychology. While Piaget linked sensation to movement as an initial step in the development of intelligence, it is Eleanor Gibson who is the champion of the perceptual cognitive theory of cognition. She pioneered the view that perception has the ability to detect order and structure, not just to organize sensory information. Her research, and those that followed her, focused on how perception guides action.[58]

The goal of perception is action.[59] Perception of the surrounding environment, which includes objects and people, serves the functional purpose of bringing about contact and interaction. The objects afford the opportunity to act, and in acting, the object and action are changed. This is the concept of *affordance*.[60] Affordance goes beyond adaptation and integration because both the object and perceiver are changed in the encounter. A jungle gym may afford a seat for one child or a place to hang upside down for another child. Perception is the means by which the child comes in contact with the world and adapts to it. The ecological view of perceptual development does not require the child to construct actions with objects as did Piaget's model. Gibson's concept of environmental affordance highlights the ecological perspective of cognition. The quality of the learning environment and the affordances that are available to

the learner can impact development of cognitive abilities. Perceptual development is further explored in Chapter 9.

Theory of Mind

Theory of mind (ToM) is a concept whereby children learn to understand human behavior.[61] It is a social cognitive theory with roots in Rochat's seven stages of self and social awareness development. The reader is referred to his description of the steps that lead the infant from an implicit self-awareness at birth to self-consciousness and finally to being able to embrace an ethical fairness toward others at age 5.[62] ToM development begins in infancy with the occurrence of joint attention. Joint attention is demonstrated when an adult and an infant mutually attend to the same object or action. Development of ToM is supported by the development of awareness of self and others during family interaction and play. Motor imitation of others' actions as seen in play around 14 months marks progression of ToM development. From there, children progress to initiating their own actions in play. Pretend play is developed by 2 years of age and requires the ability to have a mental representation of an object in the mind. The object does not have to be present to be thought of. ToM develops within the first 5 years of life. Three-year-olds are aware of others' wants, feelings, and perceptions and become attuned to norms of behavior. Preschoolers understand the role of mental states when pretending.[63] The same symbolic phenomenon that underlies pretend play also underlies ToM. Understanding the mental world of the self and others appears to be critically important for learning from others.[64]

In the last several decades, there has been an increase in studies of ToM in healthy older adults.[65,66] Different paradigms are used to study healthy elders' ability to represent another's mental state. Decision making is slower in older adults and the degree of deficits is related to deficiency in general cognition. Ruitenberg and colleagues, (2020)[66] study demonstrated changes in both the cognitive and affective components of ToM but found that the slowing did not affect the outcome of the decision.

Sociocultural Development
Behaviorist

Probably the most famous behaviorist is B. F. Skinner,[67] the father of stimulus-response (S-R) psychology, whose experiments with rats and mazes clearly showed that certain behavior can be conditioned. He applied the principles of operant conditioning to the development of human behavior and believed that the environment was the most influential factor in determining behavioral outcomes. In fact, he thought that the mind was irrelevant to understanding human behavior.[68] Skinner promoted the concept of environmental engineering as a way to shape behavior, as he was even able to condition a fear response in a child. Although the value of reinforcement is universally accepted and behavioral modification is a legitimate form of therapeutic intervention, classic conditioning is not discussed as a formative aspect of development. Behaviorists do not represent a life span view of human development because they focus on development in childhood and adolescence. According to behaviorists, all behavior is learned by observation and imitation and can be conditioned or shaped through reinforcement.

Temperament

Temperament is a person's characteristic way of responding. Temperament includes components of self-regulation and emotion. It encompasses several dimensions such as activity level, affect (both positive and negative), persistence, and inhibition. These dimensions have been distilled down from the original nine dimensions described in Thomas, Chess, and Birch's[69] original work. Three general types or clusters of temperament characteristics were identified based on their longitudinal study. These types and their characteristics are found in Table 2.5. Temperament is innate and relatively stable during infancy and the toddler years. Temperament can be influenced by the environment, which includes child-rearing practices. Thomas, Chess, and Birch[69] introduced the concept of goodness of fit.

This concept considered the infant's temperament and the parents' ability to match the environmental demands to foster mentally healthy and well-adjusted children. For example, a good fit would occur between an *easy* baby and a parent who would allow the infant to explore the environment pretty much self-directed. The majority of babies, about 40%, are categorized as *easy*. A poor fit would occur when a *difficult* baby was not directed to channel their negative energy into acceptable activities. *Difficult* babies make up about 10%, and the *slow to warm up* babies make up another 15%. The remaining infants are not able to be consistently categorized because they demonstrate a combination of characteristics. There are cultural differences in temperament. Chinese infants at 4 months are less vocal, less active, and less irritable than either their American or Irish counterparts.[70] Temperament can indirectly contribute to attachment. It may be more challenging for a mother to form an attachment to a difficult baby than to an easy baby.

Attachment

Once homeostasis is achieved in the first several months of life, the second stage of emotional development attachment begins to develop. Infants who form attachments with adults are more likely to survive. Fig. 2.10 depicts the attachment system. Ainsworth[71] described four primary types of attachment. The ideal type of attachment is called *secure* attachment. The other three types are insecure attachments and include *anxious avoidant, resistant*, and *disorganized*. These categorizations are based on how the infant responds when separated from the mother. The infant who is securely attached may or may not cry when mom leaves, is happy to see mom when she returns, and stops crying on her return. The majority (60%–65%) of babies are securely

TABLE 2.5	**Temperament in Babies**
Temperament	**Characteristics**
Easy	Infants are easy going, have a positive disposition, are adaptable, and have regular body functions.
Difficult	Infants have negative moods, withdraw in a new situation, adapt slowly or not at all, or have irregular body functions.
Slow to warm up	Infants are relatively inactive, demonstrate calm reactions to their environment, are slow to adapt to new situations, and withdraw initially but later come around.

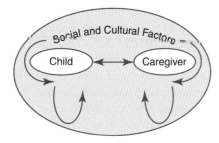

Fig. 2.10 The attachment system depicting the bidirectional nature between the caregiver and the child as they are embedded in a sociocultural context. (From Barnekow KA, Kraemer GW. The psychobiological theory of attachment: a viable frame of reference for early intervention providers. *Phys Occup Ther Pediatr.* 2005;25(1/2):3-15.)

attached. The anxious avoidant attached infant is not upset when mom leaves but gives her the cold shoulder when she returns. Approximately 20% of infants demonstrate this type of insecure attachment. The resistant attached infant gets upset and remains upset and angry even after mom returns and is difficult to console. These infants make up about 10%–15% of the population. Lastly, the disorganized or disoriented attached infants seem confused when mom leaves and when she returns, not appearing to understand what happened. These insecurely attached infants make up 5%–10% of the group. Attachment is the primary basis for interpersonal relationships. Parent-child relationships are expanded to include peer relationships. Children with secure attachments develop better peer relationships.

Social Cognitive Learning

Lev Vygotsky,[72] a Russian psychologist, thought that cognitive development could take place only as a result of social interaction. The child partners with an adult who assists the child's learning. The adult provides the tools of the particular culture such as alphabetical and numbering schemes and its concepts about distance and time. He called the support given by the other person as *scaffolding.* Anyone who has watched a building being erected can grasp this concept. In this instance, the support is given for learning and problem solving. Unlike Piaget, who thought children became little scientists on their own, Vygotsky thought the nature of cognitive development could only be understood within a cultural and social context. The *zone of proximal development* is the area of performance or level of performance that a

child can demonstrate when assisted that is not possible when left to work on their own. This zone is the potential for growth in cognitive abilities that is made possible by the assistance of a skilled adult or peer. Vygotsky thought that children could not make significant progression alone.

Play

Piaget[73] and Vygotsky[74] both appreciated the role of play in cognitive development. Play is a child's occupation.[75] Play promotes creativity and adaptation. Play is impor-tant for many reasons besides cognitive development, such as emotional development, socialization, and communication. Freud[76] and Erikson[77] used play to address wish fulfillment and coping. Culture is embodied in play. Play mirrors the socialization process of society. Mead[78] thought that children learned rules and norms through play, while Bateson[79] thought that play was important in communication but not socialization. The fact that children signal each other that they are playing is seen as a form of metacommunication. Play is not separate from reality; children know which is which, and this allows them to reflect and interpret culture.

Play fosters language and cognitive development in young children in addition to providing motivation to move. Children engage in different types of social play. A list of types of social play and their characteristics can be found in Table 2.6. The first five types were originally described by Parten[80] to identify the various levels of social interaction. Play is important in a child's life because it is a major way of learning about the world. Play provides a rich opportunity for development in all areas: physical, social-emotional, cognitive, and communication. The quality of play changes dramatically and quickly early in life. *Solitary* play occurs alone. Peer interaction may be seen as early as 6 months of age when one infant may smile or point at another infant. *Parallel* play begins soon after the first birthday and is the most prevalent form of play observed in 1- and 2-year-olds. Simple social play in which there is some interaction between the toddlers is seen between 15 and 18 months. Toys may be offered from one to the other. By age 2, young children may engage in several forms of play such as solitary, onlooker, or parallel play. *Associative* play is an example of simple social play that occurs in childhood. *Cooperative* play also begins as toddlers approach their second birthday and become children. Cooperative

TABLE 2.6 Types of Play

Type of Play	Characteristics
Solitary	Child plays alone, exploring and manipulating objects or toys without attending to others.
Onlooker	Child watches others play but does not participate except for some minimal communication.
Parallel	Child plays with one child or more but each is playing separately. Materials are not shared.
Associative	Child plays with one child or more. Materials, communication and activities are freely shared.
Cooperative	Child plays with one child or more for longer periods characterized by mutual goals, rules and turn taking.
Symbolic	Child plays using an object as if it were another object or person, such as a pretending a stick is a microphone. This is also called pretend play.

From Freiberg KL. *Human Development: A Life-Span Approach*. 3rd ed. Boston: Jones and Bartlett; 1987. Adaptation of Table 5.6, p 230.

play involves rules and taking turns being "it" or being the leader or being the seeker in hide and seek. Game playing is social play as well. This type of play becomes the norm among 3- and 4-year-olds when parallel play is seen less frequently. Howes and Matheson[81] see the transition from parallel play to cooperative play as representative of a qualitative change, from less to more involved play.

Symbolic play, also called pretend play, requires that a child be able to substitute another object for an absent object, such as when a ruler becomes a magic wand or a colander becomes a helmet. Children who demonstrate pretend play are considered socially competent.[81] Michael Casby[82,83] notes that children exhibit beginning symbolic functioning in play during their second year of life (12–18 months). At the end of the first year, sensorimotor play evolves into functional play. Children play with realistic toys; for example, a child might put a toy bottle to a doll's mouth while playing alone. Between 18 and 24 months, multiple actions may be observed such as a child pretending to comb their own hair and then the hair of another. As the child gets older, objects are used to represent other objects not present; for example, a hand can be used as a cup to give a toy bear a drink. Children will also attribute real actions and feelings to inanimate objects such as dolls or stuffed animals. At 3 years, children spend 20% of their time in pretend play, and that increases to 50% by age 4. Three- to 5-year-olds engage in sociodramatic play.[84] They exhibit complex sophisticated pretend play, sharing fantasies and using verbal strategies based on

agreed-upon rules. Play, especially pretend play, contributes unique developmental experiences that enrich the child's learning. See Table 2.7.

Other ways of describing play include the purpose of play: sensory/exploration, manipulation, imaginative/dramatic, or motor/physical play. The latter type is thought to improve the child's awareness of the body in space. Imaginative/dramatic play is symbolic play when the child can act out conflicts or become the superhero. Piaget thought that symbolic play was very important not only for the child's development of cognition but also for emotional development. To play symbolically, the child has to be able to dually represent an object. In other words, the ruler she is holding has to be thought of as a wand capable of turning the stuffed frog into a handsome prince.

Regardless of how one categorizes play, it is an integral part of cognitive, social, and linguistic development.

THEORIES OF ADOLESCENT DEVELOPMENT

The concept of adolescence includes changes that occur in the biological, psychological, and social domains.[85] There are many theories that can be applied to adolescence, but only a few will be highlighted in this section. Adolescence is a period of adaptation in all body systems. The impact of the biological, psychological, and social changes impact sexual maturation, self-regulation, gender identity, social roles, and interpersonal behavior.

TABLE 2.7   Play Development

Age	Type of Play	Purpose/Child Actions
0–6 months	Sensorimotor play: social and exploratory play	Establish attachment with caregivers
6–12 months		Explore the world
	Sensorimotor play→functional play	Learn cause and effect
12–24 months	Functional/relational play	Learn functional use of objects and to orient play toward peers
	Pretend play emerges	Play functionally with realistic toys
		Pretend one object can symbolically represent another object
2–5 years	Pretend play	Pretend dolls and animals are real
	Constructive play	Develop scripts as a basis for play
	Physical play	Draw and do puzzles
		Engage in rough and tumble play, jumping, chasing, swinging, sliding
6–10 years	Games with rules	Problem solving, think abstractly
		Negotiate rules
		Play games with friends

From Martin and Kessler. *Neurologic Interventions for Physical Therapy.* 4th ed. Philadelphia: Elsevier; 2021: 140.

Sexual Maturation

Puberty is the time of biological maturation and psychological growth. The period of psychological change often lasts longer than the period of physical growth. Adolescence is recognized as a critical period in the life span because dramatic changes occur in growth of the body and the brain. Secondary sexual characteristics develop and reproductive capacity is attained.[86] In addition to the hormonal changes that allow reproduction, hormones promote changes in the musculoskeletal and cardiopulmonary systems related to functional movement abilities. The physical changes in adolescence occur before the psychological and social changes and can be influenced by nutrition, trauma, and stress. The future of the species depends on members living to sexual maturity, reproducing, and rearing their offspring to reproductive age.

Dynamic Systems

Dynamic systems have already been discussed as a life span theory. Adolescence can be thought of a phase transition in which multiple body systems are perturbed and stable patterns of behavior are altered. "Skill is the capacity to act in an organized way in a specific context. Skills are thus both action-based and context-specific."[87] In most societies, adolescents engage in many complex skills such as driving a car, cooking, and engaging in mutually enjoyable social relationships. While the content of these skills varies from one culture to another, there is a shared expectation for a high level of skill performance.

Self-Regulation

Self-regulation is defined as the ability to control or regulate attention, emotions, or behavior depending on context.[88] Self-determination theory[89] emphasizes that self-regulation processes are needed to support choosing and achieving life goals. The theory identifies three basic psychological needs—autonomy, competence, and relatedness—as being essential for optimal development. Adolescents seek autonomy by separating from family and forming their own identity. Competence is gained by developing skills for future livelihood, sports participation, and leisure enjoyment. Relatedness is how adolescents relate to their social system (peers) and society (teachers, coaches, employers). Adolescence is a period of time that encompasses all of these needs. Independent and focused motivation are viewed as being used to guide goal-directed behavior. Problems with self-regulation are associated with sexual risk-taking and substance addictions.[90,91]

Gender Identity and Social Roles

A major theory of this period in development centers around gender identity. The American Psychological Association (APA) defines gender identity as, "A person's deeply-felt, inherent sense of self of being a boy, a man, or a male; a girl, a woman, or a female: or an alternative gender (e.g., genderqueer, gender nonconforming, gender neutral) that may not correspond to a person's sex assigned at birth or to a person's primary or secondary sex characteristics."[92]

Bussey and Bandura presented their social cognitive theory of gender role development and functioning in 1999. Since that time, research has recognized the biologic foundation of gender identity.[93,94] Gender expression is defined as external manifestations of gender such as one's name, pronouns, dress, haircut, or behavior. Gender identity is not typically affected by environmental influences but gender role may be. "Gender roles are formed in early childhood and continue to influence behavior through adolescence and adulthood…."[95] Bussey and Bandura (1999)[96] identified many external sources, such as parents, peers, media, and gendered practices of certain occupations, that could influence learning about and development of gender roles. They, however, did not think gender stereotypes played any role in guiding learning gender-congruent behavior. Social role theory[97] as a theory of gender development in childhood assumes that observational learning produces stereotypical beliefs about gender roles and behavior.

Interpersonal

Peer relationships are a prominent part of adolescent life. Cooley,[98] a sociologist from the early 1900s, provided the foundation for studying the relationship of the individual and society. Adolescents imagine how they are perceived by others and attach meaning to the assessment of their self. Symbolic thinking is required for the adolescent to develop the capacity for interpersonal communication. Group identity is important to adolescents and is marked by a search for membership in a group during early adolescence. Adolescents' group identity may be in conflict with their cultures' expectation of individuality.[99] Adolescents participate in a large number of groups and develop social networks. Brown and colleagues (2008)[100] studied the types of peer influences; some were negative as in peer pressure, while others were supportive such as modeling appropriate behavior.

Adolescents who learn to evaluate and value peer relationships gain autonomy.

THEORIES OF ADULT DEVELOPMENT

Adult development as a concept is a twentieth century phenomenon. Before that time, very little attention was paid to the longest period of human life, adulthood. Biological development is considered complete by the time a person is considered to be an adult. However, psychological and sociocultural development continues. Entrance into adulthood comes later than ever before in many countries, and most adults can expect to live longer after retirement.[101] Rethinking adult development is appropriate at this time as family life and work arrangements are changing.

Sociocultural processes are more potent than biological processes during adulthood.[102] Variables such as race, SES, ethnicity, culture, individual choices, and historical context will influence people's experiences even more in adulthood than in earlier development. People become more heterogeneous as we age.[103] Havinghurst[5] and Levinson (1986)[104] both recognized adulthood as a life phase that involved career and family formation.

Career Consolidation

George Valliant, a psychiatrist and director of the Harvard Study of Adult Development, inserted two new stages into Erikson's original eight stages: career consolidation and keeping the meaning. Career consolidation comes between intimacy and generativity. During this stage, a person chooses a career. It begins between 20 and 40 years of age, when young adults become focused on assuming a social identity within the work world. This is an extension of the person's personal identity forged in earlier stages. Valliant[105] identified four criteria that transform a "job" or "hobby" into a "career." They are competence, commitment, contentment, and compensation. Valliant drew from his 30 years of directing the Harvard Study.[106] The other stage, keeping the meaning, will be discussed later in this section.

Emerging Adulthood

Jeffrey J. Arnett[1,107] proposed a new life stage in 2000. He believed there was a period of development between the end of adolescence and the beginning of adulthood. He called it the period of emerging adulthood which begins at age 18 and ends at age 29. Emerging adulthood is characterized by being the age of (1) identity exploration, (2) instability, (3) feeling in-between, (4) self-focus, and (5) possibility. Unlike Erikson, who thinks that identity is forged in adolescence, Arnett[1] believed that the transition to knowing who you are occurs later in time due to globalization and technological changes. His belief has been supported by his own and others' research.[108-110] The events that mark the transition to adulthood, such as gaining stable work, marriage, and parenthood, are occurring later than ever. The knowledge needed requires more education and training and with that comes more stress. Emerging adults face distinct challenges. On the one hand, they are self-focused, highly content with their lives, and looking forward to the future, but at the same time are ambivalent about taking on adult roles. They see adulthood as a mixed blessing; there are rewards but there are constraints and limitations. During emerging adulthood, there is relative independence from social roles and normative expectations. Arnett (2016)[111] views this life stage as a cultural construct that can guide developmental expectations.

Established Adulthood

The structure of adulthood is less linear and predictable than previously thought. Family role expectations have changed in the last two decades.[109] Adulthood today may or may not include marriage and may or may not include parenthood. Active parenting may represent only a short phase of adult life partly due to lower fertility rates and longer life expectancy. Mehta and colleagues (2020)[112] propose a new conceptualization of the ages from 30 to 45 called *established adulthood.* They believe it is important to address research into the competing responsibilities of parenting and career progression that occur in *established adulthood. Established adulthood* (30–45 years) is different from *emerging adulthood* (18–29 years) and from *midlife* (45–65 years).

Features of *established* adulthood include being physically healthy, high life satisfaction in relationships with spouse and children, lowest for finances, and in general optimistic for the future.[113] At the core of *established adulthood* is the "career-and-care-crunch" because the two domains of adult life in all societies are work and family. The crunch is particularly problematic for women and women who are mothers, the motherhood penalty. This penalty is mediated by good and affordable child care.[113] For a more thorough discussion and comparison of *established* adulthood, see Mehta and associates (2020).[112]

Middle Adulthood

Middle adulthood or midlife is between 45 and 65 years of age. However, researchers generally consider it to be the ages between 40 and 60 with a 10-year buffer on either end. When polled, people said midlife begins at age 44 and ends at age 59.[114] Very little modern theory exists.[112] The so-called midlife crisis has never been proven to be a universal phenomenon. There are defining features of midlife such as balancing multiple roles and encountering potential life transitions related to marriage, parenthood, career changes, and retirement planning. The balancing act transpires during a period of changing physical, mental, and cognitive health that could result in some middle-aged adults putting others' needs ahead of their own. Lachman and colleagues (2015)[115] see midlife as a pivotal period characterized by gains and losses. Early life factors affect midlife and midlife affects later life outcomes. Adults in midlife are more likely to experience age-related physiological changes such as andropause (men) and menopause (women).[112] Better health in midlife is associated with health in old age.[116] Blood pressure in midlife predicted cognitive decline in old age.[117] Midlife has received less attention than other age periods, but that is changing in part due to the Midlife in the United States Study (MIDUS).[118]

Seasons of a Man's Life

Arnett is not the first to recognize the role of transitions in becoming an adult. Levinson[104] in his work on the Seasons of Life designated a 5-year period of time that bridged two developmental periods as a time of transition. The developmental periods are termed eras. There are four eras in life: preadulthood, up to 22 years; early adulthood, from age 17 to 45; middle adulthood, from age 40 to 65; and late adulthood, from age 60 to ? The transitions are the 5-year intervals between the eras: 17–22 for the early adult, 40–45 for midlife, and 60–65 for late adult.

What makes a person an adult? Is there a magic age or task to be attained that indicates when a person is an adult? Legally, you are an adult at 18 years. However, there are many 18-year-olds who would more than likely consider themselves as emerging adults. Regardless of the socioeconomic group a person belongs to, four criteria for adulthood continue to resound in the literature.[107] To be an adult, one must accept responsibility for actions, make independent decisions, be more considerate of others, and be financially independent. Maturity requires the acceptance of responsibility and empathy for others.

Social Clock

Neugarten identified the social clock theory in the 1960s as shared expectations of age-appropriate behavior. Members of society are told explicitly and implicitly when it is "appropriate" to start their first job, get married, have a baby, purchase a home, and retire.[119] She found remarkable convergence in the ideal ages for these events and behaviors. Cultures encourage people to behave in ways as defined by their social roles. Social expectations affect when transitions will occur.[120] This theory can best be understood as a fitting in with your contemporaries. Adults who follow a social clock can easily relate themselves to others, embracing their understanding of their place in society. Although age norms for many behaviors have been relaxed in recent decades, Neugarten's point is still relevant. In the social clock theory, there is a "prescriptive timetable for the ordering of life events" and how to use them to evaluate our lives.[119] Social psychology has examined the social clock in relation to aging and life course trajectories and how they affect decisions and mental health outcomes. Neugarten's theory has been affected by globalization, technology, and social media. Societies across the world are changing their perceptions about their own social clock.[121]

Keeper of Meaning

Keeper of meaning is the additional stage Valliant[105] interjected between Erikson's generativity and integrity stages. It comes near the end of generativity, so the person is in late middle adulthood. The role of the keeper of meaning is to preserve one's culture rather than care for successive generations. The focus is on conservation and preservation of society's institutions. The keeper of meaning guides groups and preserves traditions.

Culture and Well-Being

Kitayama, Berg, and Chopik (2020)[121] propose a theoretical model of how culture may affect aging dynamics. See Fig. 2.11 for a depiction of a model of aging in two

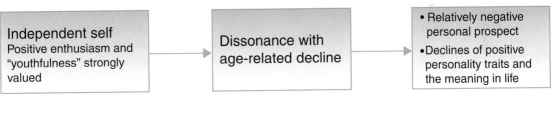

A. European American aging dynamics

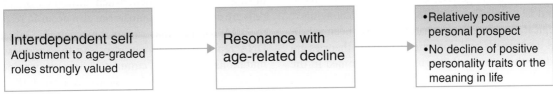

B. East Asian aging dynamics

Fig. 2.11 Schematic models of aging in two different cultural contexts: (A) In European American contexts, there is a strong push toward positivity and enthusiasm, which results in conflicts and frustration over age-related decline, which in turn leads eventually to alienation and disengagement. (B) In East Asian contexts, there is a strong push toward adjustment to age-graded roles and tasks, which results in relatively few conflicts with age-related decline, which in turn leads eventually to new meanings and engagement. (From Kitayama S, Berg MK, Chopick WJ. Culture and well-being in late adulthood: theory and evidence. *Am Psychol.* 2020;75: 567-576. Figure 1; p 569.)

cultural contexts—European American and East Asian. European Americans embrace social norms that value enthusiasm and excitement. Youthfulness is championed in this culture. However, age-related decline during late adulthood makes staying positive more challenging and could contribute to disengagement. In contrast, East Asians encounter a strong message to adjust to changes in age-related roles and tasks. Fewer conflicts of what is expected may lead to new understanding and engagement in life.

THEORIES OF AGING

Development in the Older Adult

In contrast to adulthood where there are few theories, there are a multitude of theories on aging. Aging is a lifelong process, so in reality any life span theory could contribute to this discussion. Theorists observing the later aspect of the life span hypothesize that aging occurs because of biological or physical changes in the human body. A person is aging from the moment of birth; in fact, we celebrate birthdays as a social marker of the passage of time. Aging is seen by others as the number one health problem in the United States and developing countries. As people live longer, the biology of aging becomes the primary risk factor in determining how long and how well they will live.[123] Ten leading causes of death accounted for 74% of all deaths in 2017; the majority of causes included were age-related diseases.[124]

Biophysical Theories

In 2006, Rattan hypothesized that a unified theory of biological aging involving genes, milieu, and chance was emerging.[125] Twelve years later, he states equivocally that the occurrence and accumulation of molecular damage is the basis of age-related failure of homeodynamics and is a unified explanation for biological aging.[126] Biological theories of aging had previously been subdivided into genetic and nongenetic. Genetic theories are based on the premise that aging is programmed in the cell nucleus, implying that the process of cellular aging is a *purposeful event*. Harman[127] calls cellular aging an inborn aging process (IAP) such that the human average life expectancy is limited to about 85 years. Nongenetic theories are related to environmental factors outside the cell nucleus. Here aging is viewed as part of the same continuum as the process of development—genetically controlled and probably programmed but subject to environmental influences. Explanations of aging mechanisms are more complicated than previously thought. Over 300 theories of aging have been reported. Presently, the theories fall into two categories, the *program hypotheses* and *error theories*, with a third category consisting of combinations of the two.[128]

Programmed Aging

These theories grew out of biological investigation in the 1960s. Hayflick and Moorehead[129] made a profound observation while studying human tumor viruses. When growing human cells in tissue culture, they observed a waxing and waning of cellular proliferation, followed by senescence and eventual death of the cultures. Before this time, tissue cultures had been thought to be immortal. Hayflick and Moorehead[129] interpreted their findings to mean that aging was a cellular as well as an organismic phenomenon and dramatically changed the way we viewed aging.

Hayflick[130] subsequently described, in the *Hayflick limit theory*, the number of possible life span cell replications (population-doubling potential) to be about 50. The replicative life span of specific tissue types was then linked to the age of their donor cells when cultured. The younger the donor cells, the greater was their life span. The replicative life span is also known as *replicative senescence (RS)*. In individuals with premature aging, called *progeria*, the donor cells show a lower Hayflick limit. RS has been found in other cell types such as adrenocortical cells, chondrocytes, endothelial cells, vascular smooth muscle cells, and others.[131] RS has been observed in cells of adults of all ages and those derived from embryonic tissue. The number of replications in culture varies depending on cell type.

Programmed cell death, called *apoptosis*, is apparent during early development when unwanted or unused cells are destroyed. Apoptosis can also occur in response to DNA damage that cannot be repaired. Deficits in DNA repair pathways can also lead to cancer-causing mutations. The level of cumulative damage sustained by cells determines whether *apoptosis* occurs or, if the damage is lower, senescence.[132] Senescent cells are involved in tissue repair and wound healing,[133] tumor suppression,[134] as well as in age-related diseases such as atherosclerosis, diabetes, and lung disease.[135] Senescent cells accumulate secondary to intrinsic and extrinsic stress. If the immune system does not remove the senescent cells, tissue disruption and degeneration can occur.[132]

Prevention of the accumulation of senescent cells in theory would slow the aging process.

Scientists have identified *longevity determinant genes* or *longevity assurance genes* (LAG).[136] It is thought that at least one or more genes could exert a positive influence on a person's ability to reach old age. The genetic pathways involved in longevity are those that improve repair of DNA and maintain fidelity of the information transfer in the cell. Recent studies have identified five gene polymorphisms linked to longevity and age-related disease.[137] The first is the apolipoprotein E (APOE), which in a specific variant is a risk factor for Alzheimer disease and oxidative stress. Second is ACE, a component of the renin-angiotensin system, which regulates blood pressure. Third is the forkhead box protein (FOXO). FOXO3 encodes a transcription factor which regulates stress. Klotho β-glucuronidase (KL) polymorphism plays a role in human longevity as well as a protective role in cancer.[138] Lastly, a lower frequency of the C-allele of the IL6rs1800796 locus was found in a group of long-lived Chinese compared to a control group.[139] Yan and associates found an association between IL-6 -634C/G polymorphism and osteoporosis.[140] The diversity of genes associated with aging demonstrates that there is no one universal pathway affecting lifespan.

Healthy aging depends on a complex interaction between genetic and environmental factors. Genetic biomarkers, along with lifestyle factors, can influence longevity and assess a person's risk of developing age-related disease. Many genes interact within a few biologically conserved pathways. Aging is a risk factor for both life span and health span. The aging phenotype is both individualistic and heterogenous. Essential life span of a species according to Rattan (2018)[41] is the life span "required" by evolution (50 years), which is different from an average life span (85 years) and different from the maximum life span recorded (122 years, 5 months, 14 days).[141] Survival assurance genes and the products they produce may determine a person's ability to survive and maintain health.

Error Theories

Error theories assume that aging changes occur because of influences outside the cell nucleus and involve some maladaptive response to cell, tissue, or system damage. The damage may be from external, environmental sources or from internal sources. These events eventually reach a level that is no longer compatible with life.

If the events occur randomly and represent environmental insults to the human body, they are called *stochastic changes*. The major stochastic theories include the free radical theory, cross-linkage theory, immune system theory, and the neuroendocrine system theory. In light of recent research, only one of these theories will be discussed in detail. The others will be mentioned tangentially.

The major biological theory of aging is the *free radical theory* first postulated by Harman.[142] It is also known as the *oxidative damage hypothesis*. The theory states that aging is due to the accumulation of oxidative damage to macromolecules. Macromolecules are considered DNA (nuclear and mitochondrial), RNA, protein, carbohydrates, lipids, and molecular conjugates. Reactive oxygen species (ROS) and free radicals are formed as by-products of cellular metabolism using oxygen. Mitochondria are the main generators of ROS. During electron transport in oxidative phosphorylation, electrons are leaked to oxygen. This mechanism is a major way lipids, proteins, and DNA are damaged. Both muscle and nervous system tissue are prone to oxidative damage because of their high metabolic rate and, therefore, high rate of ROS generation.[128] Mitochondria are a primary site of ATP production. As such, mitochondria play a crucial role in the aging process because of their role in not only producing ROS but also being a target of an ROS attack.[143]

Free radicals are highly charged ions with an orbiting unpaired electron. The separated electron with its high energy level attacks neighboring molecules. Free radicals have an affinity for lipid molecules, which are found in abundance in mitochondrial and microsomal membranes. These membranes are damaged by a chemical process called lipid peroxidation, which leads to structural changes and malfunctions in the cell. One of the results of the oxidative reactions within the cells is the deposition of lipofuscin, an aging pigment. Lipofuscin consists of lipid and protein, most of which has been oxidized. It accumulates in many organs with aging, particularly in postmitotic organs, such as the heart, skeletal muscle, and central nervous system, that are no longer dividing. Its formation has been postulated to be advantageous early on in the aging process, but once a critical amount of lipofuscin is formed, cell viability is threatened.[144]

In addition to forming age pigments, free radicals produce cross-linkages in some cells that can damage

DNA. If a cross-link attaches to only one strand of DNA, it can be repaired. However, if two strands of DNA are cross-linked, the strands are unable to part normally. With aging, the body's ability to repair cross-linkages declines, causing an increase in cell death related to incomplete division. Cross-links also occur in the skin with age. Cross-linkages between collagen and elastin lead to a loss of tissue elasticity and the production of wrinkles. Sun exposure can hasten this process. Loss of flexibility due to these age-related changes in collagen can be partially compensated for by diet and exercise.[145]

Oxidative stress has been implicated to have a role in several neurodegenerative disorders from Alzheimer to Parkinson disease. The brain is highly susceptible to damage from free radicals. Free radicals play a role in the formation of neuritic plaques, a structural hallmark of Alzheimer disease. Plaques are derived from beta amyloid. The amyloid is neurotoxic and leads to production of ROS that promote more aggregation of amyloid. Free radical production eventually destroys the neurons. The other structural hallmark of Alzheimer disease is the neurofibrillary tangle that contains a tau protein. This protein is also neurotoxic and causes neuron death by the accumulation of free radicals. The accumulation of ROS in the form of free radicals increases with age, regardless of the presence of pathology. The body's ability to produce antioxidants to counteract the effects of ROS declines with age. Oxidative stress is definitely involved in aging and age-related diseases.[35,191] See Chapter 8 for more age-related changes in the brain and the clinical implications of Alzheimer disease.

Immune

The immune system consists of the bone marrow, thymus gland, spleen, and lymph nodes. The first two are primary organs of immunity; the latter two are considered peripherally or secondarily responsible for developing immunity. The bone marrow and thymus are the two organs most affected by the aging process. The thymus involutes with age, which means it progressively atrophies. By age 50, it is 5%–10% of its peak mass.[146] Along with loss of peak mass, there are structural and functional changes.[147] After young adulthood, the thymus loses its ability to produce the differentiated T cells needed for cell-mediated immune responses. As the bone marrow becomes less efficient, the rate of infections, autoimmune disorders, and cancer rises. The term *immunosenescence* is used to describe the dysfunctional

immunity seen in older adults.[148] Oxidative damage has been implicated in producing the immune function decline seen with increasing age. The central nervous system and the immune system are in constant communication; what affects one affects the other. Specific cytokines, synthesized by lymphocytes, have been linked to the aging process.[149] Cytokines are hormones of the immune system.[150] The cytokine response to nonspecific inflammation has also been linked to functional decline, frailty, and even death in older adults.[148]

Neuroendocrine

The nervous system and endocrine systems work together with the immune system to maintain homeostasis. The autonomic nervous system, especially the sympathetic division, and the hormones produced by the neuroendocrine system via the pituitary affect the brain and the immune system. Neural and endocrine function can be changed by immune system responses, and in turn, endocrine and neural activity can modify immune functions. As we age, the hormones produced by the endocrine system appear to be intact and potent, although their effective interaction with target body cells is decreased. Put another way, the body's tissues are less responsive. The hypothalamic-pituitary-adrenal (HPA) interconnections act as a system to control the body functions of growth, reproduction, and metabolism. The pituitary gland controls the thyroid gland that manages the metabolic rate of the body through the secretion of thyroxine. As physiological reserve is lowered with advanced age and threatened by accumulated stress, the neuroendocrine system's initial response is adequate, but the response may persist and may be harmful. Moderate exercise and endurance training have been shown to improve immune function and to protect against the deleterious effects of stress.[151–153]

Psychological Theories
Intelligence
After peaking in early adulthood, intelligence declines through late adulthood. Horn and Cattel[154] described two dimensions of intelligence: fluid and crystallized. *Fluid intelligence* refers to learning reflective of induction, deduction, and abstract thinking, whereas *crystallized intelligence* is related to knowledge of life experiences and education or cultural knowledge. Fluid intelligence declines at some point in adulthood, whereas crystallized intelligence is maintained or may

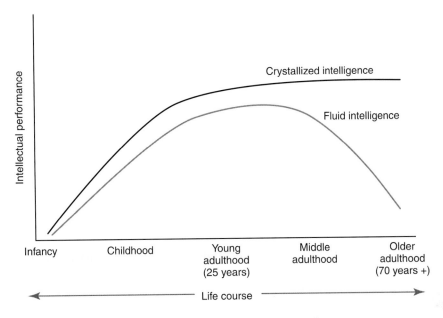

Fig. 2.12 Comparison of age-related changes in fluid and crystallized intelligence.

even increase during the adult years (Fig. 2.12). Fluid intelligence is more dependent on physiological functioning, especially the neurological system, both of which decline with advancing age.

Cognition is a complex phenomenon and is a composite of the interactions between multiple domains, including memory, information processing, and perception. Humans demonstrate age-related decline in memory, mental speed, fluid reasoning, and spatial ability.[155,156] These interactions are referred to as a general cognitive factor.[144] There appears to be more of a decline in the general factor with certain domains being selectively affected. Salthouse[157] and colleagues[158] reported that executive function (problem solving) and mental speed are more vulnerable to aging effects than other domains of cognition. During advanced aging, the majority of elderly develop diffuse plaques and neurofibrillary tangles, which may be linked to cognitive decline. Diffuse plaques are different from the neuritic plaques indicative of Alzheimer. Neurofibrillary tangles are also a hallmark of Alzheimer disease. However, they may also be found in dementia-free elderly. There can be a great deal of difference between pathology and cognitive impairment in older individuals. There is no one-to-one relationship between the degree of pathology and degree of functional decline.

Cognitive Processing Speed

Information processing theories of cognition have been used to assess the age-related differences seen in attention, reaction time, and working memory. The *processing speed theory* states that a decrease in the speed of processing operations leads to impairment in cognitive functioning.[157] Cognitive processing speed declines from midlife in healthy adults.[159] Older adults are slower to respond, with increased reaction time being well-documented.[160,161] The degree to which the response time slows depends on the difficulty of the task being performed. Attending to tasks of increasing complexity is more difficult for older than younger adults.[162,163] The decline in cognitive processing speed in the study by Ebaid and associates was not completely explained by motor performance. The results were the same whether a paper-pencil measure was used or a non-motor measure of visual perceptual processing speed. Slowed processing speed predicts driving cessation in older adults.[164]

Cognitive Reserve Theory

The theoretical construct of holding something in reserve has been applied to cognitive abilities in late adulthood. Just as Schroots and Yates[40] devised resiliency curves that mirrored the body's ability to bounce back from a stressor, Stern and colleagues (2019)[165] have discussed the neural correlates of cognitive aging. The cognitive reserve hypothesis proposes that people with more cognitive reserve can successfully sustain neuro pathology that would cause clinical dementia in those individuals with a lower cognitive ability.

Education, intelligence, and occupation are often listed as components of the cognitive reserve. Educational experiences can be thought of as enrichment. When formal education is studied as a predictor of cognitive vitality, it is usually found to have a protective effect.[166] Intelligence in childhood is highly correlated to intelligence in adulthood. Childhood intelligence is also strongly associated with the level of education attained and occupational complexity. Shimamura and colleagues[167] studied university professors and found a lower effect of aging on cognitive function. Low education level and low occupational status are risk factors for Alzheimer disease. Kramer and associates[168] also identified lifestyle and fitness as modifiers of the developmental trajectory of cognition from young to older adulthood. Modification of risk factors such as hypertension, smoking, and inactivity may slow or counter the risk of dementia. Exercise has a positive effect on cognition and neuroplasticity.[169,170] Dementia is not inevitable if you live to be 100; about 15%–25% of centenarians are functionally cognitively intact.[171] Education lowers the risk of dementia by 50% in people who have the ApoE-4 allele, the strongest genetic risk factor for Alzheimer's.[172] Many factors shape the path of brain aging. These findings support the premise of a cognitive reserve.

Sociocultural Theories

Aging may be the only thing a group of older adults have in common. Life histories and experiences are only a few of the variables present in our life course. Older adults may work for a longer period of time out of necessity. Other older adults take up volunteerism with great gusto and fervor. For those retirees who are healthy, there are many more years of leisure than ever before. Previously, selective optimization with compensation had been discussed under the psychological theories of aging but it is really a social theory of adaptation. We will begin with it and then revisit disengagement, activity, and continuity theories as well.

Selective Optimization With Compensation

This theory was originally postulated by Baltes[4] to explain why some individuals compensate for age-related declines in function. He has recently expanded this theory to encompass the life span as a way of explaining the adaptation that occurs over the entire life course. SA is viewed as optimizing gains while minimizing losses. Selection involves deciding what direction to take, making goals, and specifying outcomes. Compensation involves making a functional response in the face of a loss of a previously available means of attaining a goal.[4] For example, the pianist Arthur Rubinstein at age 80 practiced fewer pieces (selection) more frequently (optimalization), compensating for his slower speed by purposefully slowing down before rapid sequences to increase the contrast in movement speed.[173] Selective optimization with compensation (SOC) is a general model of SA. As both physical and sociocultural resources become limited with advanced age, focus is shifted to optimizing achievements and compensating for limitations. Reallocation of resources provides the best possible outcome, leading to an effective life.

Disengagement

Cumming and Henry[174] proposed the *disengagement theory*, suggesting that aging adults turned inward as a means of withdrawal from family and society. This served to ease the eventual loss of the older adult on the family. It has been suggested that mandatory retirement, which compels the older adult to withdraw from work-related roles, hastens the disengagement process. Socially, the older adult may engage in less day-to-day and face-to-face encounters. Society in some ways begins to disengage from the older adult. The theory suggests that disengagement is a mutual process.

While disengagement has a negative connotation, in actuality it may be beneficial to the older adult. Withdrawing from some social relationships may provide more time for those that are more beneficial. Investing less emotionally may make dealing with the increasing frequency of illness and death among their peer group easier. The initial research found some support for disengagement, but later research found that complete disengagement was neither normal nor natural.[175] Higher levels of social isolation are associated with being depressed while reduced social isolation is associated with living with a partner/spouse, participating in higher levels of household physical activity, and reporting better health.[176] Disengagement may occur after the loss of spouse and retirement, but many older adults return to being more actively engaged after a period of time. Disengagement is not universal for everyone in later adulthood. Presently, research is limited regarding an improvement in health through reducing social isolation.[177]

"There is a high cost associated with the essential quarantine and social distancing interventions for COVID-19" in older adults.[178] The impact of this isolation may be disproportionately amplified in persons with preexisting health issues or mental illness. These individuals were already experiencing loneliness and isolation. Older adults are functionally dependent on community and family support. Due to COVID restrictions, social networks have shrunk and access to medical care is more challenging. Social distancing should not be equated to social isolation.[178]

Activity

In sharp contrast to the disengagement theory, the *activity theory*, postulated by Neugarten and associates,[179] suggested that staying actively involved with friends, family, and society was necessary for SA. Activity was positively correlated with happiness in old age. Being active allowed for adaptation, which has always been part of life and becomes an even more important part of aging. Critics of this theory point out that not every older adult wants to be active; many look forward to slowing down and for some "less is more." The theory does not clearly delineate which activities are important to continue. Depending on life circumstances, the older adult may need to adjust to less income, increased dependency, loss or change of job role, or an inability to participate in leisure activities. Neither the disengagement theory nor the activity theory completely addresses the picture of SA.

Continuity

Continuity theory has replaced the need for debating the merits of the activity and disengagement theories. Atchley[180] described this widely accepted theory as one in which the individual seeks continuity by linking things in the past with changes in the future. For example, applying a study strategy used in college to taking on a new task at work is combining prior knowledge for future change. There are three degrees of continuity: too little, too much, and optimal.[180] Too little continuity produces an unsettled feeling that one's life is too unpredictable. Too much continuity is boring and totally predictable. The optimal amount of continuity provides sufficient challenge for change but not so much challenge that the person is overwhelmed.

Continuity can be internal or external. Internal continuity comes from those aspects of a person's personality such as temperament, emotions, and experiences unique to the individual. Internal continuity connects you to your past. External continuity comes from the environment, physical and social, and includes the roles each of us is involved in and the jobs we perform. Friendships and phasing out of employment are examples of maintaining external continuity in older adulthood. Phasing out of employment means that there will be more time for family and friends and volunteer pursuits. Continuity theory suggests that participation in familiar activities with familiar people helps preserve physical and cognitive functioning and affirm identity as individuals approach old age.[181] Internal continuity is lost in patients with Alzheimer disease who lose awareness of themselves, but external continuity allows adaptation to changing environmental demands.

The range of sociocultural theories is vast and mutilayered. Aging is viewed within the context of our relationship with the larger society and culture. Neugarten[179] described tasks that must be accomplished for SA. Some of these tasks include accepting reality and the imminence of death, coping with physical illness, and accepting the necessity of being dependent on outside support while still making independent choices that can give satisfaction. Our relationships can be defined in terms of sociocultural roles, as in SOC and continuity theory, or as a linkage to the larger group, as seen in the activity or disengagement theories.

Successful Aging

Rowe and Kahn[182] identified three components of SA based on longitudinal studies by the MacArthur Foundation. The number one component is avoiding disease and disability, number two is having a high cognitive and physical functional capacity, and number three is active engagement with life. Unlike the activity theorist, Rowe and Kahn[182] defined activity as something that holds societal value. The activity does not have to be remunerated for it to be considered productive. This model has been criticized for its lack of emphasis on psychosocial factors and not taking preexisting limitations such as a lifelong disability into consideration.[183,184] Bosnes and colleagues (2019)[185] studied lifestyle predictors of SA using a large population-based health survey. Their definition of SA was a composite of Rowe and Kahn's three operationalized concepts: being actively engaged with life, having no physical or cognitive impairment, and being free of nine specified diseases and depression. Lifestyle factors (social support, obesity, physical activity, smoking, and alcohol consumption) as midlife predictors of SA were studied as single factors and as part of a lifestyle index. Lifestyle factors predicted an overall measure of SA more than 20 years later.

Kahana and Kahana introduced a proactivity model of SA in the late 90s.[186,187] The theory has evolved to being a preventive and corrective proactivity theory (PCP)[188] that is now being used to research the challenges of late life disability.[189] The theory emphasizes the vital role of proactive and corrective behavioral adaptations to lessen the negative effects of stress due to aging. Six proactive adaptations are identified: helping others, planning for future care, self-advocacy for health care, making environmental modifications, marshaling intergenerational support, and finding strength in spiritual pursuits.[189] Self-reliance was identified as the goal of SA in an 80+ years-old group of Chinese.[190] They identified four proactive behaviors as supporting that goal: physical activity, community connectedness, financial security, and acceptance of reality.

SUMMARY

Development, as a process of change, reflects the transactional nature of our interaction with the environment and encompasses our need to survive, organize, and adapt to our surroundings. The first environment encountered is in utero where exposure to the diet, exercise habits, or stress of the mother can produce long-term health differences. As a child changes during the course of development, the people and things with which that child interacts also change. Each person's experience is different. The variables within the physical, psychological, and sociocultural environments encountered by a person need to be considered in the development of that person's functional skills. We develop a sense of identity through psychological interaction with all components of our environment. The physical, psychological, and sociocultural environment in which we develop may have an even more potent effect than previously recognized.

Erikson's stages guide the development of the child who becomes an adolescent and eventually an adult. Adolescence can be defined as being between puberty and the achievement of self-sufficiency and independence to a certain degree. The body matures but the mind is still developing, forging an identity and learning to take different perspectives. Adulthood is the longest period in most individuals' lives. Achieving adulthood and taking on adult responsibilities occurs later than ever before. The structure of work is changing, and as individuals live longer, more time may be spent during retirement as more people seek SA. Health span is becoming more of a focus in research than life span.

Theories of development have evolved over time and have been modified to reflect what we currently know about development and to provide a basis for our clinical decision making. We no longer believe that development of early functional movement is solely based on neuromaturation. Maturation plays an important role in achieving physical maturity of all body systems. We believe that the environment and the task goal shape the form of the functional movement that emerges. Movement and mobility are determinants of adaptive function and the ability to participate in all that life has to offer. We must remember that theories are subject to modification based on research; none are totally correct. As theorists of human development and clinicians seek to integrate the changes in all domains of function across the life span, the process of development of functional movement will become clearer.

REFERENCES

1. Arnett JJ. Emerging adulthood: a theory of development from the late teens through the twenties. *Am Psychol.* 2000;55:469–480.
2. Vespa J, Medina L, Armstrong DM. Demographic turning points for the United States: Population Projections for 2020 to 2060. 2020;25–1144. (From https:// www.census.gov/content/dam/Census/library/publications/2020/demo/p25-1144.pdf Accessed June 14, 2021.)
3. Baltes PB. Theoretical propositions of life-span developmental psychology: on the dynamics between growth and decline. *Dev Psychol.* 1987;23:611–626.
4. Baltes PB, Lindenberger U, Staudinger UM. Life span theory in developmental psychology. In: W Damon, RM

Lerner, eds., *Handbook of Child Psychology*. 6th ed. New York: John Wiley & Sons; 2006:569–664,

5. Havighurst R.J. *Developmental Tasks and Education*. 3rd ed. New York: David McKay Co, Inc; 1972.

6. Pew Survey 2016 Americans name the 10 most significant historic events of their lifetimes. https://www.pewresearch.org/politics/2016/12/15/americans-name-the-10-most-significant-historic-events-of-their-lifetimes/ Accessed June 23, 2021.

7. Hayflick L. New approaches to old age. *Nature*. 2000;403:365.

8. Kirkwood TBL. Why and how we are living longer? *Exp Physiol*. 2017;102(9):1067–1074. https://doi.org/10.1113/EP086205. Epub 2017 Aug 2.

9. Plomin R, von Stumm S. The new genetics of intelligence. *Nat Rev Genet*. 2018;19(3):148–159.

10. Briley DA, Tucker-Drob EM. Explaining the increasing heritability of cognitive ability across development: A meta-analysis of longitudinal twin and adoption studies. *Psychol Sci*. 2013;24:1704–1713.

11. Kail RV, Cavanaugh JC. *Human development: a life-span view*. 8th ed. Boston, MA: Cengage Learning; 2018.

12. Knopik VS, Neiderhciser J, DeFries JC, Plomin R. *Behavioral Genetics*. 7th ed. New York: Worth, 2017.

13. Brooks-Wilson AR. Genetics of healthy aging and longevity. *Hum Genet*. 2013;132:1323–1338.

14. Falah G, Giller A, Gutman D, Atzmon G. Breaking the class ceiling. *Gerontology*. 2020;66:309–314.

15. National Public Radio. https://www.npr.org/2021/02/18/968791431/american-life-expectancy--dropped-by-a-full-year-in-the-first-half-of-2020. October 14, 2021.

16. Kaeberlein M. How healthy is the healthspan concept? *GeroScience*. 2018;40:361–364. https://doi.org/10.1007/s11357-018-0036-9.

17. National Center for Health Statistics, Older Americans 2004: key indicators of well-being. (website): http://www.agingstats.gov/chartbook2004/tables-population.html Accessed March 16, 2007

18. CDC podcast cdc.gov/nchs/pressroom/podcasts/2021/20210119/EARIAS_02192_TRANSCRIPT.pdf Accessed July 24, 2021.

19. Berger SL, Kouzarides T, Shiekhattar R, Shilatifard A. An operational definition of epigenetics. *Genes Dev*. 2009;23:781–783.

20. Horvath S, Pirazzini C, Bacalini MG, et al. Decreased epigenetic age of PBMCs from Italian semisupercentenarians and their offspring. *Aging*. 2015;7:1159–1170.

21. Anderson SL, Sebastiani P, Dworkis DA, Feldman L, Perls TT. Health spa approximates life span among many supercentenarians: compression of morbidity at the approximate limit of life span. *J Gerontol A Biol Sci Med Sci*. 2012;67:395–405.

22. Sebastiani P, Nussbaum L, Andersen SL, Black MJ, Perls TT. Increasing sibling relative risk of survival to older and older ages and the importance of precise definitions of "Aging," "Life Span," and "Longevity" *J Gerontol A Biol Sci Med Sci*. 2016;71:340–346. https://doi.org/10.1093/gerona/glv020.

23. Sebastiani P, Gurinovich A, Nygaard M, et al. APOE alleles and extreme human longevity. *J Gerontol A Biol Med Sci*. 2019;74:44–51. https://doi.org/10.1093/gerona/gly174.

24. Bloom HS, Weiland C. Quantifying Variation in Head Start Effects on Young Children's Cognitive and Socio-Emotional Skills Using Data from the National Head Start Impact Study (March 31, 2015). Available at SSRN: https://ssrn.com/abstract=2594430 or https://doi.org/10.2139/ssrn.2594430 Accessed Oct 2, 2021.

25. Yamori Y. Food factors for atherosclerosis prevention: Asian perspective derived from analyses of worldwide dietary biomarkers. *Exp Clin Cardiol*. 2006;11(2):94–98.

26. World Health Organization, Global action against cancer, updated edition 2005. (website): http://www.who.int/cancer/media/GlobalActionCancerEnglfull.pdf. Accessed March 28, 2007.

27. Calcaterra V, Cena H, Regalbuto C, et al. The role of fetal, infant, and childhood nutrition in the timing of sexual maturation. *Nutrients*. 2021;13:419. https://doi.org/10.3390/nu13020419.

28. Trichopoulou A, Orfanos P, Norat T, et al. Modified Mediterranean diet and survival: EPIC-elderly prospective cohort study. *Brit Med J*. 2005;330:991 https://doi.org/10.1136/bmj.38415.644155.8F.Epub 2005 Apr 8.

29. Mentella MC, Scaldaferri F, Ricci C, Gasbarrini A, Miggiano GAD. Cancer and the Mediterranean diet: a review. *Nutrients*. 2019;11(9):2059. https://doi.org/10.3390/nu11092059.

30. Hadders-Algra M. Early human motor development: from variation to the ability to vary and adapt. *Neurosci Biobehav Rev*. 2018;90:411–427.

31. Erikson EH. *Identity, youth, and crisis*. New York: WW Norton; 1968.

32. Woelfel JR, Dudley-Javoroski S, Shields RK. Precision physical therapy: exercise, the epigenome, and the heritability of environmentally modified traits. *Phys Ther*. 2018;198:946–952.

33. Jorde LB, Carey JC, Bamshad M. *Medical Genetics*. 5th ed. Philadelphia, PA: Elsevier; 2016.

34. Khochbin Saadi (2021), Epigenetics: the genome and its environment, Encyclopedia of the Environment, [online ISSN 2555-0950]. url: https://www.encyclopedie-envi-

ronnment.org/en/life/epigenetics-genome-and-its-environment/. Accessed 7/31/2021.

35. Harman ME, Martin MG. Epigenetic mechanisms related to cognitive decline during aging. *J Neurosci Res.* 2020;98:234–246.

36. Franzago M, Fraticelli F, Stuppia L, Vitacolonna E. Nutrigenetics, epigenetics and gestational diabetes: consequences in mother and child. *Epigenetics.* 2019;14:215–235.

37. Cornwall J, Elliott JM, Walton DM, Osmotherly PG. Clinical genomics in physical therapy: where to from here? *Phys Ther.* 2018;98:733–736.

38. Brown WM. Exercise-associated DNA methylation change in skeletal muscle and the importance of imprinted genes: a bioinformatics meta-analysis. *Br J Sports Med.* 2015;49:1567–1578.

39. Lockman JJ, Thelen E. Developmental biodynamics: brain, body, behavioral connections. *Child Dev.* 1993;64:953–1050.

40. Schroots JJ, Yates RE. On the dynamics of development and aging. In: VL Bengtson, KW Schaie, eds., *Handbook of Theories of Aging.* Springer: New York;1999;417-433.

41. Rattan SIS. Biogerontology: research status, challenges and opportunities. *Acta Biomed.* 2018;89(2):291–301. https://doi.org/10.23750/abm/v89i2.7403.

42. Bugajska BE. The ninth stage in the cycle of life-reflections on E. H. Erikson's theory. *Aging & Society.* 2017;37:1095–1110.

43. Erikson EH, Erikson JM. *The Life Cycle Completed (Extended Version).* New York: WW Norton; 1997.

44. Erikson EH, Erikson JM, Kivnick HQ. *Vital involvement in old age.* WW. New York: Norton; 1986.

45. Dunkel CS, Harbke C. A review of measures of Erikson's stages of psychosocial development: evidence for a general factor. *J Adult Development.* 2017;24(1):58–76.

46. Bandura A. *Social foundation of thought and action: a social cognitive theory.* Englewood Cliffs, NJ: Prentice-Hall; 1986.

47. Maslow A. *Motivation and personality.* New York: Harper & Row; 1954.

48. Deci EL, Ryan RM. Self-determination theory: a macrotheory of human motivation, development and health. *Can Psychol.* 2008;49:182–185.

49. Ryan RM, Patrick H, Deci EL, et al. Facilitating health behavior change and its maintenance: interventions based on self-determination theory. *Eur Psychol.* 2008;10:2–5.

50. Di Dominico SI, Ryan RM. The emerging neuroscience of intrinsic motivation: a new frontier in self-determination research. *Front Hum Neurosci.* 2017;11:145. https://doi.org/10.3389/fnhum.2017.00145.

51. Bronfenbrenner U. *The ecology of human development: Experiments by nature and design.* Cambridge, Mass: Harvard University Press; 1979.

52. Chiarello LA, Catalino T. Family-centered care. In: SK Effgen, A LaForme Fiss, eds., *Meeting the Physical Therapy Needs of Children.* 4th ed. Philadelphia, PA: FA Davis; 2021:133–157.

53. Gesell A, Ilg FL, Ames LB, et al. *Infant and child in the culture of today. revised.* New York: Harper & Row; 1974.

54. Edelman GM. *Neural Darwinism.* New York, NY: Basic Books; 1987.

55. Piaget J. *Origins of intelligence.* New York: International Universities Press; 1952.

56. Cuevas L, Bell MA. Developmental progression of looking and reaching performance on the A-not-B task. *Dev Psychol.* 2010;46(5):1363–1371. https://doi.org/10.1037/a0020185.

57. Piaget J, Inhelder B. *The child's concept of space.* New York: WW Norton; 1967.

58. Pick HL, Gibson EJ. Learning to perceive and perceiving to learn. *Dev Psychol.* 1992;28:787–794.

59. Gibson EJ. *The ecological approach to visual perception.* Boston: Houghton Mifflin; 1979.

60. E.J. Gibson, 1982 The concept of affordance in development: the renaissance of functionalism. In: W.A. Collins, ed., *Minnesota Symposium on Child Psychology, Vol. 15.* Hillsdale, NJ: Erlbaum

61. Leslie AM. Pretense and representation: the origins of "theory of mind". *Psych Review.* 1987;94:412–426.

62. Rochat P. Clinical pointers from developing self-awareness. *DMCN.* 2021;63:382–386.

63. Ganea PA, Lillard AS, Turkheimer E. Preshcooler's understanding of the role of mental states and action in pretense. *J Cogn Dev.* 2004;5:213–238.

64. Carlson SM, Koenig MA, Harms MB. Theory of mind, WIREs. *Cogn Sci.* 2013;4:391–402.

65. Moran JM. Lifespan development: the effects of typical aging on theory of mind. *Behav Brain Res.* 2013;237:32–40.

66. Ruitenberg MFL, Santens P, Notebaert W. Cognitive and affective theory of mind in healthy aging. *Exp Aging Res.* 2020;46:382–395.

67. Skinner BF. *The Behavior of Organisms: An Experimental Analysis.* New York: Appleton-Century-Crofts; 1938.

68. Rejeski WJ, Fanning J. Models and theories of health behavior and clinical interventions in aging: a contemporary, integrative approach. *Clin Int Aging.* 2019;14:1007–1019.

69. Thomas A, Chess S, Birch HG. *Temperament and behavior disorders in children.* New York: University Press; 1968.

70. Kagan J, Arcus D, Snidman N, et al. Reactivity in infants: a cross-national comparison. *Dev Psychol.* 1994;30:342–345.

71. Ainsworth MS. Attachment as related to mother-infant interaction. *Adv Infancy Res.* 1995;8:1–50.

72. Vgotsky L. *Thought and Language.* Cambridge, Mass: MIT Press; 1986. (Kozulin A, translator).

73. Piaget J. *Play, dreams, and imitation in childhood.* London: Heinemann; 1951.

74. Vygotsky L. Play and its role in the mental development of the child. *Sov Psychol.* 1966;12:62–76.

75. Parham LD. Play and occupational therapy. In: LD Parham, LS Fazio, eds., *Play in Occupational Therapy.* 2nd ed. St Louis: Mosby; 2007:3–39.

76. Freud S. *Beyond the pleasure principle.* New York: Norton; 1961.

77. Erikson EH. Play and actuality. In: JS Bruner, A Jolly, K Sylva, eds., *Play: Its Role in Development and Evolution Penguin Books.* New York;1985 688–704.

78. Mead GH. *Mind, self, and society.* Chicago: University of Chicago Press; 1934.

79. Bateson G. *Steps to an ecology of mind.* New York: Ballantine Books; 1972.

80. Parten MB. Social participation among preschool children. *J Abnorm Psychol.* 1932;27:243–269.

81. Howes C, Matheson CC. Sequences in the development of competent play with peers: social and social pretend play. *Dev Psychol.* 1992;28(5):961–974.

82. Casby MW. The development of play in infants, toddlers, and young children. *Commun Disord Q.* 2003;24(4): 163–174.

83. Casby MW. Developmental assessment of play: a model for early intervention. *Commun Disord Q.* 2003;24(4):175–183.

84. Pellegrini AD. Pretend play. In: AD Pellegrini, ed., *The Role of Play in Human Development.* Oxford University Press Inc.; 2009:154–183.

85. Newman BM, Newman PR. *Development through Life: A Psychosocial Approach.* 13th ed. Boston, MA: Cengage Learning; 2018.

86. Bundy DAP, Silva ND, Horton S, et al. eds. *Child and Adolescent Health and Development.* 3rd edition. Washington, DC: The international bank for reconstruction and development/World bank; 2017Nov 20. https://doi.org/10.1596/978-1-4648-0423-6_ch9.

87. Fischer KW, Bidell TR. Dynamic development of action and thought. In: W Damon, RM Lerner, eds., *Theoretical Models of Human Development. Handbook of Child Psychology.* 6th ed. New York: Wiley; 2006:313–399.

88. Newman BM, Newman PR. *Theories of Adolescent Development.* London, UK: Academic Press; 2020.

89. Deci EL, Ryan RM. The "what" and "why" of goal pursuits: human needs and the self-determination of behavior. *Psychological Inquiry.* 2000;11:227–268.

90. Crandall A, Magnusson BM, Novilla M. Growth in adolescent self-regulation and impact on sexual risk-taking: a curve-of-factors analysis. *J Youth Adolesc.* 2018;47(4):793–806. https://doi.org/10.1007/s10964-017-0706-4.

91. Estévez A, Jáuregui P, Sánchez-Marcos I, López-González H, Griffiths MD. Attachment and emotion regulation in substance addictions and behavioral addictions. *J Behav Addict.* 2017;6(4):534–544. https://doi.org/10.15556/2006.6.2017.0866.

92. American Psychological Association, Am Psychol. 2015;70(9):832-864.

93. Korpaisarn S, Safer JD. Etiology of gender identity. *Endocrin Metab Clin N Am.* 2019;48:323–329.

94. Polderman TJC, Kreukels BPC, Irwig MS, et al. The biological contributions to gender identity and gender diversity: bringing data to the table. *Behav Genet.* 2018;48:95–108.

95. Olsson M, Martiny SE. Does exposure to counterstereotypical role models influence girls' and women's gender stereotypes and career choices? A review of social psychological research. *Fron Psychol.* 2018;9:2264 https://doi.org/10.3389/fpsyg.2018.02264.eCollection 2018.

96. Bussey K, Bandura A. Social cognitive theory of gender development and differentiation. *Psych Rev.* 1999;106:676–713.

97. Eagly AH, Wood W. Social role theory. In: P van Lange, A Kruglanski, ET Higgins, eds., *Handbook of Theories in Social Psychology.* Vol 2. Thousand Oaks, CA: Sage Publications; 2011:458–476.

98. Cooley CH. *Human Nature and the Social Order.* New York, NY: Charles Scribner's and Sons; 1909/1922.

99. Newman BM, Newman PR. Group identity and alienation: giving the we its due. *J Youth Adolesc.* 2001;30: 515–538.

100. Brown BB, Bakken JP, Ameringer SW, Mahone SD. A comprehensive conceptualization of the peer influence process in adolescence. In: MJ Prinstein, K Dodge, eds., *Understanding Peer Influence in Children and Adolescence.* New York: Guilford Press; 2008:17–44.

101. Hamm JM, Heckhausen J, Shane J, Lachman ME. Risk of cognitive declines with retirement: who declines and why? *Psychol Aging.* 2020;35:449–457.

102. Hooker K. Towards a new synthesis for development in adulthood. Res Hum Dev. 2015;12(3-4):229–236.

103. Hoare C. ed. Growing a discipline at the borders of thought. Handbook of Adult Development and Learning: A handbook of theory, research and practice. Oxford, UK: Oxford University Press; 2006;3–26.

104. Levinson DF. A conception of adult development. Am Psychol. 1986;41:3–13.

105. Valliant GE. Aging well. New York: Little, Brown; 2002.

106. Nolan RE, Kadavil N. Valliant's contribution to research and theory of adult development. Presented at the 2003 Midwestern research-to-practice conference in Adult,

Continuing, and Community Education, The Ohio State University, Columbus, OH: October 8-11, 2003.

107. Arnett JJ. Emerging adulthood in Europe: a response to Bynner. J Youth Stud. 2006;9(1):111–123.

108. Arnett JJ. Emerging Adulthood: The winding road through the late teens through the twenties. 2nd ed. New York, NY: Oxford University Press; 2014.

109. Bulher JL, Nikitin HJ. Sociohistorical context and adult social development: new directions for 21st century research. Am Psychol. 2020;75:457–469.

110. Gerstorf D, Hulur G, Drewelies J, Willis SL, Schaie KW, Ram N. Adult development and aging in historical context. Am Psychol. 2020;75:525–539.

111. Arnett JJ. Life stage concepts across history and cultures: proposal for a new field on indigenous life stages. Hum Dev. 2016;59:290–316.

112. Mehta CM, Arnett JJ, Palmer CG, Nelson LJ. Established adulthood: a new conception of ages 30 to 45. Am Psychol. 2020;75:431–444.

113. Arnett JJ. Happily stressed: the complexity of well-being in midlife. J Adult Dev. 2018;25:270–278.

114. Curkrowska-Torzewska E. Cross-country evidence on motherhood employment and wage gaps: the role of work-family policies and their interaction. Social Politics. 2017;24:178–220.

115. Lachman ME, Teshale S, Agrigoroaei S. Midlife as a pivotal period in the life course: balance growth and decline at the crossroads of youth and old age. Int J Behav Dev. 2015;39:20–31.

116. Rantanen T, Masaki K, He Q, Ross GW, Willcox BJ, White L. Midlife muscle strength and human longevity up to age 100 years: a 44-year prospective study among a decedent cohort. Age. 2012;34:563–570.

117. Launer LJ, Masaki K, Petrovitch H, Foley D, Havlik RJ. The association between midlife blood pressure levels and late-life cognitive function: the Honolulu-Asia Aging Study. JAMA. 1995;274:1846–1851.

118. Ryff CD, Krueger RF. The Oxford handbook of integrative health science. New York, NY: Oxford University Press; 2019.

119. Ferraro KF. The time of our lives: recognizing the contributions of Mannheim, Neugarten, and Riley to the study of aging. Gerontologist. 2014;54(1):127–133. https://doi.org/10.1093/geront/gnt048.

120. Peterson CC. The ticking of the social clock: adults' beliefs about the timing of transition events. Int J Aging Hum Dev. 1996;42(3):189–203. https://doi.org/10.2190/MMDD-F9YP-NPN8-720M.PMID: 8805083.

121. Helson RM, Mitchell V. Chapter 5. The Social Clock Projects in Women on the River of Life: A Fifty-Year Study of Adult Development. Berkeley: University of California Press; 2020:72–85. https://doi.org/10.1525/9780520971011-007.

122. Kitayama S, Berg MK, Chopick WJ. Culture and well-being in late adulthood: theory and evidence. Am Psychol. 2020;75:567–576.

123. Olshansky SJ. From lifespan to healthspan. JAMA. 2018;320(13):1323–1324. https://doi.org/10.1001/jama.2018.12621.

124. Heron M. Deaths: leading causes for 2017. Natl Vital Stat Rep. 2019;68:1–77.

125. Rattan SI. Theories of biological aging: genes, proteins, and free radicals. Free Radic Res. 2006;40(123):1230–1238.

126. Rattan SI. Biogerontology: research status, challenges and opportunities. Acta Biomed. 2018;89(2):291–301. https://doi.org/10.23750/abm/v89i2.7403.

127. Harman D. Free radical theory of aging: an update. Ann NY Acad Sci. 2006;10067:10–21.

128. da Costa JP, Vitorino R, Silva GM, Vogel C, Duarte AC, Rocha-Santos T. A synopsis on aging—theories, mechanisms and future prospects. Ageing Res Rev. 2016;29:90–112. https://doi.org/10.1016/j.arr.2016.06.005.

129. Hayflick L, Moorehead PS. The serial cultivation of human diploid cell strains. Exp Cell Res. 1961;24:585–621.

130. Hayflick L. The limited in vitro lifetime of human diploid cell strains. Exp Cell Res. 1965;25:614–636.

131. de Magalhaes JP, Toussaint O. Telomeres and telomerase: a modern fountain of youth? Rejuvenation Res. 2004;7:126–133.

132. de Magalhaes JP, Passos JF. Stress, cell senescence and organismal ageing. Mech Ageing Dev. 2018; 170:2–9.

133. Demaria M, Ohtani N, Youssef Sameh A, Rodier F, Toussaint W, Mitchell James R, et al. An essential role for senescent cells in optimal wound healing through secretion of PDGF-AA. Dev Cell. 2014;31: 722–733.

134. Serrano M, Lin AW, McCurrach ME, Beach D, Lowe SW. Oncogenic ras provokes premature cell senescence associated with accumulation of p53 and p16INK4a. Cell. 1997;88:593–602.

135. Munoz-Espin D, Serrano M. Cellular senescence: from physiology to pathology. Nat Rev Mol Cell Biol. 2014;15:482–496.

136. Rattan SI. The science of healthy aging: genes, milieu, and chance. Ann N Y Acad Sci. 2007;1114:1–10.

137. Guest P. New therapeutics approaches and biomarkers for increased healthspan. Adv Exp Med Biol. 2021;1286:1–13. https://doi.org/10.1007/978-3-030-55035-6_1.

138. Zhu Z, Xia W, Cui Y, Zeng F, Li Y, Yang Z, et al. Klotho gene polymorphisms are associated with healthy aging and longevity: evidence from a meta-analysis. Mech Ageing Dev. 2019;178:33–40.

139. Gulizibaer M, Hu Y, Chen F, Li H, Cheng Z, Mayila W. Association of single nucleotide polymorphisms of IL-6

gene with longevity in Uyghurs in Xinjiang. *Zhonghua Yi Xue Za Zhi.* 2015;95(42):3428–3431.

140. Yan L, Hu R, Tu S, Cheng WJ, Zheng Q, Wang JW, et al. *Genet Mol Res.* 2015;14(4):19225–19232.

141. Robine JM, Allard M. The oldest human. *Science.* 1998;279:1834–1835.

142. Harman D. A theory based on free radical and radiation chemistry. *J Gerontol.* 1956;11:298–300.

143. Akbari M, Kirkwood TBL, Bohr VA. Mitochondria in the signaling pathways that control longevity and health span. *Ageing Res Rev.* 2019;54:100940. https://doi.org/10.1016/j.arr.2019.100940.

144. Keller JN. Age-related neuropathology, cognitive decline, and Alzheimer's disease. *Ageing Res Rev.* 2006;5:1–13.

145. Peters A, Nawrot TS, Baccarelli AA. Hallmarks of environmental insults. *Cell.* 2021;184(6):1455–1468.

146. Lee IM, PaffenbargerJr RS. Association of light, moderate, and vigorous intensity physical activity with longevity. The Harvard alumni health study. *Am J Epidemiol.* 2000;151:293–299.

147. Whitbourne SK. Physical changes. In: JC Cavanaugh, SK Whitbourne, eds., *Gerontology: An Interdisciplinary Perspective.* Baltimore: Williams & Wilkins; 1999:91–122.

148. Thomas RS, Wang W, Su D-M. Contributions of age-related thymic involution to immunosenescence and inflammaging. *Immunity & Aging.* 2020;17:2. https://doi.org/10.1186/s12979-020-0173-8.

149. Fulop T, Larbi A, Dupuis G, et al. Immunosenescence and inflamm-aging as two sides of the same coin: friends or foes? *Front Immunol.* 2018;8:1960 https://doi.org/10.3389/fimmu.2017.01960.eCollection 2017.

150. Morley JE, Baumgartner RN. Cytokine-related aging process. *J Gerontol A Biol Sci Med Sci.* 2004;59(9):M924–M929.

151. Dinarello CA. Historical review of cytokines. *Eur J Immunol.* 2007;37(Suppl 1):S34–S45. https://doi.org/10.1002/eji.200737772.

152. Fleshner M. Exercise and neuroendocrine regulation of antibody production: protective effect of physical activity on stress-induced suppression of the specific antibody response. *Int J Sports Med.* 2000;21(Suppl 1):S14S19.

153. Simpson RJ, Kunz H, Agha N, Graff R. Exercise and the regulation of immune functions. *Prog Mol Biol Transl Sci.* 2015;135:355–380. https://doi.org/10.1016/bs.pmbts.2015.08.001.

154. Edwards JP, Walsh NP, Diment PC, Roberts R. Anxiety and perceived psychological stress play an important role in the immune response after exercise. *Exerc Immunol Rev.* 2018;24:26–34. PMID: 29461966.

155. Horn JL, Cattell RB. Refinement and test of a theory of fluid and crystallized intelligence. *J Educ Psychol.* 1966;57:253–270.

156. Murman DL. The impact of age on cognition. *Semin Hear.* 2015;36(3):111–121. https://doi.org/10.1055/s-0035-1555115.

157. Harada CN, Natelson Love MC, Triebel K. Normal cognitive aging. *Clin Geriatr Med.* 2013;29(4):737–752. https://doi.org/10.1016/j.cger.2013.07.002.

158. Salthouse TA. The processing-speed theory of adult age differences in cognition. *Psychol Rev.* 1996;103:403–428.

159. Salthouse TA, Atkinson TM, Berish DE. Executive function as a potential mediator of age-related cognitive decline in normal adults. *J Exp Psychol.* 2003;132:566–594.

160. Jenkins L, Myerson J, Joerding JA, Hale S. Converging evidence that visuospactial cognition is more age-sensitive than verbal cognition. *Psych Aging.* 2000;15:157–175.

161. Hong Z, Ng KK, Sim SK, et al. Differential age-dependent associations of gray matter volume and white matter integrity with processing speed in healthy older adults. *Neuroimage.* 2015;123:42–50. https://doi.org/10.1016/j.neuroimage.2015.08.

162. Tam HM, Lam CL, Juang H, et al. Age-related difference in relationships between cognitive processing speed and general cognitive status. *Appl Neuropsychol Adult.* 2015;22:94–99. https://doi.org/10.1080/232279095.2013.860602.

163. Gorus E, De Raedt R, Mets T. Diversity, dispersion and inconsistency of reaction time measures: effects of age and task complexity. *Aging Clin Exp Res.* 2006;18(5):407–417.

164. Ebaid D, Crewther SG, MacCalman K, Brown A, Crewther DP. Cognitive processing speed across the lifespan: beyond the influence of motor speed. *Font Aging Neurosci.* 2017;9:62. https://doi.org/10.3389/fnagi.2017.00062.

165. Edwards JD, Bart E, O'Connore ML, Cissell G. Ten years down the road: predictors of driving cessation. *The Gerontologist.* 2010;50:393–399.

166. Stern Y, Barnes CA, Grady C, Jones RN, Raz N. Brain reserve, cognitive reserve, compensation, and maintenance: operationalization, validity, and mechanisms of cognitive resilience. *Neurobiol Aging.* 2019;83:124–129. https://doi.org/10.1016/j.neruobiolaging.2019.03.022.

167. Stern Y, Barulli D. Cognitive reserve. *Handb Clin Neurol.* 2019;167:181–190. https://doi.org/10.1016/B978-0-12-804766-8.00011-X.

168. Shimamura AP, Berry HJM, Mangels JA, et al. Memory and cognitive abilities in university professors: evidence for successful aging. *Psychol Sci.* 1996;6:271–277.

169. Kramer AF, Bherer L, Colcombe SJ, et al. Environmental influences on cognitive and brain plasticity during aging. *J Gerontol A Biol Sci Med Sci.* 2004;59(9):M940M957.

170. Hillman CH, Erickson KI, Kramer AF. Be smart, exercise your heart: exercise effects on brain and cognition. *Nat Rev Neurosci.* 2008;9(1):58–65. https://doi.org/10.1038/nrn2298.

171. Hötting K, Röder B. Beneficial effects of physical exercise on neuroplasticity and cognition. *Neurosci Biobehav Rev.* 2013 Nov;37(9 Pt B):2243–2257. https://doi.org/10.1016/j.neubiorev.2013.04.005.Epub 2013 Apr 25.

172. Perls T. Centenarians who avoid dementia. *Trends Neurosci.* 2004;27(10):633–636.

173. Wang HX, Gustafson D, Kivipelto M, et al. Education halves the risk of dementia due to apolipoprotein ε4 allele:a collaborative study from the Swedish brain power initiative. *Neurobiol Aging.* 2011;33(5):1007–e1. https://pubmed.ncbi.nlm.nih.gov/18094706/.

174. Baltes PB, Lindenberger U, Staudinger UM. Life span theory in developmental psychology. In: W Damon, N Eisenberg, eds., *Handbook of Child Psychology.* 5th ed. New York: John Wiley & Sons; 1998:1029–1144.

175. Cumming E, Henry WE. *Growing old: the process of disengagement.* New York: Basic Books; 1961.

176. Atchley RC, Barusch AS, eds. *Social forces and aging.* 10th ed. Belmont, Calif: Wadsworth; 2004.

177. Robins LM, Hill KD, Finch CF, Clemson L, Haines T. The association between physical activity and social isolation in community-dwelling older adults. *Aging Ment Health.* 2018;22(2):175–182. https://doi.org/10.1080/13607863.2016.1232116.

178. Ibrahim AF, Tan MP, Teoh GK, Muda SM, Chong MC. Health benefits of social participation interventions among community-dwelling older persons: a review article. *Exp Aging Res.* 2021;Jul 6:1–27. https://doi.org/10.1080/0361073X.2021.1939536.Online ahead of print.

179. Hwang TJ, Rabheru K, Peisah C, Reichman W, Ikeda M. Loneliness and social isolation during the COVID-19 pandemic. *Int Psychogeriatr.* 2020;May 26:1–4. https://doi.org/10.1017/S1041610220000988.

180. Neugarten BL, Havinghurst RJ, Tobin SS. Personality and patterns of aging. In: BL Neurgarten, ed., *Middle Age and Aging.* University of Chicago Press: Chicago; 1968:173–177.

181. Atchley RC. A continuity theory of normal aging. *Gerontologist.* 1989;29:183–190.

182. Burbank PM. Psychosocial theories of aging: a critical evaluation. *Adv Nurs Sci.* 1986 Oct;9(1):73–86. https://doi.org/10.1097/00012272-198610000-00009. PMID: 3094434.

183. Rowe JW, Kahn RL. Successful aging. *Gerontologist.* 1997;37:433–440.

184. Martinson M, Berridge CJTG. Successful aging and its discontents: a systematic review of the social gerontology literature. 2014;55(1):58-69.

185. Martin P, Kelly N, Kahana B, Kahana E, Willcox BJ, Willcox DC, Poon LW. Defining successful aging: a tangible or elusive concept? *The Gerontologist.* 2015;55:14–25. https://doi.org/10.1093/geront/gnu044.

186. Bosnes I, Nordahl HM, Stordal E, Bosnes O, Myklebust TA, Almkvist O. Lifestyle predictors of successful aging: a 20 year prospective HUNT study. *PLoS ONE.* 2019;14(7):e0219200. https://doi.org/10.1371/journal.pone.0219200.

187. Kahana E, Kahana B. Conceptual and empirical advances in understanding aging well through proactive adaptation. In: V Bengtson, ed., *Adulthood and Aging: Research on Continuities and Discontinuities.* New York: Springer; 1996:18–40.

188. Kahana E, Kahana B. Contextualizing successful aging: new directions in age-old search. In: R Settersten Jr., ed., *Invitation to the Life Course: A New Look at Old Age.* Amityville, NY: Baywood Publishing Company; 2003:225–255.

189. Kahana E, Kahana B, Lee JE. Proactive approaches to successful aging. *Ageing International.* 2003;28:155–180. https://doi.org/10.1007/s12126-003-1022-8.

190. Kahana E, Kahana JS, Kahna B, Ermoshkina P. Meeting challenges of late life disability proactively. *Innovation in Aging.* 2019;3(4):1–9. https://doi.org/10.1093/geroni/igz023.

191. Chen L, Ye M, Kahana E. A self-reliant umbrella: defining successful aging among the old-old (80+) in Shanghai. *J Appl Gerontol.* 2020;39(30):242–249. https://doi.org/10.1177/0733464819842500.

Motor Development

OBJECTIVES

After studying this chapter, the reader will be able to:
1. Discuss the major theories of motor development.
2. Understand the relationship between cognitive and motor development.
3. Identify important motor accomplishments of the first six years of life.
4. Describe the acquisition and refinement of fundamental movement patterns during childhood.
5. Describe age-related changes in functional movement patterns across the life span.

INTRODUCTION

Development results from the interrelated processes of maturation, physical growth, and learning and may be observed in genetic and environmental adaptation. *Maturation* guides development genetically in the physical changes that occur during organ differentiation in the embryo, myelination of nerve fibers, and the appearance of primary and secondary ossification centers. Genes direct the timetable of physical change in all body systems. *Growth* is the process whereby changes in physical size and shape take place, as witnessed during adolescence when dramatic changes in facial and body growth occur. Growth is highly influenced by the endocrine system and nutrition. *Adaptation*, on the other hand, is the body's response to environmental stimuli. A muscle increases bulk with strength training, the immune system produces antibodies when exposed to a pathogen, and bones heal after a fracture. All of these processes illustrate adaptation.

Motor development is epigenetic. Epigenesis is a theory of development that states that a human being grows and develops from a simple organism to a more complex one through progressive differentiation. Epigenesis is the process by which environmental influences alter genetic expression. Epigenesis recognizes the role of the biological, psychological, and sociological environments that support and change the genetics of a person. Epigenetic influences begin in utero and continue throughout the life span.

Early life events can have an effect on motor development in children and adolescents. Grace and associates[1] explored early life risk factors using participants from the Western Pregnancy Cohort Study. Events experienced during pregnancy were related to motor development into late adolescence. Motor outcomes were negatively affected in both males and females by maternal preeclampsia, low maternal income, and cesarean section. Males' motor outcomes appear to be at greater risk from having a lower birthweight, and females' motor outcomes were negatively influenced by younger maternal age and smoking.

MOTOR DEVELOPMENT

Motor development is the change in motor behavior experienced over the life span. The process and the product of motor development are related to age. The study of motor development has roots in biology and psychology. Typically, researchers in motor development studied individuals of different ages performing the same task, described age differences in terms of performance, and suggesting age-appropriate standards for judging the motor performance of infants, children, teenagers, adults, and older adults. Motor development studies are really studies of motor behavior. How does motor development inform the person about the world and how does skill acquisition drive changes in perceptual, cognitive, and social domains?[2]

Motor behavior changes occur to meet our needs across the life span. Observable changes are the result of the interaction between biological and environmental factors. Biological factors are not stable over time and are evidenced by differences in rate of growth, magnitude of growth, sensory processing, flexibility, strength, and speed of response. Maturation and learning depend on each other because learning does not occur unless the system is ready to learn. The rate of maturation is affected by the amount and type of learning experiences, and the type of learning experiences is affected by the sociocultural environment. Environmentally, the variables are infinite and include physical surroundings, family structure, access to motor learning experiences, and culture. Needs are related to survival, safety, motivation, psychological development, and sociocultural expectations. Together, all of these factors produce change or adaptation in the motor behaviors of an individual.

Changes in growth are used as markers for development. Growth charts are familiar ways in which a child's height, weight, and head circumference are monitored during the course of development. Children can be classified as an early, an average, or a late maturer according to the relationship between physiological growth parameters and chronological age. Despite the smooth trajectories seen on standard growth curves, a child's growth is not continuous but episodic. Growth is episodic at all ages, with more growth occurring at night than during the day.[3] The effects of physical size and body proportion on motor skill acquisition or movement proficiency have been examined in adolescence but are only now being explored in younger age groups.[4] Changing weight and proportion of the limb segments can constrain the production of movement.[5] Infants cease reflex stepping because the limbs get too heavy, not because of any change in the nervous system.[6] Adding weights to a limb during a reaching task changes the frequency of reaching toward faraway targets because of a potential

loss of balance.[7] Infants' ability to walk down a slope is diminished when wearing a weighted shoulder pack compared to wearing a light pack.[4]

Other factors that affect how a person develops movement are genetic coding and culture. Genes code for growth and maturation. Various sets of genes are associated with newborn length and weight, adult height and weight, and rate of growth in body size.[8] Genetics can contribute to motor performance and learning although the effect varies from task to task. Children born with genetic disorders which result in intellectual disability will usually exhibit delays in motor development. Group differences are reflected in gender and in the culture in which children are raised. Males have an innate ability to develop more muscle and greater strength.[8] Why does one person become a triathlete and another a prima ballerina, whereas others have difficulty riding a bike, water-skiing, or hitting a ball? Genes and the environment contribute in a complex way to human athletic performance.[9] Achievement of motor milestones is related to later sports performance.[10] A child's experience gleaned from various child-rearing practices (including physical handling), sensory and motor feedback, and sensorimotor integration combines with a genetic predisposition to produce movement skills. As a result of the Back to Sleep campaign to decrease the incidence of sudden infant death syndrome, infants spend less time on their tummy. The lack of tummy time has been associated with delays in motor development.[11,12] Culture and child-rearing practices influence movement skill acquisition by rewarding some motor behaviors and avoiding others.

Theories of Motor Development

The two major theories of motor development are the dynamic systems theory (DST) and the neuronal group selection theory (NGST). These theories best reflect the state of our current knowledge about motor development.

Dynamic Systems Theory

According to DST, movement emerges from the interaction of multiple body systems (Fig. 3.1).[13] DST incorporates the developmental biomechanical aspects of the mover, along with the developmental status of the mover's nervous system, the environmental context in which the movement occurs, and the task to be accomplished by the movement. The acquisition of postural control

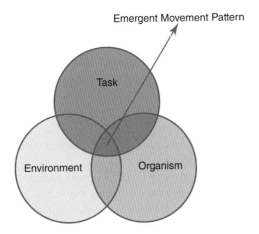

Fig. 3.1 Systems model indicating the emergent pattern of movement arising from the interaction of system elements. (From Holt KG. Biomechanical models, motor control theory, and development. *Inf Child Dev.* 2005;14:524-527.)

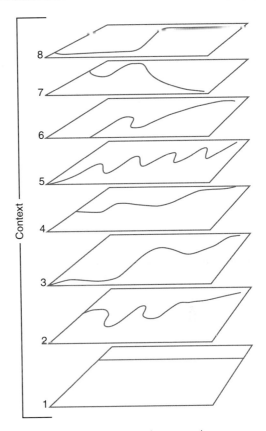

Fig. 3.2 Development as a layered system where many, parallel developing components exhibit asynchronous trajectories. (From Thelen E. Motor development: a new synthesis. *Am Psychol.* 1995;50(2):79-95.)

and balance is driven by the requirement of the specific task demands and the demands of gravity. Movement abilities associated with the developmental sequence are the result of selective motor control, which organizes movements into efficient patterns. DST is a theory of motor control and motor development. The brain and the neuromotor systems must interact to meet the developmental demands of the mover.

Several major themes that have been identified as foundational concepts in DST are:

1. Development is the result of interaction of all levels of the developing system, from the molecular to the cultural.[14] Development is represented as a layered system (Fig. 3.2). The bottom layer could represent the molecular level of a body system, followed by the tissue layer, which is further followed by a system layer, or each layer could be its own system, such as muscle, skeletal, nervous, and endocrine. The interaction among layers is continuous but occurs over different time periods. This has been described as a *nesting of time scales;*[15] each layer is part of overall development much like a child's set of stacking cups.[15] Perone and Simmering think that these time scales create each other. Research support for this concept comes from the linking of the development of motor and language systems[16,17] and development of infant visual recognition.[18]

2. Systems are *self-organized.* The behavior of a nonlinear system means that the behavior of the system is the product of how the many components interact. Components can be body systems or their products such as strength, posture, and flexibility. The interaction of components is context-dependent. "Systems organize into what are called attractor states, which are ways in which the components of a system reliably interact (e.g., crawling, walking, and running are different attractor states for locomotion)."[15] Self-organizing systems permit true novelty, so the structure of movement is emergent. For example, the stages seen in the developmental sequence represent periods of stability that emerge from the self-organization of multiple body systems. Self-organizing systems have the possibility of becoming more complex. The complexity serves the purpose of adapting to varying functional needs. A self-organizing system is able to reorganize and transition to new patterns

of movement after or during a period of instability. Phase transitions are points of instability that occur when old patterns break down and new ones appear. These transitions make adaptation possible.

3. Development is *multiply determined* and *soft assembled*. Many factors determine the form a movement takes: the mover's body size, maturation of the mover's musculoskeletal and nervous systems, and the mover's motivation, to name a few. Movement is loosely or *soft assembled*, the final product yet to be determined. The movement outcome is a product of the components within a task context. Some examples of components are strength, posture, and flexibility. These components can assist or limit emergence of movement. Soft assembly allows the infant to adapt to the changing world and learn by trial and error. Each infant learns a new movement in a different way; solutions are unique and within the context of the mover.

4. Development is *embodied.*[5] Embodiment includes the sensory information that occurs before, during, and after movement, as well as the perception of the mover as to what is happening. Sensation and perception are crucial to the integration of perception, action, and cognition. Movement happens in the context of the surrounding environment. Action or moving is a form of perception. Infants generate motor behaviors to gain perceptual information that they in turn use to learn how to make other actions possible. Sensory information can change movement. For example, walking on a treadmill turns into running when the speed is increased.

5. Development is *individualized*. Each mover is an individual with unique needs. Novice movers display incredible variability. Differences both within and between individuals are an integral component of motor development.[19] Variable movement opportunities are afforded by the mover on a daily basis as the environment changes. Each infant learns what actions are possible and which are not. Variability is inherent to development.[5]

Neuronal Group Selection

NGST proposes that motor skills result from the interaction of developing body dynamics and the structure or functions of the brain. The brain's structures are changed by how the body is used (moved). The brain's growing neural networks are sculpted to match efficient movement solutions. Three requirements must be met for neuronal selection to be effective in a motor system. First, a basic repertoire of movement must be present. Second, sensory information has to be available to identify and select adaptive forms of movement, and third, there must be a way to strengthen the preferred movement responses. Variability is a hallmark characteristic of typical motor development.[20] According to NGST, motor development occurs in two phases of variability: primary and secondary.[21,22]

The infant is genetically endowed with spontaneously generated motor behaviors. During the initial phase of variability, the nervous system spontaneously produces all kinds of possible movement combinations.[23] These self-produced movements shape the development of the nervous system via genetic coding.[22,24] This is an example of experience-expectant development. The sensory information generated by spontaneous activity prepares the nervous system to enter the next phase of variability. However, the sensory information generated by movements during this phase of variability has a limited ability to change motor behavior. The phase of primary variability is characterized by variation with little or no adaption[25] as seen in Fig. 3.3, prestructured motor commands.

Adaptation occurs during the phase of secondary variability when sensory and perceptual information is able to guide adaptation of motor behavior. This transition from primary variability to secondary variability generally occurs after 3 months of age. The exception is sucking and swallowing behavior, which are vital movements necessary for survival. The transition for this ability occurs prior to term. The process of selection of an adaptive response involves active trial and error. Motor development depends on self-generated spontaneous sensorimotor experiences which often occur during feeding and play. The ages at which secondary variability starts varies according to motor function. In general, all basic motor functions have progressed to the first stages of secondary variability around 18 months of age. These basic motor functions include posture and locomotion as well as reaching and grasping.

Fig. 3.3 illustrates rudimentary neural networks that produce initial motor behaviors. This example involves activation of postural muscles in sitting infants. Prior to independent sitting, infants demonstrate a large variation of muscle activation patterns when subjected to external perturbations, including a backward body

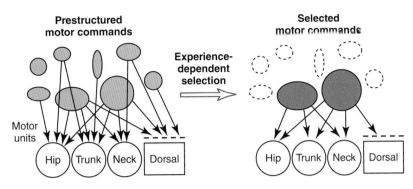

Fig. 3.3 A developmental process according to the neuronal group selection theory is exemplified by the development of postural muscle activation patterns in sitting infants. (Redrawn from Forssberg H. Neural control of human motor development. *Curr Opin Neurobiol.* 1999;9:676-682.)

sway. As indicated in Fig. 3.3, many postural muscles on the ventral side of the body are activated to counteract the backward displacement, and some dorsal muscles are inhibited, denoted by the dashes (----). With increasing age and experience, variability of the postural response decreases and a more adaptive muscle activation pattern remains. The sensory information from the experience of sitting modifies the strength of synaptic connections within and between neuronal groups with selection of some networks that predispose one action over another. As part of the secondary phase of variability, environmental and task demands become part of the neural ensemble for producing movements and actions. Spatial maps are formed and mature neural networks emerge as a product of use and sensory feedback. The maps that develop via the process of neuronal selection are preferred pathways. For example, situation-specific responses are seen in sitting where efficient responses are generated[26] and as coordinated reaching patterns emerge.[27] They become preferred because they are the ones that are used more often. Neurons that fire together wire together. Large amounts of the nervous system are interconnected in order to organize perception, cognition, emotion, and movement.

NGST supports a DST of motor control/motor development. According to NGST, the brain and nervous system are guided during development by a genetic blueprint and initial activity, which establishes rudimentary neuronal circuits. These early neuronal circuits are examples of self-organization. The use of certain circuits over others reinforces synaptic efficacy and strengthens those circuits. This is the selectivity that comes from exploring different ways of moving.

Lastly, maps are developed that provide the organization of patterns of spontaneous movement in response to mover and task demands. The linking of these early perception-action categories is the cornerstone of development.[28] Other body systems, such as the skeletal, muscular, cardiovascular, and pulmonary systems, develop and interact with the nervous system so that the most efficient movement pattern is chosen for the mover. According to this theory, there are no motor programs. The brain is not thought of as a computer and movement is not hardwired. This theory supports the idea that neural plasticity may be a constant feature across the lifespan. Neural plasticity is the ability to adapt structures in the nervous system to support desired functions. Integration of multiple systems allows for a variety of movement strategies to be used to perform a functional task. In other words, think of how many different ways a person can reach for an object or how many different ways it is possible for a person to move across a room.

The two theories, DST and NGST, agree that motor development is a nonlinear process which has many transitions that are affected by both child and environmental factors. Child factors include but are not limited to body weight, muscle power, and flexibility. Environmental factors include housing conditions, family composition, presence of toys, and a safe place to play. The theories differ in the role of genetics in the developmental process. NGST recognizes the vital contribution of genetics in determining neurodevelopmental processes while genetics plays only a limited role in DST. NGST is more in line with the complex genetic and epigenetic control of neural development.[29,30]

Influence of Cognition on Motor Development
Grounded Cognition

Grounded cognition is a concept in which cognition is embedded in the environment and the body.[31] It has also been described as embodied cognition in which intelligence develops from the interaction of the child within the environment as a result of sensorimotor experiences. This theory is similar to the perception-action theory in which the child makes use of perceptual motor experiences to develop cognition in a learning to learn paradigm. NGST and DST have been linked to development of cognition.[15,22,32] Perception and action are both required to build the brain. Movement provides sensory and perceptual information for learning within social and cultural contexts. This view of cognition is different from the traditional view where cognition exists outside of a person's everyday experiences. See Fig. 3.4 for a comparison of these two views of cognition. Researchers have identified the development of object interaction, sitting and reaching, and locomotion as models of grounded cognition.[32]

Researchers have linked motor development and subsequent cognitive ability. Diamond[33] described how the development of the prefrontal cortex and the cerebellum parallels the protracted development of the motor system. Motor experiences have a positive impact on cognition. Learning to move teaches the brain how to think. Motor development of children between birth and 4 years predicted cognitive performance at school age,[34] and achievement of gross motor milestones correlated with later cognitive outcomes.[35] Once walking emerges, toddlers experience growing autonomy and greater opportunity for perceptual learning, social interaction, and environmental exploration. In an Australian study, gross motor skills were positively associated with cognitive development in toddlers.[36]

When an infant experiences a negative environment due to prematurity, the sensory experiences that shape brain development are limited. The most negative outcomes of being born premature and having a low birth weight are impaired motor, cognitive, and language development.[37–39] Marrus and a team of investigators used resting state functional MRI to identify neural networks associated with gross motor scores and walking in a group of infants at high and low risk for autism spectrum disorder.[40] Functional connectivity of motor networks was correlated with walking at age 12 months and attention

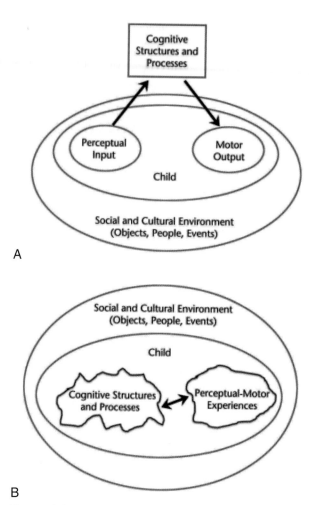

Fig. 3.4 **(A)** Traditional view of cognition. **(B)** Grounded view of cognition. (From Lobo MA, Harbourne RT, Dusing AC, et al. Grounding early intervention: physical therapy cannot be about motor skills anymore. *Phys Ther.* 2013;93:94-103.)

networks connectivity at 24 months. Their findings suggest that changes in developing brain networks explain the emergence of gross motor abilities in toddlers.

Motor development, motor control, and motor learning are influenced to varying degrees by a person's intellectual ability. Impairments in cognitive ability can affect an individual's ability to learn to move and adapt movement to tasks in varying environments. A child with intellectual disability may not have the ability to learn movement skills at the same rate as a child with average intelligence. The rate of developmental change in a child with an intellectual disability is decreased in all domains: biological, psychological, and sociological. Thus acquisition of motor skills is often as delayed as the acquisition of additional knowledge. Just as cognition can affect motor development, the motor system can affect cognition.

Developmental Concepts

The following concepts about human development are presented to help organize information on motor development. There is a sequence to early motor development; however, the sequence exhibits variability. The age of acquisition of specific motor skills is used to diagnose delayed motor performance. It is notable that a delay in only one milestone is of limited clinical value while delay in attaining multiple milestones suggests an increased risk of a problem.[41] Children who move in stereotypical ways or appear stuck in a restricted pattern of movement have been deemed to be at risk. Assessment of variability in postural control during infancy is now being used to identify motor problems.[42] Movement depends on producing sufficient force to move and learning to control and utilize those forces for action. As infants' bodies change with growth, the biomechanical constraints on action change as well.

Developmental Sequence

The developmental sequence is generally recognized to consist of the development of head control, rolling, sitting, creeping, and walking (Gesell, 1974).[43] The sequence of acquisition of motor skills has previously been known as motor milestones. The rate of change in acquiring each skill may vary from child to child within a family, among families, and among families of different cultures. Sequences may overlap as the child works on several levels of skills at the same time. For example, a child can be perfecting rolling while learning to balance in sitting. The lower-level skill does not need to be perfect before the child goes on to try something new. Some children even bypass a motor skill, such as creeping, and go on to another higher-level skill, such as walking without doing any harm developmentally. Culture and child-rearing practices influence the sequence. The attainment of typical infant motor abilities during the first year of life is found in Tables 3.1 and 3.2. Remember there are wide variations in time frames during which motor skills are typically achieved.

Cephalocaudal Development

Gesell[43] recognized that development of postural control proceeded from cephalic to caudal and proximal to

TABLE 3.1   Gross Motor Skills

Motor Skill	Age
Head control (no head lag when pulled to sit)	4 months
Roll segmentally supine to prone	6–8 months
Sit alone steadily	6–8 months
Creep reciprocally, pulls to stand	8–9 months
Cruising	10–11 months
Walk alone	12 months

From Martin ST, Kessler M. *Neurologic Interventions for Physical Therapy.* 4th ed. Philadelphia: Elsevier; 2021:78.

TABLE 3.2   Fine Motor Skills

Milestone	Age
Palmar grasp reflex	Birth
Hands together at midline	4 months
Raking	5 months
Voluntary palmar grasp	6 months
Transfer block hand to hand	7 months
Inferior pincer grasp	9–12 months
Superior pincer grasp	12 months

distal during postnatal development. Head control in infants begins with neck movements and is followed by development of trunk control. Postnatal postural development mirrors what happens in the embryo when the neural tube closes. Closure of the neural tube occurs first in the cervical area and then progresses in two directions at once, toward the head and the tail of the embryo. The infant develops head and neck and then trunk control. Overlap exists between the development of head and trunk control; think of a spiral beginning around the mouth and spreading outward in all directions encompassing more and more of the body. Development of postural control of the head and neck can be a rate-limiting factor in early motor development. If control of the head and neck is not mastered, subsequent motor development will be delayed.

Proximal to Distal Development

The body is a linked structure. The axis or midline of the body must provide a stable base for head, eye, and extremity movements to occur with any degree of control.

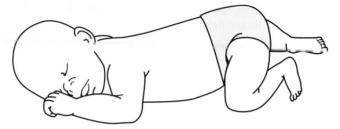

Fig. 3.5 Physiologic flexion in a newborn. (From Martin ST, Kessler M. *Neurologic Interventions for Physical Therapy.* 4th ed. Philadelphia: Elsevier; 2021:82, Fig. 4.8.)

The trunk is the stable base for head movement above and for limb movements distally. Imagine what would happen if you could not maintain an erect sitting posture without the use of your arms and you tried to use your arms to catch a ball thrown to you. You would have to use your arms for support, and if you tried to catch the ball, you would probably fall. Or imagine not being able to hold your head up. What chance would you have of being able to follow a moving object with your eyes? Early in development, the infant works to establish midline neck control by lifting the head from the prone position, then establishes midline trunk control by extending the spine against gravity, followed by establishing proximal shoulder and pelvic girdle stability through weight bearing. Proximal stability of the upper and lower extremities allows more distal control of the arms, hands, legs, and feet. In some positions where infants' head and trunk are stable, they are able to move the arms and legs freely. Reaching with the upper extremities is possible early in development but only with external trunk support, as when placed in an infant seat in which the trunk is supported.

Dissociation/Fractionation

Development proceeds from mass movements to specific movements or from simple movements to complex movements. This concept can be interpreted in several different ways. Mass can refer to the whole body, and specific can refer to smaller parts of the body. For example, when an infant moves, the entire body moves; movement is not isolated to a specific body part. The infant learns to move the body as one unit, as in log rolling, before being able to move separate parts. The ability to separate movement in one body part from movement in another body part is called dissociation. Mature movements are characterized by dissociation, and typical motor development provides many examples. When an infant learns to turn her head in all directions without trunk movement, the head is said to be dissociated from the trunk. Reaching with one arm from a prone-on-elbows position is an example of dissociation of limb movement from the trunk. While the infant creeps on hands and knees, limb movements are dissociated from trunk movement. Additionally, when the upper trunk rotates in one direction and the lower trunk rotates in the opposite direction during creeping (counterrotation), the upper trunk is dissociated from the lower trunk and vice versa. Fractionation is another term sometimes used to describe how movement is broken down or fractionated into component parts. For example, babies go from displaying a mass grasp with all fingers moving into or away from the palm to being able to isolate or fractionate movement so that only one finger is isolated as a pointer.

Biomechanical Considerations in Motor Development

Some movements are easier to perform at certain times during development. Factors affecting movement include the biomechanics of the situation, muscle strength, flexibility, level of neuromuscular maturation, and postural control. Full-term babies are born with predominant flexor muscle tone (physiologic flexion) and have a C-shaped spine. The limbs and trunk naturally assume a flexed position (Fig. 3.5). As development progresses, active movement toward extension occurs if the infant spends time in a prone position. Exposure to head lifting in prone position develops the secondary cervical curve in the spine. Without exposure to the prone position in the form of tummy time, the ability of the infant to lift and turn the head is diminished. Decreased time in prone also increases the risk of plagiocephaly, or a misshapen head is increased, because in supine, the infant tends to assume an asymmetrical head posture. The neck muscles are not strong enough to maintain the head in midline while in supine. Tummy time is essential to encourage lifting and turning of the head to strengthen the neck muscles bilaterally.

Tummy time also affords the infant opportunities to prop on elbows and push up on extended arms as preparation for weight bearing in four-point position. Gravity is conquered, sitting posture is attained, and another secondary lumbar curve develops. Adaptation of skills emerges in infancy as muscle and fat are redistributed, balance is learned, and perceptual feedback is received from the prior movement. Learning to move means learning to adapt to the current status of the body at each moment in time.[5]

Movement emerges from the interaction of all body systems, the task at hand, and the environment in which it takes place. To acquire motor skills, the mover has to control the number of planes of motion possible at a single joint and then multiple joints. Bernstein[44] thought that the new or novice mover minimized the number of independent movement elements used until control was developed. For example, in standing, the upper trunk is kept in extension by placing the arms in high guard while the lower trunk is kept stable by anteriorly tilting the pelvis. The infant is left with only having to pick up each leg at a time as if stepping in place. A little forward momentum is used to propel the new walker.

FUNCTIONAL IMPLICATIONS

The functional implication of motor development is that movement abilities change over time or across the life span. The process of motor development requires motor control and motor learning. Movement is guided by sensation and changed by sensory feedback. The goals of motor development are to acquire functional synergies that can be used to the mover's advantage, to become a competent mover, to become an efficient mover, to adapt movement to intrinsic and extrinsic demands, and lastly to achieve task goals. Movement allows for exploration, affording perception, making choices, and acquiring physical, psychological, and social skills.

Life Span Changes in Motor Development and Function
Infancy

An infant's movements are associated with reflexes for the first 3 months of life. However, a typically developing

TABLE 3.3   Primitive Reflexes

Reflex	Age at Onset	Age at Integration
Suck-swallow	28 weeks' gestation	2–5 months
Rooting	28 weeks' gestation	3 months
Flexor withdrawal	28 weeks' gestation	1–2 months
Crossed extension	28 weeks' gestation	1–2 months
Moro	28 weeks' gestation	4–6 months
Plantar grasp	28 weeks' gestation	9 months
Positive support	35 weeks' gestation	1–2 months
Asymmetrical tonic neck	Birth	4–6 months
Palmar grasp	Birth	9 months
Symmetrical tonic neck	4–6 months	8–12 months

Data from Barnes MR, Crutchfield CA, Heriza CB. *The Neurophysiological Basis of Patient Treatment.* Vol 2. Atlanta: Stokesville; 1982.

infant is not limited to reflex motor behavior. After decades of research, we know that motor behavior is not organized in terms of reflexes and that even during gestation the brain is involved in modulating motor behavior.[45]

Reflexes do play a role in pairing sensory and motor action. Reflexes occur early in developmental time, with some appearing during gestation or shortly after birth, and are integrated by 4–6 months of age. A list of primitive, or early occurring, reflexes is found in Table 3.3. Reflexes can be modified by the alertness or satiation of the infant. Some reflex behavior can also be influenced by the environment. A stepping reflex can be elicited in a newborn, but by several months of age, the reflex "disappears." Thelen and colleagues[46] proved that the reason infants no longer exhibit a stepping reflex was because their legs got too heavy to perform the movement. When weight was not an issue, as when the infants were placed in water up to their chest, they once again exhibited the ability to step.

Oral Motor Skill Development
Sucking/Swallowing/Chewing

The ability to ingest food is necessary for survival. Oral motor behaviors include sucking, biting, chewing, and swallowing. Oral reflexes are present in utero; however, most of oral motor behavior involved in rhythmical movements of sucking, swallowing, and chewing is organized by a central pattern generator in the brainstem.[47] The fetus has been shown to suck its thumb as well as to take in amniotic fluid.

At birth, sucking and swallowing have to be combined with breathing. The infant tries various combinations of when to breath relative to sucking[48] before settling into a dominant 1:1 suck-swallow ratio.[49] The adult pattern of swallowing at the cusp of inspiration and expiration gradually emerges.

Human milk is the optimal nutritional source of calcium during the first year of life.[50] Other types of food are introduced between 4 and 6 months of age. Between 5 and 8 months of age, oral motor behavior shifts from sucking to chewing. This transition is supported by growth changes in the skull and mandible, peripheral afferent input, neural maturation, and motor learning. The pharynx has elongated, and the larynx has descended, providing more space in the oral cavity. The soft palate is no longer in contact with the epiglottis. The valving of the epiglottis is needed to protect the airway during swallowing.

The infant is ready to transition to spoon feeding around the time sitting posture is more erect. Food must be chewed or masticated before swallowing. Infants rely on lateral jaw movements when chewing semisolid food.[51] By 6 months, infants can handle solid food. A rotary pattern of chewing is mastered by older children and used by adults, but its development has a protracted course.[52] Age-related changes in coordination of chewing relative to different types of food have been documented in children 9–36 months.[53] Tongue and lip movements become more coordinated in order to clean food from the lip and maintain lip closure around a spoon and drink from a cup. In the process of obtaining food, the shape of the tongue is modified. This change prepares the tongue for articulating specific speech sounds such as "p," "b," and "m" and is an example of feeding as preparation for speech.

Communication

Oral motor behavior serves a second function in development, that of communication by use of facial expressions, vocalizations, and spoken words. Facial movements begin in utero. Infants as young as 2 days old can discriminate facial expressions of emotions.[54]

Infants like human faces but imitation of movement is limited to tongue protrusion.[55] During the first year, spontaneous facial movements change considerably to support speech development. Infants learn to use quick up and down jaw movements to babble (mama, dada).[56] The first word is spoken around 12 months, and from 18 months, vocabulary increases dramatically.[57]

Motor Skill Development

Motor skill development progresses sequentially over the first year of life, with the infant able to roll, sit, crawl/creep, pull to stand, cruise, and walk by 1 year. Reaching and prehension change from swiping at objects at 5 months to discrete movement of the thumb and index finger by 10 months. Reaching and prehension are discussed at greater length in Chapter 12.

Prenatal/Neonatal

General movements (GMs) are present from early fetal life. By the end of the first trimester of fetal development, the entire neonatal repertoire of movement is present.[22] GMs involve the entire body of an infant and are present until 3–5 months postnatal age. See Fig. 3.6 for examples of GMs in a 3-month-old infant. This simple form of motility is hypothesized to be the result of a central pattern generator that begins in the brainstem and extends into the caudal part of the spinal cord.[58] GMs are characterized by complexity and variation. Think of them as the substrate for future motor actions. Goal-directed arm movements, such as manipulating clothing or fingers, take the place of GMs at 3–5 months. GMs are representative of the early developing brain and as such form the cornerstone of early development.[22] The absence of GMs is associated with cerebral palsy.[59]

Birth to 3 Months

Newborns assume a flexed posture regardless of their position because physiological flexion dominates at birth. Initially, the newborn is unable to lift the head from a prone position. The newborn's legs are flexed under the pelvis and prevent the pelvis from coming into contact with the supporting surface. If you put yourself into that position and try to lift your head, even as an adult, you will immediately recognize that the biomechanics of the situation are against you. With your hips in the air, your weight is shifted forward, thus making it more difficult to lift your head even though you have more muscular strength and control than a newborn. Although you are

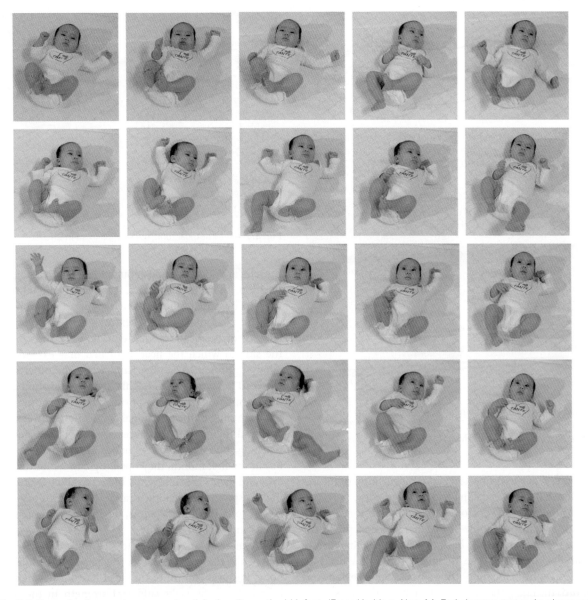

Fig. 3.6 Example of general movement activity in a 3-month-old infant. (From Hadders-Algra M. Early human motor development: from variation to the ability to vary and adapt. *Neurosci Biobehav Rev.* 2018;90:414.)

strong enough to overcome this mechanical disadvantage, the infant is not. The infant must wait for gravity to help lower the pelvis to the support surface and for the neck muscles to strengthen to be able to lift the head when in the prone position. The infant will then be able to lift the head unilaterally (Fig. 3.7) and then bilaterally. Prone is important for development of head control as it is the position that is hardest for the heavy head to lifted off the support surface.

Over the first several months, neck and spinal extensions develop and allow the infant to lift the head to one side, to lift and turn the head, and then to lift and hold the head in the midline. Tummy time is important to provide these opportunities. Just spending a few

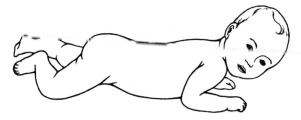

Fig. 3.7 Unilateral head lifting in a newborn. (From Martin ST, Kessler M. *Neurologic interventions for physical therapy*, 4th ed. Philadelphia: Elsevier;2021:82 Fig. 4.22.

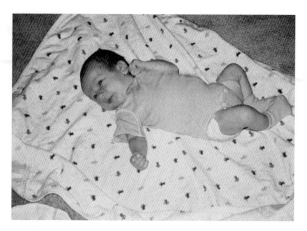

Fig. 3.9 Asymmetrical tonic neck reflex in an infant.

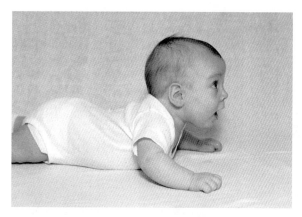

Fig. 3.8 A 3-month-old lifts head and supports some weight on forearms. (From Wong DL, Perry SE. *Maternal Child Nursing Care*. 3rd ed. St. Louis: CV Mosby; 2005:1031.)

minutes a day in prone accelerated acquisition of future motor skills such as rolling and crawling.[60,61]

As the pelvis lowers to the support surface, neck and trunk extensors become stronger. Extension proceeds from the neck down the back in a cephalocaudal direction. By 3 months of age, the infant can lift the head to 45 degrees from the supporting surface. Spinal extension affords the infant the opportunity to bring the arms from under the body to support some weight on the forearms (Fig. 3.8). This position makes it easier to extend the trunk and lift the head past 90 degrees. Weight bearing through the arms and shoulders provides greater sensory awareness to those structures and allows the infant to view the hands while in a prone position.

When in the supine position, the birth to 3-month-old infant exhibits random arm and leg movements. The limbs remain flexed and never extend completely. The head is kept to one side or the other because the neck muscles are not yet strong enough to maintain a midline position. To make eye contact, approach the infant from the side because of the asymmetrical head position. An asymmetrical tonic neck reflex may be seen when the baby turns the head to one side (Fig. 3.9). The arm on the side to which the head is turned may extend and allow the infant to see the hand while the other arm, closer to the skull, is flexed. This "fencing" position does not dominate the infant's posture, but it may provide the beginning of the functional connection between the eyes and the hand that is necessary for visually guided reaching. Initially the baby's hands are normally fisted, but in the first month, they open. By 2 to 3 months, the eyes and hands are sufficiently linked to allow for reaching, grasping, and shaking a rattle. As the eyes begin to track ever-widening distances, the infant will watch the hands and explore the body.

When an infant is pulled to sit from a supine position before the age of 4 months, the head lags behind the body. Postural control of the head has not been established. The baby lacks sufficient strength in the neck muscles to overcome the force of gravity. Primitive rolling, also known as log rolling, may be seen as the infant turns the head strongly to one side. The body may rotate as a unit in the same direction as the head moves. This turning as a unit is the result of a primitive neck righting. More discussion of the role of postural reactions in the development of postural control is presented in Chapter 11. Separation of upper and lower trunk segments around the long axis of the body is missing in primitive rolling (Fig. 3.10).

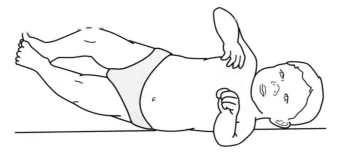

Fig. 3.10 Primitive rolling without rotation. (From Martin ST, Kessler M. *Neurologic Interventions for Physical Therapy.* 4th ed. Philadelphia: Elsevier; 2021:82, Fig. 4.25.)

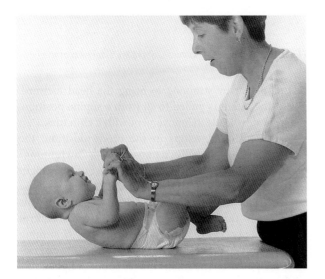

Fig. 3.11 Head in line with the body when pulled to sit. (From Martin ST, Kessler M. *Neurologic Interventions for Physical Therapy.* 4th ed. Philadelphia: Elsevier; 2021:82, Fig. 4.10.)

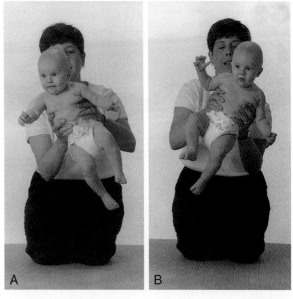

Fig. 3.12 (A and B) Head control while held upright in vertical and tilted. The head remains either in midline or tilts as a compensation. (From Martin ST, Kessler M. *Neurologic Interventions for Physical Therapy.* 4th ed. Philadelphia: Elsevier; 2021:82, Fig. 4.27.)

Four Months

The hallmark motor behaviors of the 4-month-old infant are head control and midline orientation. An infant should exhibit good head control by 4 months of age. Good head control is seen when the infant keeps the head in line with the body (ear in line with the acromion) when pulled to sit from a supine position (Fig. 3.11). When the infant is held upright in a vertical position and is tilted in any direction, the head should tilt in the opposite direction (Fig. 3.12). A 4-month-old infant, when placed in a prone position, should be able to lift and hold the head up against gravity past 45 degrees with the elbows aligned ahead of the shoulders (Fig. 3.13). Four months is critical for motor development because posture and movement change from asymmetrical to more symmetrical. Midline orientation of the head is present when the infant is at rest in the supine position (Fig. 3.14). The infant brings hands together in the midline to watch them. In fact, the first time babies get both hands to the midline and realize that the hands, to this point only viewed wiggling in the periphery, are part of their body, a real "aha" occurs. Initially, this discovery may result in hours of midline hand play. The infant can reach in the midline and bring objects to the mouth with both hands. Bimanual hand play is seen in all possible developmental positions.

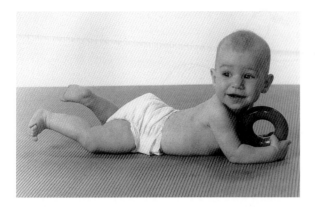

Fig. 3.13 Prone on elbows. (From Martin ST, Kessler M. *Neurologic Interventions for Physical Therapy.* 4th ed. Philadelphia: Elsevier; 2021:82, Fig. 4.23.)

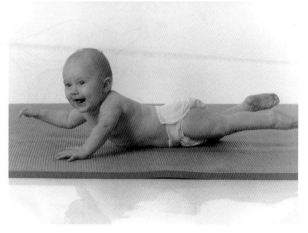

Fig. 3.15 "Swimming" posture, antigravity extension of the body.

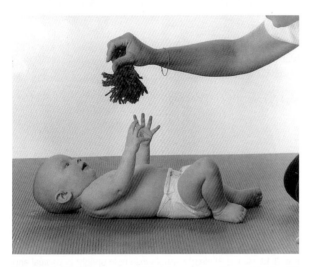

Fig. 3.14 Midline head position in supine. (From Martin ST, Kessler M. *Neurologic Interventions for Physical Therapy.* 4th ed. Philadelphia: Elsevier; 2021:82, Fig. 4.26.)

Five Months

Even though head control as defined earlier is considered to be achieved by 4 months of age, lifting the head against gravity in a supine position is not achieved until 5 months of age. At 5 months, the infant exhibits the ability to lift the head off the support surface (*antigravity neck flexion*). Antigravity neck flexion may first be noted by the caregiver when putting the baby down in the crib for a nap. As the caregiver lowers the baby toward the support surface, the infant works to keep the head from falling backwards. This is also the time when infants look as though they are trying to climb out of their car

or infant seat by straining to bring the head forward. When the infant is pulled to sit from a supine position, the head now leads the movement with a chin tuck.

As extension develops in the prone position, the infant may occasionally demonstrate a "swimming" posture (Fig. 3.15). In this position, most of the weight is on the tummy, and the arms and legs are able to be stretched out and held up off the floor or mattress. This posture is a further manifestation of extensor control against gravity. The infant plays between this swimming posture and a prone-on-elbows or prone-on-extended-arms posture. The infant makes subtle weight shifts while in the prone-on-elbows position and may attempt reaching. Movements at this stage show *dissociation* of head and limbs from the trunk. Limbs move separately in kicking, and limb and head movements also occur separately, no longer tied or yoked together.

From a froglike position in supine, the infant is able to lift the bottom off the support surface using the lower abdominals and bring the feet into the visual field. This "bottom lifting" allows the infant to reach and play with the feet, even to put them into the mouth for increased sensory awareness. This play provides lengthening for the hamstrings and prepares the baby for long sitting. The lower abdominals also have a chance to work while the trunk is supported. Moving the legs separately from the trunk is another example of dissociation.[62]

Six Months

A 6-month-old infant becomes mobile in the prone position by pivoting in a circle (Fig. 3.16). The infant is

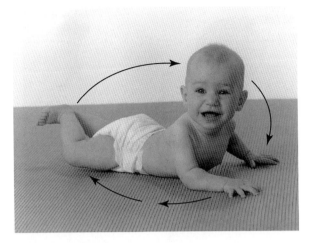

Fig. 3.16 Pivoting in prone.

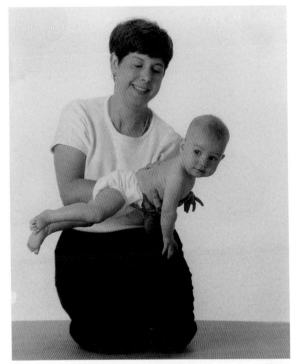

Fig. 3.18 Eliciting a Landau reflex. (From Martin ST, Kessler M. *Neurologic Interventions for Physical Therapy*. 4th ed. Philadelphia: Elsevier; 2021:82, Fig. 4.34A.)

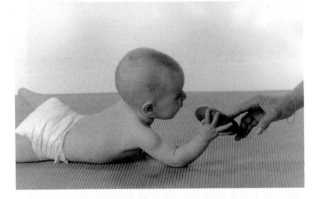

Fig. 3.17 Lateral righting reaction. (From Martin S, Kessler M: *Neurologic Interventions for Physical Therapy*. 2nd ed. St. Louis: Saunders; 2007.)

also able to shift weight onto one extended arm and to reach forward with the other hand to grasp an object. The reaching movement is counterbalanced by a lateral weight shift of the trunk that produces lateral head and trunk bending away from the side of the weight shift (Fig. 3.17). This lateral bending in response to a weight shift is called a *righting reaction*. Righting reactions of the head and trunk are discussed in Chapter 11. Maximum extension of the head and trunk is possible in the prone position along with extension and abduction of the limbs away from the body. This extended posture is called the *Landau reflex* and represents total body righting against gravity. It is mature when the infant can demonstrate hip extension when held away

from the support surface, supported only under the tummy (Fig. 3.18). The infant appears to be flying. This final stage in the development of extension can occur only if the hips are relatively adducted. Too much hip abduction puts the gluteus maximus at a biomechanical disadvantage and makes it more difficult to execute hip extension. Excessive abduction is often seen in children with low muscle tone and increased range of motion such as in Down syndrome. These children have difficulty performing antigravity hip extension.

The pull-to-sit maneuver with a 6-month-old often causes the infant to pull all the way up to standing (Fig. 3.19). The infant will most likely reach forward for the caregiver's hands as part of the task. A 6-month-old likes to bear weight on the feet and will bounce in this position if held. Back and forth rocking and bouncing in a position seem to be prerequisites for achieving postural control in a new posture.[63]

Segmental rolling. Segmental rolling or rolling with separate upper and lower trunk rotation should be accomplished by 6–8 months of age. Rolling from prone

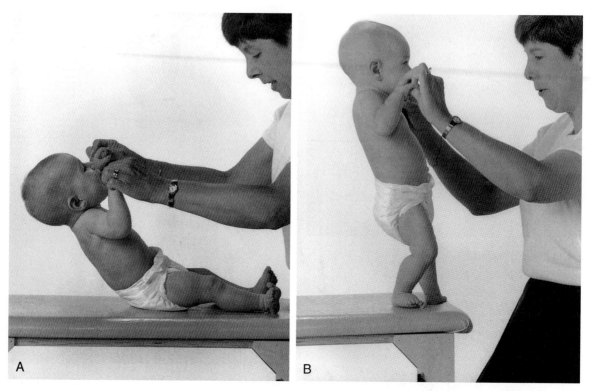

Fig. 3.19 Pull-to-sit maneuver becomes a pull-to-stand maneuver. (From Martin ST, Kessler M. *Neurologic Interventions for Physical Therapy*. 4th ed. Philadelphia: Elsevier; 2021:82, Fig. 4.37.)

to supine precedes rolling from supine to prone, because extensor control typically precedes flexor control. The prone position provides some mechanical advantage because the infant's arms are under the body and can push against the support surface. If the head, the heaviest part of the infant, moves laterally, gravity will assist in bringing it toward the support surface and will cause a change of position.

Antigravity flexion control is needed to roll from supine to prone. The movement usually begins with flexion of some body part, depending on the infant and the circumstances. If enticed with a toy, the infant may reach up and over the body for the toy with the upper extremity. Another infant may lift one leg up and over the body and allow the weight of the pelvis to initiate trunk rotation. Still another infant may begin the roll with head and neck flexion. Regardless of the body part used, segmental rotation is essential for developing transitional control. *Transitional movements* are those that allow a change of position, such as moving from prone to sitting, from a four-point

position to kneeling, and from sitting to standing (STS). Only a few movement transitions take place without trunk rotation, such as moving from the four-point position to kneeling and from STS. Individuals with movement dysfunction often have problems making the transition from one position to another smoothly and efficiently. This difficulty is often due to a lack of controlled trunk rotation. The quality of movement affects the individual's ability to perform transitional movements.

Sitting. Sitting represents a change in functional orientation for the infant. Previously the norm for achieving independent sitting was 8 months of age. However, according to the World Health Organization (WHO) (2006),[64] the mean age at which infants around the world now sit is 6.1 months (SD of 1.1). *Sitting independently* is defined as sitting alone when placed. The back should be straight, without any kyphosis (forward trunk flexion). No hand support is needed (see Fig. 3.20). The secondary lumbar curve emerges as more postural control is achieved with sitting practice. The infant does not have to assume a sitting position but is expected to free hands for reaching and manipulating objects/people. Independent sitting develops over several months as postural control of the trunk improves.

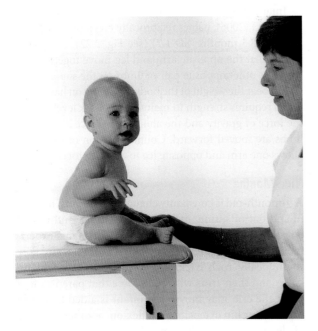

Fig. 3.20 Early sitting showing a rounding in the lumbar area. (From Martin S, Kessler M. *Neurologic Interventions for Physical Therapy*. 2nd ed. St. Louis: Saunders; 2007.)

The upright position improves processing of visual information and affords greater opportunities for object exploration. Visually, sitting provides a new vantage point for the infant by expanding the visual field (Fig. 3.21). The ability to visually attend to objects in the environment is critical for problem solving.[65] As postural stability increases in sitting, the infant has the opportunity to use both hands to explore and manipulate objects. Repetition of rhythmic upper extremity activities such as banging and shaking of objects is demonstrated during this period. Reaching becomes less dependent on visual cues as the infant uses other senses to become more aware of body relationships. The infant may hear a noise and may reach unilaterally toward the toy that made the sound.[66]

Seven Months

Functional ability in sitting improves at this age. Trunk control improves in sitting and allows the infant to free one hand for playing with objects. The infant can narrow her base of support in sitting by adducting the lower extremities as the trunk begins to be able to compensate for small losses of balance. Dynamic stability develops from muscular work of the trunk. An active trunk supports dynamic balance and complements the positional stability derived from the configuration of the base of support. The different types of sitting postures such as ring sitting, wide abducted sitting, and long sitting

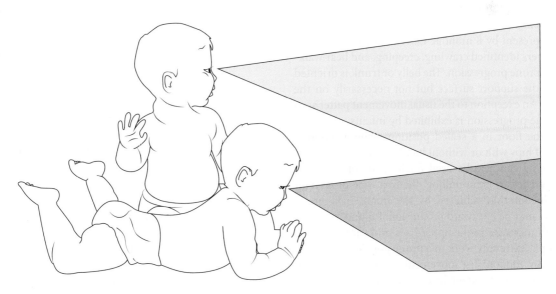

Fig. 3.21 Field of view for a sitting infant.

provide the infant with different amounts of support. When balance is lost during sitting, the infant extends one or both arms in the direction of the displacement. These upper extremity protective reactions will be seen in the forward, sideways, and backward directions over the next few months. Unilateral reach and the ability to transfer objects from hand to hand is displayed by the 7-month-old infant.

Eight Months

Sitting. Sitting is the most functional and favorite position of the infant. The infant can move into and out of sitting by pushing up from side lying. The infant's upright posture is good, and the hands are free to play with objects or extend and abduct to catch the infant if a loss of balance occurs, as happens less frequently over time. If a toy is out of reach, the infant can prop on one arm and reach across the body to extend the reach using trunk rotation and reverse the rotation to return to an upright sitting position. With increased control of trunk rotation, the body moves more segmentally and less as a whole.

Dissociation of the arms from the trunk is seen as the arms move across the midline of the body. More external rotation is evident at the shoulder (turning the entire arm from palm down, to neutral, to palm up) and allows supinated reaching to be achieved. By 8–10 months, the infant's two hands are able to perform different functions such as holding a bottle in one hand while reaching for a toy with the other.[66]

Creeping. Some form of prewalking progression is usually present by 8 months. Early motor development researchers identified crawling, creeping, and bear walking as a prone progression. The belly or trunk is oriented toward the support surface but not necessarily on the surface. An exception to the usual movement patterns in the prone progression is exhibited by infants who hitch across the floor in a seated position using a scooting action of hips with or without hand support.

Pushing can also be used for locomotion. Because pushing is easier than pulling, the first type of straight plane locomotion achieved by the infant in a prone position may be backward propulsion. Pulling is seen as strength increases in the upper back and shoulders. All this upper extremity work in a prone position is accompanied by random leg movements. These random leg movements may accidentally cause the legs to be pushed into extension with the toes flexed and may thus provide

an extra boost forward. In trying to reproduce the accident, the infant begins to learn to belly crawl or creep forward. When belly crawling, the infant may push up to hands and feet and attempt to "walk" in this position (*bear crawling/walking*).

Infants first crawl on their tummy, but according to the WHO (2006), babies reciprocally creep on hands and knees at 8.5 months (SD 1.7) (see Fig. 3.22). Reciprocal means that the opposite arm and leg move together and leave the other opposite pair of limbs on the support surface to bear the weight of the body. Creeping on hands and knees requires strength to maintain the back level against the force of gravity and the ability to balance as opposite limbs are moved forward. Counterrotation of the trunk allows one arm and opposite leg to advance together.

Nine Months

A 9-month-old is constantly changing positions, moving in and out of sitting, including side sitting, and in and out of the hands and knees position. As infants experiment more and more with the four-point position, they rhythmically rock back and forth putting weight on knees and then arms with such force that parents often think the crib may move. The infant is aided by a new capacity for hip extension and flexion, another example of dissociation of pelvic movements from trunk. The hands and knees position requires more trunk control and greater balance.

Creeping. Creeping is often the primary means of locomotion for several months, even after the infant

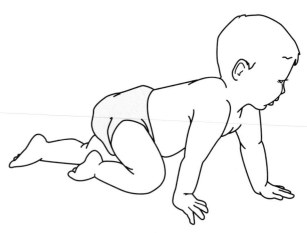

Fig. 3.22 Reciprocal creeping. (Martin ST, Kessler M. *Neurologic Interventions for Physical Therapy.* 4th ed. Philadelphia: Elsevier; 2021:82, Fig. 4.13.)

starts pulling to stand and cruising around furniture. Creeping provides fast and stable travel for the infant and allows for exploration of the environment. A small percentage of infants never creep on hands and knees according to the WHO (2006). Infants who belly crawled (belly constantly on the ground) or engaged in other forms of prone progression such as inchworm (belly off and on the ground and bear crawl/walk; hands and feet are on the ground) were twice as proficient when creeping on hands and knees compared to infants who do not display earlier forms of crawling.[2,67]

Pull to stand. When playing in the quadruped position, the infant may reach out to the crib rail or furniture and may pull up to a kneeling position. Balance is maintained by holding on with the arms rather than by fully bearing weight through the hips. The infant at this age does not have the postural control necessary to balance in a kneeling or half-kneeling (one foot forward) position. It is only after learning to walk that such control is possible for the toddler. Pulling to stand is a rapid movement transition with little time spent in either true knee standing or half-kneeling. Early standing consists of leaning against a support surface, such as the coffee table or couch, so the hands can be free to play. Legs tend to be abducted for a wider base of support, much like the struts of a tower. Knee position may vary between flexion and extension, and toes alternately claw the floor and flare upward in an attempt to assist balance. Another change in infants' field of view occurs when they transition from creeping to standing and walking (Fig. 3.23).

Ten Months

Once the infant has achieved an upright posture at furniture, she practices weight shifting by moving from side to side. While in upright standing and before cruising begins in earnest, the infant practices dissociating arm and leg movements from the trunk by reaching out or backward with an arm while the leg is swung in the opposite direction. When side-to-side weight shift progresses to actual movement sideways, the baby is cruising. Cruising is done around furniture and between close pieces of furniture. Infants perceive how large a gap they can span with their arms but not their legs.[68]

Sideways "walking" is done with arm support and may be a means of working the hip abductors to ensure a level pelvis when forward ambulation is attempted. These maneuvers always make us think of a ballet dancer warming up at the barre before dancing. In this case, the infant is warming up, practicing counterrotation in a newly acquired posture, upright, before attempting to walk (Fig. 3.24). Over the next several months, the infant will develop better pelvic and hip control to perfect upright standing before attempting independent ambulation.

Toddler

Twelve months. The infant becomes a toddler at 1 year. Most infants attempt forward locomotion by this age. The caregiver has probably already been holding the infant's hands and encouraging walking, if not placing the infant in a walker. Use of walkers continues to raise safety concerns from pediatricians and

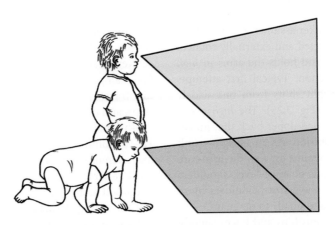

Fig. 3.23 Infants' field of view in crawling and walking. (From Adolph KE, Hoch JE, Cole WG. Development (of walking): 15 suggestions. *Trends Cogn Sci.* 2018;22:699-711, Figure 1.)

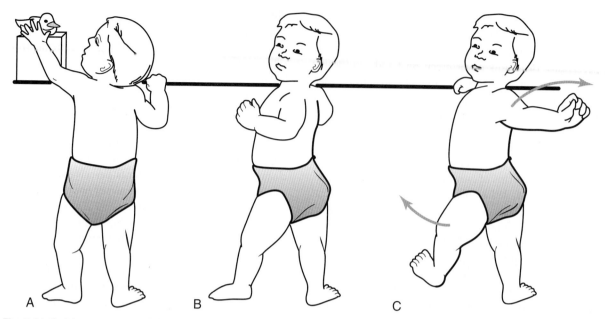

Fig. 3.24 Cruising maneuvers. **(A)** Cruising sideways, reaching out. **(B)** Standing, rotating upper trunk backward. **(C)** Standing, reaching out backward, elaborating with swinging movements of the same-side leg, thus producing counterrotation. (Redrawn by permission of the publisher from Conner FP, Williamson GG, Siepp JM: *Program Guide for Infants and Toddlers with Neuromotor and Other Developmental Disabilities*. New York: Teacher's College Press; 1978:121.)

health care professionals.[69] The American Academy of Pediatrics (AAP) reaffirmed their policy statement on injuries associated with walker use and the recommendation to not use a walker. The AAP anticipatory guidance and warning about walker use does not occur until 8–12 months.[70] Recommendations against purchase and use of baby walker should be made before 4–6 months of age.[71]

The toddler, as a new walker assumes a wide base of support, with the legs abducted and externally rotated, exhibits a lumbar lordosis and holds the arms in *high guard* with scapular adduction. Typical first attempts at walking are lateral weight shifts from one widely abducted leg to the other (Fig. 3.25). The *high guard* position results in an extended upper back that makes up for the lack of hip extension. As an upright trunk is more easily maintained against gravity, the arms are lowered to *mid guard* (hands at waist level, shoulders still externally rotated), to *low guard* (shoulders more neutral, elbows extended), and finally to no guard.

The beginning walker keeps hips and knees slightly flexed to bring the center of mass closer to the ground. Weight shifts are from side to side as the toddler moves forward by total lower extremity flexion, with the hip joints remaining externally rotated during the gait cycle. Ankle movements are minimal, with the foot pronated as the whole foot contacts the ground. Toddlers take many small steps and walk slowly. The instability of their gait is seen in the short amount of time spent in single-limb stance. As trunk stability improves, the legs come farther under the pelvis. As the hips and knees become more extended, the feet develop the plantar flexion needed for the push-off phase of the gait cycle.

New walkers engage in massive walking practice. For example, during 1 hour of free play, the average toddler travels the length of eight football fields, takes 2400 steps, and falls 17 times.[26]

The traditional age range for walking skill has been 12–18 months; however, an infant as young as 7 months may demonstrate this ability. Children demonstrate great variability in achieving this milestone. The most important motor skills to acquire are probably head control and sitting, because if an infant is unable to achieve control of the head and trunk, control of extremity movements will be difficult if not impossible. The WHO (2006) gives an average age of 12.1 months (SD 1.8) for

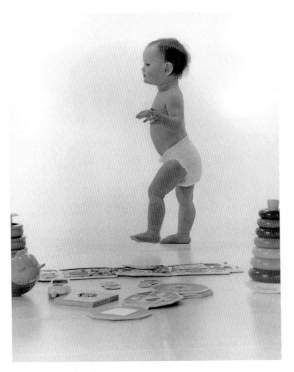

Fig. 3.25 New independent walker. (From Martin S, Kessler M. *Neurologic Interventions for Physical Therapy.* 2nd ed. St. Louis: Saunders; 2007.)

children to accomplish independent movement when standing. There are cultural and ethnic differences in the typical age of walking. African American children have been found to walk earlier (10.9 months),[72] while some Caucasian children walk as late as 15.5 months.[73] It is acceptable for a child to be ahead of typical developmental guidelines; however, delays in achieving walking may be a cause for concern.

Sixteen to eighteen months. By 16–17 months, the toddler is so much at ease with walking that a toy can be carried or pulled at the same time. With help, the toddler goes up and down the stairs, one step at a time. Without help, the toddler creeps up the stairs and may creep or scoot down on her buttocks. Most children will be able to walk sideways and backward at this age if they started walking at 12 months or earlier. The typically developing toddler comes to stand from a supine position by rolling to prone, pushing up on hands and knees or hands and feet, assuming a squat, and rising to standing (Fig. 3.26).

Most toddlers exhibit a reciprocal arm swing and heel strike by 18 months of age, with other adult gait characteristics manifested later. They walk well and demonstrate a "running-like" walk. Although toddlers may still occasionally fall or trip over objects in their path because eye-foot coordination is not completely developed, the decline in falls appears to be the result of improved balance reactions in standing and the ability to monitor trunk and lower extremity movements kinesthetically and visually. The first signs of jumping appear as a stepping off "jump" from a low object such as the bottom step of a set of stairs. Children are ready for this first step-down jump after being able to walk down a step while they hold the hand of an adult.[74] Momentary balance on one foot is also possible. Kicking is initially seen around 20 months of age for both girls and boys. The child may accidentally walk into objects before standing behind the ball and alternating the kicking foot.[75] The kick is not very functional and the child may demonstrate a loss of balance in the attempt.

Two Years

A 2-year-old's gait becomes faster; arms swing reciprocally; steps are longer; and time spent in single-limb stance increases. Many additional motor abilities emerge during this first year of childhood. A 2-year-old child can go up and down the stairs one step at a time, jump off a step with a 2-foot takeoff, kick a large ball, and throw a small one. Stair climbing and kicking are indicative of improved stability while shifting body weight from one leg to another. The child can easily step over low objects encountered in the environment. True running emerges in the second year and is characterized by a "flight" phase when both feet are off the ground at the same time. Quickly starting to run and stopping from a run are still difficult. Directional changes require a large area to make a turn. When the child first attempts to jump off the ground, one foot leaves the ground followed by the other foot, as if the child were stepping in air.

Three Years

Fundamental motor skills (FMS) are basic motor patterns that allow participation in physical activity and sport. They are generally developed from 3 to 6 years of age, although some skills take longer to mature. FMS can be subdivided into three categories: locomotion, object control (OC), and stability skills.[76] Locomotor skills include jumping, hopping, galloping, kicking, and skipping. OC includes throwing, catching, and striking with stability activities including balancing on one foot and walking

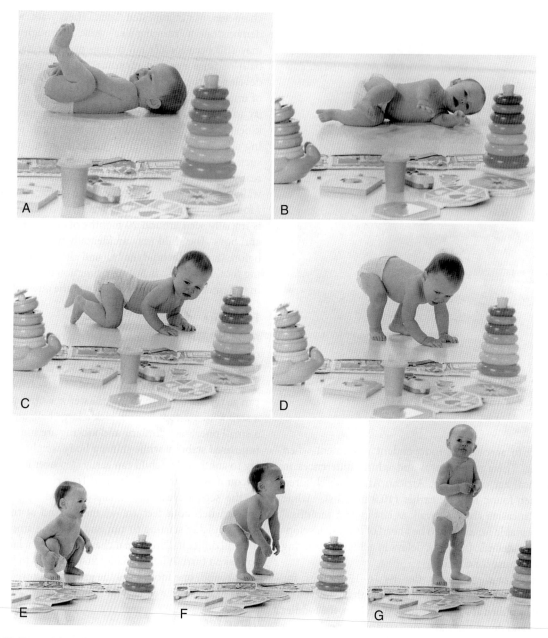

Fig. 3.26 Progression of rising to standing from supine. **(A)** Supine; **(B)** rolling; **(C)** four-point position; **(D)** plantigrade; **(E)** squat; **(F)** semisquat; and **(G)** standing.

on a narrow beam. Acquisition of these skills is described in stages as initial, emerging, and proficient. The number of stages depends on the skill being described. Fig. 3.27 depicts when 60% of children were able to demonstrate a certain developmental level for the listed FMS.

Other reciprocal actions mastered by age 3 are pedaling a tricycle and climbing a jungle gym or ladder. Walking can be started and stopped based on the demands from the environment or from a task such as playing dodgeball on a crowded playground. A

Stages of Fundamental Motor Skills

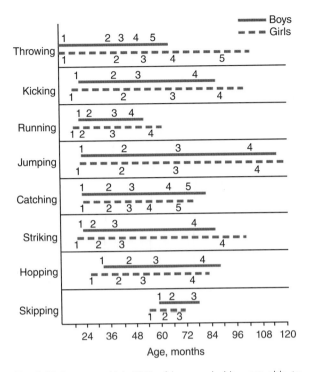

Fig. 3.27 Ages at which 60% of boys and girls were able to perform at specific developmental levels for several fundamental motor skills. Stage 1 is immature; stage 4 or 5 is mature. (Reprinted by permission from Seefledt V, Haubenstricker J. Patterns, phases, or stages: an analytical model for the study of developmental movement. In: Kelso JAS, Clark JE, eds. *The Development of Movement Control and Coordination.* New York, NY: John Wiley & Sons, Ltd; 1982:314.)

3-year-old child can make sharp turns while running and can balance on toes and heels in standing. Standing with one foot in front of the other, known as tandem standing, is possible, as is standing on one foot for at least 3 seconds. A reciprocal gait is now used to ascend stairs with the child placing one foot on each step in alternating fashion but marking time (one step at a time) when descending.

Jumping begins with a step-down jump at 18 months and progresses to jumping off the floor, jumping in place, and jumping from one place to another. Jumping over obstacles can begin with a one-foot take off or two-foot take off, the latter being more mature. Jumps can involve running and then jumping as in a running broad jump or jumping from a static start as in a standing broad jump. Jumping has many forms and is an integral part of game play. Jumping ability increases with age.

Hopping on one foot is a special type of jump requiring balance on one foot and the ability to push off the loaded foot. It does not require maximum effort. "Repeated vertical jumps from two feet can be done before true hopping can occur."[74] Most children have been jumping on two feet for a minimum of 6 months before being able to demonstrate hopping. Initially, the child hops holding the nonsupport foot in front of the support leg. Hopping one or two times on the preferred foot may also be accomplished by 3½ years of age when the child has the ability to stand on one foot and balance long enough to push off on the loaded foot. Gender differences for hopping are documented in the literature, with girls performing better than boys.[77] This may be related to the fact that girls appear to have better balance than do boys in childhood (see Chapter 11).

Four Years

A 4-year-old child should be able to hop on one foot four to six times. Improved hopping ability is seen when the child learns to use the nonstance leg to help propel the body forward. Before that time, all the work is done by pushing off with the support foot. A similar pattern is seen in arm use; at first, the arms are inactive, and later they are used opposite the action of the moving leg. Again, girls performed better than boys.

Rhythmic relaxed galloping is possible for a 4-year-old child. Galloping consists of a walk on the lead leg followed by a running step on the rear leg. Galloping is an asymmetrical gait. A good way to visualize galloping is to think of a child riding a stick horse. Toddlers have been documented to gallop as early as 20 months after learning to walk,[78] but the movement is stiff with arms held in high guard as in beginning walking.

Four-year-olds can catch a small ball using outstretched arms if it is thrown to them, and they can throw a ball overhand for some distance. Throwing begins as an accidental letting go of an object held above the horizon around 18 months of age. Over- and underhand throws can be observed in childhood with persistent gender differences. The distance a child can propel an object has been related to height, as seen in Fig. 3.28. The ability to rotate the body following a throw improves performance.

Five Years

At 5 years of age, a child can stand on either foot for 8–10 seconds, walk forward on a balance beam, hop 8–10 times on one foot, make a 2- to 3-foot standing broad jump, and some can skip on alternating feet. Skipping

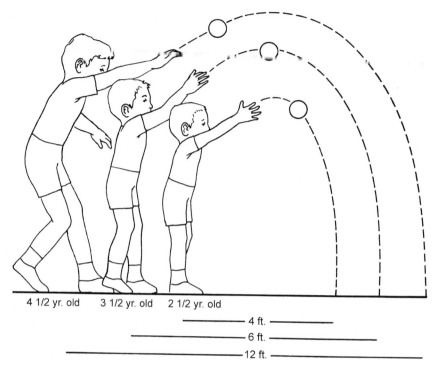

4 1/2 yr. old   3 1/2 yr. old   2 1/2 yr. old

——————— 4 ft. ———————

——————— 6 ft. ———————

——————————— 12 ft. ———————

Fig. 3.28 Throwing distance increases with age.

requires bilateral coordination. At this age, children can change directions and stop quickly while running. They can also ride a bicycle, roller-skate, somersault, and hit a target with a ball from 5 feet away. Regardless of the parameter studied, distance, velocity, or force, gender differences have been demonstrated in throwing.[79,80] Most 5-year-olds can kick a ball by stepping and then kick or run and then kick. At this age, boys' kicking is further advanced than girls in all aspects such as distance kicked and velocity generated. Girls can catch a ball with one hand that is tossed to them, whereas boys lag behind in developing this skill.[81]

Goodway and associates (2010)[82] studied gender differences in FMS in disadvantaged preschoolers residing in two geographic regions. The mean age of participants was 54.8 months. OC and locomotor skill development were studied in disadvantaged African American preschoolers in the Midwest and disadvantaged Hispanic preschoolers in the Southwest. Both groups were delayed in OC and locomotor skills. Boys performed better than girls in both regions. There was an interaction between region and gender for OC skills. Midwestern preschoolers had significantly better locomotor skills than southwestern preschoolers. Delays in childhood acquisition

of FMS may decrease participation in physical activity later in childhood. FMS competence is considered to be a prerequisite for successful engagement in sports as well as having a positive effect on health.[83]

FMS develop during early and middle childhood when the body is changing size, proportions, and composition.[8] Freitas and associates[84] assessed the effect of skeletal maturation measured by skeletal age (SA) and body size on the motor performance of children 3–6 years old. They proved their hypothesis that SA and body size would have a small influence on FMS and motor performance at this age. They recognized that differences in biological maturation exist and interact with environmental variables.

Six to Ten–Twelve Years

A 6-year-old child is well coordinated and can stand on one foot for more than 10 seconds, with eyes open or closed. This ability is important to note because it indicates that vision can be ignored and balance maintained. The 6-year-old can skip rhythmically on alternating feet, a bilateral coordination skill; throw and catch a small ball from 10 feet away; and hit a target 10 feet away. A first grader can walk on a balance beam a few inches off the floor, forward, sideways, and backwards without stepping off. Children also use alternate ways of getting around the neighborhood such as riding a bicycle, skate boarding, or roller skating.

It is not uncommon to see young children demonstrate a mature pattern of movement at one age and a less mature pattern at a later age. Regression of patterns is possible when a child attempts to combine skills. For example, a child who can throw overhand while standing may revert to underhand throwing when running. Alterations between mature and immature movement are an example of individual variation in motor development. In a study of dual task coordination, children were able to couple walking and clapping like adults by 8 years of age but were not successful in coordinating galloping and clapping by age 10.[85] Between 6 and 10 years of age, most children master the adult forms of running, throwing, and catching, but not all.

Patterns of movement learned in game playing help form the basis for later sports skills. Throughout the process of engaging in motor activities and learning FMS, the nervous, muscular, and skeletal systems are maturing, and the body is growing in height and weight. Power develops slowly in children because strength and speed within a specific movement pattern are required. Being proficient in FMS is related to participation in organized sports and active recreation in middle childhood.[86] Nine-year-old girls and boys were found to demonstrate different patterns of motor skill competence. Girls' locomotor skills were positively correlated with intensity of participation in gymnastics while boys' locomotor and OC skills were positively correlated with intensity of participation in team sports.[86] Participation in team sports has been associated with improved motor coordination and cardiovascular fitness.[87] Proficiency in OC in childhood has been found to be predictive of participation in moderate to high levels of physical activity in adolescence.[88] Children with higher levels of motor competence in middle childhood have a greater opportunity to engage in a broader range of activities, sports, and games.

Adolescence

The onset of puberty occurs 2 years earlier in girls than in boys. Static strength increases in females during adolescence, but the gains are not as great as in males. Although strength changes are related to skeletal maturity, such as peak height velocity (PHV) (rate of fastest growth), motor performance is not.[89,90] Although females demonstrate

an increase in motor performance to around 14 years of age,[79,91] performance on tasks is highly variable during the remainder of adolescence. The variability is probably due to a complex interaction of strength, PHV, and the onset of menses. Motivation, interest, and attitudes toward physical activity may also be factors.

The onset of puberty can have a short-term positive effect on motor performance of boys, which is related to an increase in adrenergic hormones. Boys who mature early demonstrate greater strength and endurance than do boys who have not yet matured. The height growth spurt seen in adolescent males is marked by rapid gain in strength. The acceleration peaks around 14 years of age and stops at about 18 years of age. Motor performance peaks during late adolescence, which for males occurs around 17–18 years of age.

Adolescents may continue to gain prowess in motor skills with practice. Parameters of performance such as power, speed, accuracy, form, and endurance can be changed. Lean body mass (LM) and biological maturation as measured by PHV and bone age (BA) have been associated with strength and power in young athletes.[92] Almeida-Neto and colleagues[93] found that PHV, BA, and LM are strong predictors of upper limb strength and upper and lower limb power in both male and female adolescent athletes. The amount of change is highly variable and depends on practice and innate ability. The maximum degree of skill possible on most tasks is related to individuals' satisfaction with their performance within the limits of cognitive, structural (physical), or sociocultural factors.[94] This perception of motor competence can be a positive motivator.

Motor competence has been studied as used as a measure of fitness in children and adolescents.[95,96] Motor competence is defined by some as the level at which children can execute FMS.[97,98] Others define it more generally as "mastery of physical skills and movement patterns that enable enjoyable participation in physical activities."[81] Fitness for health and performance-related fitness change quickly during adolescence.[81] However, females improve less rapidly than males during adolescence in both health and performance-related fitness, plateauing around age 15. See Chapter 13 for more about health and fitness.

Adulthood

Physical performance generally peaks in adulthood.[99] Spirduso[100] examined the effect of age on sport-specific abilities. Generally, peak performance of sports requiring explosive bursts of power or speed over time occurs in the person's early 20s. Older athletes (over 30 years) have triumphed over younger athletes as a result of training and a competitive edge in swimming. For example, Dara Torres won three silver medals at the age of 41; Anthony Ervin won gold at age 35; and Michael Phelps won at age 31. The physical demands of the task, such as power, speed, or endurance, must be taken into consideration. The average age of Olympians competing in Tokyo in 2021 was 27 years, up from 23 in the 1980s.[101] Motor performance in adulthood is variable, and with increasing age, the variability increases even more.

Older Adulthood

Spirduso and associates[102] described a continuum of physical function among older adults (see Fig. 3.29). The highest level of physical performance is represented by the physically elite. They represent the growing number of master athletes who are defined as "exercise-trained individuals who compete in athletic events at a high level well beyond a typical athletic retirement age."[103] They may also be working in high risk or physically demanding jobs past usual retirement age. The next group are the physically fit who participate in moderate physical work and enjoy active hobbies and endurance sports but do not compete. The physically independent group of older adults do not engage in exercise for health benefits but perform light physical work, some hobbies, and engage in low physically demanding activities such as golf, vacation travel, and driving. Independence in basic activities

of living (BADLs) and instrumental activities of daily living (IADLs) is characteristic of this group.[104] Physically frail elderly are described as able to do light housekeeping activities, some IADLs and all BADLs. Many of these individuals are homebound. As older adults become less able to perform BADL, they move toward greater levels of physical dependency and disability.

Sports participation does decline in older age. The reason why some older adults play sports was a question asked by researchers in a recent systematic review.[105] Older adults gave many reasons for participating such as maintaining health, developing social relationships, and feeling and being part of a community. Competition appears to motivate older adults to engage and challenge their own limitations and set goals to achieve. The researchers concluded that sports participation in older adults contributes to successful aging. The top five sports for older people based on participation rates are golf, tennis, lawn bowling, track and field, and swimming.[106] In the United States, pickleball, a combination of badminton, tennis, and table tennis, is one of the fastest growing sports in the older adult community. In a survey, respondents stated their primary motivation to participate in this new sport was to master the difficult training techniques and to be competitive.[107]

Master athletes have been touted to be exemplars for successful aging. Master athletes are those who train regularly and compete. Those who train for endurance are exceedingly fit and very physically active.[108] As a group, master athletes compete in team-based sports as well as swimming, cycling, and long- and short-distance

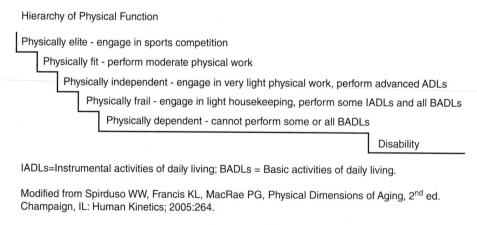

Hierarchy of Physical Function

Physically elite - engage in sports competition

Physically fit - perform moderate physical work

Physically independent - engage in very light physical work, perform advanced ADLs

Physically frail - engage in light housekeeping, perform some IADLs and all BADLs

Physically dependent - cannot perform some or all BADLs

Disability

IADLs=Instrumental activities of daily living; BADLs = Basic activities of daily living.

Modified from Spirduso WW, Francis KL, MacRae PG, Physical Dimensions of Aging, 2nd ed. Champaign, IL: Human Kinetics; 2005:264.

Fig. 3.29 Continuum of physical function of older adults. (Adapted from Spirduso W, Francis K, MacRae PG. *Physical Dimensions of Aging.* Champaign, IL: Human Kinetics; 2005, Fig. 11.1.)

running. The number of aging master athletes has increased and participation in master's competition has grown to 4000 individuals from 80 countries in 2016.[103] Geard and associates reviewed the evidence regarding master athletes and successful aging.[109] While there is a wealth of evidence to support the physical functioning of master athletes, their psychological and sociological functioning has not been sufficiently explored to conclude that master athletes are truly an example of successful aging. Geard et al.[109] concluded that the lack of consensus of the definition of successful aging makes it difficult to generalize findings in this group.

Age-Related Changes in Movement Patterns Beyond Childhood

Functional movement competence begins in childhood and continues throughout the life span. Research shows a developmental order of movement patterns across childhood and adolescence with trends toward increasing symmetry with increasing age.[110] Mature movement patterns have always been associated with efficiency and symmetry. Early in motor development, patterns of movement appear to be more homogeneous and follow a fairly prescribed developmental sequence. As a person matures, movement patterns become more symmetrical. With aging, movement becomes more asymmetrical and less homogeneous.

According to the ICF mobility activities are those that involve changing position or location.[111] Such activities are crucial for independent living and include transitions such as rising from a bed, moving from STS, and rising from supine to standing. Walking on level ground and stairs will be explored in Chapter 11.

Rising from a bed. Bed mobility is essential for all individuals. Ford-Smith and VanSant[112] studied adults from 30 to 50 years of age performing trials of rising from a bed. The younger group of adults, 30 to 39 years of age, tended to grasp and push with their arms, roll to sit, and asynchronously lift legs so that one touched the floor before the other. In the older group, 50 to 59 years of age, synchronous coming to sit and synchronous leg lifting were preferred (see Fig. 3.30). The authors commented that in the older group, the pattern appeared to be almost two separate tasks: coming to sit and coming to stand from sitting.

Sitting to standing. Moving from STS is a critical part of daily activities of life. STS is a very demanding

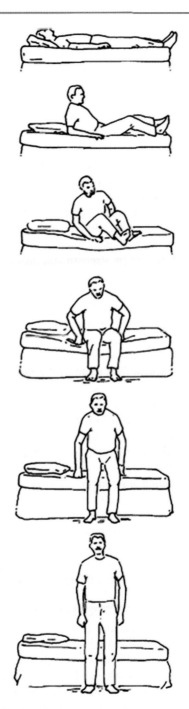

Fig. 3.30 Rising from bed. (Adapted from Ford-Smith CD, VanSant AF. Age differences in movement patterns used to rise from a bed in the third through fifth decades of age. *Phys Ther.* 1993;73:300-307.)

task which requires leg muscle strength and power, coordination, and balance. Sloot and associates[113] studied the effect of age on STS balance and found that older adults were more conservative, meaning they stayed more statically balanced than younger individuals during STS. Older adults kept their center of mass (COM) within their base of support (BoS) from the seat lift-off to stand while younger adults began seat off with their COM outside their BoS. The researchers concluded that the older adults were compensating for decreased physical ability or confidence in their balance. Dynamic balance as they measured it was not affected.

Tests of STS measure functional abilities and are often used to assess fall risk. Older adults are slower to come to stand than young adults. Timed up-and-go and five-time sit-to-stand test depend on strength and muscle power of the individual. Alcazar and colleagues[114] found that the sit-to-stand muscle power test could reliably assess muscle power in older adults. Velocity and power were determined mathematically based on body mass and height, chair height, and time needed to complete five STS repetitions. The authors concluded that the test is more clinically relevant than traditional time values for STS. Individuals who are obese use different strategies to come to stand. Bollinger and associates[115] found that excess body weight accounted for the kinematic changes in strategy, not knee extensor torque. Older adults who have difficulty visually orienting to an upright posture may also incur difficulties with sit-to-stand.[116]

Rising from supine to standing. Descriptive research of the progression used by adults to move from supine to standing changes with age. Individuals in their 20s use symmetrical patterns. With increasing age, increasing asymmetry is seen.[117] By age 70–80 years, older adults demonstrated more upper extremity and trunk movements than at younger ages and required more time to complete the action.[118] The researchers found that a shorter time to rise was related to lower age, greater knee extension strength, and greater hip and ankle range of motion (flexion and dorsiflexion, respectively). However, older adults who maintain their strength and flexibility rise to standing faster and more symmetrically than do those who are less strong and flexible.[118]

Getting up from the floor has been identified as a risk factor for falls for over two decades.[119,120] Individuals who are unable to rise from the floor safely may be at greater risk for serious injury. Rising from the floor can be utilized to determine safe and appropriate living arrangements.[121,122] Being able to rise from the floor has also been shown to be a predictor of mortality.[123] Cattuzzo and associates'[124] thorough systematic review of supine-to-stand studies includes children, adults, and older adults. Children's supine-to-stand abilities correlated with motor competence,[125] as did young adults.[126] Klima et al.[127] studied community-dwelling adults over the age of 60 years and described that 90% rolled with an asymmetrical squat sequence to rise from the floor. Time to rise was significantly greater in older healthy subjects over 60 years than in younger adults 20–50 years of age. Schwickert and colleagues[128] identified seven different movement components used by adults and older adults in a lie-to-stand-to-walk transfer. Older adults used more complex strategies to achieve upright. Based on the review of studies by Cattuzzo and colleagues,[124] supine to stand is a task applicable to all ages. Furthermore, it may provide a useful way to assess functional motor competence across the life span, as well as be a general marker for health status.

SUMMARY

Motor development includes the change in motor behavior over the life span and the sequential, continuous, age-related process of change. It is determined by the merging of our genetic predisposition for movement and our experiences. Movement emerges from the dynamic interaction of multiple components and systems to meet intrinsic or extrinsic demands. GMs seen in the newborn form the cornerstone of early development and represent the status of the developing brain.

The two major theories of motor development are the DST and neuronal group selection. They are both predicated on the interaction of multiple layered systems. NGST recognizes that genetics plays a larger role in determining the motor outcomes of development than DST. NGST recognizes that the environment both internal and external can have a far-reaching effect on gene expression in every body system. Both theories recognize that movement development is an integral part of cognitive development.

Motor behavior is embedded in the environment. Environmental experiences further shape developmental change. Perception and cognition are required to plan and guide movements adaptively in order to achieve the goals of everyday life. Movement cannot be separated from the environmental, social, and cultural contexts in which it occurs. Nor can it be separated from the physical body in which the movement is produced. The body structure changes over time and so does the functionality of that body.

Functional tasks are defined by the age and social and psychological expectation of the individual or society. An infant's function is to overcome gravity and learn to move into the upright position. The toddler explores the world in an upright position, and the child acquires fundamental movement patterns of running, jumping, hopping, and skipping. Exploring the environment provides sensory information that informs and predisposes the child to acquire cognitive and linguistic skills. Self-care skills are mastered by the time a child enters school.

The level of motor competence can affect participation in physical activity and sports. Sports skills build on FMS learned and perfected in childhood and adolescence. Work and leisure skills become more salient in late adolescence and adulthood. Golf, pickle ball, swimming, and tennis are activities that are enjoyed in retirement. Older adults continue to participate in physical activities/exercise for pleasure or maintenance of mobility while others such as master athletes continue to participate in competitions. Every period of the life span has different functional expectations that are driven by the mover; the task; and the social, physical, and psychological environments. Knowledge of motor development across the life span is critical for therapists to ascertain the most appropriate therapeutic strategies for people to function optimally regardless of age, occupation, or disability.

REFERENCES

1. Grace T, Bulsara M, Robinson M, Hands B. Early life events and motor development in childhood and adolescence: a longitudinal study. *Acta Pediatr.* 2016;105(5):E219–E227.
2. Adolph KE, Franchak JM. The development of motor behavior. *Wiley Interdiscip Rev Cogn Sci.* 2017;8(1–2). https://doi.org/10.1002/wcs.1430.
3. Lampl M, Thompson AL. Growth chart curves do not describe individual growth biology. *Am. J Hum Biol.* 2007;19:643–653.
4. Adolph KE, Avolio AM. Walking infants adapt locomotion to changing body dimensions. *J Exp Psychol.* 2000;26(3):1148–1166.
5. Adolph KE, Hoch JE. Motor development: embodied, embedded, enculturated, and enabling. *Annu Rev Psychol.* 2019;70:141–164.
6. Thelen E, Fishern DM. Newborn stepping: an explanation for a disappearing reflex. *Dev Psychol.* 1982;18:760–775.
7. Rochat P, Goubet N, Senders SJ. To reach or not to reach? Perception of body effectivities by young infants. *Infant Child Dev.* 1999;8:129–148.
8. Malina RM, Bouchard C, Bar-Or O. *Growth, Maturation and Physical Activity.* 2nd ed. Champaign, IL: Human Kinetics; 2004.
9. Smith L, van Jaarsveld CHM, Llewellyn CH, et al. Genetic and environmental influences on developmental milestones and movement: results from the Gemini Cohort Study. *Res Q Exerc Sport.* 2017;88:401–407.
10. Ridgway CL, Ong KK, Tammelin TH, et al. Infant motor development predicts sports participation at age 14 years: northern Finland birth cohort of 1966. *PLoS One.* 2009;4(8):e6837. https://doi.org/10.1371/journal.pone.0006837.
11. Liao PJ, Zawacki L, Campbell SK. Annotated bibliography: effects of sleep position and play position on motor development in early infancy. *Phys Occup Ther Pediatr.* 2005;25:149–160.
12. Pin T, Eldridge B, Galea MP. A review of the effects of sleep position, play position, and equipment use on motor development. *Dev Med Child Neurol.* 2007;49: 858–867.
13. Thelen E, Smith LB. *A Dynamic Systems Approach to the Development of Cognition and Action.* Cambridge, MA: The MIT Press; 1994.
14. Thelen E, Smith LB. Dynamic systems. In: Damon W, Lerner RM, eds. *Handbook of Child Psychology.* 6th ed. New York: John Wiley & Sons; 2006:258–312.
15. Perone S, Simmering VR. Applications of dynamic systems theory to cognition and development: new frontiers. *Adv Child Dev Behav.* 2017;52:43–80.
16. Iverson JM. Developing language in a developing body: the relationship between motor development and language development. *J Child Lang.* 2010;37(2): 229–261.
17. Oudgenoeg-Paz O, Volman JM, Leseman PM. First steps into language? Examining the specific longitudinal relations between walking, exploration and linguistic skills. *Front Psychol.* 2016;27(7):1458.
18. Perone S, Spencer JP. Autonomous visual exploration creates developmental change in familiarity and novelty seeking behaviors. *Front Psychol.* 2013;4:648.
19. Karimi-Aghdam S. Zone of proximal development (ZPD) as an emergent system: a dynamic systems theory perspective. *Integr Psychol Behav Sci.* 2017;51:76–93.

20. Dusing SC. Postural variability and sensorimotor development in infancy. *Dev Med Child Neurol.* 2016; 58(Suppl 4):17–21.

21. Edelman GM. *Neural Darwinism: The Theory of Neuronal Group Selection.* Oxford, UK: Oxford University Press; 1989.

22. Hadders-Algra M. Early human motor development: from variation to the ability to vary and adapt. *Neurosci Biobehav Rev.* 2018;90:411–427.

23. Leighton AH, Lohmann C. The wiring of developing sensory circuits—from patterned spontaneous activity to synaptic plasticity mechanism. *Front Neural Circuits.* 2016;10:71.

24. Greenough WT, Black JE, Wallace CS. Experience and brain development. *Child Dev.* 1987;58:539–559.

25. Hadders-Algra M. Variation and variability: key words in human motor development. *Phys Ther.* 2010;90:1823–1837.

26. Adolph KE, Cole WG, Komati M, et al. How do you learn to walk? Thousands of steps and dozens of falls per day. *Psychol Sci.* 2012;23:1387–1394.

27. Hadders-Algra M. Typical and atypical development of reaching and postural control in infancy. *Dev Med Child Neurol.* 2013;55(Suppl 4):5–8.

28. Edelman GM. *Neural Darwinism.* New York: Basic Books; 1987.

29. Lv J, Xin Y, Zhou W, et al. The epigenetic switches for neural development and psychiatric disorders. *J Genet Genomics.* 2013;40:339–346.

30. Gilmore JH, Santelli RK, Gao W. Imaging structural and functional brain development in early childhood. *Nat Rev Neurosci.* 2018;19(3):123–137.

31. Barsalou LW. Grounded cognition: past, present, and future. *Top Cogn Sci.* 2010;2:716–724.

32. Lobo MA, Harbourne RT, Dusing SC, et al. Grounding early intervention: physical therapy cannot be about motor skills anymore. *Phys Ther.* 2013;93:94–103.

33. Diamond A. Close interrelation of motor development and cognitive development and of the cerebellum and prefrontal cortex. *Child Dev.* 2000;71:44–56.

34. Piek JP, Dawson L, Smith LM, et al. The role of early fine and gross motor development on later motor and cognitive ability. *Hum Mov Sci.* 2008;27(5):668–681.

35. Ghassabian A, Sundaram R, Bell E, et al. Gross motor milestones and subsequent development. *Pediatrics.* 2016;138:e2015–e4372.

36. Veldman SLC, Santo R, Jones RA, et al. Associations between gross motor skills and cognitive development in toddlers. *Early Hum Dev.* 2019;132:39–44.

37. Pitcher JB, Schneider LA, Drysdale JL, et al. Motor system development of the preterm and low birthweight infant. *Clin Perinatol.* 2011;38:605–625.

38. LeBarton ES, Iverson JM. Associations between gross motor and communicative development in at-risk infants. *Infant Behav Dev.* 2016;44:59–67.

39. Leisman G, Moustafa AA, Shafir T. Thinking, walking, talking: integratory motor and cognitive brain function. *Front Public Health.* 2016;4:94.

40. Marrus N, Eggebrecht AT, Todorov A, et al. Walking, gross motor development, and brain functional connectivity in infants and toddlers. *Cereb Cortex.* 2018;28:750–763.

41. Peterson MC, Kube DA, Palmer FB. Classification of developmental delays. *Semin Pediatr Neurol.* 1998;5:2–14.

42. Novak I, Mogran C, Adde L, et al. Early, accurate diagnosis and early intervention in cerebral palsy: advances in diagnosis and treatment. *JAMA Pediatr.* 2017;171990:897–907.

43. Gesell A, Ames LB, et al. *Infant and Child in the Culture of Today, Rev.* New York: Harper & Row; 1974.

44. Bernstein N. *The Coordination and Regulation of Movements.* Oxford, UK: Pergamon; 1967.

45. Hadders-Algra M. Neural substrate and clinical significance of general movements: an update. *Dev Med Child Neurol.* 2018;60:39–46.

46. Thelen E, Fisher DM, Ridley-Johnson R. The relationship between physical growth and a newborn reflex. *Infant Behav Dev.* 1984;7:479–493.

47. Barlow SM. Oral and respiratory control for preterm feeding. *Curr Opin Otolaryngol Head Neck Surg.* 2009;17:179–186.

48. Kelly BN, Huckabee ML, Jones RD, et al. The first year of human life: coordinating respiration and nutritive swallowing. *Dysphagia.* 2007;22:37–43.

49. Vice FL, Gewolb IH. Respiratory patterns and strategies during feeding preterm infants. *Dev Med Child Neurol.* 2008;50:467–472.

50. American Academy of Pediatrics Committee on Injury and Poison Prevention. Injuries associated with infant walkers. *Pediatrics.* 2012;129:e561.

51. Gisel EG. Effect of food texture on the development of chewing of children between 6 months and two years of age. *Dev Med Child Neurol.* 1991;33:69–79.

52. Wilson EM, Green JR, Weismer G. A kinematic description of the temporal characteristics of jaw motion for early chewing: preliminary findings. *J Speech Lang Hear Res.* 2012;55(2):626–638.

53. Simione M, Loret C, Le Reverend B, et al. Differing structural properties of foods affect the development of mandibular control and muscle coordination in infants and young children. *Physiol Behav.* 2018;186:62–72.

54. Addabbo M, Longhi E, Marchis IC, et al. Dynamic facial expressions of emotions are discriminated at birth. *PLoS One.* 2018;13(3):e093868.

55. Meltzoff AN, Murray L, Simpson E, et al. Re-examination of Oostenbroek et al. (2016): evidence for neonatal tongue protrusion. *Dev Sci.* 2018;21(4):e12609.

56. Green JR, Moore CA, Higashikawa M, et al. The physiologic development of speech motor control: lip and jaw coordination. *J Speech Lang Hear Res.* 2000;43:239–255.

57. Kuhl PK. Early language learning and literacy: neuroscience implications for education. *Mind Brain Educ.* 2011;5(3):128–142.

58. Hadders-Algra M. Putative neural substrate of normal and abnormal general movements. *Neurosci Biobehav Rev.* 2007:1181–1190.

59. Einspieler C, Prechtl HFR, Bos AF, et al. *Prechtl's Method on the Qualitative Assessment of General Movements in Preterm, Term and Young Infants.* London: Mac Keith Press; 2008.

60. Majnemer A, Barr RG. Influence of supine sleep positioning on early motor milestone acquisition. *Dev Med Child Neurol.* 2005;47:370–376.

61. Dudek-Shriber L, Zelazy S. The effects of prone positioning on the quality and acquisition of developmental milestones in four-month-old infants. *Pediatr Phys Ther.* 2007;19:48–55.

62. Conner FP, Williamson GG, Siepp JM. *Program Guide for Infants and Toddlers with Neuromotor and Other Developmental Disabilities.* New York: Teacher's College Press; 1978.

63. Thelen E. Rhythmical stereotypies in infants. *Anim Behav.* 1979;27(3):699–715.

64. WHO Multicentre Growth Reference Study Group WHO Motor Development Study: windows of achievement of six gross motor milestones. *Acta Paediatr Suppl.* 2006;450:86–95.

65. Bornstein MH, Hahn CS, Bell C, et al. Stability in cognition across early childhood: a developmental cascade. *Psychol Sci.* 2006;17:151–158.

66. Duff SV. Prehension. In: Cech D, Martin S, eds. *Functional Movement Development Across the Life Span.* 2nd ed. Philadelphia: WB Saunders; 2002.

67. Adolph KE, Vereijken B, Denny MA. Learning to crawl. *Child Dev.* 1998;69:1299–1312.

68. Adolph KE, Berger SE, Leo AJ. Developmental continuity? Crawling, cruising, and walking. *Dev Sci.* 2011;14:306–318.

69. Sims A, Chounthirath T, Yang J, Hodges NL, Smith GA. Infant walker-related injuries in the United States. *Pediatrics.* 2018;142(4):e20174332.

70. American Academy of Pediatrics. Movement: 8–12 months. https://www.healthychildren.org/English/ages-stages/baby/ Pages/Movement-8-to-12-Months.aspx. Accessed November 29, 2021.

71. Schecter R, Das P, Milanaik R. Are baby walker warnings coming too late? Recommendations and rationale for anticipatory guidance at earlier well-child visits. *Glob Pediatr Health.* 2019;6 https://doi.org/10.1177/2333794X19876849. 2333794X19876849.

72. Capute AJ, Shapiro BK, Palmer FB, et al. Normal gross motor development the influences of race, sex, socio-economic status. *Dev Med Child Neurol.* 1985;27:635–643.

73. Bayley N. *Bayley Scales of Infant Development.* 3rd ed. San Antonio, TX: Pearson; 2005.

74. Wickstrom RL. *Fundamental Movement Patterns.* 3rd ed. Philadelphia: Lea & Febiger; 1983.

75. Gabbard C. *Lifelong Motor Development.* 4th ed. San Francisco: Benjamin/Cummings; 2004.

76. Lubans DR, Morgan PJ, Cliff DP, et al. Fundamental movement skills in children and adolescents: review of associated health benefits. *Sports Med.* 2010;40(12):1019–1035. https://doi.org/10.2165/11536850-000000000-00000.

77. Hakebeeke TH, Caflisch J, Chaouch A, et al. Neuromotor development in children, Part 3: motor performance in 3- to 5-year-olds. *Dev Med Child Neurol.* 2013;55(3):248–256. https://doi.org/10.1111/dmcn.12034

78. Whithall J. A developmental study of the inter-limb coordination in running and galloping. *J Mot Behav.* 1989;21:409–428.

79. Butterfield SA, Angell RM, Mason CA. Age and sex differences in object control skills by children ages 5 to 14. *Percept Mot Skills.* 2012;114:261–274. https://doi.org/10.2466/10.11.25.PMS.114.1.261-274.

80. Angell RM, Butterfield, Tu S, et al. Children's throwing and striking: a longitudinal study. *J Mot Learn Dev.* 2018;6(2):315–332.

81. Goodway JD, Ozmun JC, Gallahue DL. *Understanding Motor Development: Infants, Children, Adolescents, Adults.* Burlington, MA: Jones & Barlett Learning; 2021.

82. Goodway JD, Robinson LE, Crowe H. Gender differences in fundamental motor skill development in disadvantaged preschoolers from two geographical regions. *Res Q Exerc Sport.* 2010;81:17–24. https://doi.org/10.1111/apa.13380.

83. Robins LE, Stodden DF, Barnett LML, et al. Motor competence and its effect on positive developmental trajectories of health. *Sports Med.* 2015;45:1273–1284. https://doi.org/10.1007/s40279-015-0351-6.

84. Freitas DL, Lausen B, Maia JA, et al. Skeletal maturation, fundamental motor skills and motor performance in preschool children. *Scan J Med Sci Sports.* 2018;28:2358–2368. https://doi.org/10.1111/sms.13233.

85. Getschell N, Whitall J. How do children coordinate simultaneous upper and lower extremity tasks? The development of dual task coordination. *J Exp Child Psychol.* 2003;85:120–140.

86. Field SC, Temple VA. The relationship between fundamental motor skill proficiency and participation in organized sports and active recreation in middle childhood. *Sports (Basel)*. 2017;5:43. https://doi.org/10.3390/sports5020043.

87. Vandendriessche JB, Vandorpe BFR, Vaeyens R. Variation in sport participation, fitness and motor coordination with socioeconomic status among Flemish children. *Pediatr Exerc Sci*. 2012;24:113–148.

88. Barnett LM, van Beurden E, Morgan PJ, Brooks LO, Beard JR. Childhood motor skill proficiency as a predictor of adolescent physical activity. *J Adol Health*. 2009;44:252–259.

89. Freitas DL, Lausen B, Maia JA, et al. Skeletal maturation, fundamental motor skills and motor coordination in children 7-10 years. *J Sports Sci*. 2015;33:924–934. https://doi.org/10.1080/02640414.2014.977935.

90. Freitas DL, Lausen B, Maia JA, et al. Skeletal maturation, body size, and motor coordination in youth 11-14 years. *Med Sci Sports Exerc*. 2016;48:1129–1135. https://doi.org/10.1249/MSS.0000000000000873.

91. Almeida-Neto PF, Bulhões-Correia A, Matos DE. DG, et al. Relationship of biological maturation with muscle power in young female athletes. *Int J Exerc Sci*. 2021;14:696–706.

92. Almeida-Neto PF, de Matos DG, Pinto VCM, et al. Can the neuromuscular performance of young athletes be influenced by hormone levels and different stages of puberty? *Int J Environ Res Public Health*. 2020;17:5637. https://doi.org/10.3390/ijerph17165637.

93. Almeida-Neto PF, de Medeiros RCDSC de Matos DG, et al. Lean mass and biological maturation as predictors of muscle power and strength performance in young athletes. *PLoS One*. 2021;16:e0254552. https://doi.org/10.1371/journal.pone.0254552.

94. Higgins S. Motor skill acquisition. *Phys Ther*. 1991;71:123–139.

95. Luz C, Rodrigues LP, Meester AD, Cordivil R. The relationship between motor competence and health-related fitness in children and adolescents. *PLoS ONE*. 2017;12(6):e0179993. https://doi.org/10.1371/journal.pone.017993.

96. Schmutz EA, Leeger-Aschmann CS, Kakebeeke TH, et al. Motor competence and physical activity in early childhood: stability and relationship. *Front Pub Health*. 2020;8:39. https://doi.org/10.3389/fpubh.2020.00039.

97. True L, Pfeiffer KA, Dowda M, et al. Motor competence and characteristics within the preschool environment. *J Sci Med Sport*. 2017;20:751–755. https://doi.org/10.1016/jsama.2016.11.019.

98. Haywood K, Getchell N. *Life Span Motor Development*. 5th ed. Champaign, IL: Human Kinetics Publishers; 2009.

99. Westerterp KR. Changes in physical activity over the lifespan: impact on body composition and sarcopenic obesity. *Obes Rev*. 2018;19(Suppl 1):8–13. https://doi.org/10.1111/obr.12781.

100. Spirduso WW. *Physical Dimensions of Aging*. Champaign, IL: Human Kinetics; 1995.

101. Berkowitz B., Galocha A. Olympians are probably older—and younger—than you think. https://www.washingtonpost.com/sports/olympics/2021/07/31/oldest-youngest-olympians/ Accessed December 10, 2021.

102. Spirduso WW, Francis KL, MacRae PG. *Physical Dimensions of Aging*. 2nd ed. Champaign, IL: Human Kinetics; 2005.

103. Tanaka H. Aging of competitive athletes. *Gerontology*. 2017;63:488–494.

104. Shumway-Cook A, Woollacott M. *Motor Control: Translating Research into Clinical Practice*. 5th ed. Philadelphia, PA: Wolters Kluwer; 2017.

105. Stenner BJ, Buckley JD, Mosewich AD. Reasons why older adults play sport: a systematic review. *J Sport Health Sci*. 2020;9:530–541.

106. Australian Sports Commission. *AusPlay-Participation data for the sports sector*. Canberra, AUS: Australian Sport Commission; 2016.

107. Buzzelli AA, Draper JA. Examining the motivation and perceived benefits of pickleball participation in older adults. *J Aging Phys Act*. 2020;28:180–186. https://doi.org/10.1123/japa.2018-0413.

108. Tanaka H, Seals DR. Endurance exercise performance in masters athletes: age-associated changes and underlying physiological mechanisms. *J Physiol*. 2008;586:55–63. https://doi.org/10.1113/jphysiol.2007.141879.

109. Geard D, Reaburn PRJ, Rebar AL, Dionigi RA. Masters athletes: exemplars of successful aging? *J Aging Phys Act*. 2017;25:490–500. https://doi.org/10.1123/japa.2016-0050.

110. VanSant AF. Age differences in movement patterns used by children to rise from a supine position to erect stance. *Phys Ther*. 1988;68:1130–1138.

111. International Classification of Functioning, Disability, and Health. *ICF Short Version*. World Health Organization; 2001.

112. Ford-Smith CD, VanSant AF. Age differences in movement patterns used to rise from a bed in the third through fifth decades of age. *Phys Ther*. 1993;73:300–307.

113. Sloot LH, Millard M, Werner C, Mombaur K. Slow but steady: similar sit-to-stand balance at seat-off in older vs younger adults. *Front Sports Act Living*. 2020;l2:548174. https://doi.org/10.3389/fspor.2020.548174.

114. Alcazar J, Losa-Reyna J, Rodriguez-Lopez C, et al. The sit-to-stand muscle power test: an easy, inexpensive

and portable procedure to assess muscle power in older people. *Exp Gerontol.* 2018;112.38–43. https://doi.org/10.1016/j.exger.2018.08.006.

115. Bollinger LM, Walaszek M, Seay RF, Ransom A. Knee extensor torque and BMI differently relate to sit-to-stand strategies in obesity. *Clin Biomech (Bristol, Avon).* 2019;62:28–33. https://doi.org/10.1016/j.clinbiomech.2019.01.002.

116. Almajid R, Tucker C, Wright WG, Vasudevan E, Keshner E. Visual dependence affects the motor behavior of older adults during the Timed Up and Go (TUG) test. *Arch Gerontol Geriatr.* 2020;87:104004. https://doi.org/10.1016/j.archger.2019.104004. Epub 2019 Dec 19.

117. VanSant AF. Rising from a supine position to erect stance: description of adult movement and a developmental hypothesis. *Phys Ther.* 1988;68:185–192.

118. Thomas RL, Williams AK, Lundy-Ekman L. Supine to stand in elderly persons: relationship to age, activity level, strength, and range of motion. *Issues Aging.* 1998;21:9–18.

119. Bergland A, Laake K. Concurrent and predictive validity of "getting up from lying on the floor." *Aging Clin Exp Res.* 2005;17:181–185. https://doi.org/10.1007/BF03324594.

120. Bergland A, Wyller TB. Risk factors for serious fall related injury in elderly women living at home. *Inj Prev.* 2004;10:308–313. https://doi.org/10.1136/ip.2003.004721.

121. Ardali G, Brody LT, States RA, Godwin EM. Reliability and validity of the Floor Transfer Test as a measure of readiness for independent living among older adults. *J Geriatr Phys Ther.* 2019;42:136–147. https://doi.org/10.1519/JPT.0000000000000142.

122. Ardali G, States RA, Brody LT, et al. Characteristics of older adults who are unable to perform a floor transfer: considerations for clinical decision-making. *J Geriatr Phys Ther.* 2020;43:62–70.

123. Brito LB, Ricardo DR, Araújo DS, et al. Ability to sit and rise from the floor as a predictor of all-cause mortality. *Eur J Prev Cardiol.* 2014;21:892–898.

124. Cattuzzo MT, de Santana FS, Safons MP, et al. Assessment in the supine-to-stand task and functional health from youth to old age: a systematic review. *Int J Environ Res Public Health.* 2020;17:5794.

125. Duncan MJ, Lawson C, Walker LJ, et al. The utility of the supine-to-stand test as a measure of functional motor competence in children aged 5-9 years. *Sports (Basel).* 2017;5:67.

126. Nesbitt D, Molina SL, Sacko R, et al. Examining the feasibility of supine-to-stand as a measure of functional motor competence. *J Mot Learn Dev.* 2018;6:267–286.

127. Klima DW, Anderson C, Smarah D, et al. Standing from the floor in community-dwelling older adults. *J aging Phys Act.* 2016;24:207–213.

128. Schwickert L, Oberle C, Becker C, et al. Model development to study strategies of younger and older adults getting up from the floor. *Aging Clin Exp Res.* 2016;28:277–287.

4

Motor Control and Motor Learning

OBJECTIVES

After studying this chapter, the reader will be able to:
1. Define motor control, motor learning, and neural plasticity.
2. Understand the relationship among motor control, motor learning, and motor development.
3. Discuss theories of motor control and motor learning.
4. Discuss the role of experience and feedback.
5. Understand the age-related changes in motor control and motor learning.

INTRODUCTION

Motor skills and abilities are acquired during the process of motor development through motor control and motor learning. After an initial pattern of movement is established, it can be varied to suit the purpose of the task or the environment in which the task occurs. Early motor development as described in Chapter 3 displays a fairly predictable sequence of skill acquisition through childhood. However, the manner in which these skills are used functionally exhibits considerable variability. Individuals rarely perform even the same movement in exactly the same way every time. Variability must be part of any model used to explain how posture and movement is controlled.

Any movement system must be able to adapt to the changing demands of the individual mover and the environment in which the movement takes place. The mover must be able to learn from prior movement experiences and recognize when a movement strategy is successful or unsuccessful. Theories of motor control emphasize various developmental aspects of posture and movement. Development of postural control and balance is embedded in the development of motor control. The individual cannot learn to control posture and develop balance without moving. Therefore an understanding of

the relationship among motor control, motor learning, and motor development is fundamental to assessing human movement systems. Motor development, motor control, and motor learning contribute to the ongoing process of change throughout the life span of every person who moves.

MOTOR CONTROL

Motor control is the ability to maintain and change posture and movement. It is the result of a complex set of neurologic and mechanical processes. Motor control begins with the control of self-generated movements and proceeds to the control of movements relative to changing task and environmental demands. The relationship of the mover, task, and the environment is depicted in Fig. 4.1. As body systems mature, movement emerges. The perceptual consequences of self-generated movements drive motor development.[1] Learning to move requires active participation of the mover and is spurred by natural curiosity about the environment. Motor control allows the nervous system to direct what muscles should be used, in what order, and how quickly, to solve a movement problem.

Motor abilities of a person change over time and the motor solutions to any given motor problem may also change. For example, gravity is a problem for the infant developing head control, whereas a set of stairs may be an obstacle for a toddler. A person's motivation to move may also change over time and may affect the intricacy of the movement solution. A young child encountering a set of stairs sees a toy at the top stair. Depending on age, ability, and motivation, many solutions are possible. How many solutions can you develop? Consider all three components of motor control—the task, the environment, and the mover.

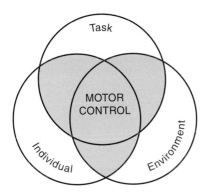

Fig. 4.1 Movement emerges from an interaction between the individual, the task, and the environment. (From Shumway-Cook A, Woollacott MH. *Motor Control: Theory and Practical Application.* 4th ed. Baltimore: Williams and Wilkins; 2012.)

Motor Control Time Frame

Motor control happens not in the space of days or weeks, as is seen in motor development, but in fractions of seconds. Fig. 4.2 illustrates a comparison of time frames associated with motor control, motor learning, and motor development. Motor control occurs because of physiologic processes that happen at cellular, tissue, and organ system levels. Physiologic processes have to happen quickly to produce timely and efficient movement. It is not helpful if you cannot respond quickly enough to prevent a loss of balance. Individuals with movement dysfunction may exhibit appropriate patterns of movement but lack timing or they may have impaired sequencing of muscle activation, producing a muscle contraction at the wrong time. These are examples of deficits in motor control.

Role of Sensation in Motor Control

Sensory information plays an important role in motor control. Initially, sensation cues reflexive movements in which few cognitive or perceptual abilities are needed. A sensory stimulus produces a reflexive motor response. Touching the lip of a newborn produces head turning, whereas stroking an outstretched leg produces withdrawal. Sensation is a cue for motor behavior in the seemingly reflex-dominated infant. As voluntary movement emerges during motor development, sensation provides feedback accuracy for hand placement

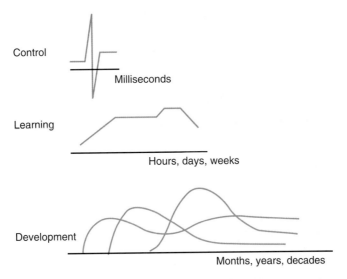

Fig. 4.2 Time scales of interest from a motor control, motor learning, and motor development perspective.

during reaching and later for creeping. Sensation from weight bearing reinforces developmental postures, such as prone on elbows and hands and knees. Sensory information is crucial to the mover when interacting with objects and maneuvering within an environment. Fig. 4.3 depicts how sensation provides the necessary feedback for the body to know whether a task such as reaching or walking was performed and how well the task was accomplished. Sensory experience contributes to the development of postural control and motor skill acquisition.

Role of Feedback

Feedback is a very crucial feature of motor control. Feedback is defined as sensory or perceptual information received as a result of movement. There is intrinsic feedback, or feedback produced by the movement. Sensory feedback can be used to detect errors in movement. Feedback and error signals are important for two reasons. First, feedback provides a means to understand the process of self-control. Reflexes are initiated and controlled by sensory stimuli from the environment surrounding the individual. Motor behavior generated from feedback is initiated as a result of an error signal produced by a process within the individual. The highest level of many motor hierarchies is volitional, or self-control of function, but there has been very little explanation of how it operates.

Second, feedback also provides the fundamental process for learning new motor skills. Intrinsic feedback

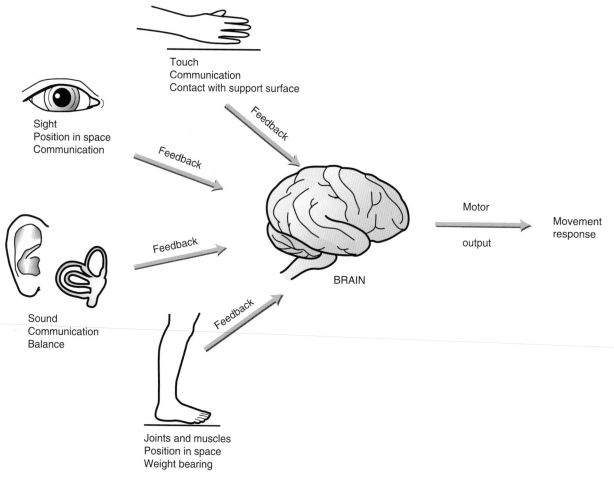

Fig. 4.3 Sources of sensory feedback.

comes from any sensory source from inside the body such as from proprioceptors or outside the body when the person sees that the target was not hit or the ball was hit out of bounds.[2] Extrinsic feedback is extra or augmented sensory information given to the mover by some external source.[2] A therapist or coach may provide enhanced feedback of the person's motor performance. For this reason, feedback is a common element in motor control and motor learning theories.

MOTOR CONTROL THEORIES

Early theories of motor control were presented in the 1800s with Sherrington and others proposing a reflex/hierarchical theory to explain the production of movement. Specific anatomical levels of the nervous system were deemed responsible for development of postural control and balance. The reflex was seen as the basic unit of motor control in this model. While reflexes are used as a measure of neurologic maturity in preterm and term infants, reflexes are not chained together as was once proposed to produce voluntary movement. Reflexes present in the infant are also referred to as primitive, not because they are not sophisticated but because they occur early in the human life span.

Tonic reflexes are associated with the brain stem of the central nervous system (CNS) in this model because they produce changes in muscle tone and posture. Examples of tonic reflexes exhibited by infants are the tonic labyrinthine reflex and the asymmetrical tonic neck reflex. In the latter, when the head is turned to the right, the right arm extends and the left arm flexes. The tonic labyrinthine reflex produces increased extensor tone when the infant is supine and increased flexor tone in the prone position. Most infantile reflexes are integrated by 4–6 months of age (see Table 3.1). Exceptions do exist. Integration is the mechanism by which less mature responses are incorporated into voluntary movement.

Nervous system maturation is seen as the ultimate determinant of postural control in the reflex/hierarchical theory of motor control. Righting reactions, an example of reactive postural responses, utilize sensory information to orient the head in space and body relative to the support surface. Equilibrium reactions are complex postural responses that respond to slow perturbations of balance. They continue to be present even in adulthood. These reactive postural responses involve the head and trunk and provide the body with an automatic way to respond to movement of the center of gravity within and outside of the body's base of support. See Chapter 11 for a description of various reactions as they relate to reactive postural control. Extremity movements in response to quick displacement of the center of gravity out of the base of support are called protective reactions. These serve as a back-up system should righting or equilibrium responses fail to compensate for a loss of balance.

MOTOR PROGRAM THEORY

Motor program theory was developed to challenge the notion that all movements are generated by chaining of reflexes because even slow movements occur too fast for sensory input to influence them.[3] A motor program is a memory structure that provides instructions for the control of actions. For efficient movement to occur in a timely manner, an internal representation of movement actions must be available. "Motor programs are associated with a set of muscle commands specified at the time of action production, which do not require sensory input."[4] Schmidt[5] expanded motor program theory to include the notion of a generalized motor program or an abstract *neural representation* of an action, distributed among different systems. Being able to mentally represent an action is part of developing motor control.[6]

Movement is affected by the ability of the mind to understand the rules of moving. Children around the age of 5 years begin to develop the ability to imagine motion or mentally represent action.[6] This is termed *motor imagery* (MI). MI is functionally equivalent to motor planning. The areas of the brain involved in idea formation can be active in triggering movement. Children's motor abilities are positively associated with their MI (Gabbard et al., 2012).[7] Motor control improves from childhood to early adulthood and declines toward late adulthood.[8]

The term motor program may also refer to a specific neural circuit called a central pattern generator (CPG), which is capable of producing a coordinated pattern of movement, such as in walking. CPGs exist in the human spinal cord. Stepping pattern generators are located in each leg that controls stepping movement at the hip and knee.[9] Postural control of the head and trunk as well as voluntary control of the ankle are required for walking. Sensory feedback adjusts timing and reinforces muscle activation.[10] Older adults exhibit altered muscle activation during fast goal-directed movements compared to young adults. The difference is related to an altered motor plan.[11] End point control is required for fast and accurate movements such as moving the foot from the gas to the brake. With increasing age, errors increase which are thought to be related to changes in timing of the motor plan.[12–14] Older adults choose a motor plan that is detrimental to end-point control, which in the example may have significant safety ramifications.

SYSTEMS THEORIES

Systems theories are the dominant and preferred way to describe the relationship between the brain and spinal cord centers that control posture and movement.[15] Systems theory is predicated on a distributed control of movement. Although the CNS is organized in a hierarchical fashion to a certain degree, the direction of control is not simply from the top down.[3,16] For example, lower levels of the nervous system can assume control over higher levels depending on the goals and constraints of the task. Distributive theory is attributed to a Russian physiologist Nicolai Bernstein,[17] whose work was done in the 1930s but not translated until 1967. Bernstein proposed that other systems contributed to movement as depicted in Fig. 4.4.

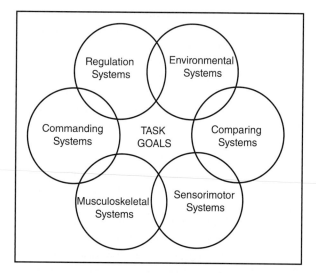

Fig. 4.4 Systems model of motor control. (From Horak B. Assumptions underlying motor control for neurologic rehabilitation. In: Lister M, ed. *Contemporary Management of Motor Control Problems: Proceedings of the II STEP Conference.* Alexandria, VA: Foundation for Physical Therapy; 1991:11–28.)

The brain undergoes anatomical growth during development, which includes cell proliferation, migration, and differentiation,[18] as well as functional and organizational changes in response to environmental and task demands. The cortex can initiate movement, but it is not the only neural structure able to do so. Other neural structures such as the basal ganglia, cerebellum, and spinal cord can initiate or control movement. Because the nervous system has the ability to self-organize, it is feasible that several systems within the nervous system are engaged in resolving movement problems; therefore, solutions typically are unique to the context and goal of the task at hand.[16,17] "The control shifts among the systems depending on the task, environment, and internal state of the person."[19] The advantage of a systems model is that it can account for the flexibility and adaptability of motor behavior in a variety of environmental conditions.

Another systems theory was identified by Horak[16] as the task-oriented theory. Functional goals, as well as environmental and task constraints, play a major role in determining movement.[16] The context within which a movement takes place provides a foundation for developing intervention strategies based on task goals aimed at improving motor skills. Teaching task-oriented skills requires that the environment and the person's motivation are considered.

Body systems, other than the nervous system, are involved in the control of movement. The most obvious ones are the muscular and skeletal systems. As a mechanical system, the muscles have viscoelastic properties while tendons do not. The skeleton is a linked structure so that controlling which joint moves and which joint or joints is/are stabilized produces a *degrees of freedom* problem. There are multiple levels of redundancy within the CNS. Bernstein[17] suggested that a key function of the CNS was to control this redundancy by minimizing the degrees of freedom or the number of independent movement elements that are used. For example, muscles can fire in different ways to control particular movement patterns or joint motions. In addition, many different kinematic or movement patterns can be executed to accomplish one specific outcome or action. During the early stages of learning novel tasks, the body may produce very simple movements, often "linking together two or more degrees of freedom"[3] and limiting the amount of joint motion by holding some joints stiffly via muscle co-contraction. As an action or task is learned, we first hold our joints stiffly through muscle coactivation, and then, as we learn the task, we decrease coactivation and allow the joint to move freely. This increases the degrees of freedom around the joint.[20]

Certainly, an increase in joint stiffness used to minimize degrees of freedom at the early stages of skill acquisition may not hold true for all types of tasks. In fact, different skills require different patterns of muscle activation. For example, Spencer and Thelen[21] reported that muscle coactivity increases with learning of a fast vertical reaching movement. They proposed that high-velocity movements actually result in the need for muscle coactivity to counteract unwanted rotational forces. However, during the execution of complex multijoint tasks, such as walking and rising from sitting to standing, muscle coactivation is clearly undesirable and may in fact negatively affect the smoothness and efficiency of the movements. The resolution of the degrees of freedom problem varies depending on the characteristics of the learner as well as on the components of the task and environment. Despite the various interpretations of Bernstein's original hypothesis,[17] the resolution of the degrees of freedom problem continues to form the underlying basis for a systems theory of motor control.

DYNAMIC SYSTEMS THEORY

A dynamic system is any system that changes over time.[22] Development of control of the body systems involved in movement occurs asynchronously. However, all systems of the body interact with each other and with the environment in which the movement takes place on an ongoing basis. The interface of the mover, the task, and the environment is where the movement pattern emerges to best fit the needs at that time. Not only are the body systems involved in movement maturing over time, but so is the psychological understanding of the mind and body maturing to provide motivation, ideation, and an understanding of how things work. The common solutions to early movement dilemmas, such as gravity and changing body proportions that are the developmental sequence, support this view of motor control. A further discussion of dynamic systems theory as it relates to motor development is found in Chapter 3.

Role of Feedback in Systems Theory

To control movements, the individual needs to know whether the movement has been successful. In a closed-loop model of feedback, sensory information is used as feedback to the nervous system to provide assistance with the next action. A person engages in closed-loop feedback when playing a video game that requires guiding a figure across the screen. This type of feedback provides self-control of movement. A loop is formed from the sensory information that is generated as part of the movement and is fed back to the brain. This sensory information influences future motor actions. Errors that can be corrected with practice are detected, and performance improves. This type of feedback is shown in Fig. 4.5.

By contrast, in an open-loop model of feedback, movement is cued either by a central structure, such as a motor program, or by sensory information from the periphery. The movement is performed without feedback. For example, when a baseball pitcher throws a favorite pitch, the movement occurs too fast to allow feedback. Errors are detected after the fact. An example of action triggered by an external sensory source is what happens when the fire alarm sounds. The person hears the alarm and moves without thinking about moving. This type of feedback model is also shown in Fig. 4.5 and is thought to be the way in which fast movements are controlled. Another way to think of the difference between open- and closed-loop feedback can be exemplified by someone who learns to play a piano piece. The piece is played slowly while learning and receiving closed-loop feedback, but once it is learned, the student can sit down and play the piece through quickly from beginning to end.

Use of Sensory Information

Movement occurs within an environmental context. First, sensation is paired with movement reflexively, after which sensation can be used to learn movement by using feedback that is received. Finally, sensation can cue movement in a feedforward manner. Sensory information most pertinent to motor control comes from three key sources: somatosensory (proprioceptive and tactile), visual, and vestibular processes. Sensory processing improves through childhood and adolescence, as does the integration of sensory information for planning and executing movements. Vision is extremely important for postural control and balance early in life. The vestibular system provides information about the infant's relationship to gravity and head movements. Proprioception of the upper limb is particularly important in the development of accuracy of motor performance in children.

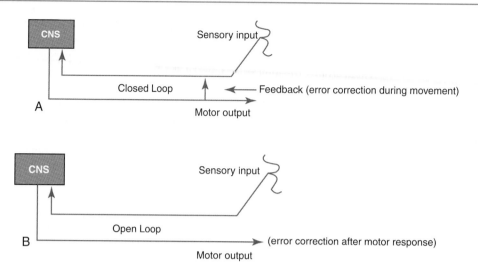

Fig. 4.5 (**A, B**) Models of feedback. (Redrawn from Montgomery PC, Connolly BH. Motor Control and Physical Therapy: Theoretical Framework and Practical Application. Hixson, TN: Chattanooga Group; 1991.)

Depending on the type of task employed, studies have shown that proprioceptive abilities are stable by age 8 or that proprioceptive ability continues to improve well into adolescence.[23,24] Loss of proprioceptive sensibility in older adults has functional consequences for movement.[25] The effects of these sensory systems relative to posture and balance are discussed in Chapter 11.

Optimization Principles

Optimization theory suggests that movements are specified to optimize a select cost function. Cost functions are those kinematic (spatial) or dynamic (force) factors that influence movement at an expense to the system. Motor skill development or relearning is aimed at achieving select objectives while minimizing cost to the system. Reducing such cost while meeting task demands and accommodating to task constraints theoretically solves the degrees of freedom problem and enhances movement efficiency.

Flash and Hogan[26] theorized that the cost function being reduced during point-to-point reaching movements is *jerk* (rate of change in acceleration). This results in a straighter hand path, as exemplified in a 1997 study by Konczak and Dichgans (Fig. 4.6).[27] These authors found that the distance the hand traveled during reaching movements in young infants was initially prolonged with a noticeable curvature in the sagittal hand path or paths. However, with practice, the distance the hand

traveled was reduced, the hand path became straighter, and the overall movement was smoother. Hypothetically, optimization principles drive the nervous system toward greater efficiency within the confines of task demands, environmental constraints, and performer limitations.

As children and adults struggle to achieve functional gains during development or during recovery from neural injury, they may appear to use inefficient movement strategies, at least from an outside view. In actuality, they may be expressing the most efficient movements available to them given their current resources. For example, a child with hemiplegic cerebral palsy may have the physical constraints of shoulder or wrist weakness and reduced finger fractionation (isolation). In an effort to reduce cost to the system while meeting task demands, the child may use a "flexion synergy," in which elbow flexion is used in combination with shoulder elevation and lateral trunk flexion to reach for objects placed at shoulder height. This flexion synergy is a strategy that seems to reduce the number of movement elements yet allows for successful attainment of the target object. Although this strategy may be useful in a specific situation, it may become habitual and may not be effective in performing a wide range of tasks. Researchers have found that children with hemiplegic cerebral palsy as a result of right hemisphere damage have deficits in using proprioceptive feedback to recognize arm position.[25]

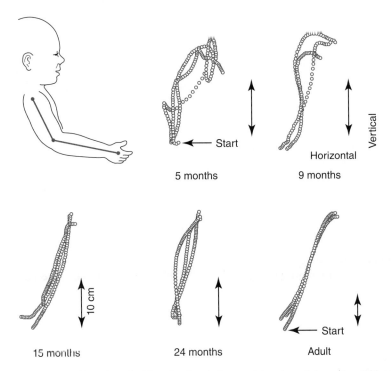

Fig. 4.6 Progressive smoothing of sagittal hand paths during reaching, from infancy to adulthood. (Redrawn from Konczak J, Dichgans J. The development toward stereotypic arm kinematics during reaching in the first 3 years of life. *Exp Brain Res.* 1997;117:346–354.)

AGE-RELATED CHANGES IN MOTOR CONTROL

The development of motor control is thought to be linked to the development of the ability to form a mental representation of movement, which has been studied using a MI paradigm. MI is an active cognitive process whereby representation of an action is internally reproduced in working memory.[28] This internal representation occurs without motor output. MI has frequently been used to study how adults plan and control movements.[29] Studies in children have increased significantly over the last two decades.[30]

Children

In a review article, Spruijt, van der Kamp, and Steenbergen[30] collated the most recent studies of children's MI abilities. Studies indicate that such abilities emerge between 5 and 7 years of age and continually improve during childhood.[6,31,32] A relationship exists between the ability to mentally represent an action by forming internal models and MI. Gabbard and colleagues[31] defined MI as way in which a child could use an internal model of movement to predict the sensory consequence of a motor action. MI improves when the mover observes the action to be performed.[33] Using a water tilting task, Frick and colleagues[34] tried to determine if motor or visual information about movement of water in a glass that was tilted would make it easier to perform the task successfully. Movement of the glass provided information to the youngest children studied who were 5 years old. The experimental setups are shown in Fig. 4.7. Funk and colleagues also noted that motor processes guided 5- and 6-year-old children in performing a mental rotation task. Gabbard[6] concluded that by the age of 5, children appear to be able to use mental imagery to represent actions.

MI is refined around 9 years of age, but development continues to progress in adolescence. Guilbert and colleagues[31] were able to demonstrate that the refinement of MI between 5 and 9 years was associated with an increased ability to utilize proprioceptive information along with visual and auditory information. Crognier and associates[35] compared actual and imagined arm pointing in children (9–11 years), adolescents (14 years), and adults (21 years). Their results showed age-dependent improvement in MI ability. See Fig. 4.8 for the experimental setup.

Feedforward or predictive motor control develops rapidly between 6 and 10 years of age.[36] The connection between MI and motor action gets stronger with age and represents the maturation of neural networks involved in motor execution. As children age, they improve in their ability to generate internal models of movement that are scaled to their intrinsic biomechanics. Caeyenberghs and fellow researchers studied a cross section of children from 7 to 12 years of age to assess their development of MI using a radial pointing task and a hand rotation task.[36] There was a strong relationship between MI and motor skills with clear age differences.

Adolescents and Adults

The ability to generate accurate mental images of actions improves and is refined with age. Adolescents and adults show changes in MI that could not be accounted for by general cognitive changes. Choudhury and associates[37] assessed movement execution time in adolescents and adults while performing two different hand movements and while imagining performing the same two different hand movements. There was a definite tight correlation between the time it took to perform the real and the imagined movements. The ability to form motor images was better in adults than adolescents. The researchers attributed this difference to the fact that the adolescent brain is experiencing ongoing maturation of the parietal cortex thought to be involved with storage and modification of internal models of action (Van de Walle de Ghelcke et al., 2021).[38] The parietal cortex, prefrontal cortex, motor cortices, cerebellum, and basal ganglia are involved in MI and motor execution.[39] Adolescents

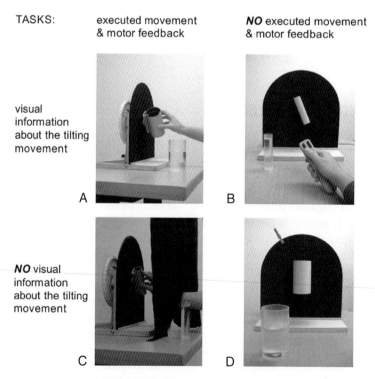

Fig. 4.7 Experimental setups for the different tasks: (**A**) Manual tilting task—experiment 1; (**B**) remote control task—experiment 2; (**C**) blind tilting task—experiment 3; (**D**) judgment task—experiment 4. (From Frick A, Daum MM, Wilson M, et al. Effects of action on children's and adult's mental imagery. *J Exp Child Psych.* 2009;104:34–51.)

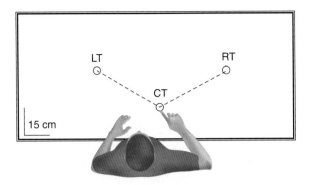

Fig. 4.8 Experimental device (top view). Children, adolescent, and young adults performed horizontal pointing toward two different targets, each 60 degrees on right *(RT)* and left *(LT)* of the central target *(CT)*. Inertial resistance was low moving from CT-RT and high moving from CT-LT. (From Crognier L, Skoura X, Vinter A, et al. Mental representation of arm motion dynamics in children and adolescents. *Plos One.* 2013;8(8):e73042.)

with dyslexia have impaired MI which is consistent with their concomitant sensorimotor deficits (Van de Walle de Ghelcke et al., 2021).[38]

Brandwayn and colleagues[40] studied the effect of type of motor activity on cognitive functions such as attention, praxis, and executive function in college students. They used MI as one type of physical activity along with gross motor and fine motor activities using novel and routine tasks. No significant differences were found. MI is credited for advancements in sport performance and rehabilitation.[41] MI studies are prevalent in the neurologic and orthopedic rehabilitation literature.[42-44]

Older Adults

Saimpont and associates[45] reviewed studies of MI in healthy adults aged 55 and older. They concluded there were no changes in the MI ability of older adults to imagine simple-usual movements. There were some changes in the mental simulation of difficult-unusual movements. In a comparison of young adults (M = 22 years) and older adults (M = 66 years), Gabbard and Cordova[46] found that estimation of reach using MI and actual functional reach was overestimated by the younger group and underestimated by the older group. Changes in MI have been reported for adults age 64 and older.[32,47] Young elderly (64 years of age) compensate by increasing neural activation of the occipitotemporal region of the brain during MI.

Skoura and associates[48] showed that young and older adults displayed similar timing for a walking and pointing task that was imagined or performed. However, the groups were dissimilar in the timing of a stand-sit-stand task. Both young and older adults demonstrated a shorter time for the imagined task than for the stand-sit-stand task. The authors thought that this was related to the fact that when actually performing the movement, the sit-to-stand part of the task was performed more quickly than the stand-to-sit portion of the task. They surmised that occurred because of a lack of visual information regarding movement into backward space.

Nicholson and associates[49] conducted a systematic review to determine if MI training improves balance and mobility in older adults. Twelve articles were included. All trials included at least three sessions of MI. All participants were at least 60 years of age and had no neurological conditions. There was evidence that MI improved balance, gait speed, and Timed Up and Go scores, but the quality of evidence was low to very low.

MOTOR LEARNING

Across the life span, individuals are faced with new motor challenges and must learn to perform new motor skills. Infants must learn how to hold up the head, roll over, sit, crawl, and eventually walk. Each skill takes time to master and occurs only after the infant has practiced each skill in several different ways. The young child then masters running, climbing on furniture, walking up stairs, jumping, and playing ball. The school-age child takes these tasks further to specifically kick a soccer ball into a net, throw a ball into a basketball hoop, ride a bike, or skateboard. As teens and adults learn new sports, they refine their skills, becoming more efficient at turning while on snow skis or pitching a baseball into the strike zone with more force. Adults also learn to efficiently perform tasks related to their occupation. These tasks vary widely from one occupation to another and may include efficient computer keyboarding, climbing up a ladder, or lifting boxes. Older adults may need to modify their motor skill performance to accommodate for changes in strength and flexibility. For example, older adult golfers may change their stance during a swing or learn to use a heavier golf club to maximize the distance of their drive. Often injury or illness requires an individual to relearn how to sit up, walk, put on a shirt, or get into or out of a car. The method each individual uses to learn new movements demonstrates the process of motor learning. Motor learning examines how an individual learns or modifies a motor task. As discussed in the section on motor control, characteristics of the task, the learner, and the environment will impact the performance and learning of the skill. With motor learning, general principles apply to individuals of any age, but variations also have been found between the motor learning methods used by children, adults, and older adults.

Definition and Time Frame

Motor learning is defined as the process that brings about a permanent change in motor performance as a result of practice.[2] The time frame of motor learning falls between the milliseconds of motor control and the years involved in motor development. Hours, days, and weeks of practice are part of motor learning. It takes an infant the better part of a year to overcome gravity and learn to walk. The perfection of some skills take years; ask anyone trying to improve a batting average or a soccer kick. Olympic caliber athletes spend years perfecting their motor performance. Even though motor development, motor control, and motor learning take place within different time frames, these time frames do not preclude one or the other processes from taking place. In fact, it is possible because of these different time frames, the processes are mutually compatible.

THEORIES OF MOTOR LEARNING

There are two theories of motor learning that have generated a great deal of study about how we control and acquire motor skills. Both theories use programs to explain how movements are controlled and learned: they are Adams' closed-loop theory of motor learning[50] and Schmidt's schema theory.[51] The two theories differ in the amount of emphasis placed on open-loop processes that can occur without the benefit of ongoing feedback.[52] Schmidt incorporated many of Adams' original ideas when formulating his schema theory in an attempt to explain the acquisition of both slow and fast movements. Intrinsic and extrinsic feedback, as defined earlier in this chapter, are both important factors in these two theories.

Adams' Closed-Loop Theory

The name of Adams' theory emphasizes the crucial role of feedback. The concept of a closed loop of motor control is one in which sensory information is funneled back to the central nervous system for processing and control of motor behavior. The sensory feedback is used to produce accurate movements.

The basic premise of Adams' theory is that movements are performed by comparing the ongoing movement with an internal reference of correctness that is developed during practice. This internal reference is termed a *perceptual trace*, which represents the feedback one would receive if the tasks were performed correctly. Through ongoing comparison of the feedback with the perceptual trace, a limb may be brought into the desired position. To learn the task, it would be necessary to practice the exact skill repeatedly, strengthening the correct perceptual trace. The quality of performance is directly related to the quality of the perceptual trace. A perceptual trace, formed as the learner repeatedly performs an action, is made up of a set of intrinsic feedback signals that arise from the learner. Intrinsic feedback here means the sensory information that is generated through performance, for example, the kinesthetic feel of the movement. As a new movement is learned, correct outcomes reinforce development of the most effective, correct perceptual trace, while perceptual traces leading to more incorrect outcomes are discarded. The perceptual trace becomes stronger with repetition and more accurately represents correct performance as a result of feedback.

With further study, limitations of the closed-loop theory of motor learning have been identified. One limitation is that the theory does not explain how movements can be explained when sensory information is not available. The theory also does not explain how individuals can often perform novel tasks successfully, without the benefit of repeated practice and the perceptual trace. The ability of the brain to store individual perceptual traces for each possible movement has also been questioned, considering the memory storage capacity of the brain.[51]

Schmidt's Schema Theory

Schmidt's schema theory was developed in direct response to Adams' closed-loop theory and its limitations. Schema theory is concerned with how movements that can be carried out without feedback are learned, and it relies on an open-loop control element, the motor program, to foster learning. The *motor program* for a movement reflects the general rules to successfully complete the movement. These general rules, or schema, can then be used to produce the movement in a variety of conditions or settings. For example, the general rules for walking can be applied to walking on tile, on grass, going up a hill, or on an icy sidewalk. The motor program provides the spatial and temporal information about muscle activation needed to complete the movement.[52] The motor program is the schema, or abstract memory, of rules related to skilled actions.

According to schema theory, when a person produces a movement, four kinds of information are stored in short-term memory:

1. The initial conditions under which the performance took place (e.g., the position of the body, the kind of surface on which the individual carried out the action, or the shapes and weights of any objects that were used to carry out the task)
2. The parameters assigned to the motor program (e.g., the force or speed that was specified at the time of initiation of the program)
3. The outcome of the performance
4. The sensory consequences of the movement (e.g., how it felt to perform the movement, the sounds that were made as a result of the action, or the visual effect of the performance)

These four kinds of information are analyzed to gain insight into the relationships among them and to form two types of schema: the recall schema and the recognition schema.

The *recall schema* is used to select a method to complete a motor task. It is an abstract representation of the relationship among the initial conditions surrounding performance, parameters that were specified within the motor program, and the outcome of the performance. The learner, through the analysis of parameters that were specified in the motor program and the outcome, begins to understand the relationship between these two factors. For example, the learner may come to understand how far a wheelchair travels when varying amounts of force are generated to push the chair on a gravel pathway. The learner stores this schema and uses it the next time the wheelchair is moved on a gravel path.

The *recognition schema* helps assess how well a motor behavior has been performed. It represents the relationship among the initial conditions, the outcome of the performance, and the sensory consequences that are perceived by the learner. Because it is formed in a manner similar to that of the recall schema, once it is established, the recognition schema is used to produce an estimate of the sensory consequences of the action that will be used to adjust and evaluate the motor performance of a given motor task.

In motor learning, the motor behavior is assessed through use of the recognition schema. If errors are identified, they are used to refine the recall schema. Recall and recognition schema are continually revised and updated as skilled movement is learned. Limitations of the schema theory have also been identified. One limitation is that the formation of general motor programs is not explained. Another question has arisen from inconsistent results in studies of effectiveness of variable practice on learning new motor skills, especially with adult subjects.

STAGES OF MOTOR LEARNING

It is generally possible to tell when a person is learning a new skill. The person's performance lacks the graceful, efficient movement of someone who has perfected the skill. For example, when adults learn to snow ski, they generally hold their bodies stiffly, with knees straight and arms at their side. Over time, as they become more comfortable with skiing, they will bend and straighten their knees as they turn. Finally, when watching the experienced skier, the body fluidly rotates and flexes/extends as the skier maneuvers down a steep slope or completes a slalom race. The stages associated with mastery of a skill have been described and clearly differentiate between the early and later stages of motor learning. Two models of motor learning stages are described below and in Table 4.1.

In the early stages of motor learning, individuals have to think about the skill they are performing and may even "talk" their way through the skill. For example, when learning how to turn when snow skiing, the novice skier may tell herself to bend the knees as initiating the turn, then straighten the knees through the turn, and then bend the knees again as the turn is completed. The skier might even be observed to say the words "bend, straighten, bend" or "down, up, down" as turns are performed. Early in the motor learning process, movements tend to be stiff and inefficient. The new learner may not always be successful in completing the skill or might hesitate, making the timing of movements inaccurate.

In the later stages of motor learning, the individual may not need to think about the skill. For example, the skier automatically goes through the appropriate motions with appropriate timing as in making a turn down a steep slope. Likewise, the baseball player steps

TABLE 4.1 Stages of Motor Learning

Model	Stage 1	Stage 2	Stage 3
Fitts' stages of motor learning[53]	Cognitive stage Actively think about goal Think about conditions	Associative stage Refine performance Error correction	Autonomous stage Automatic performance Consistent, efficient performance
"Neo-Bernsteinian" model of motor learning[20]	Novice stage Decreased number of degrees of freedom	Advanced stage Release some degrees of freedom	Expert stage Uses all degrees of freedom for fluid, efficient movement
General characteristics	Stiff looking Inconsistent performance Errors Slow, nonfluid movement	More fluid movement Fewer errors Improved consistency Improved efficiency	Automatic Fluid Consistent Efficient Error correction

up to the plate and does not think too much about how to hit the ball. The batter automatically swings at a ball that comes into the strike zone. If either the experienced skier or batter makes an error, the person will self-assess the performance and try to correct.

Fitts' Stages

In analyzing acquisition of new motor skills, Fitts[53] described three stages of motor learning. The first stage is the *cognitive phase* where the learner has to consciously consider the goal of the task to be completed and recognize the features of the environment to which the movement must conform.[54] In a task such as walking across a crowded room, the surface of the floor and the location and size of people within the room are considered regulatory features. If the floor is slippery, a person's walking pattern is different than if the floor is carpeted. Background features such as lighting or noise may also affect task performance. During this initial cognitive phase of learning, an individual tries a variety of strategies to achieve the movement goal. Through this trial-and-error approach, effective strategies are built upon and ineffective strategies are discarded.

At the next stage of learning, the *associative phase*, the learner has developed the general movement pattern necessary to perform the task and is ready to refine and improve the performance of the skill. The learner makes subtle adjustments to adjust errors and to adapt the skill to varying environmental demands of the task. For example, a young baseball player may learn to be more efficient

and consistent in hitting the ball by choking up on the bat. During this phase, the focus of the learner switches from "what to do" to "how to do the movement."[5]

In the final stage of learning, the *autonomous phase*, the skill becomes more "automatic" because the learner does not need to focus all of their attention on the motor skill. The person is able to attend to other components of the task, such as scanning for subtle environmental obstacles. At this phase, the learner is better able to adapt to changes in features in the environment. The young baseball player will be relatively successful at hitting the ball when using different bats or if a cheering crowd is present.

"Neo-Bernsteinian" Model

This model of staging motor learning considers the learners' ability to master multiple degrees of freedom as they learn the new skill.[17,20] Within this model, the initial stage of motor learning, the *novice stage*, is when the learner reduces the degrees of freedom that need to be controlled during the task. The learner will "fix" some joints so that motion does not take place and the degree of freedom is constrained at that joint. For example, think of the new snow skier who holds the knees stiffly extended while bending at the trunk to try to turn. The resultant movement is stiff looking and not always effective. For example, if the slope of the hill is too steep, or if the skier tries to turn on an icy patch, a fall may be the result rather than a turn. The second stage in this model, the *advanced stage*, is seen when the learner allows more joints to participate in the task, in essence releasing some of the degrees of freedom. Coordination is improved as agonist and antagonist muscles around the joint can work together to produce the movement, rather than co-contracting as they did to "fix" the joint in earlier movement attempts. The third stage of this model, the *expert stage*, is when all degrees of freedom necessary to perform a task in an efficient, coordinated manner are released. Within this stage, the learner can begin to adjust performance to improve the efficiency of the movement by adjusting the speed of the movement. Considering the skier, the expert may appreciate that by increasing the speed of descent, a turn may be easier to initiate.

IMPORTANT ELEMENTS OF THE MOTOR LEARNING PROCESS

Effects of Practice

As defined earlier in this chapter, motor learning is a permanent change in motor behavior resulting from practice. Motor learning theorists have studied the effects of practice on learning and whether certain types of practice make initial learning easier. Practice is therefore a key component of motor learning. Some types of practice make initial learning easier but make transferring that learning to another task more difficult. The more closely the practice environment resembles the actual environment where the task will take place, the better the transfer of learning. This is known as task-specific practice. Therefore if you are going to teach a person to walk in the physical therapy gym, this learning may not transfer to walking at home, where the floor is carpeted. Many rehabilitation facilities have an Easy Street (mock or mini-home, work, and community environment) in which to practice, which helps simulate actual conditions. Providing therapy in the home setting is an excellent opportunity for motor learning. Many factors need to be considered when designing the practice component for learning different tasks. The amount of practice and a practice schedule should be considered. The order in which tasks are practiced can also influence learning, as can whether a task is practiced as a whole skill or is broken down into its parts.

Massed Versus Distributed Practice

The difference between massed and distributed practice schedules is related to the proportion of rest time and practice time during the session. In *massed practice*, greater practice time than rest time occurs in the session. The amount of rest time between practice attempts is less than the amount of time spent practicing. In *distributed practice* conditions, the amount of rest time is longer than the time spent practicing. In some clinical settings, tasks may be more safely learned with a distributed practice schedule than massed practice, especially tasks in which a person might fatigue. If the learner becomes too fatigued and is at risk for injuring themselves or not being able to maintain correct form during an activity, it is better to give her a rest period. In contrast, some tasks such as picking up a coin or buttoning a button do not take excessive energy and may be better learned with less rest between trials. One example of how massed practice is used in rehabilitation is the use of constraint-induced movement therapy (Clinical Implications Box 4.1). Constraint-induced therapy can be considered a modified form of massed practice in which learned nonuse is overcome by shaping or reinforcement.[55] In an individual with hemiplegia, the uninvolved arm or hand is constrained, thereby necessitating use of the involved (hemiplegic) upper extremity in functional tasks.

Random Versus Blocked Practice

Another consideration in structuring a practice session is the order in which tasks are practiced. *Blocked practice* occurs when the same task is repeated several times in a row. One task is practiced several times before a second task is practiced. *Random practice* occurs when a variety of tasks are practiced in a random order, with any one skill rarely practiced two times in a row. Fig. 4.9 shows the difference between blocked and random practice. *Mixed practice* sessions may also be useful in some situations, where episodes of both random and blocked practice are incorporated into the practice session.

In most instances of learning functional and skilled tasks, it has been shown that adults learn better from random practice situations. Adult learners' retention and transfer of motor skills is stronger following random practice (Fig. 4.10).[71] Blocked practice may help someone improve form on a task in an isolated setting but does not seem to translate into performing that skill in a natural situation. For example, in learning to play tennis, it would be better to practice forehand and backhand strokes and volleying in a random order—similar to how they will really occur in a game—rather than

CLINICAL IMPLICATIONS BOX 4.1
Constraint-Induced Movement Therapy: Use of Massed Practice for Improvement of Upper Extremity Function in the Patient With Hemiplegia

Constraint-induced movement therapy (CIMT) and modified CIMT (mCIMT) have been used with individuals with hemiplegia. CIMT involves both constraint of the noninvolved upper extremity of an individual with hemiplegia and repetitive practice of skilled activities or functional tasks. The intense, repetitive practice in this therapeutic approach reflects the use of massed practice strategies in rehabilitation.

In both CIMT and mCIMT, massed practice of tasks by the involved upper extremity of the patient with hemiplegia is completed while the noninvolved extremity is constrained. Practice refers to the repetitive performance of a functional skill. Shaping is also incorporated into the practice session. Shaping incorporates the motor learning concept of part practice as a task is learned in small steps, which are individually mastered. Successive approximation of the completed task is made until the individual is able to perform the whole task. Both repetitive practice and shaping approaches to functional task mastery are included in constraint-induced therapy.

The majority of the research has investigated mCIMT in adults with hemiplegia. Evidence indicates that mCIMT is effective in improving use of the involved arm for functional tasks.[56] Initially, constraint of the upper extremity was maintained for 90% of waking hours, and practice sessions of 6 hours per day were recommended. Modified approaches have decreased the percent of time a person wears a constraint during the day and the hours of practice. Lin[57] has demonstrated improved motor control

strategies during goal-directed reaching tasks, implying that the mCIMT improved reaction time and use of feedforward motor control strategies. Optimal dosage of mCMIT is still unclear. Previous reviews support a significant effect of CIMT,[58,59] but Corbetta and colleages[60] found CIMT was associated with only limited improvements in motor function.

CIMT has also been used for children with hemiplegia from infancy through adolescence. CIMT and/or bimanual training are both recommended in clinical practice guidelines for early intervention and suspected unilateral cerebral palsy.[61,62] The recommendation suggests short intervals of CIMT (30–60 min of supervised therapist-supervised home programs for 6 weeks) in early infancy.[61] Intensity should be increased with age. Both CIMT and bimanual training improve arm function in children with unilateral cerebral palsy.[63–66] Home training is essential when using CIMT.[67,68] Parents need to be involved in selecting the best approach for their child. Some children may tolerate the constraint more easily than others. Activities are selected to reflect a child's interests and maintain attention, incorporating both games and functional activities. Massed practice contributes to cortical reorganization. The earlier the intervention, the greater the activity-dependent neural plasticity.[69] Despite the evidence, only 23% of therapists reported using CIMT and/or bimanual training as an intervention for children with asymmetrical arm function.[70]

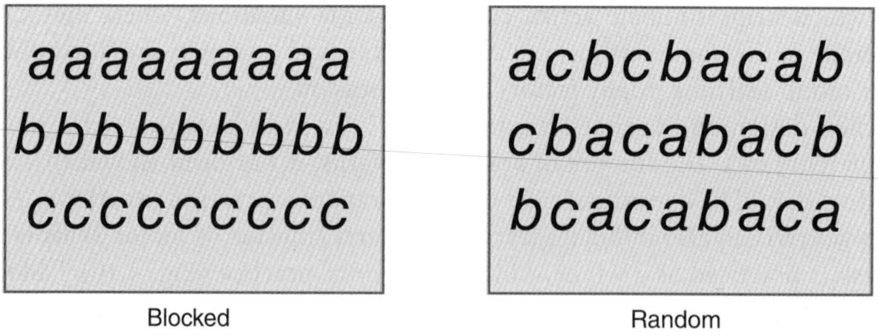

Blocked	Random
aaaaaaaaa bbbbbbbbb ccccccccc	acbcbacab cbacabacb bcacabaca

Fig. 4.9 Sample practice schedules for reach-to-grasp activity illustrate blocked and random practice: *a,* reach and grasp for a paper cup; *b,* reach and grasp for a coffee mug; *c,* reach and grasp for a glass.

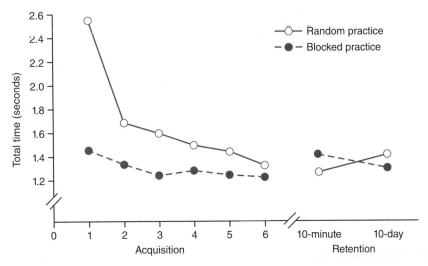

Fig. 4.10 Effect of blocked versus random practice on acquisition and retention of a motor skill. Although blocked practice led to better performance during acquisition, random practice led to greater learning as measured by retention tests. (Adapted with permission from Shea JB, Morgan RL. Contextual interference effects on the acquisition, retention, and transfer of a motor skill. *J Exp Psychol.* 1979;5(2):179–187.)

practice forehand strokes for 50 trials, then backhand strokes for 50 trials. It has been suggested that in random practice, when the learner shifts from one task to another, thinking needs to focus on the different strategies that must be performed to complete each task. Random practice seems to be best for skilled learners because it allows them to derive a range of solutions to the task that can be used at a later time.

Blocked practice does seem to have a place in the early stages of learning brand-new skills that have never been done. Blocked practice may be most appropriate in the early cognitive stages of motor learning, for children and individuals with cognitive impairments.[72–74] Adolescents with Down syndrome appear to benefit more from blocked practice than random practice.[72] Impact of practice method on motor learning in children will be further discussed later in this chapter.

Constant Versus Variable Practice

Constant practice occurs when an individual practices one variation of a movement skill several times in a row. An example would be repeatedly practicing standing up from a wheelchair or throwing a basketball into a hoop. *Variable practice* occurs when the learner practices several variations of a motor skill during a practice session. For example, a rehabilitation patient may practice standing up from the wheelchair, standing up from the bed, standing up from the toilet, and standing up from the floor. A child might practice throwing a ball into a hoop, throwing a ball at a target on the wall, throwing a ball underhand, throwing a ball overhand, or throwing a ball to a partner all within the same session. Variable practice training is useful in helping the learner generalize a motor skill over a wide variety of environmental settings and conditions. Learning is felt to be enhanced by the variable practice because the strength of the general motor program rules, specific to the new task, would be increased. This mechanism is also considered one way that an individual can attempt a novel task because the person can incorporate rules developed for previous motor tasks to solve the novel task.

Whole Versus Part Task Training

A task can be practiced as a complete action (*whole task practice*) or broken up into its component parts (*part practice*). Continuous tasks such as walking, running, or stair climbing are more effectively learned with whole task practice. It has been demonstrated that if walking is broken down into part practice of a component, such as weight shifting forward over the foot, the learner demonstrates improvements in weight shifting behaviors but does not generalize this improvement into the walking sequence.[75]

Skills that can be broken down into discrete parts may be most effectively taught using part practice training. For example, a patient learning how to independently transfer out of a wheelchair might be first taught how to lock the brakes on the chair, then how to scoot forward in the chair. After these parts of the task are mastered, the patient might learn to properly place her feet, lean forward over the feet, and finally stand. Similarly, when learning a dressing task, a child might first be taught to pull a shirt over her head and then push in each arm. Once these components are completed, the focus might be on learning how to fasten buttons or the zipper.

Open and Closed Tasks

Movement results when the mover and the environment interact to perform a specific task. Tasks to be learned can be classified as open or closed. Open tasks are those done in an environment that changes over time, such as playing softball, walking on uneven terrain, or driving a car. Closed tasks are skills that have set parameters that stay the same, such as walking across a carpeted floor, holding an object, or reaching for a target. These tasks appear to be processed differently. Which type of task involves more processing of perceptual information? Open tasks require the mover to constantly update movements and pay attention to the need to adjust for incoming information about the softball, movement of traffic, or the support surface. Would a person have fewer motor problems with open or closed tasks? Closed tasks with set parameters pose fewer problems. Have you ever brushed your teeth while still being half asleep? Gentile developed an entire taxonomy of tasks that you might find useful.[76] Remember that open and closed tasks are different from open- and closed-loop processing used for motor control or motor learning.

OPTIMAL THEORY

The OPTIMAL theory of motor learning is so named because it stands for optimizing performance through intrinsic motivation and attention for learning.[77] These researchers propose that because motor behavior is embedded in culture, it has a social context that can be used to influence motor learning behavior. They assume that attention and motivation influence motor behavior in the same way as it influences personal behavior. The literature on the effect of motivation and attention on motor learning has shown that a focus on positive expectations will enhance motor learning. By providing the learner autonomy, such as allowing choices of task, practice, or environment, motor learning is enhanced. Adolescents learning to hit a ball with a racket toward a target who were supported psychologically exhibited task learning.[78] Young adults in an autonomy-supportive group outperformed young adults in an autonomy-controlling group when learning a stepping sequence task.[79] Older adults allowed to choose when to stop practicing a speed cup stacking task outperformed a group that had a predetermined number of practice trials.[80] The external focus is put on the intended movement effect rather than on the body movements needed to improve motor learning. Ten-year-old children improved motor skill learning when feedback was focused on their ability to change performance results rather than on their inherent ability.[81] An external focus of attention resulted in superior performance of a classical ballet pirouette in a group of 10-year-old ballet students.[82] The theory has been successfully applied to motor learning in children with autism, intellectual disability, adults with Parkinson disease, and older adults with balance issues (Reis, 2018).[83–86]

Feedback

Feedback is a critical component of motor learning. As discussed in the motor learning theory section, two types of feedback guide learning: intrinsic feedback and extrinsic feedback. When structuring the learning session, a therapist will want the learner to experience the type of intrinsic feedback that will best help the learner learn the task or general motor programs necessary for efficient performance of the skill. In structuring the motor learning session, the therapist must consider how to structure the extrinsic feedback provided to enhance learning.

Terminal Versus Concurrent Feedback

Information given during task performance is known as *concurrent feedback*. Coaches, therapists, and educators often use concurrent feedback by altering sensory input, providing manual cues, or giving verbal information to facilitate specific movements. Concurrent feedback has several purposes: to help guide the learner to feel the desired movement pattern, to enhance execution of a certain pattern of movement by encouraging activation of specific musculature, and to assist the individual in successfully accomplishing a goal. Similar to other types of extrinsic feedback, when concurrent feedback is used too frequently, it may actually impede learning because the learner may

TABLE 4.2   Examples of Feedback Given After Task Performance

Knowledge of Results	Knowledge of Performance
Outcome of Success or Failure	**Task Execution**
"You walked across the room!"	"You did not keep your elbow straight."
"That task took you 1 minute 30 seconds to complete."	"You are not bearing as much weight on your right side when you walk."
"You scored 5 points out of 8!"	"You were looking at your feet."

become dependent on it. Furthermore, the person providing the feedback becomes a part of the performer's environment. Therefore the performer still needs to learn how to move effectively when the feedback is removed.

Feedback can also be provided less frequently. Feedback that is provided less than 100% of the time is called *intermittent feedback*. *Faded feedback* can also be given, in which the frequency of feedback is greater in the early stages of learning a task and then decreases as the learner progresses in learning the task. Another schedule of giving feedback is *summarized feedback*, in which feedback is given after several trials. These various feedback schedules decrease a performer's reliance on external feedback and may ultimately enhance learning of a motor skill.[87]

Feedback can also be given at the completion of a motor task and is called *terminal feedback*. Terminal feedback is usually categorized into two forms: knowledge of results (KR) and knowledge of performance (Table 4.2). *KR* is information related to the outcome, whether successful or not. We know whether we have been successful in picking up a cup or walking across the room. KR feedback appears to be most effective if provided in a faded or summary feedback schedule, with too much immediate feedback of performance outcome detrimental to learning.[52] *Knowledge of performance* pertains to information received regarding execution of the task and typically relates to the type or quality of the movement. Although KR is useful at any time during the learning process, knowledge of performance should be used selectively. Because a learner is thinking so hard about performing a task in the early stages of learning, providing detailed information can be confusing and may be detrimental to long-term learning.

Key concepts related to providing concurrent or terminal feedback for any population include (1) use of feedback that is specific to the task and the learner's needs; (2) minimizing use of excessive feedback; and (3) encouragement of active problem solving that allows time to self-assess, rather than rely on feedback.

AGE-RELATED CHANGES IN MOTOR LEARNING

Motor learning strategies must meet the needs of the learner to be effective. Children learn differently than adults. Nervous system development/maturation in children may influence a child's ability to learn and master some motor skills.[88] Self-produced movements provide sensorimotor experiences that are crucial to learning to move.[89,90] Cognitive development may influence how a child can receive and process information. Movement provides sensation and perception that supports cognitive development. When working with children, adults, and older adults, therapists need to consider the unique needs of each learner to design optimal motor learning sessions and provide the most useful extrinsic feedback. Both practice and feedback components of the motor learning tasks are important considerations in designing and implementing motor learning strategies for each individual person.

Children practice, practice, practice when learning a new motor skill. For example, when learning to walk, an infant covers a distance equal to 29 football fields daily.[91] A typical 14-month-old is reported to take more than 2000 steps per hour.[92] These two examples lend support to use of block practice to learn and retain a new skill. Infants demonstrate inherent variability in performing tasks. Surprisingly, learning in one posture, such as sitting, does not carry over to standing. Learning to function in upright posture does not generalize to other actions such as walking down a ramp.[89,93] Adolph's work supports the dynamic systems theory that developing a level of skill in one posture does not automatically transfer to another posture. Knowing how to crawl on a slope does not transfer to walking down a slope. The infant is constantly problem solving to meet challenges of the task and the environment.

As young children are learning new gross motor tasks, blocked practice appears to lead to better transfer and performance of the skill. Del Rey and colleagues[74] had typically developing children (approximately 8 years old) practice an anticipation timing task at different speeds in either a blocked or random order and then tested them on a transfer test with the new coordination pattern. The researchers found that blocked practice led to better performance on the transfer task than did random practice. In Frisbee throwing experiments, accuracy in throwing the Frisbee at a target was improved by blocked practice in children, although adults improved accuracy the most with random practice.[94,95] The contextual interference provided by random practice schedules does not appear to help children learn new motor skills.[96]

Although most of the literature on children supports a blocked or mixed schedule for learning whole body tasks, some researchers have found that typically developing children may learn skilled or sport-specific skills if a variable practice schedule is used.[97–99] This variable practice schedule combines blocked and random practice elements and allows the child to benefit from practicing the new skill with elements of contextual interference. Vera and associates[97] found that 9-year-old children performed the skill of kicking a soccer ball best following blocked or combined practice, but only children in a combined practice situation improved in dribbling the soccer ball. Similarly, Douvis[98] examined the impact of variable practice on learning the tennis forehand drive in children and adolescents. Adolescents did better than children on the task, reflecting the influence of age and development, but both age groups did the best with variable practice. The variable practice sessions allowed the tennis players to use the forehand drive in a manner that more resembled the actual game of tennis, where a player may use a forehand drive, then a backhand drive.

Feedback

Feedback plays an important role in motor learning for infants and children. Infants in an imitation experiment demonstrated strongest responses when their mothers offered demonstration and verbal praise related to completion of play tasks. Infants as young as 10 months of age have demonstrated the use of intrinsic, proprioceptive input in learning new tasks.[100] In these experiments, infants were exposed to the task of using a cane to pull an out-of-reach toy closer. Infants who physically practiced the task appeared to perceive the cane could be used as a tool to reach a toy, but infants who only watched as someone else pulled the cane to obtain a toy did not seem to react to the cane as a tool that could be used to obtain a toy.

Children differ from adults in the type and frequency of feedback that best supports their motor learning. In children, if KR is too specific, it confuses the child and interferes with learning.[52,101] When learning a new motor task, it appears that children benefit more from more constant feedback than they do from reduced feedback. A group of 10-year-olds learning a new task in a 100% feedback group had better consistency in a retention test compared with 10-year-olds who received reduced (62% faded) feedback.[102] Because of developmental differences in information processing abilities and memory, children may require the increased level of feedback. In looking at the type of extrinsic feedback provided, children also appear to benefit from feedback addressing internal requirements of a task rather than external results. In a dart-throwing learning situation, adults benefited more from feedback about the darts and target than about their form (e.g., hand position, elbow activity) during dart throwing. Children in this same experiment improved the most in dart throwing when they received feedback on specific hand, elbow, and arm activity to be used during dart throwing.[103] A child's ability to benefit from more internally focused, proprioceptive, or kinesthetic feedback than from information related to the task outcome may also reflect the child's developmental ability in processing sensory information and information processing.

Practice that simulates the demands of competition was found to improve elite junior tennis players' serving skills after a 6-week intervention.[104,105] The researchers observed that increased task representation led to fewer differences between practice performance and match performance. Specificity of learning to make free throws in basketball by high school players was dependent on the type of visual condition used during skill acquisition.[106] Participants trained using either full vision or viewing only the target. Delayed retention performance was significantly decreased when participants were tested using a visual condition that differed from what they used to learn the skill. For example, if a participant who practiced using full vision was tested in the target only condition, performance dropped significantly. Learning a sport skill, in this case, free throws in basketball, is specific to the source of the sensory information available during practice. These findings support the use of condition-specific practice.

Motor Learning and Older Adults

Very broadly speaking, aging affects motor learning. The deficits in processing and encoding sensorimotor information are thought to contribute to the decline in the ability to learn motor skills in older adults (Roig et al., 2014).[107] However, the deficit is not the only reason for a decline. Aging increases the susceptibility to impaired memory consolidation, which can reduce motor skill learning after practice (Roig et al., 2104).[107] Mooney et al.[108] studied activation and inhibition of motor areas in the brain in young and older adults. They concluded that learning and retaining novel motor skills was maintained with advanced age. Cirillo[109] in a mini-review discussed the importance of movement in the form of regular physical activity as a way to maintain brain health and function. Despite the fact that older adults can learn novel tasks, the structural plasticity in the motor cortex may be less than young adults. Exercise appears to play a role in enhancing motor learning. Both moderate- and high-intensity exercises have been shown to improve motor skill acquisition and motor cortex plasticity, respectively.[110,111] Acute exercise has been used to improve motor memory consolidation.[112]

There are presently a handful of studies suggesting that older adults have:

- Deficits in sequence motor learning.
- Deficits in learning new technology but not in benefits of practice.
- Deficits in learning effortful bimanual coordination patterns with preserved or enhanced use of augmented feedback. Older adults do respond when a task has salience and the new task to be learned is related to previous learning.

Sequential Learning

Performing learned or learning new motor sequences is important functionally. Clearly, linking motor acts such as rolling, sitting up, standing up, and walking play a major role in daily life. However, motor sequence learning is typically evaluated by the use of more rudimentary acts such as pointing to different targets on a computer screen or pressing different sets of buttons on a keypad. The relationship between the sensorimotor organization of sequences of actions like those performed during activities of daily living and those being tested in a motor learning experiment remains to be established. Irrespective of this issue, a recent well-designed laboratory-based study on sequential motor learning did find that older adults were slower to perform a novel sequential action and that it may have been due to how older persons organize subsequences of complex movements.[113]

At least one example of learning a functional sequence exists in the literature. Tunney and associates[114] provided healthy younger and older adults with a 10-step sequence for performing a car transfer using a standard walker. This sequence was practiced in (first) four-step and (second) six-step trials. Subjects were scored on a final trial and 48 hours later by a physical therapist based on the number of steps followed or completed. Older adults' scores were significantly lower immediately after practice and at 48 hours as compared with younger adults. The authors took this as evidence that older adults do not acquire and maintain a functional motor skill as accurately as younger adults. All subjects were healthy, did not need to use a walker to ambulate or transfer, and were equally successful in actually transferring into the car. It is unclear if the measure of learning matched the outcome of the to-be-learned task. Did the 10-step procedure map, in an ecologically valid way, onto the subjects' natural performance and, therefore, their learning? Was following the 10-step procedure actually necessary? In the following section, it will be shown that guided attention, such as attending to key aspects of a task, may be more useful for learning a complex motor sequence than using a guided action in which a person follows a specific step-by-step process.

Practice

It is clear that older adults are able to improve motor performance with practice.[115-117] For example, an early study suggested that benefits of blocked versus random practice were tied to a participant's general level of physical activity: those with higher levels of physical activity were able to benefit from random practice.[118] This suggests that individual differences may interact with practice schedules. Jamieson and Rogers[117] evaluated the effects of blocked and random practice on learning to use an ATM machine in younger and older adults. While older adults were slower and less accurate in menu selections and more likely to forget the receipt or cash, both younger and older adults benefited from random practice. Random practice was also superior to blocked practice. Additionally, older adults were able to transfer learning to a novel ATM scenario.

More recently, Hickman and associates[119] studied guided action versus guided attention training in learning to use a new technology—a hydroponic garden control system. Both younger and older adults were able to follow the guided action information (step-by-step training materials), and this method offered benefits in performance. However, groups that originally received guided attention training, which assisted in remembering what to do more generally, benefited more when step-by-step training materials were not provided. This effect was found in both older and younger adults.

With respect to massed versus distributed practice, at least one study has demonstrated benefits of distributed over massed practice for older adults. Kausler and associates[120] had subjects perform a set of 16 motor tasks under distributed or massed practice conditions. Distributed practice resulted in better recall of these tasks. As with previously cited studies, older adults demonstrated performance decrements when compared with younger adults.

In summary, older adults tend to perform to-be-learned tasks with slower speeds and greater error, yet they seem to benefit equally, as compared with younger adults, from practice schedules conducive to motor learning.

Feedback

KR has been shown to be equally effective in motor learning when younger and older adults are compared. For example, Swanson and Lee[121] had younger and older subjects learn a continuous movement comprising a three-step spatial sequence with the upper extremity. While older adults exhibited decrements in movement accuracy and consistency during acquisition trials, both groups benefited from KR similarly. Wishart and Lee[122] expanded this result to include KR provided at 100% frequency of trials and in a fading fashion. They found that for this type of task, younger and older adults used KR in a similar way to learn. More recently, using an isometric force production task, van Dijk and associates[123] found that KR or kinetic feedback was similarly beneficial to younger and older adults.

When tasks are complex and deviate from preferred patterns, there appears to be a difference with respect to how older adults use extrinsic information. In a series of studies, an examination was undertaken to determine the role of feedback in assisting acquisition and maintenance of automatic versus effortful bimanual coordination patterns with the upper extremities.[124–126] First, so-called automatic (in-phase), bimanual coordination patterns are performed equally well by younger and older adults with only a small decrement in accuracy (error) and stability (standard deviation) with increasing pacing speeds.[125] On the other hand, effortful patterns (antiphase upper extremity movements) tended to show a greater decrement in accuracy and stability by older adults.

A 90-degree bimanual coordination pattern is considered complex and effortful because it is not purely in-phase (0 degree difference between two limbs) and not purely antiphase (180 degrees "out-of-phase"). Swinnen and associates[124] examined the acquisition of this pattern in older and younger adults. During acquisition, both groups tended toward the less effortful patterns of in-phase and antiphase. However, older adults had more difficulty (greater absolute deviation from required phase) and exhibited greater variability in maintaining the 90-degree phase pattern by the end of the acquisition trials. Augmented visual feedback in real time benefited both groups. These researchers also examined learning under blindfolded and normal vision (nonaugmented) conditions as a means to determine the extent to which subjects were dependent upon the augmented visual feedback. Older subjects exhibited more difficulties in these nonaugmented conditions, suggesting that they may have become more dependent on the augmented visual feedback. But this could also have been explained by the possible reduced quality of sensory information associated with aging.

A follow-up study by Wishart and associates[126] compared concurrent versus terminal feedback in this 90-degree phase bimanual coordination pattern. Older adults gained more from the concurrent feedback than younger adults relative to the terminal feedback condition. Taking this series of findings collectively, it appears older adults are able to use KR for learning new motor skills, but on the other hand, the utility of feedback in learning complex coordination patterns may lie in its nature and extent.

NEURAL PLASTICITY

Neural plasticity is the ability of the nervous system to change. Although it has always been hypothesized that the nervous system adapts throughout the life span, there is ample evidence to indicate that the adult brain maintains the ability for reorganization or plasticity.[127] Previously, it was thought that plasticity was limited to the developing nervous system. Activity-dependent changes in neural circuitry usually occur during a specific time in a development or critical period, when the organism is sensitive to the effects of experience.[128] *Critical periods* are times when neurons compete for synaptic sites. Plasticity provides the mechanism for the nervous system to make structural changes in response to internal and external demands. Motor behavior and learning appear to modulate neurogenesis throughout life.

Experience is critical for development. In the course of typical prenatal and postnatal development, the infant is expected to be exposed to sufficient environmental stimuli (visual, vestibular, and auditory) at appropriate times to complete the development of these sensory systems (see Chapter 9). If an infant is not exposed to the proper quality and quantity of input within the critical time period, development of these systems will not proceed normally. Neural plasticity also allows the nervous system to incorporate unpredictable and idiosyncratic information from environmental experiences. Unique experiences depend on the context in which development occurs and can encompass cultural differences in child rearing, social expectations, and physical differences in climate. Lebeer[129] refers to this as *ecological plasticity*. What each child learns depends on the unique physical, psychologic, and social challenges encountered. Motor learning, as a part of motor development, is an example of *activity-dependent* neural plasticity. Experiences of infants in different cultures may result in alterations of motor skill acquisition. Similarly, not every child experiences the same words, but every child does learn language. *Activity-dependent* plasticity drives changes in synapses or neuronal circuits as a result of experience or learning.

Experience can drive recovery of function following injury to the nervous system. Change in function is thought to be the result of activity which produces cortical reorganizations. This change is also called use-dependent cortical reorganization. Kleim and Jones[130] summarized the existing research on activity-dependent neural plasticity and recommended 10 principles for neurorehabilitation. These are in keeping with the principles of motor learning involving repetition and task-specific practice.

SUMMARY

Motor control and motor learning are continually occurring during a person's life time. Movement emerges from the interaction between all body systems, the task, and the environment. Theories of motor control emphasize various developmental aspects of posture and movement. Systems theory recognizes that control of movement is distributed throughout the nervous system in order to provide the most efficient solution to a movement problem. Motor control adapts to the individuals' functional task needs, available physical attributes, and psychological and social/cultural environment. Development of motor control can be tracked by age-related changes in MI, which is the ability to form a mental representation of movement. Functional movement is possible because of motor control and motor learning.

Motor learning has occurred when performance of a motor behavior has permanently changed as a result of practice. Motor skills are acquired over time. Individuals progress through stages of learning, from the stiff, awkward cognitive stage through the expert stage where fluid movement seems to occur automatically. Motor skill learning depends on feedback and practice. Clinicians must make decisions as to how much practice is necessary, how practice sessions should be structured, and how to maximize the most effective forms of feedback. Motor learning of functional tasks is considered to be complete when an individual can easily perform the task in a variety of environments or situations (generalization) and can consistently perform the task over several sessions. The overall motor learning process is similar in individuals of all ages, but some differences exist in which forms of practice and feedback best enhance learning in children, adults, and older adults.

REFERENCES

1. Anderson DI, Campos JJ, Rivera M, et al. The consequences of independent locomotion for brain and psychological development. In: Shephard RB, ed. *Cerebral Palsy in Infancy*. London, UK: Churchill Livingston; 2014:199–224.
2. Schmidt RA, Wrisberg CA. *Motor Learning and Performance*. 5th ed. Champaign, IL: Human Kinetics; 2013.
3. Gordon J. Assumptions underlying physical therapy intervention. In: Carr JA, Shephard RB, eds. *Movement Science: Foundations for Physical Therapy in Rehabilitation*. Rockville, MD: Aspen; 1987:1–30.
4. Wing AM, Haggard P, Flanagan J. *Hand and Brain: The Neurophysiology and Psychology of Hand Movements*. New York: Academic Press; 1996.
5. Schmidt R. *Motor Control and Learning*. Champaign, IL: Human Kinetics; 1988.
6. Gabbard C. Studying action representation in children via motor imagery. *Brain Cogn*. 2009;71(3):234–239.
7. Gabbard C, Caçola P, Bobbio T. The ability to mentally represent action is associated with low motor ability in children: a preliminary investigation. *Child Care Health Dev*. 2012;38:390–393.
8. Casamento-Moran A, Fleeman R, Chen Y-T, et al. Neuromuscular variability and spatial accuracy in children and older adults. *J Electromyogr Kinesiol*. 2018;41:27–33.
9. Yang JF, Lamont EV, Pang MY. Split-belt treadmill stepping in infants suggest autonomous pattern generators for the left and right leg in humans. *J Neurosci*. 2005;25: 6869–6876.
10. Knikou M. Neural control of locomotion and training-induced plasticity after spinal and cerebral lesions. *Clin Neurophysiol*. 2010;121:1655–1668.
11. Casamento-Moran A, Chen Y-T, Lodha N, Yacoubi B, Christou EA. Motor plan differs for young and older adults during similar movements. *J Neurophysiol*. 2017;117:1483–1488.
12. Chen Y-T, Kwon M, Fox EJ, Christou EA. Altered activation of the antagonist muscle during practice compromises motor learning in older adults. *J Neurophysiol*. 2014;112:1010–1019.
13. Kwon M, Chen Y-T, Fox EJ, Christou EA. Aging and limb alter the neuromuscular control of goal-directed movement. *Exp Brain Res*. 2014;232:1759–1771.
14. Delmas S, Choi YJ, Komer M, et al. Older adults use a motor plan that is detrimental to endpoint control. *Sci Rep*. 2021;11(1):7562.
15. Shumway-Cook A, Woollacott M. *Motor Control: Translating Research Into Clinical Practice*. 5th ed. Philadelphia, PA: Wolters Kluwer; 2017.
16. Horak B. Assumptions underlying motor control for neurologic rehabilitation. In: Lister M, ed. *Contemporary Management of Motor Control Problems: Proceedings of the II STEP Conference*. Alexandria, VA: Foundation for Physical Therapy; 1991:11–28.
17. Bernstein N. *The Coordination and Regulation of Movements*. Oxford, UK: Pergamon; 1967.
18. Guarnieri FC, de Chevigny A, Falace A, Cardoso C. Disorders of neurogenesis and cortical development. *Dialogues Clin Neurosci*. 2018;20(4):255–266.
19. Latash LP, Latash ML, Meijer OG. 30 years later: the relation between structure and function in the brain from a contemporary point of view (1996), part II. *Motor Control*. 2000;4:125–149.
20. Vereijken B, van Emmerik REA, Whiting HTA, et al. Freezing degrees of freedom in skill acquisition. *J Mot Behav*. 1992;24:133–142.
21. Spencer JP, Thelen E. A multimuscle state analysis of adult motor learning. *Exp Brain Res*. 1997;128:505–516.
22. Heriza C. Motor development: traditional and contemporary theories. In: Lister M, ed. *Contemporary Management of Motor Control Problems: Proceedings of the II STEP Conference*. Alexandria, VA: Foundation for Physical Therapy; 1991:99–126.
23. Hay L, Redon C. The control of goal-directed movements in children: role of proprioceptive muscle afferents. *Hum Mov Sci*. 1997;16:433–451.
24. Goble DJ, Lewis CA, Hurvitz EA, et al. Development of upper limb proprioceptive accuracy in children and adolescents. *Hum Mov Sci*. 2005;24:155–170.
25. Goble DJ, Coxon JP, Wenderoth N, et al. Proprioceptive sensibility in the elderly: degeneration, functional consequences and plastic-adaptive processes. *Neurosci Biobehav Rev*. 2009;33:271–278.
26. Flash T, Hogan N. The coordination of arm movements: an experimentally confirmed mathematical model. *J Neurosci*. 1985;5:1688–1703.
27. Konczak J, Dichgans J. The development toward stereotypic arm kinematics during reaching in the first 3 years of life. *Exp Brain Res*. 1997;117:346–354.
28. Decety J, Grezes J. Neural mechanisms subserving the perception of human actions. Trends Cogn Sci. 1999;3: 172–178.
29. Munzert J, Lorey B, Zentgraf K. Cognitive motor processes: the role of motor imagery in the study of motor representations. *Brain Res Rev*. 2009;60(2):306–326.
30. Spruijt S, van der Kamp J, Steenbergen B. Current insights in the development of children's motor imagery ability. *Front Psychol*. 2015;6:787.
31. Guilbert J, Jouen F, Molina M. Motor imagery development and proprioceptive integration: which sensory reweighting during childhood? *J Exp Child Psychol*. 2018;166:621–634.
32. Gabbard C, Cacola P, Cordova A. Is there an advanced aging effect on the ability to mentally represent action? *Arch Gerontol Geriatr*. 2011;53(2):206–209.

33. Conson M, Sara M, Pistoia F, Trojano L. Action observation improves motor imagery: specific interactions between simulative processes. *Exp Brain Res.* 2009;199:71–81.

34. Frick A, Daum MM, Wilson M, et al. Effects of action on children's and adult's mental imagery. *J Exp Child Psychol.* 2009;194:34–51.

35. Crognier L, Skoura X, Vinter A, Papaxanthis C. Mental representation of arm motion dynamics in children and adolescents. *PLos One.* 2013;8(8): e73042.

36. Caeyenberghs K, Tsoupas J, Wison PH, et al. Motor imagery development in children. *Dev Neuropsychol.* 2009;34(1):103–121.

37. Choudhury S, Charman T, Bird V, et al. Development of action representation during adolescence. *Neuropsychologia.* 2007;45:255–262.

38. Van de Walle de Ghelcke A, Skoura X, Edwards MG, Quercia P, Papaxanthis C. Action representation deficits in adolescents with developmental dyslexia. *J Neuropsychol.* 2021;15:215–234.

39. Fadiga L, Craighero L. Electrophysiology of action representation. *J Clin Neurophysiol.* 2004;21:157–169.

40. Brandwayn N, Restrepo D, Marcela Martinez-Martinez A, Acevedo-Triana C. Effect of fine and gross motor training or motor imagery, delivered via novel or routine modes, on cognitive function. *Appl Neuropsychol Adult.* 2020;27:450–467.

41. MacIntyre TE, Madan CR, Moran AP, et al. Motor imagery, performance and motor rehabilitation. *Prog Brain Res.* 2018;240:141–159.

42. Taube W, Lorch M, Zeiter S, Keller M. Non-physical practice improves task performance in an unstable, perturbed environment: motor imagery and observational balance training. *Front Hum Neurosci.* 2014;8:972.

43. Taube W, Mouthon M, Leukel C, et al. Brain activity during observation and motor imagery of different balance tasks: an fMRI study. *Cortex.* 2015;64:102–114.

44. Moukarzel M, Guillot A, Di Rienzo F, Hoyek N. The therapeutic role of motor imagery during the chronic phase after total knee arthroplasty: a pilot randomized controlled trial. *Eur J Phys Rehabil Med.* 2019;55(6):806–815.

45. Saimpont A, Malouin F, Tousignant B, Jackson PL. Motor imagery and aging. *J Mot Behav.* 2013;45(1):21–28.

46. Gabbard C, Cordova A. Association between imagined and actual functional reach (FR): a comparison of young and older adults. Arch Gerontol Geriatr. 2013;56(3): 487–491.

47. Zapparoli L, Saetta G, De Santis C, et al. When I am (almost) 64: the effects of normal ageing on implicit motor imagery in young elderlies. *Behav Brain Res.* 2016;303: 137–151.

48. Skoura X, Papaxanthis C, Vinter A, et al. Mentally represented motor actions in normal aging: I. Age effects on the temporal features of overt and covert execution of actions. *Behav Brain Res.* 2005;165:229–239.

49. Nicholson V, Watts N, Chani Y, Keogh JWL. Motor imagery timing improves balance and mobility outcomes in older adults: a systematic review. *J Physio.* 2019;65:200–207.

50. Adams JA. A closed-loop theory of motor learning. *J Mot Behav.* 1971;3:110–150.

51. Schmidt RA. A schema theory of discrete motor skill learning. *Psychol Rev.* 1975;82:225–260.

52. Schmidt RA, Lee TD, Winstein CJ, Wulf G, Zelaznik HN. *Motor Control and Learning: A Behavioral Emphasis.* 6th ed. Champaign, IL: Human Kinetics; 2019.

53. Fitts PM. Categories of human learning. In: Melton AW, ed. *Perceptual-Motor Skills Learning.* New York: Academic Press; 1964:243–285.

54. Gentile AM. Skill acquisition: action, movement, and neuromotor processes. In: Carr JA, Shepherd RB, Gordon J, eds. *Movement Science: Foundations for Physical Therapy in Rehabilitation.* Rockville, MD: Aspen; 1987: 93–154.

55. Taub E, Miller NE, Novack TA, et al. Technique to improve chronic motor deficit after stroke*Arch Phys Med Rehabil.* 741993347–354.

56. Kwakkel G, Veerbeek JM, van Wegen E, Wolf SL. Constraint-induced movement therapy after stroke. *Lancet Neurol.* 2015;14(2):224–234.

57. Lin KC. Effects of modified constraint-induced movement therapy on reach-to-grasp movements and functional performance after chronic stroke: a randomized controlled study. *Clin Rehabil.* 2007;21:1075–1086.

58. Corbetta D, Sirtori V, Moja L, Gatti R. Constraint-induced movement therapy in stroke patients: systematic review and meta-analysis. *Eur J Phys Rehabil Med.* 2010;46(4):537–544.

59. Shi YX, Tian JH, Yang KH, Zhao Y. Modified constraint-induced movement therapy versus traditional rehabilitation in patients with upper-extremity dysfunction after stroke: a systematic review and meta-analysis. *Arch Phys Med Rehab.* 2011;92:972–982. https://doi.org/10.1016/j.apmr.2010.12.036.

60. Corbetta D, Sirtori V, Castellini G, Moja L, Gatti R. Constraint-induced movement therapy for upper extremities in people with stroke. *Cochrane Database Syst Rev.* 2015;10:CD004433. https://doi.org/10.1002/14651858.CD004433.pub3.

61. Morgan C, Fetters L, Adde L, et al. Early intervention for children aged 0 to 2 years with or at high risk of cerebral palsy: international clinical practice guideline based on systematic reviews. *JAMA Pediatr.* 2021;175(8):846–858. https://doi.org/10.1001/jamapediatrics.2021.0878.

62. Jackman M, Sakzewski L, Morgan C, et al. Interventions to improve physical function for children and young

people with cerebral palsy: international clinical practice guideline. *Dev Med Child Neurol.* 2021; Sep 21 https://doi.org/10.1111/dmcn.15055. Online ahead of print.

63. Eliasson AC, Nordstrand L, Ek L, et al. The effectiveness of Baby-CIMT in infants younger than 12 months with clinical signs of unilateral-cerebral palsy; an explorative study with randomized design. *Res Dev Disabil.* 2018;72:191–201. https://doi.org/10.1016/j.ridd.2017.11.006.

64. Hoare BJ, Wallen MA, Thorley MN, et al. Constraint-induced movement therapy in children with unilateral cerebral palsy. *Cochrane Database Syst Rev.* 2019;4 (4):CD00419.. https://doi.org/10.1002/14651858. CD004149.pub3.

65. Chamudot R, Parush S, Rigbi A, Horovitz R, Gross-Tsur V. Effectiveness of modified constraint-induced movement therapy compared with bimanual therapy home programs for infants with hemiplegia: a randomized controlled trial. *Am J Occup Ther.* 2018;72(6): https://doi.org/10.5014/ajot.2018.025981. 7206205010p1-7206205010p9.

66. Ouyang R, Yang C, Qu Y, et al. Effectiveness of hand-arm bimanual intensive training on upper extremity function I children with cerebral palsy: a systematic review. *Eur J Paediatr Neurol.* 2020;25:17–28.

67. Sakzewski L, Ziviani J, Boyd RN. Efficacy of upper limb therapies for unilateral cerebral palsy: a meta-analysis. *Pediatrics.* 2014;133(1):e175–e204.

68. Chen Y-T, Pinto Neto O, de Miranda Marzullo AC, et al. Age-associated impairment in endpoint accuracy of goal-directed contractions performed with two fingers is due to altered activation of the synergistic muscles. *Exp Gerontol.* 2012;47:519–5126. https://doi.org/10.1016/j.exger.2012.04.007.

69. Kolb B, Harker A, Gibb R. Principles of plasticity in the developing brain. *Dev Med Child Neurol.* 2017;59(12):1218–1223.

70. Gmmash AS, Effgen SK. Early intervention services for infants with or at risk for cerebral palsy. *Pediatri Phys Ther.* 2019;31(3):242–249.

71. Chua L-K, Dimapilis MK, Iwatsuk T, Abdollahiour R, Lewthwaite R, Wulf G. Practice variability promotes an external focus of attention and enhances motor skill learning. *Hum Mov Sci.* 2019;64:307–319. https://doi.org/10.1016/j.mov.2019.02.015.

72. Edwards IM, Elliot D, Lee TD. Contextual interference effects during skill acquisition and transfer in Down syndrome adolescents. *Adapt Phys Activ Q.* 1986;3:250–258.

73. Herbert EP, Landin D, Solmon MA. Practice schedule effects on the performance and learning of low- and high-skilled students: an applied study. *Res Q Exerc Sport.* 1996;67:52–58.

74. Del Rey P, Whitehurst M, Wughalter E, et al. Contextual interference and experience in acquisition and transfer. *Percept Mot Skills.* 1983;57:241–242.

75. Winstein CJ, Gardner ER, McNeal DR, et al. Standing balance training: effect on balance and locomotion in hemiparetic adults. *Arch Phys Med Rehabil.* 1989;70:755–762.

76. Gentile AM. A working model of skill acquisition with application to teaching. *Quest.* 1972;17(1):3–23. https://doi.org/10.1080/00336297.1972.10519717.

77. Wulf G, Lewthwaite R. Optimizing performance through intrinsic motivation and attention for learning: the OPTIMAL theory of motor learning. *Psychon Bull Rev.* 2016;23:1382–1414. https://doi.org/10.3758/s13423-015-0999-9.

78. Kaefer A, Chiviacowsky S. Relatedness support enhances motivation, positive affect, and motor learning in adolescents. *Hum Move Sci.* 2021;79:102864. https://doi.org/10.1016/j.humov.2021.102864.

79. Levac D, Driscoll K, Galvez J, Mercado K, O'Neil L. OPTIMAL practice conditions enhance the benefits of gradually increasing error opportunities on retention of a stepping sequence task. *Hum Mov Sci.* 2017;56(Pt B):129–138.

80. Lessa HT, Chiviacowsky S. Self-controlled practice benefits motor learning in older adults. *Hum Mov Sci.* 2015;40:372–380. https://doi.org/10.1016/j.humov.2015.01.013.

81. Chiviacowsky S, Drews R. Effect of generic versus non-generic feedback on motor skill learning in children. *PLos One.* 2014;9(2):e88989. https://doi.org/10.1371/journal.pone.0088989.

82. Teixeira da Silva M, Lessa HT, Chiviacowsky S. External focus of attention enhances children's learning of a classical ballet pirouette. *J Dance. Med Sci.* 2017;21(4):179–184. https://doi.org/10.12678/1089-313X.21.4.179.

83. Chiviacowsky S, Wulf G, Avila L. An external focus of attention enhances motor learning in children with intellectual disabilities. *J Intellect Disabil Res.* 2013;57:627–634. https://doi.org/10.1111/j.1365-2788.2012.01569.x.

84. Chiviacowsky S, Wulf G, Lewthwaite R, Campos T. Motor learning benefits of self-controlled practice in persons with Parkinson's disease. *Gait Posture.* 2012;35:601–605. https://doi.org/10.1016/j.gaitpost.2011.12.003.

85. Chiviacowsky S, Wulf G, Wally R. An external focus of attention enhances balance learning in older adults. *Gait Posture.* 2010;32:572–575. https://doi.org/10.1016/j.gaitpost.2010.08.004.

86. Reis E. Physical therapy for people with autism: PTs explain why their role-nonexistent not so long ago- is vitally important today. *PT in Motion.* 2018;10(6):26–34.

87. Winstein CJ, Pohl PS, Lewthwaite R. Effects of physical guidance and knowledge of results on motor learning: support for a guidance hypothesis. *Res Q Exerc Sport*. 1994;65(4):316–324.

88. Savion-Lemieux T, Bailey JA, Penhune VB. Developmental contributions to motor sequence learning. *Exp Brain Res*. 2009;195:293–306.

89. Adolph KE, Franchak JM. The development of motor behavior. *Wiley Interdiscip Rev Cogn Sci*. 2017;8(1-2). https://doi.org/10.1002/wcs.1430.

90. Hadders-Algra M. Early human motor development: from variation to the ability to vary and adapt. *Neurosci Biobehav Rev*. 2018;90:411–427.

91. Adolph KE, Vereijken B, Shrout PE. What changes in infant walking and why. *Child Dev*. 2003;74:475–497.

92. Adolph KE. Learning to move. *Curr Dir Psychol Sci*. 2008;17(3):213–218.

93. Berger SE, Adolph KE. Learning and development in infant locomotion. *Prog Brain Res*. 2007;164:237–255.

94. Pinto-Zipp G, Gentile AM. Practice schedules in motor learning: children vs. adults. *Soc Neurosci Abstr*. 1995; 21:1620.

95. Jarus T, Goverover Y. Effects of contextual interference and age on acquisition, retention and transfer of motor skill. *Percept Mot Skills*. 1999;88:437–447.

96. Perez CR, Meira CM, Tani G. Does the contextual interference effect last over extended transfer trials? *Percept Mot Skills*. 2005;10(1):58–60.

97. Vera JG, Alvarex JC, Medina MM. Effects of different practice conditions on acquisition, retention, and transfer of soccer skills by 9-year-old schoolchildren. *Percept Mot Skills*. 2008;106(2):447–460.

98. Douvis SJ. Variable practice in learning the forehand drive in tennis. *Percept Mot Skills*. 2005;101(2): 531–545.

99. Granda VJ, Montilla MM. Practice schedule and acquisition, retention and transfer of a throwing task in 6-year-old children. *Percept Mot Skills*. 2003;96: 1015–1024.

100. Sommerville JA, Hildebrand EA, Crane CC. Experience mattes: the impact of doing versus watching on infants' subsequent perception of tool use events. *Dev Psychol*. 2008;44(5):1249–1256.

101. Newell KM, Kennedy JA. Knowledge of results and children's motor learning. *Dev Psychol*. 1978;14:531–536.

102. Sullivan KJ, Kantak SS, Burtner PA. Motor learning in children: feedback effects on skill acquisition. *Phys Ther*. 2008;88:720–732.

103. Emanuel M, Jarus T, Bart O. Effect of focus of attention and age on motor acquisition, retention, and transfer: a randomized trial. *Phys Ther*. 2008;88(2):251–260.

104. Krause LM, Buszard T, Reid M, Pinder R, Farrow D. Assessment of elite junior tennis serve and return practice: a cross-sectional observation. *J Sports Sci*. 2019;37 (24):2818–2825. https://doi.org/10.1080/02640414.201 9.1665245.

105. Krause LM, Farrow D, Pinder R, Buszard T, Kovalchik S, Reid M. Enhancing skill transfer in tennis using representative learning design. *J Sports Sci*. 2019;37(22): 2560–2568. https://doi.org/10.1080/02640414.2019.16 47739.

106. Moradi J, Movahedi A, Salehi H. Specificity of learning a sport skill to the visual condition of acquisition. *J Mot Beh*. 2014;46(1):17–23. https://doi. org/10.1080/00222895.2013.838935.

107. Roig M, Ritterband-Rosenbaum A, Lundbye-Jensen J, Nielsen JB. Aging increases the susceptibility to motor memory interference and reduces off-line gains in motor skill learning. *Neurobiol Aging*. 2014;35:1892–1900.

108. Moody RA, Cirillo J, Byblow WD. Neurophysiological mechanisms underlying motor skill learning in young and older adults. *Exp Brain Res*. 2019;237(9):2331–2344. https://doi.org/10.1007/s00221-019-05599-8.

109. Cirillo J. Physical activity, motor performance and skill learning: a focus on primary motor cortex I healthy aging. *Exp Brain Res*. 2021; Sep 9. https://doi.org/10.1007/ s00221-021-06218-1.

110. Statton MA, Encarnacion M, Celnik P, Bastian AJ. A single bout of moderate aerobic exercise improves motor skill acquisition. 2015;10. e0141393. https://doi. org/10.1371/journal.pone.0141393.

111. Anderson SC, Curtin D, Hawi Z, et al. Intensity matters: high-intensity interval exercise enhances motor cortex plasticity more than moderate exercise. *Cereb Cortex*. 2020;30(1):101–112. https://doi.org/10.1093/cercor/ bhz075.

112. Thomas R, Johnsen LK, Geertsen SS, et al. Acute exercise and motor memory consolidation: the role of exercise intensity. *Plos One*. 2016;11. https://doi. org/10.1371/journal.pone.0159589. e0159589.

113. Shea CH, Park JH, Braden HW. Age-related effects in sequential motor learning. *Phys Ther*. 2006;86(4): 478–488.

114. Tunney N, et al. Aging and motor learning of a functional motor task. *Phys Occup Ther Geriatr*. 2003;21(3): 1–16.

115. Salthouse TA, Somberg BL. Skill performance: effects of adult age and experience on elementary processes. *J Exp Psychol Gen*. 1982;111:176–207.

116. Hertzog CK, Williams MV, Walsh DA. The effect of practice on age differences in central perceptual processing. *J Gerontol*. 1976;31:428–433.

117. Jamieson BA, Rogers WA. Age-related effects of blocked and random practice schedules on learning a new technology. *J Gerontol B Psychol Sci Soc Sci*. 2000;55B(6): P343P353.

118. Del Rey P. Effects of contextual interference on the memory of older females differing in levels of physical activity. *Percept Mot Skills.* 1982;55:171–180.

119. Hickman JM, Rogers WA, Fisk AD. Training older adults to use new technology. *J Gerontol B Psychol Sci Soc Sci.* 2007;62B(Special Issue I):77–84.

120. Kausler DH, Wiley JG, Phillips PL. Adult age differences in memory for massed and distributed repeated actions. *Psychol Aging.* 1990;5:530–534.

121. Swanson LR, Lee TD. Effects of aging and schedules of knowledge of results on motor learning. *J Gerontol.* 1992;47(6): P406P411.

122. Wishart LR, Lee TD. Effects of aging and reducing relative frequency of knowledge of results on learning a motor skill. *Percept Mot Skills.* 1997;84:1107–1122.

123. van Dijk H, Mulder T, Hermens HJ. Effects of age and content of augmented feedback on learning an isometric force-production task. *Exp Aging Res.* 2007;33(3): 341–353.

124. Swinnen SP, Verschueren SMP, Bogaerts H, et al. Age-related deficits in motor learning and differences in feedback processing during the production of a bimanual coordination pattern. *Cogn Neuropsychol.* 1998; 15(5):439–466.

125. Wishart LR, Lee TD, Murdoch JE, et al. Effects of aging on automatic and effortful processes in bimanual coordination. *J Gerontol B Psychol Sci Soc Sci.* 2000;55B(2): P85P94.

126. Wishart LR, Lee TD, Murdoch JE. Age-related differences and the role of augmented visual feedback in learning a bimanual coordination pattern. *Acta Psychol (Amst).* 2002;110(2–3):247–263.

127. Nguyen L, Murphy K, Andrews G. Cognitive and neural plasticity in old age: a systematic review of evidence from executive functions cognitive training. *Ageing Res Rev.* 2019;53:100912. https://doi.org/10.1016/j.arr.2019.100912.

128. Johnston MV. Plasticity in the developing brain: implications for rehabilitation. *Dev Disabil Res Rev.* 2009;15 (2):94–101. https://doi.org/10.1002/ddrr.64.

129. Lebeer J. How much brain does a mind need? Scientific, clinical, and educational implication of ecological plasticity. *Dev Med Child Neurol.* 1998;40:352–357.

130. Kleim JA, Jones TA. Principles of experience-dependent neural plasticity: implications for rehabilitation after brain damage. *J Speech Lang Hear Res.* 2008;51: S225–S239.

5

Skeletal System Changes

OBJECTIVES

After studying this chapter, the reader will be able to:

1. Describe the structures and components of the skeletal system.
2. Identify the function of bone and cartilage in supporting posture and movement.
3. Discuss unique structural and functional characteristics of the skeletal system in the developing fetus, infant, child, adolescent, adult, and older adult.
4. Relate the age-related characteristics of the skeletal system to functional movement abilities and risk factors.
5. Incorporate consideration of life span development of the skeletal system into patient assessment and treatment planning.

The ability to walk, run, lift, and manipulate objects is influenced by the strength and resilience of the skeletal system. A young infant cannot walk, climb stairs, push a stroller, or tie shoes. Not only do infants lack the experience and practice necessary for these tasks, their immature skeleton does not provide a structural framework on which these movements can take place. Older adults may not have the spring in their step, power in their tennis serve, or manual dexterity they enjoyed when they were younger. The changes in the skeletal system that occur with aging may contribute to decreased efficiency of movement. Across the life span, the skeletal system evolves and influences our ability for unrestricted movement.

The skeletal system, as discussed in this chapter, consists of the bony skeleton and cartilage. The skeleton provides a structure on which muscles can work. The size and shape of the bones, mechanics of joint articulations, and location of muscular attachments form an efficient system of levers and struts. Joints allow bones to articulate with each other, and the shape of the joint contributes to efficiency of movement. Cartilage acts as a shock absorber and protects joint surfaces from wear and tear. We better appreciate the contribution of the skeletal system to functional movement when we understand the role of its components and their changing properties throughout development.

COMPONENTS OF THE SKELETAL SYSTEM

Cartilage

Cartilage, a type of connective tissue, can tolerate mechanical stress and acts as a supporting structure in the body. It provides a mechanism for shock absorption, acts as a sliding surface for the joints, and plays a role in the development and growth of bone. During fetal development, a cartilage model is laid down from which the long bones of the body will develop. The ends of immature long bones and some sites of muscular attachment also contain cartilage plates, which are sites of bone growth.

Three types of cartilage exist, each meeting different functional needs (Fig. 5.1). *Hyaline cartilage* is the most abundant and rigid. It is found at the articular surfaces

HYALINE CARTILAGE

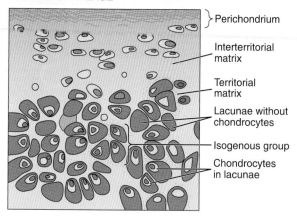

- Perichondrium
- Interterritorial matrix
- Territorial matrix
- Lacunae without chondrocytes
- Isogenous group
- Chondrocytes in lacunae

FIBROCARTILAGE

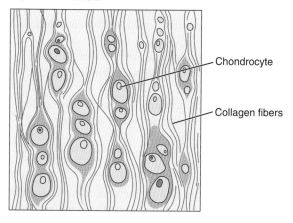

- Chondrocyte
- Collagen fibers

ELASTIC CARTILAGE

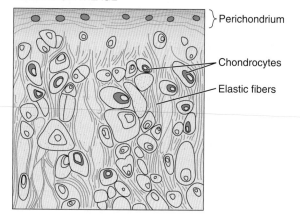

- Perichondrium
- Chondrocytes
- Elastic fibers

Fig. 5.1 Diagram of the types of cartilage. (From Gartner LP, Hiatt JL. *Color Textbook of Histology*. 2nd ed. Philadelphia: WB Saunders; 2001:130.)

of joints and the walls of respiratory passages, such as the trachea and bronchi. Hyaline cartilage also makes up the fetal model of the future long bones and can be found at the epiphyseal growth plates of immature bone. *Fibrocartilage* is found at the acetabulum, intervertebral disks, menisci, and tendinous insertions. It is more pliable than hyaline cartilage but still provides strength and support to the skeletal system. Fibrocartilage fibers are arranged parallel to the stress forces that the tissue experiences. *Elastic cartilage* is the most pliable cartilage and can be found at the larynx, ear, and epiglottis, where it provides support with flexibility.

Hyaline cartilage covers the ends of the bones that make up synovial joints, and in this capacity, it is called *articular cartilage*. It is responsible for facilitating motion at the joints and can tolerate a variety of loading forces. Synovial fluid and the compression of fluids from within the surface of the articular cartilage contribute to lubrication of the joint. Articular cartilage provides a low friction surface and allows joints to move freely through older adulthood.[1,2] Years of microtrauma, isolated instances of more severe joint trauma, and aging of the cartilaginous tissue eventually result in a breakdown of articular cartilage, which contributes to the development of *osteoarthritis* (OA) for many older adults.

Properties

Cartilage consists of water, proteoglycans, collagen fibers, and cartilage cells (*chondrocytes*). The proteoglycans and collagen fibers make up the extracellular collagen matrix surrounding the chondrocytes. Differences in the extracellular matrix and amount of water in the tissue help to differentiate the three types of cartilage. For example, the water content of articular cartilage is 60%–80% and contributes to the ability of the tissue to absorb shock.[1] Fibrocartilage consists of a high density of collagen fibers which contribute to its strength. The collagen matrix contributes to the stiffness and resilience of the collagen and helps to bind water within the cartilage.[3]

Cartilage has no nerve supply and no vascular supply of its own. Oxygen and nutrients must be obtained from surrounding tissues. Most cartilage is covered by a layer of dense connective tissue called the *perichondrium*. The perichondrium is vascularized and supplies nutrients to the cartilage via diffusion. Articular cartilage is not covered with perichondrium and depends on diffusion of nutrients from synovial fluid and subchondral bone. In articular cartilage, periods of compression and decompression facilitate the exchange of fluids: during decompression, osmotic forces allow nutrients to diffuse into the cartilage, and during compression, fluids and waste products can be squeezed out.[2] Both processes are necessary to maintain adequate nutrition of the cartilage. Health of the articular cartilage is promoted through use, or the loading of the cartilage.[4] In the absence of mechanical loading, atrophy of the articular tissue may be seen. The atrophied articular cartilage may be less able to withstand weight-bearing and movement forces, leading to further degeneration of the cartilage.[3,4]

Formation

Cartilage is derived from embryonic mesoderm, as is other connective tissue. Cartilage growth occurs through two different processes: interstitial growth and appositional growth. Interstitial growth occurs within the cartilage through mitotic division of the existing chondrocytes. It occurs in the early phases of cartilage development to increase tissue mass, at the epiphyseal plates of long bones, and at articular surfaces. In appositional growth, new cartilage is laid down at the surface of the perichondrium. In this process, chondroblasts of the perichondrium, which are precursors to chondrocytes, form an extracellular matrix and develop into mature chondrocytes. Nonarticular cartilage loses the capacity for interstitial growth early and then undergoes only appositional growth.

In the formation of articular cartilage, three structurally and functionally different layers form. In the surface layer, collagen fibers of the extracellular matrix weave together and form a loop parallel to the joint surface. This layer serves to protect the deeper layers of the cartilage. In the middle layer, collagen fibers are arranged obliquely and provide protection from compressive forces. Collagen fibers in the deepest layers are arranged perpendicular to the joint surface and further protect from compressive forces. This structural arrangement helps the cartilage to retain water and maintain mechanical function.[2]

With use and age, cells of the articular surface are worn away, the cartilage thins, and eventually the surface changes. Cartilage repair depends on interstitial growth and the ability of chondrocytes to synthesize and maintain the extracellular matrix. Articular cartilage has the ability to repair itself, undergo limited mitosis, metabolize nutrients, and maintain its matrix

even during aging. Aging cartilage is more limited than younger cartilage in its ability to repair because of a decrease in the number of cartilage cells with aging[5] and possibly because of a decreased ability to synthesize a new extracellular matrix.[3–5] For example, with rest, a young individual with chondromalacia is able to recover from articular cartilage damage. In the older individual, similar cartilage degeneration cannot be repaired, and OA results.

The factors that limit healing in cartilage are the limited ability of mature chondrocytes to divide and the avascularity of cartilage. Some repair can occur only in cartilage with perichondrium where limited new cartilage cells are produced.[1] Damaged articular cartilage is replaced by dense connective tissue or fibrocartilage, whose mechanical properties are not optimal for providing low-friction joint motion under high mechanical loads. The effects of aging and wear and tear over time result in a worn, less efficient articular surface.

Aging

The composition of articular cartilage changes with age. Aging changes in articular cartilage increase the risk of articular cartilage degeneration and include fibrillation of the articular surface and decrease in the size and aggregation of proteoglycan aggrecans. There is an increase in collagen and protein cross-linking which causes loss of tensile strength and increased stiffness. There are changes in the composition of the cellular matrix of the chondrocyte, less effective chondrocyte repair ability, calcification of cartilage, loss of water concentration, and increased fibrillation.[3,6] The cellular matrix changes include changes in water concentration and loss of some of the protein molecules that contribute to the stiffness and resilience of articular cartilage. As cartilage loses its stiffness and tensile strength, it is more susceptible to injury.[7]

Increased cross-linkage of collagen fibers, elastin fibers, and protein causes the extracellular matrix to become more rigid and eventually calcify, making diffusion of nutrients more difficult. If cartilage nutrition cannot be maintained, chondrocytes die. Calcification is seen when calcium phosphate crystals enter the cartilage matrix.[1,3] When cartilage is damaged in the adult, blood vessels also develop at the site of injury to assist in healing, but this blood supply leads to calcification rather than repaired cartilage.[1] Decreased numbers of cells are seen throughout the cartilage, especially at weight-bearing surfaces. Repeated exposure to mechanical loading wears away the cartilage and compromises its ability to protect the articulating bony surfaces. The extracellular matrix of the articular cartilage becomes hard and brittle, resulting in decreased resiliency, strength, and efficiency. Friction increases during joint movement with the thinning, fraying, and cracking of articular cartilage.

With age, cartilage becomes dehydrated, poorly nourished, and thinner. It is less able to withstand stresses placed upon it, and when damage occurs, the cartilage cannot repair itself effectively. Over time, this is one mechanism that is thought to lead to OA.[4] Another theory relates the cause of OA to wear and tear on the articular cartilage from lifelong stresses.[7] OA was originally considered strictly a mechanical issue from the "wear and tear" of the joint over time. A growing body of evidence from molecular studies now demonstrates that abnormal gene expression that is regulated by epigenetic mechanisms plays an important role in the pathogenesis of OA.[8] Epigenetics is defined as the modification of gene expression without changes in the underlying DNA sequence.

Bone

The bony skeleton accounts for 14% of older adult weight, 15% of the weight of the newborn, and 17% of young adult weight. It also accounts for 97%–98% of the total height. Intervertebral disks contribute to the remaining height. In humans, bone has several functions, including (1) protection of vital organs, (2) support of body weight, (3) storage for minerals, (4) structural leverage for movement, and (5) bone marrow storage.[9]

Bony protection of the central nervous system is provided by the skull, which forms a vault around the brain, and by the vertebral column, which encases the spinal cord. The rib cage protects the lungs and heart. The bones of the vertebral column, shoulder girdle, pelvic girdle, upper extremities, and lower extremities are arranged to effectively support the body weight in upright postures. Joints functionally connect the bones, enhancing their support functions or fostering efficient articulations. Muscles are strategically attached to this bony framework, allowing efficient movement to occur with muscular contraction.

In addition to providing protection and support, bone is a storage site for materials used by the body. Bone marrow, which is important in the formation of blood cells, is stored in bone. Calcium, phosphate, and other ions are stored in bone as crystalline salts. These salts contribute to the strength of the bone and its ability to withstand the compressive forces of weight bearing. The stored minerals are also used to maintain blood mineral levels when changes in diet or metabolic demand occur. If the blood levels of calcium and phosphate drop, these minerals are accessed from the bone. Likewise, after a meal, calcium is deposited in bone or excreted rather than increased in blood levels.

The structure of bone, as well as its stiffness and strength, allows it to meet the functional demands of everyday activities. Throughout development, bone must be produced and maintained in sufficient quantity to withstand a lifetime of weight bearing, movement, and functional activity.

General Structure and Form

Bone is a connective tissue composed of bone cells and bone matrix. These elements are held together by a ground substance. The bone matrix is a hard, calcified substance made up of collagen fibers and mineral salts. It surrounds the primary bone cell, the *osteocyte*, which functions to maintain the nutrition and mineral content of the bone matrix. Two other types of bone cells are the *osteoblast*, which is active in the formation of new bone, and the *osteoclast*, which is associated with the resorption of bone. Osteoblasts are found on the surface of bone and synthesize new bone matrix. As they are encased in sufficient bone matrix, they become osteocytes. Osteoclasts are found in areas of bone resorption, where they break down the bone matrix and release minerals into the circulation.[9]

The external surface of bone, except at articular surfaces, is covered with periosteum. The periosteum is made up of collagen fibers and bone-forming cells, which provide a source of osteoblasts. The internal surface of bone, the *endosteum*, is thinner than the periosteum but also supplies osteoblasts for bone growth and repair. Both surfaces are vascularized and play a role in nutrition of bone.

All bones are made up of two types of bone tissue: *compact bone* (also called *cortical bone* or *lamellar bone*) and *cancellous bone* (also called *trabecular or spongy bone*) (Fig. 5.2). Compact bone, which is hard and dense, represents the majority of bone in the human skeleton. It makes up the shaft of long bones and provides a thin outer covering for areas of cancellous bone. Compact

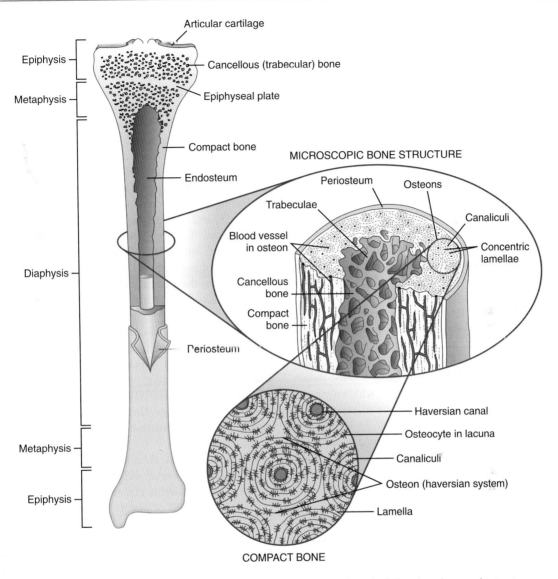

Fig. 5.2 The structural components of a long bone with cross sections depicting the microscopic structure and enlarged view of compact bone with haversian system.

bone is dense and stiff, which allows it to resist bending and torsional forces. Compact bone supports the body weight, protects vital organs, provides a lever system for movement, and stores/releases calcium.[10] Cancellous bone, made up of loosely woven strands of bone tissue (*trabeculae*), represents only about 20% of bone in the human skeleton. It is found at the ends of the long bones and surrounds the inner bone marrow cavity of the shaft. The open spaces of the cancellous bone house

the bone marrow, minerals, and vessels that nourish the bone. With a rich supply of red bone marrow, cancellous bone is a site for production of blood cells and a source for stem cells.[10] The structure of the trabeculae of the cancellous bone provides more flexibility than compact bone, making the cancellous (trabecular) bone more responsive to compressive forces.[11] Cancellous bone is made up of large amounts of water, fat, and bone marrow. This composition allows the cancellous bone to provide shock absorption for the mechanical load placed upon the joints and transfers the load to the cortical bone.[12]

Compact bone is formed when thin plates of bone (*lamellae*) are arranged concentrically around a channel containing blood vessels and nerves (*haversian canals*). This vascular channel is formed when new bone matrix surrounds existing blood vessels. Four to 20 lamellae surround a haversian canal, making up an osteon (*haversian system*). Osteons provide a mechanism to maintain nutrition of the bone. They are continuously being destroyed and rebuilt throughout the life span.

Fig. 5.2 shows compact bone surrounding a portion of cancellous bone within one of the long bones of the human skeleton. The shaft of the long bones contains a marrow cavity. This structure allows the load-bearing compact bone to form the outer ring of the shaft of the bone and moves the load-bearing function away from the center of the bone. Because of this structure, the long bones provide a light-weight structure that can effectively resist bending, torsional, and compressive forces. In adulthood, through the activity of osteoclasts and osteoblasts, the size of this central canal and the radius of the long bone increase (see Fig. 5.3), which mechanically increases the ability of the bone to resist forces placed on it.[11,12]

Cancellous bone formation is influenced by mechanical forces exerted upon the tissue. Thickness and directional alignment of the trabeculae develop based upon the mechanical stresses experienced by the tissue.[13] Remodeling of cancellous bone continues across the life span in relation to the forces placed upon the bone. Bones of the spine, wrist, and hip are made up of a high proportion of cancellous bone. As we age, loss of cancellous bone occurs earlier than that of cortical bone. It is not surprising then that the wrist, spine, and hip are frequent sites of fracture in older adults with osteoporosis.

The general form of each bone, its muscular attachments, and its anatomic relationships are all genetically determined. Heredity and the mechanical stresses placed on developing bone dictate the shape, size, and structure of the mature bone. Bone mass, girth, cortical thickness, curvature, density, and arrangement of trabeculae are influenced by the mechanical stresses produced during functional activities. Heredity also appears to influence bone mass as evidenced by the racial differences in skeletal weight, bone size, bone metabolism, and bone mineral content of adults of different races. Bone size, bone mineral density, and bone strength of non-Hispanic Black children, adolescents, and adults are greater than in non-Hispanic White individuals.[14–17] Asian individuals appear to have lower bone mineral density than non-Hispanic White populations.[18,19] Racial and ethnic differences in bone size and density become apparent in childhood in non-Hispanic White, non-Hispanic Black, and Hispanic populations in the United States.[19,20] Bone metabolism also appears to vary between racial groups, with less bone turnover in non-Hispanic Black populations.[19]

The development and maintenance of bone shape, thickness, and size appear to be related to the forces placed upon the bone and influenced further by hormonal and nutritional factors. In considering the influences of mechanical loads upon bone tissue development, two theoretical models should be considered: Wolff's law and the mechanostat theory.[21] The relationship between bone structure and the mechanical loads it experiences was identified by J. Wolff in 1892. According to *Wolff's law* of bone transformation, the structure of bone will change in response to the mechanical loads placed on it, according to certain mathematical laws. Weight bearing and the pull of muscular attachments on bone during activities direct the arrangement of collagen fibers within bone trabeculae in the same direction as the stress forces.

The *mechanostat theory* explains how mechanical input is used to develop effective load-bearing bones.[22] As mechanical strain is placed upon the bone by muscle pull or the pull of gravity in weight-bearing positions, the bone adapts to effectively support the body. As mechanical forces are placed on the bone, osteoblast function is stimulated, and new bone is laid down on the periosteal surface and in the trabeculae. Likewise, when bone is not exposed to mechanical strain, because of bed rest, space flight, or immobility, osteoclast activity is favored, and bone is resorbed from the endosteal surface and the trabeculae. It is thought that the osteoclast is the cell that detects the mechanical forces placed on the bone because the osteoclast is surrounded by fluid and displaced by compression. The osteoclast and its dendrites then trigger the response by the osteoblasts. If insufficient compression is placed upon the osteoclast, it is thought that nutrition to the osteocyte is compromised and the cell dies, triggering the osteoclast function.[23] In addition to the mechanical forces on the bone, the mechanostat theory also considers the hormonal

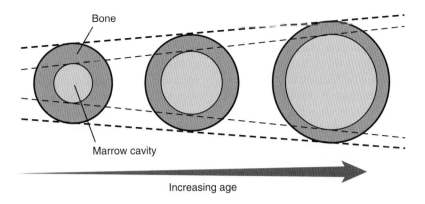

Bone

Marrow cavity

Increasing age

Fig. 5.3 Schematic approximates the effect of appositional bone growth over time, which leads to an increase in the diameter of bone. Bone thickness decreases, and the width of the marrow cavity increases because resorption is greater than production.

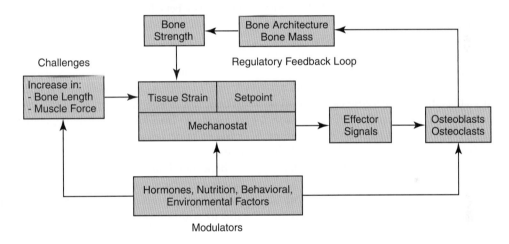

Fig. 5.4 A functional model of bone development based on the mechanostat theory. (From Rauch F, Schoenau E. The developing bone: slave or master of its cells and molecules? *Pediatr Res.* 2001;50(3):309-314.)

and nutritional influences on bone growth (Fig. 5.4).[22–24] Based on the mechanostat theory, mechanical strain and hormonal and nutritional factors all influence the shape, size, and density of the bone. These theories support the importance of physical activity, especially in weight bearing, on optimizing bone development, bone density, and bone strength.

As discussed earlier, nutrition and hormones are important factors in the growth and development process of bone. Throughout life, nutrition influences the effectiveness with which bone can be formed and maintained. People who do not have sufficient protein, calcium, vitamin D, and vitamin C in their diet experience

abnormal bone growth. Protein makes up a significant component of bone and is also important for utilization of insulin-like growth factor-1 (IGF-1) hormone in bone development. Dietary protein is important for bone remodeling and maintaining bone health across the life span. Amino acids provided by dietary protein intake are important for developing and maintaining bone structure. Levels of dietary protein appear to have a positive influence on bone mineral density in children, adults, and older adults. Across the life span, inadequate dietary protein interferes with collagen production by the osteoblasts, leading to poor calcification of the bone matrix. Protein deficiency can result in bone absorption from the endosteal surface and thinning of trabecular bone.[24-27]

Vitamins C and D play an important role in bone development, and deficiencies in these vitamins can contribute to bone malformation in children, as well as osteoporosis. Vitamin C is important in collagen synthesis to support bone development. In vitamin C deficiency, the cartilage formed for bone growth lacks collagen. In severe vitamin C deficiency (scurvy), decreased rate of growth at the cartilage growth plates of the long bones results in deficient bone formation. In animal studies, vitamin C has been found to support development of osteoclasts, stimulating bone formation, reducing osteoblast activity, and increasing bone mineral density, suggesting that vitamin C supplementation may be a resource for treating osteoporosis.[28,29] Vitamin D also contributes to osteoblast development and decreases bone resorption due to osteoclast activity.[30] Vitamin D is also important in the absorption of calcium in the gastrointestinal tract.[31] Vitamin D deficiency in children and adolescents causes rickets, as well as osteomalacia in adults. In rickets, bone growth in the region of the cartilage growth plate is distorted because calcification of the cartilage is deficient.[32] Osteomalacia results in softening of existing bone, due to impaired mineralization. Vitamin D deficiency is an ongoing problem globally, especially for individuals with decreased exposure to sunlight and for dark-skinned populations.[32]

The role of hormones, such as growth hormone (GH), insulin-like growth factor-1 (IGF-1), thyroid hormones, and sex hormones, in bone development is evident both before and after puberty. Before puberty, thyroid function, GH, and IGF-1 hormonal activity regulate bone growth.[33] During and after puberty, the sex steroid hormones begin playing a major role.[22,33] A rapid growth period accompanies the hormonal changes of adolescence. Low levels of estrogen are needed for the pubertal growth spurt of bone in both boys and girls.[34] During puberty, girls also demonstrate greater growth in cortical bone than boys, which may be related to increased sensitivity to estrogen, providing girls with increased bone storage to support gestational and lactation roles.[11,22] In contrast, accelerated loss of bone mineral content occurs immediately after menopause, again related to hormonal changes in the body. Estrogen loss plays a major role in the accelerated rate of bone loss for women in the 4–8 years after menopause.[33,35] Decreases in both circulated estrogen and testosterone play a role

in bone loss for men.[33,35] Parathyroid hormone and calcitonin also influence bone resorption because they respond to serum calcium levels. Because bone serves as the storage site for calcium, as the concentration of calcium in the blood changes, calcium in the bone is accessed through stimulation of calcium-regulating hormones. The parathyroid hormone is sensitive to serum calcium levels. If the serum calcium level gets low, then the parathyroid hormone signals for bone resorption, which will increase the amount of circulating calcium. If serum calcium levels get too high, calcitonin will signal that no further calcium needs to be resorbed from the bone, and osteoblast activity will decrease.

Development

In embryological development, bone forms from the mesoderm. Fetal bone is made of *primary* or *woven bone tissue*. Woven bone consists of an irregular array of collagen fibers and is less mineralized than mature bone. As osteons form, mineralization of the bony matrix increases, and mature bone tissue replaces woven bone. A similar process can be seen throughout development as new, woven bone is laid down and other bone tissue is resorbed. Therefore, woven bone, mature bone, and areas of bone resorption are all found in adult bone tissue.

Bone develops through one of two different processes: intramembranous ossification or endochondral ossification. *Intramembranous ossification* takes place directly within mesenchyme tissue, beginning near the end of the embryonic period and proceeding rapidly. Mesenchymal cells produce an organic matrix called *osteoid*, which is composed of collagen fibers. Calcium phosphate crystals accumulate on the collagen fibers, resulting in ossification. In this process, numerous ossification centers are formed, which fuse into cancellous bone tissue. With time, some of this cancellous bone will become compact bone. The skull, carpals, tarsals, and part of the clavicle are formed by intramembranous ossification.

In *endochondral ossification*, a hyaline cartilage model of the bone is laid down first and then replaced by bone in an orderly fashion. Endochondral bone growth is seen in the long bones of the body and is the method by which bones increase in length. The parts of the long bone (see Fig. 5.2) are defined as the following:

- Diaphysis: the shaft of the long bone; the portion of bone formed by the primary center of ossification

- Epiphysis: the ends of the long bone; the portions formed by secondary centers of ossification
- Epiphyseal plate: the bone's growth zone, which is composed of hyaline cartilage
- Metaphysis: the wider part of the shaft of the long bone, adjacent to the epiphyseal plate, which consists of cancellous bone during development; in adulthood, it is continuous with the epiphysis.

Endochondral bone development is illustrated in Fig. 5.5. Primary centers of ossification form at the center of the diaphysis. First, a bony collar is laid down around the center of the diaphysis via intramembranous ossification of the perichondrium. Cartilage cells in the central diaphysis then become hypertrophied and are destroyed. As the remaining cartilage matrix becomes calcified, the area is infiltrated by osteoblasts and capillaries. The osteoblasts lay down ossified bone matrix. Ossification proceeds toward the ends of the diaphysis. Secondary ossification centers form in the epiphysis. Ossification radiates in all directions from the secondary ossification center. Endochondral ossification is also seen in the vertebrae, as depicted in Fig. 5.6.

A growth (epiphyseal) plate, composed of hyaline cartilage, is formed between the diaphysis and epiphysis. This is the site of longitudinal bone growth. Interstitial growth of the hyaline cartilage continues at the surface of the epiphysis. The new cartilage undergoes endochondral ossification in the metaphysis. As the bone approaches its adult length, chondrocyte formation slows while endochondral ossification at the metaphysis continues. The epiphyseal plate narrows and eventually closes.

Mechanical loading of the epiphyseal plate affects longitudinal bone growth. The growth plate is usually aligned perpendicular to the load that crosses it, and formation of new bone is stimulated as tension or compression forces are applied.[9] Unequal forces along the epiphyseal plate may stimulate a change of direction of bone growth, whereas torsional forces at the growth plate may result in rotational changes. The changes in angle of inclination between the femoral neck and shaft change with age, providing an example of directional change in normal bone development. The angle of inclination is approximately 135–150 degrees in infancy, 125 degrees in the adult, and 120 degrees in the older adult (Fig. 5.7).[36] The torsional changes in the femur, from retroversion prenatally to 25–30 degrees of anteversion at birth and 10–15 degrees of anteversion

in the adult,[37] are also a result of mechanical loading (Fig. 5.7).[38] It should also be noted that shearing forces applied across the epiphyseal plate may contribute to displacement of the growth plate. Therapeutically, this is an important consideration when working with individuals whose skeleton has not reached maturity because displacement of the epiphyseal plate interferes with normal growth.

Cartilaginous growth plates are found not only at the ends of long bones but also at points of muscular attachment, where they are called traction *epiphyses* or *apophyses*. Muscle contraction places a traction force on the bone and stimulates bone growth. This is demonstrated at the proximal femur. Fig. 5.8 reflects the effects of muscle pull on the greater trochanter and lesser trochanter of the femur. The greater trochanter has broad muscular attachments, whereas the lesser trochanter has only one muscular attachment. The traction force exerted by the muscular activity stimulates varying degrees of bone growth at these locations, helping shape the developing bone into its mature form. Muscle weakness can affect bone growth, as demonstrated in Fig. 5.8, as well as bone length. Children with brachial plexus injuries at birth and with childhood onset hemiplegia demonstrate less bone growth of the involved upper extremity as compared with the upper extremity without neurological impairment, resulting in limb length inequality.[39-41]

Bones grow not only in length but also in diameter. New bone is laid down on the outer surface of the bone and is absorbed from the inner surface, determining the thickness of the bone and the size of the marrow cavity within the bone. This process is called *appositional growth* and continues throughout life, but the proportion of bone formation to resorption varies. In childhood and adolescence, formation is greater than resorption, increasing bone diameter and thickness. Throughout early and middle adulthood, equilibrium between the two processes maintains bone size. In later adult life, resorption exceeds formation, resulting in loss of bone mass. Because resorption occurs at the inner surface of the bone, the marrow cavity becomes larger, and the bony shell surrounding it becomes thinner (Fig. 5.3). Muscle weakness can also affect appositional bone growth.

Bone is an adaptable tissue, responding to hormonal demands and the mechanical stresses placed on it. To maintain bone mass and architecture, a balance must be achieved between these two processes. Good nutrition

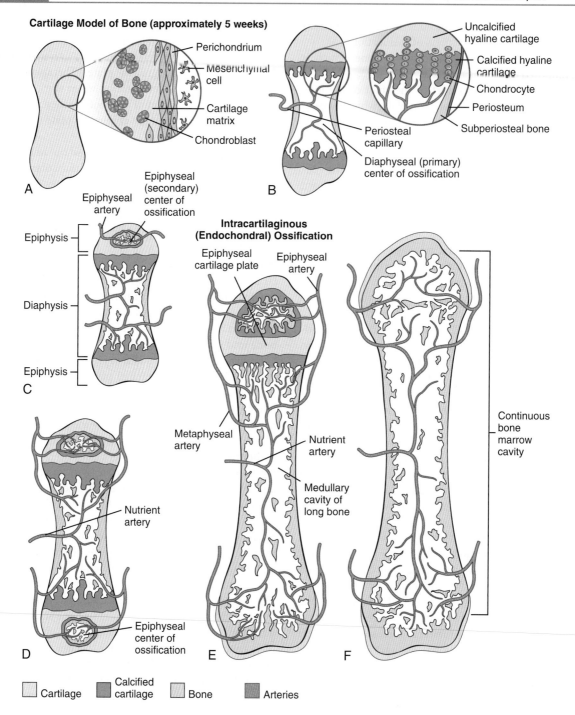

Fig. 5.5 Stages in endochondral ossification of a long bone. (**A**) Cartilage model. (**B**) Periosteal stage; cartilage begins to calcify. (**C**) Vascular mesenchyme enters the calcified cartilage matrix and divides the cartilage matrix into two zones of ossification; blood vessels and mesenchyme enter the upper epiphyseal cartilage. (**D**) The epiphyseal center of ossification develops in the cartilage. A similar center of ossification develops in the lower epiphyseal cartilage. (**E**) Intracartilaginous ossification; the lower epiphyseal plate disappears. (**F**) Next, the upper epiphyseal plate disappears, forming a continuous bone marrow cavity.

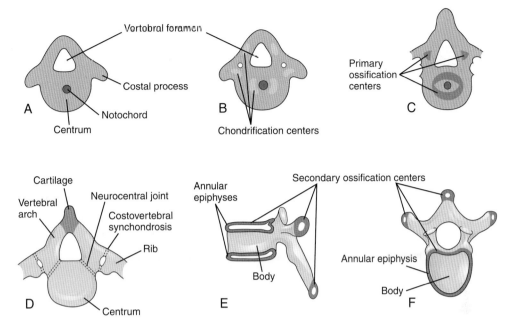

Fig. 5.6 Stages of vertebral development. (**A**) Precartilaginous vertebra at 5 weeks. (**B**) Chondrification centers in a mesenchymal vertebra at 6 weeks. (**C**) Primary centers of ossification in a cartilaginous vertebra at 7 weeks. (**D**) A thoracic vertebra at birth, consisting of three bony parts. Note the cartilage between the halves of the vertebral neural arch and between the arch and the centrum. (**E** and **F**) Two views of a typical thoracic vertebra at puberty showing the location of the secondary centers of ossification. (From Moore KL, Persaud TVN. *The Developing Human.* 6th ed. Philadelphia: WB Saunders; 1998:413.)

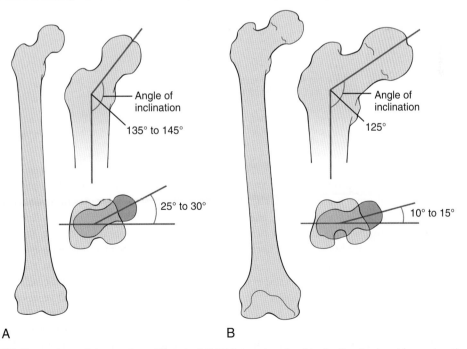

Fig. 5.7 Comparison of the newborn (**A**) and adult (**B**) femoral angle of inclination (top) and femoral angle of torsion (bottom). The enlarged views of the femoral angle of torsion show a superior perspective, looking down from the head/neck of femur to the femoral condyles.

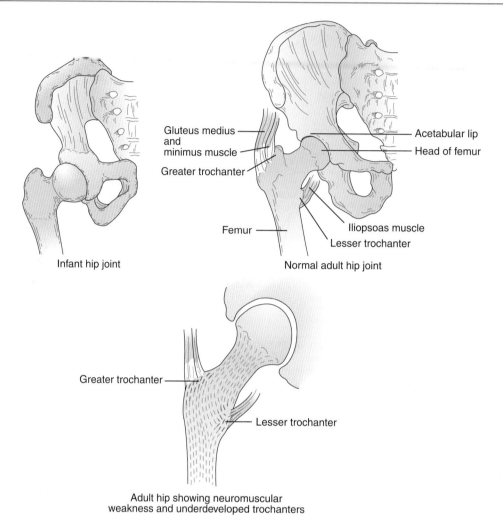

Infant hip joint

Gluteus medius and minimus muscle
Greater trochanter
Femur

Acetabular lip
Head of femur
Iliopsoas muscle
Lesser trochanter

Normal adult hip joint

Greater trochanter
Lesser trochanter

Adult hip showing neuromuscular weakness and underdeveloped trochanters

Fig. 5.8 The muscular attachments to an immature bone help to shape bone growth. Compared with the hip joint of a normal adult, a hip joint of an adult with neuromuscular weakness shows an underdeveloped trochanter.

and exercise are important throughout the life span to build and maintain maximal bone mass and structural competence of the skeleton. Many studies of the effect of exercise on bone mass suggest that increased functional loading results in increased bone mass, whereas decreased functional loading results in bone loss.[42-47] The role of exercise on bone development at various stages of the life span will be discussed later in this chapter.

Aging

As discussed, adaptation of bone through remodeling continues throughout life. Skeletal maturity, however,

as measured by closure of the epiphyseal plate, occurs within the first two decades of life. Maximal bone mass, which is the total bone growth in length and thickness, is thought to be obtained during the late 20s or early 30s.[42,43] Time of peak bone mass is difficult to specify because factors such as sex and race influence when peak bone mass is reached.[14,43] Females appear to reach peak bone mass earlier (18–20 years of age) than males (20–24 years of age) at the femoral neck, hip, and lumbar spine, supporting that peak bone mass is attained at different sites at different times.[48,49] The age at which bone resorption begins to exceed bone formation is also not consistently reported in the literature. Bone mineral density generally begins to decrease in the fifth decade for women and in the sixth decade for men.[43,50] It also appears that cancellous bone loss may begin earlier than cortical bone loss.[33,35,51] Bone loss appears to vary between racial groups[14,15] and with gender.[33,35,51] Although bone loss appears to be less severe in Black adults than it is in White adults, this may be reflective of the greater bone mass attained during bone growth in this racial group.[14–18] Women also appear to lose more bone mass than men, related to accelerated bone loss during menopause, when estrogen is no longer present to slow bone resorption. Testosterone levels of men also enhance calcium absorption in the intestinal tract, which diminishes the amount of calcium reabsorbed from the bone to maintain serum calcium levels.[33,35,51] A decrease in mass eventually results in a more fragile bone, which is less able to withstand mechanical forces such as compression and bending, which can lead to spontaneous fracture.

Other changes involved in the aging of bone include cross linkage, architectural rearrangement of collagen fibers, and excessive mineralization of trabecular bone. Fibrils are arranged more longitudinally. Osteons become shorter and narrower as the haversian canals become wider. Excessive mineralization of bone occurs as bone matrix deteriorates, because as the bone becomes more porous, more sites for mineral deposition are provided. These changes increase the brittleness of bone and compromise its ability to withstand mechanical loads.

Throughout life, the body must maintain the necessary serum calcium level. Osteoporosis can be accelerated due to reduced calcium intake over time secondary to dietary choices, or even as a result of medication interactions that decrease calcium absorption in the small intestine.[52,53] Intestinal absorption of calcium declines with age, thereby increasing the amount of calcium that must be retrieved from the bone to meet the needs of the body. Vitamin D is essential for calcium absorption. Deficiencies in vitamin D will also impair normal differentiation and proliferation of bone cells, setting the stage for this chronic disease. Older adults are faced with the challenges of maintaining a well-balanced diet in conjunction with maintaining adequate activity levels out of doors (to produce vitamin D), making them especially susceptible to long-term bone demineralization and fracture as a result of this combination.[54,55] As a result, bone mass is gradually lost because bone resorption frequently occurs faster than new bone can be formed. The loss of bone tissue during remodeling leaves the bone thinner and more susceptible to injury. The increased brittleness due to internal changes in bone structure also increases the risk of fracture.

Joints

The joints provide the functional connection between bones. The primary purpose of most joints is to enable a wide range of movement. Within the joint, bones can be connected by ligaments, tendons, muscles, other connective tissue structures, and the joint capsule. Two types of joints are found in the mature skeletal system: synarthroses and diarthroses.

Synarthrosis joints allow minimal to no movement and provide areas of stability to the skeleton. The sutures of the skull and tibiofibular joint are examples of this type of joint. The articulation between the bones consists of connective tissue, which may be replaced by bone during aging.

Diarthrosis joints allow movement. The joint capsule functionally connects two adjoining bones to form a cavity that is filled with synovial fluid, which bathes the joint surfaces with nutrition and provides a cushion between the bones (Fig. 5.9). Diarthrodial joints are found in several shapes and sizes; their shape and form help define the type of movement that can be produced at the joint. For example, hinge joints, such as the elbow, allow movement in one axis only, whereas a ball-and-socket type of joint, such as the hip, allows a wide range of motion in multiple axes.

Joint movement becomes stiffer and less flexible because the amount of lubricating fluid inside the joints decreases and the cartilage becomes thinner. Inactivity causes the cartilage to shrink and stiffen, reducing joint mobility. In addition, it has been demonstrated that aging induces structural degenerative changes to capsular, fascial, and ligamentous structures. These changes occur mainly as a result of the decrease in elastic fibers responsible for resistance.[56] There appears to be a significant interrelation among ligament degeneration, synovitis, joint cartilage degradation, and dysbalanced subchondral bone remodeling. Ligament degeneration accompanies joint cartilage degradation and includes chondroid metaplasia, cyst formation, heterotopic ossification, and mucoid and fatty degenerations.[57]

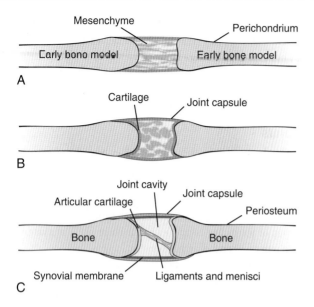

Fig. 5.9 Development of synovial joints. (**A**) Mesenchyme collects in the space between early bone models. (**B**) Differentiation of mesenchyme into cartilage and joint capsule; beginning of cavitation. (**C**) Formation of joint cavity and structure.

SKELETAL SYSTEM DEVELOPMENT

Skeletal system development follows a pattern of maturation that begins before birth and continues through the last decades of life.

Prenatal Period

As discussed earlier, bone and cartilage are differentiated from the mesoderm layer early in the gestational period. Development of bone, via either intramembranous or endochondral ossification, begins in the embryonic period (third to eighth gestational weeks). By the fifth week of gestation, mesenchymal models of bones appear in the extremities, with upper extremity development preceding lower extremity development. In the sixth week, mesenchymal cells have differentiated into chondroblasts, which form the cartilage model of the long bones. Primary centers of ossification appear as early as the seventh to eighth week (Fig. 5.10); by the 12th week of gestation, they have appeared in almost all the bones of the extremities.[58] The diaphyses are fairly well ossified by birth, but the epiphyses remain cartilaginous. A few secondary ossification

centers begin to appear late in fetal development (Figs. 5.10 and 5.11).

Vertebral development also begins in the embryonic period. Cartilage models of the vertebrae are formed from mesenchymal cells located around the notochord. By the seventh to eighth gestational week, three ossification centers have formed in the vertebrae model. These bony parts remain connected by cartilage at birth (see Fig. 5.5).[58]

After the early models of bone are present, joint formation occurs, and by the early fetal period, most joints have been formed. In articular joints, mesenchyme differentiates into the joint capsule, ligaments, tendons, and menisci. Depressions then begin to form in the mesenchyme, resulting in formation of the joint cavity and bursae (see Fig. 5.9). Once the joint is formed, intrauterine movement is important for ongoing joint development.[59]

The confined intrauterine environment in the later weeks of gestation limits the positioning options of the fetus and applies forces to the fetal skeletal system. Intrauterine molding of the developing skeletal system can occur and results in deformities such as congenital hip dislocation, tibial bowing, metatarsus adductus, calcaneus varus, and extreme ankle dorsiflexion. Some of these deformities will spontaneously improve in the first few years of life. Others, such as congenital hip dislocation, require early orthopedic management, applying corrective mechanical forces to the skeleton during infancy.

Functionally, early intramembranous ossification of the skull serves to protect the developing brain. The bones of the skull are not fused, as evidenced by the "soft spots," called *fontanelles*. Expansion and molding of the cranium accommodate brain growth. The lack of fusion of the bones of the skull also allows adaptation of the cranium to the intrauterine environment and passage through the birth canal.

Infancy and Childhood

Infancy and childhood are times of bone growth, modeling, and remodeling. Two periods of rapid growth in bone mineral density are seen in childhood, first from 1 to 4 years of age and again at puberty, preceded by similar growth spurts in body mass.[43] Bone mineral content increases more in the 2–3 years surrounding peak height velocity than at any other time in life, with 20%–30% of peak bone density and bone mineral content reported

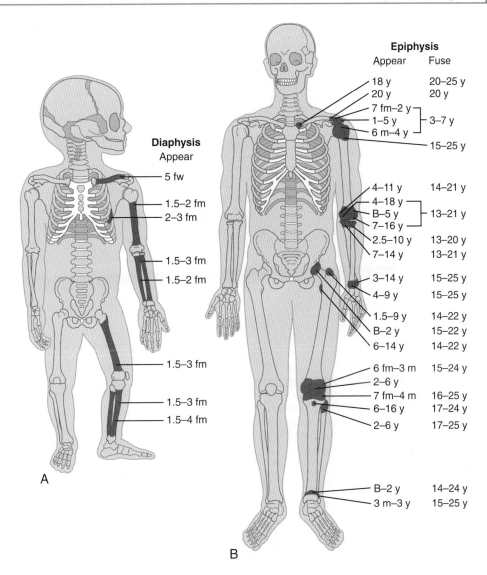

Diaphysis
Appear

— 5 fw

— 1.5–2 fm
— 2–3 fm

— 1.5–3 fm
— 1.5–2 fm

— 1.5–3 fm

— 1.5–3 fm

— 1.5–3 fm
— 1.5–4 fm

A

Epiphysis

Appear	Fuse
18 y	20–25 y
20 y	20 y
7 fm–2 y	
1–5 y	3–7 y
6 m–4 y	
	15–25 y
4–11 y	14–21 y
4–18 y	
B–5 y	13–21 y
7–16 y	
2.5–10 y	13–20 y
7–14 y	13–21 y
3–14 y	15–25 y
4–9 y	15–25 y
1.5–9 y	14–22 y
B–2 y	15–22 y
6–14 y	14–22 y
6 fm–3 m	15–24 y
2–6 y	
7 fm–4 m	16–25 y
6–16 y	17–24 y
2–6 y	17–25 y
B–2 y	14–24 y
3 m–3 y	15–25 y

B

Fig. 5.10 Appearance of primary and secondary ossification centers. (**A**) Appearance of diaphyses. (**B**) Appearance and fusion of epiphyses. *B*, Birth; *fm*, fetal months; *fw*, fetal weeks; *m*, postnatal months; *y*, years. (From Graca JC, Noback CR: Revised on the basis of Augier, 1931.)

in this time frame.[11,42,43,51,60] Children attain 50%–60% of their peak bone mass by puberty and up to 90% (in boys) and 95% (in girls) before age 20.[43,61] Before puberty, both boys and girls demonstrate similar, linear increases in peak bone mineral density and bone mineral content,[22] but after peak height velocity is reached, increases are greater for boys than girls (Fig. 5.12).[11,43,60,62] The increased testosterone levels in boys contribute to the increased level of bone formation.[51] Both bone mineral density and bone mineral content are influenced by height and weight in childhood, with bone mineral content most influenced by these factors.[43,62] Factors that may contribute to the sex differences in bone mineral content and density are related to differences in bone shape and geometry, calcium intake and absorption, hormone production, and physical activity levels.

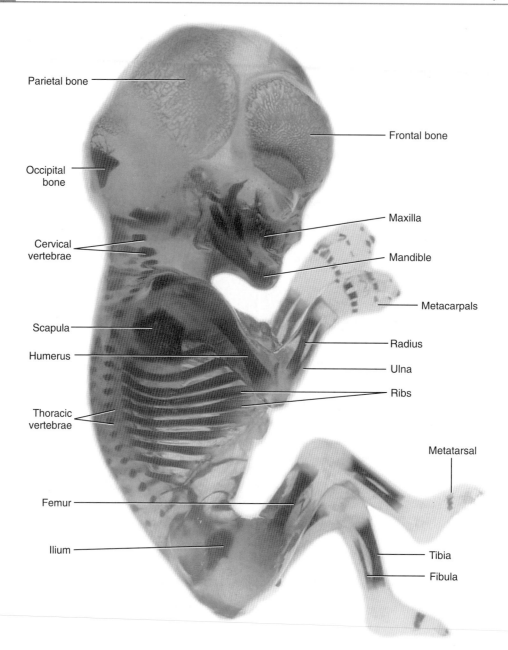

Fig. 5.11 Electron micrograph of a 12-week human fetus shows the progression of ossification from the primary centers that are endochondral in the appendicular and axial parts of the skeleton except for most of the cranial bones. (From Moore KL, Persaud TVN. *Before We Are Born: Essentials of Embryology and Birth Defects.* 5th ed. Philadelphia: WB Saunders; 1998:395.) Courtesy of Dr. Gary Geddes, Lake Oswego, Ore.

Dynamic Bone Growth

Through childhood, both endochondral and appositional bone growth are dynamic processes. As mentioned, the diaphyses of the long bones are fairly well ossified at birth. Secondary ossification centers in the epiphyses continue to appear through adolescence (see Fig. 5.10). Throughout infancy and early childhood, bone growth occurs rapidly. Physical activity has been

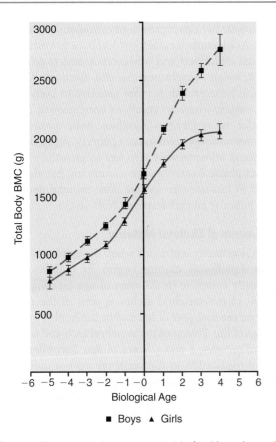

Fig. 5.12 Total bone mineral content *(g)* of subjects in yearly age increments; younger than (negative) and older than (positive) age of peak bone velocity. (From Whiting SJ, Vatanparast H, Baxter-Jones A, et al. Factors that affect bone mineral accrual in the adolescent growth spurt. *J Nutr.* 2004;134(3):696S-700S.)

demonstrated to increase bone mineral content and bone mineral density in prepubertal children.[42,43,48,60,63] Participation in physical activity, especially high-impact activities, is most beneficial in children in the years immediately preceding peak height velocity.[42,44,48,60,64] Participation in physical activity before puberty fosters growth in both muscle and bone mass. As children then continue to be active, especially in high-impact activities such as jumping, bone growth is stimulated both by weight-bearing forces and the mechanical pull of the muscles. Physical activity and sports place forces on the growing bone that impact length, size, curvature, and shape of the bone, all of which are important for optimal bone function across the life span.[48,60] Exercise programs, including high-impact activities such as jumping and soccer, have been shown to increase site-specific

bone mineral density in children through early stages of puberty,[46,65,66] regardless of ethnicity.[67]

Areas of Bone Growth

During infancy and childhood, many changes are seen in the size, shape, angulation, rotation, and proportions of the skeleton. The head and trunk of the newborn infant make up a proportionally larger part of the total skeleton than in the adult. During childhood, the growth of the axial skeleton does not contribute as much to a child's increasing height as does the growth of the lower extremities. The lower extremities and pelvis undergo angular, rotational, and length changes as the infant learns to move. At birth, the ilia and sacrum are more upright than they are in the adult. Once the infant starts walking, the curvature of the sacrum increases, the ilia thicken, and the acetabular depth increases.[68] The femoral angle of inclination decreases (see Fig. 5.6), creating a better lever arm for force production of the hip abductors. The femoral angle of torsion also changes (see Fig. 5.6), decreasing the amount of anteversion from birth to adulthood. Different rates of growth in the three epiphyseal zones of the proximal femur contribute to the angular and rotational changes of the bone.[69] By 8 years of age, the proximal femur has attained its adult form.[70]

Angular and torsional changes also take place in the tibia and ankle/foot complex. External tibial torsion increases from the newborn period to adulthood. The relationship between the femur and tibia changes from a position of genu varum (bow-legged) in infancy to one of genu valgus (knock-knee) by 3 years of age. The degree of valgus increases until approximately 7 years of age and then decreases to 5–6 degrees.[71] In adolescence, girls have demonstrated a stable valgus angle of approximately 5.5 degrees, while in boys the valgus angle decreases slightly to approximately 4.5 degrees.[72] The newborn's foot also is in a position of varus at the calcaneus and forefoot, which slowly decreases until adult values are reached. Slight forefoot varus may persist until 2 years of age. Weight bearing and the torsional forces of muscles actively contracting during creeping (four-point), standing, and walking contribute to these changes.

Not only does the lower extremity skeleton undergo transformation as the infant develops functional movement skills, but also changes are seen in the spine. In the newborn, the anteroposterior spinal curve is relatively concave. The cervical lordosis is present at birth, possibly because of early ossification of the occipital bone, but it becomes more evident by 3 months of age, when the infant has developed head control. The lumbar lordosis develops as the infant learns to sit. Iliopsoas muscle tightness from fetal positioning combined with antigravity work in prone, four-point, and kneeling positions may contribute to development of the lumbar lordosis.[73] When spinal deformities occur, such as scoliosis and kyphosis, bracing the immature skeleton places mechanical forces upon the growing spine to assist in correcting or minimizing the problem.

Adolescence

During adolescence, bone continues to grow and remodel in response to mechanical loading stresses. Physical activity, body weight, and caloric and calcium intake contribute to the growth of bone, formation of bone matrix, and bone mineralization.[43,44,60,62,74] Calcium absorption is also more efficient during puberty, especially in black teens.[42] The adolescent experiences sudden increases in height and weight, with growth of the trunk exceeding the lower extremities. The adolescent growth spurt of girls begins at an average of 12 years of age, preceding that of boys by approximately 2 years. A growth spurt in bone width is seen through adolescence in boys and up to age 14 in girls.[9] In general, boys enter puberty later than girls, and their pubertal growth spurt lasts longer than girls, contributing to greater height, bone mass, and bone size in boys as compared with girls.[51] Lean body mass is related to increases in cortical bone mass in both boys and girls, while fat mass is only related to increased cortical bone mass in girls.[75,76] Rapid bone growth frequently outpaces increases in muscle length, resulting in decreased flexibility. Injuries can result if adolescents do not modify their activities to accommodate these changes in flexibility.

Hormonal influences on growing bone change with puberty as the sex hormones, androgens and estrogen, influence bone growth and bone mineral acquisition.[42] Hormones, nutrition, and physical activity all affect the mechanostat and therefore influence bone growth during adolescence.[11] Androgens increase bone size by stimulating appositional growth in boys, while estrogen may contribute to increased cortical bone density in girls.[11,22] Estrogen appears to reduce bone resorption at the endosteal surface, while allowing bone to be laid down at the periosteal surface.[75] Hormonal influences

also appear to impact growth of cancellous (trabecular) bone. As mentioned earlier, cortical bone growth is seen through childhood and adolescence and is related to height, weight, weight bearing, and mechanical forces. Cortical bone growth is more sensitive to body height than weight, whereas cancellous bone growth is more sensitive to weight.[43] Cancellous bone growth also becomes more apparent in later puberty, suggesting that hormonal influences are also key to growth.[11,43] High-impact physical activity such as jumping has also been found to increase site-specific bone mineral density in early puberty[6] and adolescence.[46,77,78]

Attainment of Skeletal Maturity

Skeletal maturity is attained when the epiphyseal plates close. Epiphyseal closure begins in childhood and is usually complete by 25 years of age (see Fig. 5.10). Fusion of the vertebral arches is seen in the cervical spine in the first year of life and in the lumbar spine by 6 years of life. Fusion of the vertebral arch and centrum occurs between 5 and 8 years of age. Secondary centers of ossification in the vertebrae do not unite until the 25th year.[58] Fusion of the epiphyses occurs earlier in girls than in boys and has been linked to the fact that estrogen levels are higher in girls than in boys.[34] When skeletal maturity is reached, 95% of peak bone mass is present. The remaining 5% of peak bone mass is attained through appositional bone growth and continued thickening of the trabeculae.[51]

Adulthood

After the epiphyses have closed, the bones no longer lengthen. Throughout adulthood, only bone remodeling occurs. Weight bearing and muscle contraction continue to stimulate bone remodeling and to increase bone density.[79] Adequate nutritional and calcium intake also supports appropriate mineralization of the remodeled bone. Both men and women attain their maximal bone mass by their late 20s or early 30s.[49,61,80,81] Bone formation and resorption remain balanced until 30–50 years of age in men and 38–48 years of age in women, with the variation reported based on ethnicity.[82] After that time, bone loss is greater than bone replacement. In the adult skeleton, cortical bone loss has been reported to begin in the fourth decade and cancellous bone loss to begin in the third decade of life.[33,51]

Several different estimates of the amount of bone loss with aging are reported in the literature. Women lose

1% of bone mass per year before menopause.[80,83] For the 4–8 years after menopause, bone loss is accelerated in women, but after this time, the rate of loss returns to 0.5%–1% per year.[80] Men are reported to lose 0.5% of bone mass per year. This loss translates into a decline in bone strength, which increases the risk for spontaneous fractures and functional motor deficits. In general, women begin to lose bone mass at an earlier age and faster rate than men.[50]

Physical activity also plays a role in bone mass during adulthood. Individuals who have been physically active through childhood and adolescence have a greater peak bone mass as they enter adulthood, and these individuals also show greater bone mass throughout adulthood than their peers who were not as active in childhood and adolescence. Participation in exercise programs does increase muscle mass in adulthood and therefore muscles can generate greater force on the bone. Appositional bone growth is stimulated by weight-bearing and strength-training exercise programs, especially those that include high-impact activities.[84–87]

Fibrous cartilage changes also become apparent in adulthood. The intervertebral disk begins to undergo changes at approximately 30 years. The nucleus pulposus loses the ability to absorb water and becomes dehydrated, impacting on the ability to function effectively in shock absorption. Structurally, small tears also appear around the annulus fibrosis, and the structural integrity of the intervertebral disc is compromised. Water loss continues slowly in older adulthood, during which the annulus fibrosus also undergoes further fibrotic changes. The intervertebral disc becomes flattened and less resilient. Considering the early changes in the disc, it is not surprising that a high incidence of back pain is reported between the ages of 30 and 50 years.[80,88]

Older Adulthood

With aging, the skeletal system becomes progressively more compromised. Loss of bone mass continues in older adulthood and can be related to osteopenia, osteomalacia, or osteoporosis. *Osteopenia* occurs when either organic or inorganic components of bone fail to develop. *Osteomalacia* refers to abnormal mineralization of the bone matrix because of calcium, vitamin D, and phosphate deficiencies.[32] It affects both recently formed and well-established bone, decreasing the amount of mineral per unit of bone matrix. *Osteoporosis* refers to a reduction in bone mass because of decreased formation of

new bone or increased resorption while bone chemistry is normal. Age-related bone loss may be related to hormonal changes, dietary changes, and the decreased activity level of older adults.[89,90] Decreased estrogen levels in both women and men are primarily responsible for loss of bone mineral density in older adults.[33,50] Estrogen and testosterone also appear to enhance calcium absorption from the intestine, minimizing the signaling of bone resorption in response to serum calcium levels.[91] In women, the ability of estrogen to decrease bone resorption at the endosteal surface is also lost. Deficiencies in vitamin D also contribute to bone loss in older adults, possibly related to development of high parathyroid hormone levels.[33,91] Vitamin D metabolism is also affected by decreased levels of calcitonin. In addition, the diet may contain lower amounts of calcium, vitamins, and minerals.[92]

Maintaining physical activity levels and participation in weight-bearing and strength-training exercise programs can help maintain levels of bone mineral density for older adults.[85,86,93–97] Continued functional loading of the skeletal system appears to help balance bone formation and resorption. Site-specific increases in bone mineral density have been demonstrated in older adults participating in exercise programs.[84,85,98–100] As with other age groups, weight-bearing activities were more effective than non–weight-bearing activities in bone growth. Strength training was also effective, but power training, which included both a speed component and a resistance component, was the most effective at improving bone density.[101]

FUNCTIONAL IMPLICATIONS OF SKELETAL SYSTEM ISSUES

Changes in the skeletal system affect its effectiveness at all age levels, requiring special concern with relation to functional activities (Table 5.1). In infants, congenital bone malformations or positional deformities may occur and impact development of an efficient, effective skeleton. In adolescence, not only do conditions such as idiopathic scoliosis impact on posture and functional ability, but also rapid growth of the skeleton may leave the teen vulnerable to avulsion fractures or injury to the cartilage growth plates in the bone. Osteoporosis and OA are common problems for older adults. When therapists understand the processes underlying these two disorders, they can develop individualized prevention

TABLE 5.1   Age-Related Skeletal System Concerns Related to Physical Activity

Age Period	Skeletal System Concern
Prenatal	Intrauterine molding late in gestation
	Congenital hip dysplasia
	Congenital limb deficiency
Newborn	Epiphyseal infection
Childhood	Epiphyseal injury; growth plate fracture
	Apophyseal avulsion
	Greenstick fracture
Adolescence	Scoliosis
	Epiphyseal injury
	Apophyseal avulsion
	Stress fracture
Adulthood	Back pain secondary to disc changes
Older adulthood	Osteoporosis
	Osteoarthritis

programs that will help limit the functional losses experienced by older adults (see Clinical Implications Box 5.1: Osteoporosis Prevention: A Lifelong Process).

Childhood and Adolescence

The dynamic quality of bone growth in childhood is also very useful in the management of skeletal abnormalities. Mechanical forces can contribute to the spontaneous correction of some skeletal abnormalities and the responsiveness of others to orthopedic treatment in children. The infant born with congenital bony deformities, such as congenital hip dysplasia, metatarsus adductus, or club foot, may benefit greatly from early orthopedic intervention. Corrective forces can be applied with casting or taping procedures, which when combined with muscle activity will correct bony alignment. Congenital plagiocephaly, which may occur secondary to positioning or torticollis (where the head is turned persistently to the side), may also self-correct as the infant develops head control and spends quality play time in a prone position. New parents are often given information on the importance of "tummy time" to enhance muscular control of the head and neck and development of symmetrical skull shape. If plagiocephaly is more severe, infants often wear orthotic helmets to help mold the skull into a more symmetrical shape.

Abnormal skeletal development also occurs if unbalanced muscle action around a joint is present, as in cerebral palsy or spina bifida. For example, bone growth will proceed in response to the strong adduction and internal rotation forces exerted by muscles at the hip of the child with cerebral palsy. This abnormal force interferes with normal development of the acetabulum, femoral torsion, and the femoral neck/shaft angle. The hip can become unstable, and the risk for dislocation is increased.

The epiphysis is an active site for new bone formation and plays an important role in early skeletal development. During periods of rapid growth, forces acting on the epiphysis can have dramatic effects. Injury or infection to the epiphysis can result in abnormal bone growth and limb length deficiencies.[106] The newborn infant is especially susceptible to infection of the epiphysis because the epiphyseal plate is very thin at this age and does not provide a significant barrier between the metaphysis and the epiphysis. Blood vessels easily cross the growth plate, allowing infection to be spread from the metaphysis to the epiphysis. As the epiphyseal plate becomes thicker, the blood vessels can no longer cross it, eliminating the possibility for transmission of infection. Fractures of the epiphyseal plate are also seen in children because the cartilaginous growth plates within the bone are not as resistant to stress as adult bone. The growth plate is also weaker than the surrounding tissue. Even though many of these fractures heal well with rest and medical management, those injuries where the growth plate alignment is altered leave the child at risk for growth abnormalities and development of bone deformities. Children are most susceptible to growth plate fractures as they enter the period of peak height velocity growth.[106] During this rapid growth spurt, the epiphysis is less stable than the joints, making epiphyseal injury likely when the joint area is involved. Apparent joint sprains in this age group should be critically evaluated to rule out involvement of the epiphysis.

Structural differences between growing and adult bone also make children more susceptible to injuries such as plastic deformation of the bone, greenstick fractures, and apophyseal avulsion (avulsion of muscle tendon from its insertion). In general, growing bone is less dense and more porous than adult bone. As a result, it is more sensitive to both compressive and tensile stress. The cortex of the metaphysis is also thinner than that

CLINICAL IMPLICATIONS BOX 5.1
Osteoporosis Prevention: A Lifelong Process

Osteoporosis is a common, costly condition of older adults that results in bone fracture, pain, and disability. The best way to prevent or minimize risk for osteoporosis is to maximize the amount of bone tissue present in adulthood. Peak bone mass is attained in young adulthood and can be enhanced by several factors throughout childhood. These factors include dietary intake of adequate amounts of calories, calcium, and vitamin D; physical activities that provide weight-bearing and mechanical strain stimuli to the bone and muscle; and maintenance of appropriate body weight. Research has shown that the effects of increased physical activity in increasing bone mineral concentration and bone mineral density are greatest in prepubertal children.[11,43,48,49,60,74,85,102–105]

- For this reason, it is important to begin preventive measures for osteoporosis in early childhood and continue across the life span. Health care providers can guide their patients of all ages to the most effective methods that will optimize bone growth and minimize the risk of osteoporosis.

Osteoporosis prevention strategies for individuals of all ages include the following:

- Regular, ongoing physical activity that begins in childhood and continues throughout adulthood.
- Participation in a variety of diverse movement activities that provide different patterns of mechanical strain.

Moderate- to high-impact activities are recommended for children and adolescents. Low- to moderate-impact activities are recommended for middle-aged and older adults.

- Participation in weight-bearing exercise at least three to five times per week, for 10–45 minutes per session.
- Exercise that increases strength, flexibility, and coordination. Muscle strength gains positively influence bone density, and improved flexibility and coordination also decrease the likelihood of falls in older adults.
- Eating a well-balanced diet to support the energy demands of the growing body and to provide appropriate vitamins and minerals for bone growth and maintenance.
- Intake of appropriate levels of calcium from the diet to enhance mineralization of the developing bone and to maintain appropriate levels of blood calcium.
- Maintaining optimal body weight. Increased body weight, especially of lean muscle mass, has been associated with increased bone mass.
- Ensuring optimal hormonal function, periods of amenorrhea should be avoided and delayed puberty should be managed medically. Appropriate levels of estrogen are necessary to trigger the adolescent growth spurt and to optimize bone growth.
- Avoiding periods of immobilization when bone density is rapidly lost.

of the diaphysis, making it less resistant to compressive forces. The periosteum, however, is thicker than in adult bone and less readily torn, resulting in fewer displaced fractures.

Skeletal system problems such as scoliosis often become obvious and may progress rapidly during adolescence. Idiopathic scoliosis, which is a lateral curvature of the spine of unknown origin, can occur through childhood but is most common in adolescence and can be seen in 2%–4% of the population. Curves are generally mild; boys and girls are equally represented. Only a small percentage of scoliotic curves progress to greater than 15 degrees, more often in girls.[107,108]

Stress fractures and apophyseal avulsion fractures are also seen, especially in the adolescent athlete when activity or training level changes. These injuries are related to overuse and stress on the system beyond the ability for self-repair. Common sites for growth plate injury and stress fracture in the adolescent are the proximal humerus, distal radius, lumbar spine, tibia,

and fibula. Young baseball players or those children who play overhead sports are at risk for humerus or shoulder injuries.[106] Gymnasts or other athletes performing repetitive activities that place an axial load on an extended spine are at risk for lumbar spondylolysis, a stress fracture of the pars interarticularis.[109] Gymnasts also frequently report distal radius fractures.[106] Long-distance runners frequently have stress fractures at the tibia.[110]

Apophyseal avulsion fractures occur when traction forces are applied at the apophysis and it is pulled away from the bone. Common sites for avulsion fractures are the anterior superior iliac spine, anterior inferior iliac spine, lesser trochanter, and ischium.[111] Osgood-Schlatter disease may also be associated with avulsion of the apophysis at the tibial tuberosity after a traction injury. The definite cause of this disease is unknown, but it affects adolescent boys (12–15 years of age) and girls (8–12 years of age).[112] Physical conditioning programs, thorough preseason screening examinations,

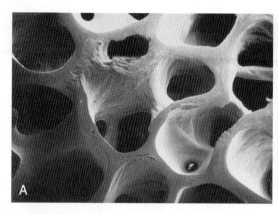
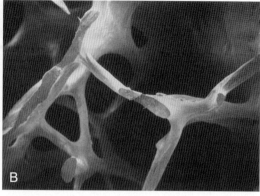

Fig. 5.13 Electron micrograph of normal (**A**) and osteoporotic (**B**) bone. (From Dempster DW, Shane E, Horbert W, et al. A simple method for corrective light and scanning electron microscopy of human iliac crest bone biopsies. *J Bone Miner Res.* 1986;1:16-21, with permission of the American Society of Bone and Mineral Research.)

and appropriate supervision during athletic activities are impor-tant to prevent these stress-related injuries.

Cartilage injury can also be seen in adolescence. Chondromalacia of the patella, with softening and fibrillation of the cartilage, results from stress on the kneecap. Rotational or angular malalignment of the patella is usually seen. Restriction of overactivity allows the cartilage to repair itself.

Osteoporosis

Osteoporosis can be classified into two main groups by considering the factors affecting bone metabolism. The two groups are primary osteoporosis and secondary osteoporosis. Primary osteoporosis, the most common, can also be divided into two subgroups: involutional osteoporosis type I and involutional osteoporosis type II. Type I is also known as postmenopausal osteoporosis, caused by the deficiency of estrogen, mainly affecting the trabecular bone, making women more susceptible to this type of osteoporosis than men. Type II is also caused by senile osteoporosis and is related to bone mass lost due to aging of cortical and trabecular bone mass, which can occur in both sexes. Secondary osteoporosis has clearly definable etiologic mechanisms, includes a collection of different diseases, and can be caused by medication side effects or sedentary lifestyle changes.[90]

Osteoporosis is defined as having bone density more than 2.5 standard deviations below that of a reference range for young women[113] and leaves the older adult at risk for bone fracture. Both older men and older women can develop osteoporosis, but it is more common in women. Risk for osteoporosis appears to be greatest for non-Hispanic White and Asian populations, as compared to non-Hispanic Black and Hispanic populations.[18] As previously discussed, primary prevention against development of osteoporosis and fractures in older adulthood is thought to be development of the maximum possible peak bone mass through childhood and young adulthood. Participation in load-bearing physical activity and good nutrition contribute to maximizing peak bone mass and maintaining bone health across the life span. Physical inactivity related to aging, long periods of bed rest, and exposure to weightless environments have been identified as factors that contribute to osteoporosis. Cigarette smoking, alcohol use, and long-term use of corticosteroids are also risk factors for osteoporosis.[90,113] The individual most at risk for the development of osteoporosis is a White woman who has gone through menopause.

The clinical features of osteoporosis are pain, loss of height, kyphosis, and decreased function, because bone is unable to withstand the compression forces of weight bearing. When the amount of bone mass is no longer sufficient to support the body during activity, spontaneous fracture may result (Fig. 5.13). The most frequent sites for spontaneous fracture secondary to osteoporosis are the spine, proximal femur, and wrist. These sites are also made up of primarily cancellous (trabecular) bone, which loses bone mineral density, especially immediately after menopause.[51] Anterior compression fractures of the vertebrae result in wedge-shaped vertebrae and lead to kyphotic posturing. Central collapse of adjacent vertebra leads to fish-shaped vertebrae, decreasing the disk space and skeletal height. In general, the microfractures related to osteoporosis cause pain and lead to a flexed posture.

Osteoporosis caused by the progressive loss of bone mass with aging is referred to as *senile*, or *involutional, osteoporosis*. Type 2 involutional osteoporosis, related to decreased intestinal absorption of calcium, occurs in both men and women and affects both cortical and cancellous bone. Type 1 involutional osteoporosis occurs in the 4–8 years after menopause[35] and affects primarily cancellous bone.[51] When estrogen secretion decreases with menopause, the bone is thought to become more sensitive to the parathyroid hormone, increasing the rate of bone resorption.

Good nutrition and a lifelong commitment to exercise may influence the maximum bone mass attained in early adulthood and maintenance of that bone mass. Participation in moderate- to high-impact physical activities (jumping, skipping, dancing) appears to have the greatest impact on bone growth in the prepubertal years.[11,43,48,60,85,102–104]

- Exercise programs may effectively slow or prevent the bone loss associated with aging or even slightly increase the bone mass at the sites of bone loading (such as the lumbar spine or femoral neck).[85,98–100,102,104,114]
- In the planning of exercise programs, weight-bearing and strengthening activities should be included.[93] The most effective type of exercise program for maintaining bone health in adults and older adults includes low- to moderate-impact weight-bearing activities, such as walking, jogging, and stair climbing.[102,104,114] A program that includes this variety of weight-bearing activity places a variety of stresses on the bone and is more effective than just walking. Resistance training, a form of strengthening exercise, has also been found to be effective in maintaining bone health in adults.[86,102,104] Power training, in which resistance training is performed with fast movements rather than slow movements, appears to be most effective in maintaining bone mineral density.[101] Spinal extension exercises should be emphasized because flexion exercises may be problematic, contributing to anterior wedging and compression fractures of the vertebrae.[115] For older adults, the exercise program should also focus on balance and flexibility to help decrease risk for falls.

Osteoarthritis

OA is an age-related condition characterized by joint pain during movement and weight bearing, limited joint range of motion, and loss of physical function, which ultimately limits participation in important life activities. Development of OA is related to the degeneration of articular cartilage, which occurs with age. As mentioned earlier, chondrocytes in articular cartilage are dependent upon mechanical loading for nutritional purposes. Abnormal mechanical loading can also contribute to degeneration of the articular cartilage.[116] Inflammatory processes within the joint also appear to play a role in the development of OA.[117] Over 300 million people in the world were affected by OA in 2017,[118] which is also reported to be a common cause of pain and disability in the elderly.[6] The cartilage thins, and clefts and cracks form, leaving the surface uneven and unable to efficiently provide frictionless joint motion. Calcification of the cartilage is also seen with age and in response to injury.[1] Underlying bone, which is innervated, becomes exposed to mechanical stress, resulting in pain. Bony spurs or outgrowths covered with hyaline cartilage may also develop in the joint. The individual with OA experiences pain with movement and limited range of motion.

Treatment for OA has traditionally been limited to the protection of affected joints from undue stress, minimization of joint range-of-motion limitations, and relief of pain. Mesenchymal stem cell treatments appear to address the inflammatory process within the joint and may offer another effective treatment of OA.[117] Antiinflammatory medications offer some relief. Weight loss in overweight individuals will also help decrease pain by lessening the loading of the joint. Individuals with OA benefit from participation in exercise programs that include aerobic, resistance, and functional exercises.[119] The exercises should address improvement in muscle strength, preservation of joint range of motion, and improved efficiency when performing everyday tasks so that loading forces on the cartilage are equalized. High-impact exercises should be avoided because they put high loads on the cartilage and may increase tissue destruction. When conservative treatment approaches do not relieve symptoms, surgical debridement of the joint surface or joint replacement is considered.

SUMMARY

Cartilage, bones, and joints are the essential components of the skeletal system that develop over a lifetime and have the capacity to increase or limit physical ability to function. Together, these elements provide a structural base on which movement can take place. Optimal, healthy development of the skeletal system depends not only on genetics and nutrition but also on an active lifestyle. The mechanical stresses of everyday functional activities and exercises help the system achieve its most efficient form and maintain its stability. The time period in which physical activity and exercise can make the most impact upon peak bone mass development is in the 2–3 years before peak height velocity. The changes in bone architecture and in the mechanical properties of the tendons and ligaments can lead to an increase in injury and decreased function for the older adult. Sedentary behavior, pain, and dysfunction lead to poor health outcomes. As a result of these physical changes in the older population, exercise and adequate activity remain critically important in maintaining proper skeletal health. With a proactive response to exercise and nutrition, many of the adverse changes seen in the skeletal system can be better managed. This is critically important in maintaining the functional independence of the elderly population and in reducing fall risk that could lead to fracture. Lifelong commitment to good nutrition and exercise helps the attainment of maximal bone mass and maintenance of a strong skeletal system well into older adulthood.

DISCUSSION QUESTION: Osteoporosis is a progressive loss of bone mass seen with aging. Please review the developmental process of bone and discuss how bone development influences the development of osteoporosis at each of the following ages.

Age	Developmental Characteristics of Bone	Influence on Bone Density/ Osteoporosis	Prevention Ideas?
Infancy			
Childhood			
Adolescence			
Adulthood			
Older adulthood			

REFERENCES

1. Ross MH, Kaye GI, Pawlina W. *Histology: A Text and Atlas.* 4th ed. Baltimore: Lippincott Williams & Wilkins; 2003.
2. Fox AJ, Bedi A, Rodeo SA. The basic science of articular cartilage: structure, composition and function. *Sports Health.* 2009;1(6):461–468.
3. Ahmed MS, Matsumura B, Cristian A. Age-related changes in muscles and joints. *Phys Med Rehabil Clin N Am.* 2005;16:19–39.
4. Bullough PG. The role of joint architecture in the etiology of arthritis. *Osteoarthritis Cartilage.* 2004;12:S2S9.
5. Bobacz K, Erlacher L, Smolen J, et al. Chondrocyte number and proteoglycan synthesis in the aging and osteoarthritic human articular cartilage. *Ann Rheum Dis.* 2004;63:1618–1622.
6. Li Y, Wei X, Zhou J, Wei L. The age-related changes in cartilage and osteoarthritis. *BioMed Research International.* 2013 https://doi.org/10.1155/2013/916530.Article ID 916530.
7. Martin JA, Buckwalter JA. Aging, articular cartilage chondrocyte senescence and osteoarthritis. *Biogerontology.* 2002;3:257–264.
8. Zhang M, Theleman JL, Lygrisse KA, Wang J. Epigenetic mechanisms underlying the aging of articular cartilage and osteoarthritis. *Gerontol.* 2019;65:387–396.
9. Malina RM, Bouchard C, Bar-Or O. *Growth, Maturation and Physical Activity.* 2nd ed. Champaign, IL: Human Kinetics; 2004.
10. Singh A.P. Cortical bone and Cancellous Bone. www.boneandjoint.com. Accessed 9/22/2021.
11. Kontulainen SA, Hughes JM, Macdonald HM, et al. The biomechanical basis of bone strength development during growth. *Med Sport Sci.* 2007;51:13–32.

12. Ott SM. Cortical or trabecular bone: what is the difference. *Am J Nephrol*. 2018;47:37–375

13. Ruimermen R, Hilbers P, van Reitbergen B, Huiskis R. A theoretical framework for strain-related trabecular bone maintenance and adaptation. *J Biomech*. 2005;38: 931–941.

14. Berenson AB, Rahman M, Wilkinson G. Racial difference in the correlates of bone mineral content/density and age at peak among reproductive-aged women. *Osteoporos Int*. 2009;20:1439–1449.

15. Melton III LJ, Marquez MA, Achenbach SJ, et al. Variations in bond density among persons of African heritage. *Osteoporos Int*. 2002;13:551–559.

16. Pollock NK, Laing EM, Taylor RG, et al. Comparisons of trabecular and cortical bone in late adolescent black and white females. *J Bone Miner Metab*. 2011;22(2):655–665.

17. Vásquez E, Shaw BA, Gensburg L, et al. Racial and ethnic differences in physical activity and bone density: National Health and Nutrition Examination Survey, 2007-2008. *Prev Chronic Dis*. 2013;10:130183.

18. Thomas PA. Racial and ethnic differences in osteoporosis. *J Am Acad Orthop Surg*. 2007;15(Suppl 1):S26–S30.

19. Jorgetti V, dos Reis LM, Ott SM. Ethnic differences in bone and mineral metabolism in healthy people and patients with CKD. *Kidney International*. 2014;85: 1283–1289.

20. Wetzsteon RJ, Hughes JM, Kaufman BC, et al. Ethnic differences in bone geometry and strength are apparent in childhood. *Bone*. 2009;44:970–975.

21. Frost HM. Bone "mass" and the "mechanostat": a proposal. *Anat Rec*. 1987;219:1–9.

22. Schoenau E. From mechanostat theory to development of the "Functional Muscle-Bone-Unit". *J Musculoskelet Neuronal Interact*. 2005;5(3):232–238.

23. Hughes JM, Petit MA. Biological underpinnings of Frost's mechanostat thresholds: the important role of osteocytes. *J Musculoskelet Neuronal Interact*. 2010;10(3):128–135.

24. Bass SL, Eser P, Daly R. The effect of exercise and nutrition on the mechanostat. *J Musculoskelet Neuronal Interact*. 2005;5(3):239–254.

25. Bourrin S, Toromanoff A, Ammann P, et al. Dietary protein deficiency induces osteoporosis in aged male rats. *J Bone Miner Res*. 2000;15(8):1555–1563.

26. Heany RP, Layman DK. Amount and type of protein influences bone health. *Am J Clin Nutr*. 2008;87(suppl): 1567S–1570S.

27. Darling AL, Millword DJ, Lanham-New SA. Dietary protein and bone health: towards a synthesized view. *Proceedings of the Nutrition Society*. 2021;80:165–172.

28. Choi HK, Kim GJ, Yoo HS, et al. Vitamin C activates osteoblastogenesis and inhibits osteoclastogenesis via Wnt/?-Catanin/ATF4 signaling pathways. *Nutrients*. 2019,11.506.

29. Brezinska O, Lukasik Z, Makowska J, Walczak K. Role of Vitamin C in osteoporosis development and treatment—a literature review. *Nutrients*. 2020;12:2394.

30. Zaria A, Morovat A, Javaid K, Brown CP. Vitamin D receptor expression in human bone tissue and dose-dependent activation in resorbing osteoclasts. *Bone Research*. 2016;4:16030.

31. Bickle DD. Vitamin D and bone. *Curr Osteoporors Rep*. 2012;10(2):151–159.

32. Uday S, Wolfgang H. Nutritional rickets and osteomalacia in the 21st century: revised concepts, public health and prevention strategies. *Cur Osteoporos Rep*. 2017;15:293–302.

33. Riggs BL, Khosla S, Melton III LJ. Sex steroids and the construction and conservation of the adult skeleton. *Endocr Rev*. 2002;23(3):279–302.

34. Cutler GB. The role of estrogen in bone growth and maturation during childhood and adolescence. *J Steroid Biochem Mol Biol*. 1997;61(3-6):141–147.

35. Khosla S, Riggs L. Pathophysiology of age-related bone loss and osteoporosis. *Endocrinol Metab Clin North Am*. 2005;34:1015–1030.

36. Zaghloul A, Mohamed EM, Maaty MT, El-Saied GE, Hammad A. Computing measurements of femoral neck shaft angle in children and adolescents from Nile Delta. *Ortho and Rheum Open Access J*. 2020;17(1):555954.

37. Kong M, Hongsik J, Lee CH, Chun SW, Yoon C, Shin H. Change of femoral anteversion angle with intoeing gait measured by three-dimensional computed tomography reconstruction: one-year follow-up study. *Ann Rehabil Med*. 2018;42(1):137–144.

38. Scorcelletti M, Reeves ND, Rittweger J, Ireland A. Femoral anteversion: significance and measurement. *Journal of Anat*. 2020;237:811–826.

39. Bae DS, Ferretti M, Waters PM. Upper extremity size differences in brachial plexus birth palsy. *Hand*. 2008;3:297–303.

40. Demir SO, Oktay F, Uysal H, et al. Upper extremity shortness in children with hemiplegic cerebral palsy. *J Pediatr Orthop*. 2006;26(6):764–768.

41. Uysal H, Demir SO, Oktay F, et al. Extremity shortness in obstetric brachial plexus lesion and its relationship to root avulsion. *J Child Neurol*. 2007;22(12):1377–1383.

42. Loud KJ, Gordon CM. Adolescent bone health. *Arch Pediatr Adolesc Med*. 2006;160:1026–1032.

43. Ondrak KS, Morgan DW. Physical activity, calcium intake and bone health in children and adolescents. *Sports Med*. 2007;37(7):587–600.

44. Proia P, Amato A, Drid P, Korovljev D, Vasto S, Baldassaon S. The impact of diet and physical activity on bone

health in children and adolescents. *Fronteirs in Endocrinology*. 2021;12:704647.

45. Zhao R, Zhang M, Zhang Q. The effectiveness of combined exercise interventions for preventing post menopausal bone loss: a systematic review and meta-analysis. *J Orthop Sports Phys Ther*. 2017;47(4):241–251.

46. Noguira RC, Weeks BK, Beck BR. Exercise to improve pediatric bone and fat: a systematic review and meta-analysis. *Med Sci Sport Exercise*. 2014;46(3):610–621.

47. Simus V, Hing W, Pope R, Climstein M. Effects of water-based exercise on bone health on middle-aged and older adults: a systematic review and meta-analysis. *Open Access Journal of Sports Medicine*. 2017;8:39–60.

48. Greene DA, Naughton GA. Adaptive skeletal responses to mechanical loading during adolescence. *Sports Med*. 2006;35(9):723–732.

49. Xue S, Kemal O, Lu M, Lix LM, Leslie WD, Yang S. Age at attainment of peak bone mineral density and its associated factors: the National Health and Nutrition Survey 2005–2014. *Bone*. 2020;131:115163. https://doi.org/10.1016/j.bone.2019.115163.

50. Alswat KA. Gender disparities in osteoporosis. *J Clin Med Res*. 2017;9(5):382–387.

51. Riggs BL, Melton III LJ, Robb RA, et al. Population-based study of age and sex differences in bone volumetric density, size, geometry, and structure at different skeletal sites. *J Bone Miner Res*. 2004;19:1945–1954.

52. National Institutes of Health (US). Dietary supplement fact sheet: calcium. Web site. https://ods.od.nih.gov/factsheets/Calcium-HealthProfessional/ Accessed January 4, 2022.

53. Choi YS, Joung H, Kim J. Evidence for revising calcium dietary reference intakes (DRIs) for Korean elderly. *FASEB J*. 2013;27(1065):28.

54. Tian L, Yang R, Wei L, Liu J, Yang Y, Shao F, Ma W, Li T, Wang Y, Guo T. Prevalence of osteoporosis and related lifestyle and metabolic factors of postmenopausal women and elderly men. *Medicine (Baltimore)*. 2017;96(43):e8294.

55. Yang YJ, Kim J. Factors in relation to bone mineral density in Korean middle-aged and older men: 2008-2010 Korea National Health and Nutrition Examination Survey. *Ann Nutr Metab*. 2014;64:50–59.

56. Barros EM, Rodriques CJ, Rodriques NR, Oliveira RP, Barros TE, Rodriques AJ. Aging of the elastic and collagen fibers in the human cervical interspinous ligaments. *Spine J*. 2002;2(1):57–62.

57. Schulze-Tanzil G. Intraarticular ligament degeneration is interrelated with cartilage and bone destruction in osteoarthritis. *Cells*. 2019;8(9):990 https://doi.org/10.3390/cells8090990. Published 2019 Aug 27.

58. Moore KL, Persaud TVN. 2008 *Before We Are Born: Essentials of Embryology and Birth Defects*. 7th ed. Philadelphia: WB Saunders 2008.

59. Shea CA, Murphy P, Rolfe BA. The importance of foetal movement for co-ordinated cartilage and bone development in utero. *Bone Joint Res*. 2015;7:105–116. https://doi.org/10.1302/2046-3758.47.2000387.

60. Vincente-Rodriguez G. How does exercise affect bone development during growth? *Sports Med*. 2006;36(7):561–569.

61. Anderson J. Calcium, phosphorus, and human bone development. *J Nutr*. 1996;1261153S–1158S.

62. Whiting SJ, Vatanparast H, Baxter-Jones A, et al. Factors that affect bone mineral accrual in the adolescent growth spurt. *J Nutr*. 2004;134:696S–700S.

63. Janz KF, Letuchy EM, Eichenberger Gilmore JM, et al. Early physical activity provides sustained bone health benefits later in childhood. *Med Sci Sport Exercise*. 2010;42(6):1072–1078. https://doi.org/10.1249/MSS.ob013e3181c619b2.

64. Bierhals IO, Assuncao MC, Vaz JdS, et al. Growth from birth to adolescence and bone mineral density in young adults: the 1993 Pelotas birth cohort. *Bone*. 2020;130:115108. https://doi.org/10.1016/j.bone.2019.115108.

65. Hind K, Burrows M. Weight-bearing exercise and bone mineral accrual in children and adolescents: a review of controlled trials. *Bone*. 2007;40:14–27.

66. MacKelvie KJ, Petit MA, Khan KM, et al. Bone mass and structure are enhanced following a 20-year randomized controlled trial of exercise in prepubertal boys. *Bone*. 2004;34:755–764.

67. MacKelvie KJ, McKay HA, Petit MA, et al. Bone mineral response to a 7-month randomized controlled, school-based jumping intervention in 121 prepubertal boys: associations with ethnicity and body mass index. *J Bone Miner Res*. 2002;17:834–844.

68. Sinclair D, Dangerfield P, eds. *Human Growth After Birth*. 6th ed. New York: Oxford University Press; 1998.

69. Bernhardt DB. Prenatal and postnatal growth and development of the foot and ankle. *Phys Ther*. 1988;68:1831–1839.

70. Ogden JA. Development and growth of the hip. In: Katz JF, Siffert RS, eds. *Management of Hip Disorders in Children*. Lippincott: Philadelphia: JB Lippincott; 1983.

71. Baruah RK, Kumar S, Harikrishnan SK. Developmental pattern of tibiofibular angle in healthy North-East Indian children. *J Child Orthop*. 2017;11(5):339–347. https://doi.org/10.1302/1863-2548.11.170047.

72. Cahuzac JP, Vardon D, Sales de Gauzy J. Development of the clinical tibiofemoral angle in normal adolescents. A study of 427 normal subjects from 10 to 16 years of age. *J Bone Joint Surg Br*. 1995;77(5):729–732.

73. LeVeau BF, Bernhardt DB. Developmental biomechanics. *Phys Ther.* 1984;64:1874–1882.

74. Gordon CM, Zemel BS, Wren TAL, Leonard MB, Bachrach LC, Rauch F, Gilsanz V, Rosen CJ, Winer KK. The determinants of peak bone mass. *Journal of Pediatrics.* 2017;180:261–269.

75. Sayers A, Tobias JH. Fat mass exerts a greater effect on cortical bone mass in girls than boys. *J Clin Endocrinol Metab.* 2010;95(2):699–706.

76. Ashby RL, Adams JE, Roberts SA, Mughal MZ, Ward KA. The muscle-bone unit of peripheral and central skeletal sites in children and young adults. *Osteoporo Int.* 2011;22(1):121–132. https://doi.org/10.1007/s00198-110-1216-3.

77. Petit MA, McKay HA, MacKelvie KJ, et al. A randomized school-based jumping intervention confers site- and maturity-specific benefits on bone structural properties in girls: a hip structural analysis study. *J Bone Miner Res.* 2002;17(3):363–372.

78. DeBar LL, Ritenbaugh C, Ickin M, et al. A health plan-based lifestyle intervention increases bone mineral density in adolescent girls. *Arch Pediatr Adolesc Med.* 2006;160:1269–1276.

79. Whitbourne SK. *The Aging Body—Physiological Changes and Psychological Consequences.* New York: Springer-Verlag; 1985.

80. Goodman CC, Fuller KS. *Pathology: Implications for the Physical Therapist. 3rd ed.* Philadelphia: WB Saunders; 2009.

81. Lu J, Shin Y, Yen MS, Sun SS. Peak bone mass and patterns of change in total bone mineral density and bone mineral contents from childhood into young adulthood. *J Clin Densiton.* 2016;19(2):180–191. https://doi.org/10.1016/j.jocd.2014.08.001.

82. Malkin I, Karasik D, Lifshits G, et al. Modelling of age-related bone loss using cross-sectional data. *Ann Hum Biol.* 2002;29(3):256–270.

83. Raab DM, Smith EL. Exercise and aging: effects on bone. *Top Geriatr Rehabil.* 1985;1:31–39.

84. Bailey CA, Kukuljan S, Daly RM. Effects of lifetime loading history on cortical bone density and its distribution in middle aged and older men. *Bone.* 2010;47:673–680.

85. Guadalupe-Grau A, Fuentes T, Guerra B, et al. Exercise and bone mass in adults. *Sports Med.* 2009;39(6):439–468.

86. Kelley GA, Kelley KS, Tran ZV. Resistance training and bone mineral density in women: a meta-analysis of control trials. *Am J Phys Med Rehabil.* 2001;80:65–77.

87. Nikander R, Kannus P, Rantalainen T, et al. Cross-sectional geometry of weight-bearing tibia in female athletes subjected to different exercise loadings. *Osteoporos Int.* 2010;21(10):1687–1694.

88. Koeller W, Muehlhaus S, Meier W, et al. Biomechanical properties of human intervertebral discs subjected to axial dynamic compression: influence of age and degeneration. *J Biomech.* 1986;19:807–816.

89. Demontiero O, Vidal C, Duque G. Aging and bone loss: new insights for the clinician. *Ther Ad Musculoskel Dis.* 2012;4(2):61–76. https://doi.org/10.1177/1759720X114.30858.

90. Sözen T, Özışık L, Başaran NÇ. An overview and management of osteoporosis. *Eur J Rheumatol.* 2017;4(1):46–56. https://doi.org/10.5152/eurjrheum.2016.048.

91. Siddiqui JA, Partridge NC. Physiological bone remodeling: Systemic regulation and growth factor involvement. *Physiology.* 2016;31:233–245. https://doi.org/10.1152/physiol.00061.2014.

92. Spirduso WW. *Physical dimensions of aging.* Human Kinetics: Champaign, Ill; 1995.

93. Cousins JM, Peti MA, Paudel ML, et al. Muscle power and physical activity are associated with bone strength in older men: the osteoporotic fractures in men study. *Bone.* 2010;47:205–211.

94. Hamilton CJ, Swan VJD, Jamal SA. The effects of exercise and physical activity participation on bone mass and geometry in postmenopausal women: a systematic review of pQCT studies. *Osteoporos Int.* 2010;21:11–23.

95. Hamilton CJ, Thomas SG, Jamal SA. Associations between leisure physical activity participation and cortical bone mass and geometry at the radius and tibia in a Canadian cohort of postmenopausal women. *Bone.* 2010;46:774–779.

96. Souminen H. Physical activity and health: musculoskeletal issues. *Adv Physiother.* 2007;9:65–75.

97. Smith C, Tacey A, Mesinovic J, Scott G,D, Lin X, Brennan-Speranza TC, Lewis JR, Duque G, Levinger I. The effects of acute exercise on bone turnover in middle-aged and older adults: a systematic review. *Bone.* 2021;143:115766. https://doi.org/10.1016/j.bone.2020.115766.

98. Bravo G, Gauthier P, Roy PM, et al. Impact of a 12-month exercise program on the physical and psychological health of osteopenic women. *J Am Geriatr Soc.* 1996;44:756–762.

99. Prior JC, Barr SI, Chow R, et al. Physical activity as therapy for osteoporosis. *Can Med Assoc J.* 1996;155:940–944.

100. Muir JM, Ye C, Bhandari M, Adachi JD, Thebane L. The effect of regular physical activity on bone mineral density in post-menopausal women aged 75 and over: a retrospective analysis from the Canadian multicenter osteoporosis study. *BMC Musculoskeletal Disorders.* 2013;14:253.

101. Stengel SV, Kemmler W, Pintag R, et al. Power training is more effective than strength training for maintaining bone mineral density in postmenopausal women. *J Appl Physiol*. 2005;99:181–188.

102. Beck BR, Snow CM. Bone health across the lifespan—exercising our options. *Exerc Sport Sci Rev*. 2003;31(3):117–122.

103. Corteix D, Lespessailles E, Peres SL, et al. Effect of physical training on bone mineral density in prepubertal girls: a comparative study between impact loading and non-impact loading sports. *Osteoporosis Int*. 1998;8:152–158.

104. Nikander R, Sievanen H, Heinonen A, et al. Targeted exercise against osteoporosis: a systematic review and meta-analysis for optimising bone strength throughout life. BMC Med (serial online) www.biomedcentral.com/1741-7015/8/47

105. Marin-Puyalto J, Maestu J, Gomez-Cabello A, et al. Frequency and duration of vigorous physical activity bouts are associated with adolescent boys' bone mineral status: a cross-sectional study. *Bone*. 2019;120:141–147.

106. Caine D, DiFiori J, Maffulli N. Physeal injuries in children's and youth sports: reasons for concern? *Br J Sports Med*. 2006;40:749–760.

107. Horne JP, Flannery R, Usman S. Adolescent idiopathic scoliosis: diagnosis and management. *Am Fam Physician*. 2014;89(3):193–198.

108. Konieczny MR, Senyurt H, Krauspy R. Epidemiology of adolescent idiopathic scoliosis. *J Child Orthop*. 2013;7:3–9. https://doi.org/10.1007/s11832-012-0457-4.

109. Tawfic S, Phan K, Mobbs RJ, Rao PJ. The incidence of pars interarticularis defects in athletes. *Global Spine Journal*. 2020;10(1):89–101. https://doi.org/10.1177/2192568218823695.

110. Gallo RA, Plakke M, Silvis ML. Common leg injuries of long-distance runners: anatomical and biomechanical approach. *Sports Health*. 2012;4(6):485–495.

111. Shiller J, DeFroda S, Blood T. Lower extremity avulsion fractures in the pediatric and adolescent athlete. *J Am Acad Orthop Surg*. 2017;25:251–259. https://doi.org/10.5435/JAAOS-D-15-00328.

112. Guldhammer C, Rathleff SK, Jensen HP, Holden S. Long term prognosis and impact of Osgood-Schlatters disease 4 years after diagnosis: a retrospective study. *The Orthopedic Journal of Sports Medicine*. 2019;7(10): https://doi.org/10.1177/2325967119878136.2325967119878136.

113. World Health Organization (WHO), 2007. WHO Scientific Report on the assessment of osteoporosis at primary health care level. Geneva, Switzerland.

114. Benedetti MG, Furlini G, Zati A, Mauro GL. The effectiveness of physical exercise on bone density in osteoporotic patients. *Biomed Research International*. 2018;Volume 2018 https://doi.org/10.1155/2018/4840531. Article ID 4840531:10 pages.

115. Wong CC, McGirt MJ. Vertebral compression fractures: a review of current management and multimodal therapy. *Journal of Multidisciplinary Healthcare*. 2013;6:205–214.

116. Zheng L, Zhang Z, Sheng P, Moshberi A. The role of metabolism in chondrocyte dysfunction and progression of osteoarthritis. 2021. *Ageing Research Reviews*. 66:101249. https://doi:10.1016/j.arr.2020.101249.

117. van den Bosch MHJ. Osteoarthritis year in review 2020: Biology. *Osteoarthritis and Cartilage*. 2021;29:143–150.

118. Kloppenberg K, Berenbaum F. Osteoarthritis year in review 2019: epidemiology and therapy. *Osteoarthritis and Cartilage*. 2020;28:242–248.

119. Skou ST, Petersen BK, Abbott JH, Patterson B, Barton C. Physical activity and exercise therapy benefit more than just symptoms and impairments in people with hip and knee osteoarthritis. *J Ortho Sports Phys Ther*. 2018;48(6):439–447.

6

Muscle System Changes

OBJECTIVES

After studying this chapter, the reader will be able to:

1. Define the basic characteristics of skeletal muscle morphology and organization.
2. Describe the basic physiology of skeletal muscle contraction.
3. Discuss the development changes in skeletal muscle across the life span.
4. Identify the functional implications of age-related changes in skeletal muscles.

Muscle is the largest tissue mass in the body. There are three types of muscles: voluntary (skeletal), involuntary (smooth), and cardiac. These three types of muscle are further divided into two subtypes of muscle: striated and nonstriated. Smooth muscle is the single example of the nonstriated type and is found in the walls of the digestive system, urinary bladder, and blood vessels. Smooth muscle contraction in these structures decreases their diameter.

Cardiac and skeletal muscles are composed of striated muscle. Cardiac muscle is a special form of striated muscle found only in the heart. Its arrangement of contractile proteins is identical to that of skeletal muscle, but the arrangement of fibers is different. Cardiac cells are joined together by specialized intercellular junctions that are visible in the light microscope as dark heavy lines between the cells. The cells are irregularly shaped and usually contain a single, centrally placed nucleus.

Skeletal muscle, the focus of this chapter, is generally considered the main energy-consuming tissue of the body and provides the propulsive force to move about and to perform physical activities. Skeletal muscles in the trunk, such as the oblique abdominal muscles, provide protection and support for internal organs. Skeletal muscle is also known as voluntary, striated, striped, or segmental muscle. It is vascularized and innervated.

Approximately 20% of the energy produced during muscle contraction is used to produce movement; the remainder is lost as heat. Heat generation helps maintain body temperature. For example, when a person is cold, they shiver and the muscle activity provides heat to the body.

There are more than 600 skeletal muscles in the human body, making up approximately 40% of the body weight.[1,2] On a microscopic level, muscle cells are considered to be cylindrical. They range from 1 to 40 μm in length and from 10 to 100 μm in diameter. The cells are multinucleated, with the nuclei located at the periphery of the cell or just beneath the *sarcolemma*, or plasma membrane. External to the sarcolemma is a highly glycosylated layer of collagen fibers called the *external lamina*; it is the external lamina that completely ensheaths each cell. This layer also contains proteins that function as enzymes.

ORGANIZATION OF MATURE SKELETAL MUSCLE

Skeletal muscle is organized from macroscopic to microscopic levels. A muscle's function is determined in large part by the muscle architecture. Architectural differences between muscles are the best predictors of force production.[3] There are many different muscle designs.[4] Muscles are usually categorized into one of three types: longitudinal, unipennate, and multipennate. In one type, called the parallel or longitudinal architecture, muscle fibers are arranged parallel to the force generating axis such as seen in the biceps. In a second type called the unipennate architecture, the fibers are arranged at a single angle relative to the force generating axis, such as is present in the vastus lateralis. In the third type, the multipennate, fibers are arranged at varying angles relative to the force generating axis, such as seen in the gluteus medius. Muscle architecture also includes the length of the fibers within the muscle and the cross-sectional area of the muscle.[3,5] Muscle design reflects the functional use pattern of that muscle.

The entire muscle is encased in a thick connective sheath of collagen fibers called the *epimysium*. Extensions of this sheath extend into the interior of the muscle, subdividing it into small bundles or groups of myofibers called fascicles. Each bundle or fascicle is surrounded by a layer of connective tissue called the *perimysium*. Within the fascicle, each individual muscle myofiber is surrounded by a layer of connective tissue called the *endomysium*. The endomysium is rich in capillaries and, to a lesser extent, nerve fibers. All connective tissue coverings ultimately come together at the tendinous junction; the tendon transmits all contractile forces generated by the muscle fibers to the bone. The elasticity of the tendon contributes to the control of the force and power of the muscle contraction.[6]

Each individual myofiber is filled with cylindric bundles of myofibrils that are made up of myofilaments. Myofibrils are the contractile structures of muscle. Filaments of actin and myosin are arranged in parallel groupings, anchored by the Z disk (Fig. 6.1). Actin and myosin are contractile proteins. Actin, the thinner filament, originates at the Z disk; myosin is the thicker filament. During muscle contraction, as two Z disks move closer together, the actin and myosin filaments slide over each other. The area from one Z disk to the next Z disk constitutes a sarcomere, which is the basic contractile unit of the muscle fiber (Fig. 6.1). Striations, the alternating light and dark pattern in the sarcomere seen under a light microscope, reflect the amount of overlap of the actin and myosin filaments. Myofibrils also contain the regulatory proteins, tropomyosin and troponin, and accessory proteins, titin and nebulin. Titin and nebulin maintain the alignment of the actin and myosin filaments within the sarcomere. Tropomyosin and troponin are both involved in muscle contraction. Troponin is a Ca^{2+} binding protein complex attached to tropomyosin.[5,6]

A sagittal section of a muscle bundle depicted in Fig. 6.2 shows the arrangement of the *sarcoplasmic reticulum* (SR), a system of membranous anastomosing channels intimately associated with the surface of each myofibril. At the feet of the SR are voltage-sensitive receptor proteins: the ryanodine receptor (RyR) and calcium-ATPase (Ca-ATPase). Calcium (Ca^{2+}) stored in the SR is necessary for muscle contraction. RyR senses an action potential and opens the calcium channels to allow calcium to be released into the region of the myofilament. The *transverse tubular system* (T-tubules) contains tubules that are extensions of the sarcolemma going deep into the interior of the muscle fiber. The function of the T-tubules is to extend the wave of depolarization that initiates muscle contraction throughout all the myofibrils of the muscle. The Ca-ATPase pumps calcium back into the SR, allowing the muscle to relax. RyR and Ca-ATPase are two key calcium regulatory proteins involved in the excitation-contraction coupling process.[7]

Excitation-Contraction Coupling

Excitation-contraction coupling is the mechanism that links plasma membrane stimulation with cross-bridge force production. The muscle receives a neural signal and converts that signal into mechanical force after synapsing at the *neuromuscular junction*. Fig. 6.3 illustrates the expansion of an axon into a motor end plate that comes to rest in a depression of the surface of the myofiber. The chemical signal comes from the release of acetylcholine (ACh).

Muscle action potentials produced by the excitation-contraction coupling initiate calcium signals. The calcium signals activate a contraction-relaxation cycle. *Contraction* refers to the activation of the cross-bridge cycle. Ca^{2+} activates the attractive forces between the filaments of actin and myosin by binding to troponin (Fig. 6.4). However, the process of contraction will only continue if there is energy; this energy is derived from the high-energy bonds of adenosine triphosphate (ATP), which are degraded to adenosine diphosphate (ADP). In the presence of Ca^{2+} and ATP, the heads of the myosin molecules form cross-bridges with active sites on the thin filaments of actin (see Fig. 6.4). The resulting energy produces a conformational change in

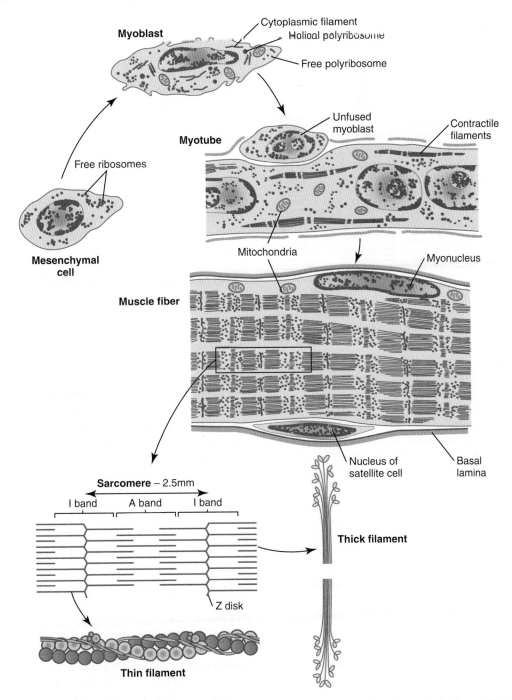

Fig. 6.1 A skeletal muscle fiber showing important subcellular elements. (Modified from Carlson BM. *Human Embryology and Developmental Biology.* 4th ed. St Louis: Mosby; 2009.)

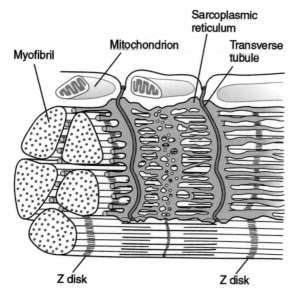

Fig. 6.2 Transverse tubule sarcoplasmic reticulum system. (From Porterfield JA, DeRosa C. *Mechanical Low Back Pain: Perspectives in Functional Anatomy.* 2nd ed. Philadelphia: WB Saunders; 1998:57.)

the myosin head region that exerts a directional force on the actin filament. As a result, the actin filaments are drawn toward the center of the sarcomere, overlapping the myosin filament. The net result is a shortening of the sarcomere, or contraction of the muscle. One ATP is needed for each cross-bridge cycle. After cross-bridge formation during the contraction phase of excitation-contraction coupling, relaxation occurs. Ca-ATPase pumps the calcium back into the SR, lowering the calcium levels and producing muscle relaxation. The concentration of calcium must drop to allow the unbinding of Ca^{2+} from troponin. The filaments slide back to their initial position assisted by elastic connective tissues within the muscle and titin. In summary, ACh initiates the excitation-contraction coupling, and calcium binding to troponin initiates muscle contraction. A muscle twitch is synonymous with a single contraction-relaxation cycle in a skeletal muscle fiber. For more detailed information on muscle control and force generation, see Mukund and Subramaniam.[5]

Muscle Fiber Types

Muscle fibers can be described based on speed as type I or type II. Muscle fibers can also be classified according

to their metabolic abilities. All human muscles are a mixture of three fiber types: I, IIa, and IIx.[8-10] Each of the fiber types has unique protein profiles, and type II fibers also have glycolytic enzymes.[10,11] *Type I muscle fibers are* classified as slow oxidative because they use slow glycolysis and oxidative phosphorylation to produce ATP. Slow-twitch, type I fibers have a small diameter, with large amounts of oxidative enzymes and an extensive capillary density. Type I fibers are best suited for activities required in repetitive, lower-force contractions and are considered fatigue resistant. Only slow fibers are found in the extraocular and middle ear muscles. Most "postural" muscles, such as those associated with the spinal column or the lower extremities, are composed predominantly of slow-twitch, or type I, fibers. Force is maintained economically by having lower myosin CA-ATPase activity than the fast-twitch fibers. The soleus muscle has a preponderance of slow-twitch muscle fibers and therefore is considered a postural muscle used for prolonged lower extremity activity to support the body against gravity.

Type II muscle fibers are classified as fast oxidative-glycolytic fibers. Type IIa and IIx fiber types vary in contractile speed and force generation.[5] Type IIa fibers use both oxidative (aerobic) and glycolytic (anaerobic) metabolism. These fiber types are found in some ocular muscles and demonstrate fine, fast movements almost continuously. When glucose is quickly broken down without oxygen present, large amounts of lactate are produced along with ATP. Type IIx fibers have a high capacity for glycolytic metabolism and can rapidly shorten. Fast-twitch fibers are suited for short bursts of powerful activity, although type IIa fibers are more fatigue resistant. The contractile speed and twitch duration of type IIa are between those of type I and type IIx fibers. The gastrocnemius muscle has a preponderance of fast-twitch fibers. This gives the muscle its capacity for very forceful and rapid contractions, which are used for jumping. The reader is advised that much of the muscle research related to aging was done before the change in nomenclature of the subcategories of type II fibers. Prior to 1995, Type IIx fibers were called Type IIb;[11] therefore, references continue to be made to type IIb fibers instead of type IIx in some of the cited studies.

Motor Unit

The functional unit of a muscle is the *motor unit*, which is defined as a single nerve cell body and its axon plus

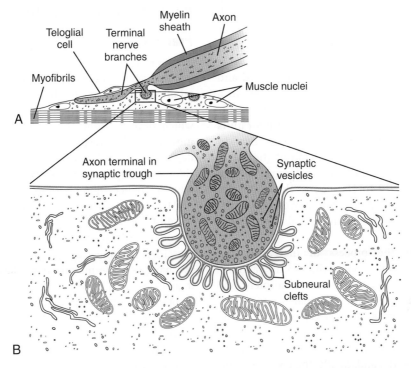

Fig. 6.3 Neuromuscular junction: different views of the motor end plate. (**A**) Longitudinal section through the end plate. (**B**) Electron micrographic appearance of the contact point between one of the axon terminals and the muscle fiber membrane, representing the rectangular area shown in A. (Modified from Fawcett DW. *Bloom and Fawcett: Textbook of Histology*. 11th ed. Philadelphia: WB Saunders; 1986:290.)

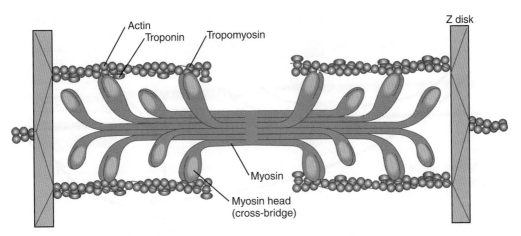

Fig. 6.4 A single sarcomere is depicted showing the cross-bridge structure created by the myosin heads and their attachment to the actin filaments. The proteins troponin and tropomyosin are also shown. Troponin is responsible for exposing the actin filament to the myosin head, thereby allowing cross-bridge formation, that is, a contraction. (Modified from Berne RM, Levy MN. *Principles of Physiology*. 2nd ed. Mosby; 1996.)

all muscle fibers innervated by the axon's branches. All the muscle fibers of a motor unit are of the same fiber type. Each muscle fiber receives innervation from one neuron. The intensity of a muscle contraction is graded by the number of motor units recruited and the rate of firing. The number of muscle fibers in a motor unit varies according to the muscle. For example, in the large muscles of the lower limb, motor units range in size from approximately 500 to 1000 fibers. In contrast, the small muscles in the hand or the extraocular muscles have motor units that range in size from approximately 10 to 100 fibers. These muscles are capable of producing very fine movements, such as typing, tying a bow, or making small adjustments of the eye.

Recruitment is the process of increasing the number of motor units contracting within a muscle at a given time.[8] The process of recruitment follows the size principle, with the small motor units being recruited before the larger motor units. The small motor neurons innervated by slow oxidative type I fibers are fired first, followed by fast oxidative-glycolytic, type IIa, and, finally, the fast glycolytic type IIx fibers.

SKELETAL MUSCLE DEVELOPMENT

Prenatal

To understand some of the age-related changes in skeletal muscle, it is important to study the events of skeletal muscle development. The muscular system develops from mesoderm, except for the muscles of the iris, which develop from neuroectoderm.[12] The events of mesenchymal tissue differentiation into muscle fiber are depicted in Fig. 6.5. The important cell types to be considered are myogenic precursor cells, myoblasts, myotubes, myofibers, fibroblasts, and satellite cells.[5,13]

Myogenic precursor cells are derived from the myotome of the somite. The somites are paired masses of mesoderm, which develop in the embryonic period. The muscles (myotomes), bony segments (sclerotomes), and overlying skin (dermatomes) are derived from somites that lie on either side of the neural tube. Each segmental myotome separates into an epaxial and a hypaxial division. Myoblasts from the epaxial division become the extensor muscles of the neck and vertebral column (Fig. 6.6). Myoblasts from the hypaxial division become the accessory muscles of the neck and the lateral and ventral trunk muscles. The muscles of the extremities develop

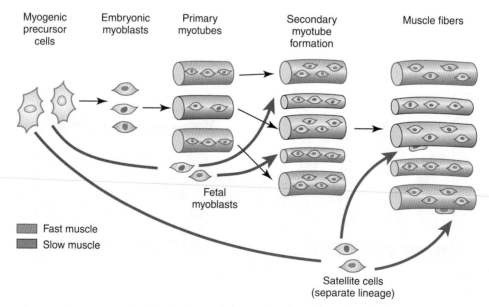

Fig. 6.5 Stages in the formation of primary and secondary muscle fibers. A family of embryonic myoblasts contributes to the formation of the primary myotubes, and fetal myoblasts contribute to secondary myotubes. The origin of satellite cells is still unresolved. (From Carlson BM. *Human Embryology and Developmental Biology*. 4th ed. St Louis: Mosby; 2009:250.)

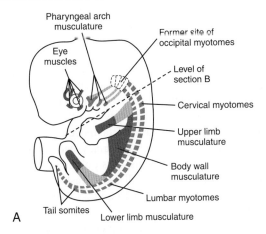

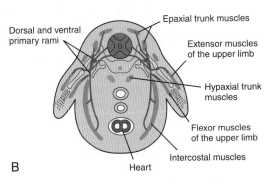

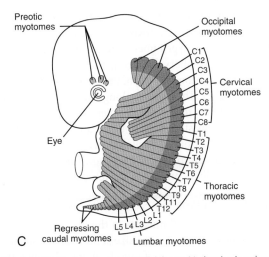

Fig. 6.6 (A) Sketch of an embryo (about 41 days), showing the myotomes and developing muscular system. **(B)** Transverse section of the embryo, illustrating the epaxial and hypaxial derivatives of a myotome. **(C)** Six-week embryo showing the myotome regions of the somites that give rise to most skeletal muscles. (Moore KL, Persaud TVN, Torchia MG, eds. The Developing Human; Clinically Oriented Embryology. 11th ed. Philadelphia: Elsevier; 2020)

from myoblasts located within the limb region that surrounds the developing bones (in situ). Some of the precursor myogenic cells in the limb buds come from somites.[12]

Muscle-specific genes in these premuscle mesenchymal cells are turned on by regulatory factors. Exposure to growth factors produces *myoblasts*, which are spindle-shaped cells with centrally placed elongated nuclei. While these cells do begin to produce actin and myosin, their biggest role developmentally is to fuse together to form large, multinucleated cylinders called myotubes. They align into chainlike configurations parallel to the long axis of the limb. Following fusion, the multinucleated embryonic muscle cell contains a varying number of nuclei ranging up to several hundred. Cellular fusion via disintegration of the plasma membranes of adjacent myoblasts and myotubes is at present the explanation for how striated muscle cells become multinucleated.[5]

Myotubes are immature multinucleated muscle cells. Nuclei are centrally located in these elongated cylindrical cells. Contractile proteins actin and myosin are rapidly synthesized and become evident as striated fibrils in the peripheral cytoplasm. Other regulatory proteins, such as troponin and tropomyosin, are also synthesized. In the fetal period, myotubes fuse to form *myofibers*. *Myofibers* are mature multinucleated muscle cells more commonly called muscle fibers. Myofibers contain the characteristic striations, or sarcomeres, of skeletal muscle. The peripheral migration of the nuclei marks the differentiation of the myotube into a muscle fiber. Most skeletal muscle tissue is developed before birth.[12,14]

Fibroblasts are the flattened, irregularly shaped cells found in association with the developing myofibers. During the early stages of development, these cells provide an extracellular matrix on which the connective tissue framework of a muscle is developed. Fibroblasts form the perimysium and epimysium.

The last cell type to be discussed is the *satellite cell*, which is muscle-specific stem cells. Satellite cells begin to form late in the embryonic period.[5,15] These mononucleated, spindle-shaped cells are closely associated with the surface of the myofibers. They are found between the basal lamina and the muscle fiber (see Figs. 6.1 and 6.5). Skeletal muscle after birth is a postmitotic tissue but can grow and regenerate because of the function of the satellite cells. Satellite cells play an integral role in normal muscle growth after birth and in the repair of muscle following injury.[16]

The role of the satellite cells during normal postnatal growth is to supply nuclei to the enlarging fibers. Although myoblasts constitute a rapidly proliferating cell population during embryonic development, once incorporated into the syncytium of a myofiber, they no longer replicate DNA or divide. The nuclei are permanently postmitotic once they become part of the syncytium. Nevertheless, when myofibers increase in size during growth, the number of nuclei increases, in some cases more than 100 times. This increase in myonuclei depends on the satellite cells associated with the fiber. These cells are continually dividing. After a mitotic division, one or both of the daughter cells fuse with the fiber, thereby injecting an additional nucleus into the syncytium. Likewise, in the event of massive injury to the muscle, myofibers usually die. New muscle fibers can be formed by surviving satellite cells. Activated by stress, the satellite cells repeat the embryonic events leading to muscle formation.[17] The damaged muscle is repaired or replaced by the division of the satellite cells. New daughter cells also contribute to the satellite cell population of the muscle, maintaining a pool of stem cells available for future muscle repair.[16,18]

Control of Muscle Development and Differentiation

Primary myotubes are developed from embryonic myoblasts. Differentiation into both slow (type I) and fast fiber types (type II) begins in the fetal period[15,19] This differentiation occurs before the motor nerve axons have contacted the newly formed muscle. Early motor neurons are present by the time the secondary myotubes are formed because they are derived from fetal myoblasts. Therefore, it was thought that the secondary myotubes required nervous input for their formation and differentiation.[13] Recent evidence suggests that differentiation of myotubes into types of myofibers is not dependent on innervation during the fetal period, but is regulated by regulatory proteins, and a variety of myogenic regulatory factors.[15,19] The composition of contractile proteins determines the phenotype of muscle fibers. There are qualitative differences in the contractile proteins found in slow and fast muscle fibers, with different forms (isoforms) of those proteins being present from the fetal to neonatal periods and on to maturity.[13] Embryonic forms of myosin are present by 15 weeks of gestation, as well as troponin. The fetal muscle has a less-developed sarcomere structure and contracts slower and with less force than adult muscle tissue.[20] At 27 weeks of gestation, slow forms of fetal myosin are present. Embryonic and neonatal myosins disappear just after birth and are replaced with adult-like fast and slow myosins.[15] Both type I and type IIA muscle fibers are noted just before birth, and type IIX fibers are seen in the first week after birth.[21]

The formation of the myoneural junction is initiated with the development of ACh receptors in the periphery of the myotubes at approximately 8 weeks of gestation. This coincides with the earliest fetal movement observed in the intercostal muscles.[22] Prenatally, each motor end plate receives multiple axons. This polyneuronal innervation ensures that there will be at least one axon for every muscle fiber. Between 16 and 25 weeks of gestation, there is a dying back of extra connections and thus a transition to mononeuronal innervation indicative of the classic motor unit.[22] During the last half of gestation, there is also a tremendous increase in the number and size of muscle fibers. The increase in number is primarily from secondary myotubes. During the fetal period, when significant skeletal muscle growth is occurring, animal studies of large mammals have shown that maternal undernutrition or overnutrition can impact skeletal muscle and muscular adiposity. Overnutrition appears to increase intramuscular adiposity and can impact skeletal muscle insulin resistance.[19]

Changes in Fiber Types

Muscle is developed from two distinct lineages: the primary and secondary myotubes. Generally, primary myotubes become type I fibers, and secondary myotubes become type II fibers.[15] During the secondary myogenesis stage, secondary myotubes can fuse with primary myotubes. This fusion, along with environmental cues, contributes to the development of heterogeneous motor units consisting of both type I and type II muscle fibers.[14,15] Studies have concluded that between 31 and 37 weeks of gestation, type II fibers constitute about 25% of the muscle fibers present in the fetus.[23]

Infancy and Childhood

The growth of skeletal muscles in the first year of life is the result of an increase in the size of the individual fibers and possibly the number of muscle fibers. Although the greatest increase in the number of muscle fibers occurs before birth, an increase in muscle fiber number does occur during the first year of postnatal development. After birth, the growth of the muscle comes mainly from an increase in the size of the individual fibers and from satellite cell activity.[14,19]

Differentiation of muscle fibers continues into postnatal life. In the first weeks after birth, immature neuromotor junctions are eliminated and more specific innervation of fast and slow myofibers is seen.[15] Muscle fiber bundles in skeletal muscle contain a heterogeneous mix of fiber types, allowing the muscle to respond to the muscle activity required.[14,15,24] Training can influence the fiber-type composition of skeletal muscle to meet the demands of the activity.[15,24] Genetics, nutrition, and lifestyle may also influence fiber-type distribution.[24] Proportions of different types of fibers also vary considerably among individuals for a given skeletal muscle. For example, a standard deviation of about 15% is observed in the percentage of type I fibers in the vastus lateralis muscle of young men (the mean is about 50%) according to Malina, Bouchard, and Bar-Or.[23] Lexell and colleagues[25] did not find adult distribution of type I fibers in the vastus lateralis muscle of children from 5 to 15 years of age. However, a later study observed the adult distribution in 16-year-olds, which might suggest a change occurs relative to puberty.[26] Changes in fiber-type differentiation continue postnatally, even into the period preceding young adulthood. It appears that the remodeling of motor units postnatally may be related to genetic profiles of the fiber type, transcription factors, and epigenetic gene expression.[15]

Muscle maturation occurs in childhood. Contractile properties of muscle are measured by maximal twitch tension, time to peak tension, and half-relaxation times. Soleus muscle relaxation time was studied as a measure of muscle dynamics in children 3–10 years of age.[27] Researchers found that a child's muscles are initially slow to relax after contraction but that relaxation speed doubles between 3 and 10 years of age. These values reach adult rates at age 10. In further examination of this phenomenon, the investigators found that the speed of contraction improved because of the ability of the muscle to relax more quickly.[28] A possible mechanism for the change in muscle dynamics with age may be a change in the calcium reuptake mechanism of the SR.

Strength gains in children follow a typical growth curve for height and weight. Changes in strength are associated with increases in muscle size and muscle maturation. There are several characteristics of strength that may determine how strong someone will be at a given age, including the cross-sectional area of the muscle, the age of the individual, the gender of the individual, the body size or type, and the fiber type and size of the muscle being assessed. Muscle mass is gained before strength.[29] Muscle makes up only 25% of the lean body mass at birth and increases to 40%–45% at maturity.[30] Children are stronger than infants, and adolescents are stronger than children. In absolute terms, whether assessed cross-sectionally or longitudinally, muscle strength increases linearly with chronological age from childhood to age 12 or 13[31] and is mainly determined by the muscle's cross-sectional area. Tonson and associates[32] demonstrated that maximal isometric strength of the forearm flexors of three age groups—children, adolescents, and adults—was found to be proportional to the size of the muscle regardless of the age of the subject.

Muscle strength and mass increase significantly in childhood. Physical activity contributes to an increase in skeletal muscle mass and muscle strength in children.[33] Mean levels of isometric strength increase gradually between 3 and 6 years of age. Minimal gender differences are present in muscle strength gain during childhood.[31,34] Static strength in boys continues to increase linearly from 6 to 13 years, followed by a spurt that continues through the late teens. Wiggin and associates[35] reported normative data of quadriceps and hamstring strength as measured by isokinetic dynamometry in children 6–13 years old. Height was considered the best predictor of strength. Isokinetic dynamometry is being shown to be the most valid clinical means of measuring strength in children.[35]

Adolescence and Adulthood

Puberty marks an increase in growth of the musculoskeletal systems. As the skeleton grows, the muscles have to lengthen to reestablish the appropriate length-tension relationship. The resting length of a muscle affects the amount of tension that can be generated. At rest, the majority of skeletal muscles are near the optimal length for force production. Separation of the attachments of the muscles as the skeleton grows appears to be a strong stimulus for muscle growth.[36] Muscles add sarcomeres and fibrils to achieve a new length.[29] During puberty, increases in muscle strength are seen, with greater muscle growth in males than females because of the effects of steadily rising levels of testosterone.

Strength in Relation to Age and Muscle Mass

Strength is seen to increase linearly between the ages of 6 and 18 years (Fig. 6.7). Boys have a strength spurt during the adolescent years, which is due to a rise in hormone production. The rise in testosterone begins 1 year before peak height velocity (PHV). This spike occurs at the same time as the divergence of strength between boys and girls.[37] Although testosterone is the most likely reason why males increase muscle mass and strength more than females, other hormones play a role. Growth hormones, insulin, and thyroid hormones are important for somatic and muscle growth. Levels of amino acids,

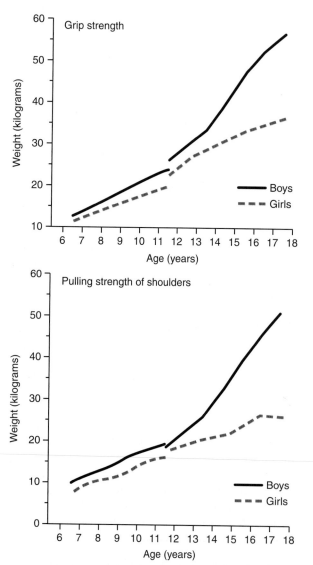

Fig. 6.7 Mean grip strength and pulling strength between 6 and 18 years of age. (From Malina RM, Bouchard C, Bar-Or O. *Growth, Maturation and Physical Activity.* 2nd ed. Champaign, IL: Human Kinetics; 2004:219.)

carbohydrates, and growth factors also stimulate muscle growth during puberty.[34] With increasing age, the percentage of girls whose performance on strength tests equals or exceeds that of boys declines considerably. After age 16, the strength of an average boy is greater than that of a very strong girl. Peak strength velocity occurs about a year after PHV.[37] Although growth studies generally stop at age 18, strength continues to increase into the 20s, especially for men.

Testosterone levels are related to fat-free body mass and strength. Testosterone stimulates muscle protein synthesis and whole-body protein synthesis, allowing increases in the amount of muscle mass. Size and number of muscle fibers, satellite cells, and myonuclei, as well as the biogenesis of mitochondria and expression of myoglobin, lead to increased muscle strength in the presence of testosterone in adolescent boys. Testosterone seems to have the biggest influence early in puberty, and the influence of testosterone weakens in late puberty.[33]

Strength appears to peak during young adulthood.[33] While there is some slowing of contraction during middle adulthood, it is not until the sixth decade (the 50s) that muscle strength begins a more steady decline and begins to effect function.[38,39] There is a 30% decline in muscle strength from age 50 to 70 years and a more rapid decline after 70 years of age.[40] While studies vary slightly, the loss of muscle mass generally occurs by 40 years of age.[41] "Normal" loss is about 1% per year, but may accelerate in later years and in severe instances can lead to a loss of approximately 50% muscle mass by the eighth to ninth decade of life.[42] In summary, the two major influences upon the loss of muscle mass and function with age are muscle fiber atrophy and muscle fiber loss.

The decrease is evident in both isometric and dynamic strength, but relatively speaking, eccentric strength is better maintained in older adults than concentric strength.[43–46] Loss of strength in older men and women is greater than can be explained by loss of muscle mass alone.[47] The effect of age on strength is seen in Fig. 6.8.

Researchers agree that the rate of decline in muscular strength with age appears greater in the lower body than in the upper body.[48] Studies of women indicate that muscle strength, both static and dynamic, decreases with age.[43] Women are weaker than men in muscular strength.[43] Women also demonstrate a decrement in strength earlier than men.[49] There is a curvilinear relationship between maximum voluntary isometric strength and age in healthy adults.[50,51] The curvilinear

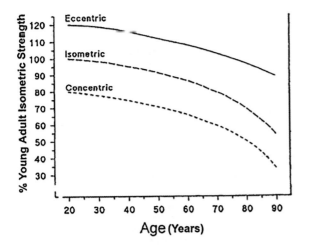

Fig. 6.8 Effect of age on maximal strength throughout the human life span. The shape and height of the schematic curves are based on Vandervoort's gerontology research and depend on the type of strength being measured: isometric, concentric (muscle allowed to shorten while contracting), or eccentric (active muscle being lengthened by external load). (From Vandervoort AA. Aging of the human neuromuscular system. *Muscle Nerve* 2002;25:17–25.)

relationship is also seen with changes in eccentric and concentric strength in older adults (Fig. 6.8). Some of the strength loss in individuals may be related to the activity or fitness level of the individual. If an individual remains active, the amount of muscle strength lost may be less (Table 6.1). Lifelong-trained older adults have been found to be stronger than age-matched untrained older adults.[52]

Older Adulthood

Sarcopenia

Muscle mass is stable until approximately age 40 and a slow, continuous loss of muscle mass begins, which accelerates by 70 years of age.[41] The greater decline in strength relative to decline in muscle mass seems to be accounted for by the significant decline in the quality of muscle.[47] In those older adults who are lifelong trained, muscle mass and strength may be relatively preserved but not to the extent that loss of muscle mass and strength can be prevented with aging.[52]

The age-related loss of muscle called *sarcopenia* literally means "loss of flesh." Sarcopenia is the loss of skeletal muscle mass, quality, and strength that is seen during normal aging, often accompanied by increased intramuscular and body fat levels.[41] The European Working Group on Sarcopenia in Older People (EWGSOP2) met in 2018 to update the definition of sarcopenia. "Sarcopenia is a progressive and generalized skeletal muscle disorder that is associated with increased likelihood of adverse outcomes including falls, fractures, physical disability, and mortality."[53] EWGSOP2 emphasizes that health care providers have ever-increasing abilities for preventing, delaying, treating, and sometimes even reversing sarcopenia by way of early and effective interventions such as exercise and nutritional counseling.[53,54] Individuals are considered sarcopenic if their lean body mass is <2 SD below the mean compared with a sample of healthy young adults. Wiedmer and colleagues[41] report that 23%–30% of adults over 60 years of age were sarcopenic, based on appendicular lean mass. Iannuzzi-Sucich et al.[55] found similar rates in a population of older, community-dwelling adults. They concluded that sarcopenia is common in adults over 65, with body mass index (BMI) being a strong indicator of muscle mass. A larger BMI was associated with less lean muscle mass. Risk factors for sarcopenia include age, gender, and level of ongoing physical activity.[56] The reduction in muscle mass is most prominent in the lower extremities and is characterized by a preferential atrophy of type 2 muscle fibers.[41,56,57]

Sarcopenia is a commonly recognized cause of loss of strength and functional abilities in older adults. Understanding sarcopenia is important because the condition has high personal, social, and economic burdens when not addressed. Sarcopenia increases mobility problems,[58] risk of falls and fractures,[59,60] and impairs the ability to independently perform activities of daily living (ADL).[61] Sarcopenia is also associated with cardiac disease,[62] respiratory disease,[63] and cognitive impairment.[64] Sarcopenia can also contribute to a lowered quality of life[65] with loss of functional independence or admission to a long-term care facility.[66] Weak muscles hasten the loss of independence and everyday instrumental activities of daily living (IADLs) such as cleaning, shopping, walking, and driving. Higher rates of physical disability have been demonstrated in those individuals with sarcopenia. Baumgartner and associates[67] found a fourfold higher rate of disability in men and a 3.6 higher rate of disability in women in their study compared to those with more muscle mass. Janssen et al.[68] found a prevalence of severe sarcopenia in women than in men over 60 years of age, which was then associated with a greater

TABLE 6.1	Strength Changes in Older Adulthood	
Easier to Maintain	**Harder to Maintain**	
Muscles used in activities of daily living	Muscles used infrequently in specialized activities	
Isometric strength	Dynamic strength	
Eccentric contractions	Concentric contractions	
Slow-velocity contractions	Rapid-velocity contractions	
Repeated low-level contractions	Power production	
Strength using small joint angles	Strength using large joint angles	
Strength in males	Strength in females	

From Spirduso WW: Physical dimensions of aging, Champaign, IL 1995, Human Kinetics.

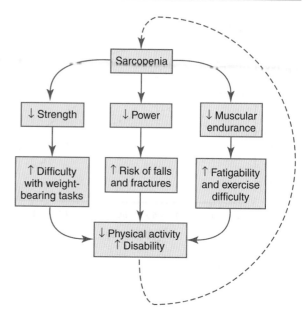

Fig. 6.9 A model of the functional consequences of age-related sarcopenia and positive feedback loop by which the end result of reduced physical activity further exacerbates progression of the disorder. ↓ indicates decrease; ↑ indicates increase. (From Hunter GR, McCarthy FP, Bamman MM. Effects of resistance training on older adults. *Sports Med.* 2004;34(5):329–348.)

amount of impairment and disability. A model of the potential functional consequences of age-related sarcopenia is seen in Fig. 6.9.

The degree of muscle loss associated with aging may be partially related to the activity level of the individual. Adults who do not regularly participate in strength training can expect to lose 4–6 pounds of muscle per decade, which is usually replaced with fat.[69] Intervention strategies to minimize risk for and functional impact of sarcopenia focus on exercise and nutrition. Exercise can increase skeletal mass and function and is thought to increase the number of available satellite cells and the number of type II muscle fibers. Exercise may also decrease inflammation and decrease fat infiltration into the muscle. Nutritional interventions focus on including sources of protein in the diet.[41]

Mechanisms of Muscle Loss

The etiology of sarcopenia is multifactorial[70–73] as seen in Fig. 6.10.[41] Loss of muscle mass has been associated with muscle disuse, oxidative stress, inflammatory effects, changes in the nervous system (especially the motor unit), hormonal changes, decreased protein synthesis, and changes in muscle structure and function. Functional decline in older adults has a strong inverse relationship with physical activity.[41,74]

Oxidative Stress and Inflammatory Effects

Oxidative stress and inflammation in muscle tissue have been implicated in the loss of muscle power and mass that is characteristically seen with aging.[5,41,75] Oxidative stress is characterized by increased levels of skeletal muscle reactive oxygen species (ROS). Oxidation is the precursor to inflammation and is simply the interaction between oxygen molecules and human tissue.[76–78] When oxygen is metabolized, it creates "free radicals," which steal electrons from other molecules, causing cellular damage. Oxidative processes stimulate inflammation and the cascade of biochemical reactions associated with it. The cytological changes seen in muscle tissue represent some of the adverse effects of the body's inflammatory reaction to oxidation. An imbalance occurs between anabolic and catabolic intracellular signaling pathways and an increase in oxidative stress both play important roles in muscle abnormalities.[76]

Aging results in chronic low-grade inflammation that is associated with increased risk for chronic conditions including cardiovascular dysfunction, diabetes, and kidney disease, poor physical functioning, and mortality. While transient inflammation is necessary for recovery from injury and exercise, the hypothesis is that the excessive inflammation in aging may also be caused by an exaggerated acute-phase response that may be

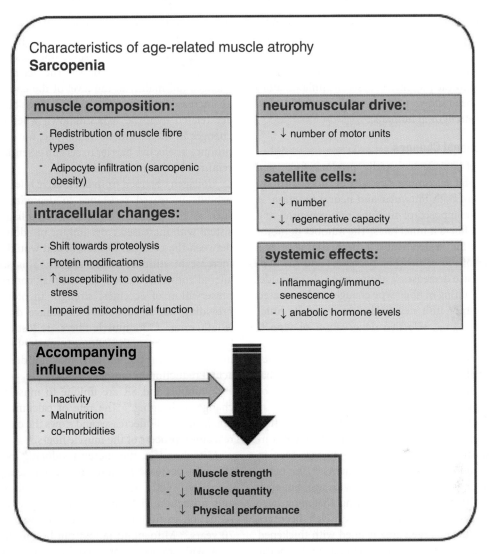

Fig. 6.10 Major characteristics of sarcopenia comprise several components from the cellular level to neuromuscular innervation and systemic effects. This complex mixture of components might, in combination with other accompanying situations, lead to the major features of sarcopenia.

a cause or consequence of a delayed recovery from an insult that promotes inflammation.[79] Physical exercise can result in free radical-mediated damage to muscle tissue. While low levels of ROS are needed for normal force production, higher levels are detrimental and can result in weakness and fatigue.[80] Exercise is thought to be protective of muscle function, but the recommendation is to rest for 48 hours between strength training episodes to allow the inflammation to decrease.[81]

The increase in inflammatory mediators that normally occurs with exercise is transient. Chronically elevated levels of these inflammatory mediators because of age and disease are not beneficial. The mechanism whereby inflammation contributes to the overall loss of muscle mass and strength with aging continues to be investigated. Higher levels of inflammatory markers (interleukin 6 and C-reactive protein) have been found to be associated with a greater risk of losing muscle strength in older women and men.[82] The risk is 2–3 times greater for more than a 40% loss over a 3-year period of time. Inflammatory factors may play a role in the onset and progression of sarcopenia.[83] Chronic inflammation, as demonstrated by the presence of systemic inflammatory markers, has been shown to be inversely related to muscle mass and strength in humans.[84]

Neural Functional Changes

The ability of muscle to rapidly produce force and therefore exhibit maximum strength declines with age due to a loss of both muscular and neural function. A motor unit is composed of an alpha motor neuron and all the muscle fibers it innervates. The number of motor units innervating skeletal muscle decreases with age. The number of motor neurons decreases and the axonal cell body size decreases.[41] Motor units also remodel with aging, resulting in fiber-type changes and increased size of the motor unit negatively impacting its function.[42,78] With aging, selective denervation of type II fibers occurs with reinnervation by slow motor neurons.[78,85] Physiologically, they become slow motor units. The functional significance of the reorganization is that the nervous system may have to alter its strategies for controlling muscle force.

Changes in one part of the motor unit affect other parts of the motor unit. Motor end plates remodel continuously during normal aging, with changes seen in presynaptic and postsynaptic components.[86] The number of synaptic vesicles is increased with age, but they are found in tight clusters, suggesting that they have undergone agglutination. The synaptic cleft becomes enlarged, and the enlarged area is filled with thickened basal lamina. In addition, the functional folds appear unfolded, and the plasma membrane of the muscle fiber appears thickened.[87]

Changes in Skeletal Muscle Structure and Function

Structural changes are seen in the muscle itself. The overall decrease in muscle function can be attributed to a combination of muscular, tendonous, and neural factors. The changes in muscle architecture, tendon mechanical properties, excitation-contraction coupling, and single-fiber contractility combine to decrease overall muscle function. Muscle architecture changes include a decrease in pennation angle of muscle fibers; decreased fascicle length; an increase in intramuscular fat and connective tissue; and a decrease in muscle thickness.[87]

As we age, the amount of connective tissue increases, mostly at the level of the endomysium. In addition, the basement membrane increases in thickness around both the capillary and the myofiber. The net result of these changes (all mainly at the level of the endomysium) is an increase in diffusion distances, possibly producing age-related hypoxia. It is unknown whether chemical changes in the basement membrane, for example, may produce a selective barrier to certain essential molecules required by the muscle fibers.

Collagen obtained from old muscle is less soluble and exhibits increased resistance to degradative enzymes such as collagenase. Changes in the collagen are consistent with increased cross-linking or additional bonds between the collagen molecules and would explain the increase in stiffness of old muscle. This stiffness and altered connective tissue content may contribute to the preservation of eccentric strength in older adults by providing increased passive resistance during muscle lengthening.[72,88] As muscle fibers are lost and replaced by fat and collagen, the volume or girth of the muscle as measured anthropometrically may not demonstrate an actual reduction in muscle mass.

T-tubules and SR are unique to muscle fibers and change with aging.[89] The rate of calcium release and uptake in the SR decreases and slows the contractile and relaxation process of the muscle fibers.[46]

Mitochondria, the energy-producing parts of muscle cells, decrease in number and efficiency. Aging is associated with decreased skeletal muscle function and mitochondrial function, leading to a 25%–30% reduction in functional capacity between ages 30 and 70 years.[90] Mitochondria loss can be intimately linked to a wide range of processes associated with aging including senescence and inflammation, as well as the more generalized age-dependent decline in tissue and organ function.[91] Mitochondrial dysfunction is thought to be closely related to the biological aging of muscles.[92] Therapeutic benefits of exercise training are associated with the suppression of aging-related mitochondrial dysfunction. Exercise may inhibit mitochondrial dysfunction and thereby ameliorate age-related complications.[49]

Increased apoptosis, or the process of programmed cellular death, may be a contributing factor to muscle aging. In apoptosis, biochemical events lead to characteristic changes in cellular morphology. Specifically, in relation to muscle tissue, it appears nuclear fragmentation may lead to cellular death and subsequent tissue atrophy. Apoptosis is different from necrosis, which involves some form of cellular trauma, and the resulting apoptotic bodies are engulfed and removed by phagocytic cells before they can cause damage to surrounding tissue.[93]

Satellite cell number and function also decrease with age.[5,16,18] The number of satellite cells decreases, especially those related to type II muscle fibers.[94] Satellite cells also appear to demonstrate less ability to regenerate, diminishing the renewing pool of cells.[78] Diminished regenerative capacity may be the result of age-related DNA damage to the satellite cell or telomere attrition.[41]

Changes in Muscle Protein Synthesis

Older adults demonstrate decreased muscle protein synthesis. This decline affects three processes involved in muscle contraction: ATP production, excitation-contraction coupling, and cross-bridge cycling.[70] A decline in mitochondrial protein production and activity results in decreased oxidative capacity by limiting the amount of ATP available for muscle contraction. The decline in muscle proteins has been associated with age-related loss in muscle strength and aerobic exercise tolerance.[95] The decline in protein synthesis in muscle has been related to declines in insulin-like growth factor, testosterone, and dehydroepiandrosterone sulfate.[70] The degradation of excitation-contraction coupling that occurs with age also contributes to the loss of strength seen in sarcopenia. Uncoupling occurs because two key proteins are altered, resulting in a slower release of calcium through the ryanodine receptor. The functional result is that it takes longer to produce a contraction and longer to relax after a contraction in older adults. The cross-bridging cycle is unable to produce as much strength with age due to structural and chemical changes in myosin, the muscle protein that contributes most to muscle mass.[70] Evidence indicates that physical activity prevents some muscle loss by mechanically loading specific cells in muscle cell membranes that promote protein synthesis.[96]

Dietary intake of protein stimulates muscle protein synthesis, but evidence indicates that the skeletal muscle of older adults demonstrates resistance to muscle protein synthesis. Decreased muscle protein synthesis in older adults is also impacted by levels of growth hormone and insulin growth factor 1 (IGF-1). Insulin typically limits muscle protein breakdown. Older adults, with increased lipid deposition in muscle, demonstrate insulin resistance and inflammation in muscle tissue.[42,78] These factors, as well as oxidative stress, also contribute to muscle protein breakdown.[41,42]

Many older adults do not ingest the recommended daily allowance (RDA) for protein, which is 0.8 g/kg/day. Evans[97] suggests that this minimum RDA may not be sufficient to maintain muscle mass with exercise. Boirie[98] suggested that dietary supplementation with certain amino acids, institution of changes in patterns of protein ingestion, as well as increases in the amount of dietary protein could counteract some of the age-related loss of muscle in older adults. Combining exercise with the dietary intake of protein is also important.[41,78] Even with dietary and exercise interventions, older adults demonstrate diminished muscle protein synthesis, as compared to younger adults.[42,78]

Changes in Contractile Properties

The ability of muscle to generate force and power is reduced with age. Declines in strength and power are related to the loss of the fast-twitch, type II muscle fibers, decreased muscle mass, altered muscle quality, and neuromuscular changes that occur with age.[99] Muscle quality is the relationship between muscle mass, strength, and speed. It encompasses all the factors governing rapid force development (RFD), such as motor unit firing rate, amount of type II fibers, reduced tendon stiffness, and reduced pennation angle of the muscle fibers.[52,99] Decline in RFD in older adults occurs because of the preferential decline in the cross-sectional area of type II muscle fibers.[38]

As we age the size of type I muscle fibers decreases although not to the same extent as type II. The size of type II (both IIA and IIX) also decreases, along with myosin protein synthesis and overall protein metabolism. Older adults do not develop force as rapidly as young adults because of the loss of type II muscle fibers. Type II muscles can intrinsically develop more force because they have a larger cross-sectional area and a fast cross-bridge cycling rate compared with type I muscles.[89,100] A selective loss of type II fibers could explain why muscles generate force more slowly but also relax more slowly. Diminished speed of contraction impacts muscle power.

Muscle power reductions are seen earlier than decreases in muscle strength in older adults.[99,101] Loss of muscle power with aging has a greater influence on loss of motor function than loss of muscle strength.[87,99,102,103] Motor unit firing rates appear to generally be reduced with aging, but the changes seem to be task and muscle specific. Not all muscles are equally affected by age.

Force control is lessened in older adults because of the greater number of low threshold (type I) motor units compared with the number found in younger adults. The force-velocity curve is shifted secondary to aging (Fig. 6.11). This occurs because the older muscle is less able to generate force at all contraction speeds. For an excellent review of aging and force-velocity relationship of muscles, the reader is referred to Raz et al. (2010).[104]

Older adults have less difficulty with eccentric contractions than with concentric contractions. Concentric actions decline the greatest with eccentric contractions and eccentric strength being relatively preserved.[46] Loss of eccentric strength is 10%–30% less than concentric strength, with women showing greater preservation then men.[45,104] Maintenance of eccentric strength seems to be related to both mechanical and cellular factors. From a mechanical perspective, older skeletal muscle is stiffer than younger muscle because of increased noncontractile components (fat and connective tissue) within the muscle-tendon unit. This stiffness provides a mechanical advantage in eccentric contraction, where a stretch of the muscle fibers stimulates contraction. From a neurologic perspective, eccentric muscle contraction does not stimulate as strong an antagonist response as concentric contraction, allowing for more force to be generated.[44,45]

FUNCTIONAL IMPLICATIONS

Changes occurring in the development of skeletal muscle tissue across the life span have functional and clinical implications for muscle strength, endurance, power, and function. Clinical Implications Box 6.1: Muscle Strength Acquisition Across the Life Span outlines markers for promoting strength and related training and exercise programs along the developmental continuum.

Muscle strength is an expression of muscular force, or the individual's capacity to develop tension against an

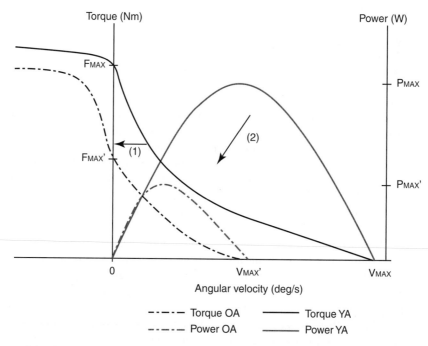

Fig. 6.11 A summary of the changes to the force-velocity and power-velocity relationship with age based on data from the studies referenced in this review. With increased age, the force-velocity and power-velocity curves shift downward and to the left. F_{max}, Young adults' peak isometric torque; $F_{max'}$, older adults' peak isometric torque; *OA*, older adults; $P_{max'}$, older adults maximal power; $V_{max'}$, older adults' maximum contraction velocity; *YA*, young adults. (From Raz IS, Bird SR, Shield AJ. Aging and the force-velocity relationship of muscles. *Exp Gerontol.* 2010;45:81–90.)

CLINICAL IMPLICATIONS BOX 6.1
Muscle Strength Acquisition Across the Life Span

Strength acquisition follows a general growth curve as seen in other anthropometric measures, such as height and weight. Muscle strength in children increases linearly before puberty, and accelerates at puberty. In middle adulthood muscle strength begins to decline, and the decrease in strength increases further in older adulthood.

Children
- Children can increase strength and endurance as a result of regular participation in a program of progressive resistance training.[105–107]
- Strength training programs should be well supervised and well designed with the child's age, level of motor proficiency, and current level of strength.[108]
- A properly designed resistive exercise program does not negatively impact the growth and development of youth.[76,106]
- Recommendations regarding resistance training in children and adolescents are available from the Canadian Society for Exercise Physiology,[109] the American Academy of Pediatrics,[106] and several other international groups.[108]
- Benefits of resistance training for children include improved bone mineral density, strengthening of tendons, improved motor skill performance/motor competency, improved balance, and decreased musculoskeletal injury.[110] It also improves lipid profiles, insulin sensitivity (in overweight children), and positively influences psycho-social health and well-being.[106,108]

Adolescents
- Muscle strength increases rapidly in puberty and is non-linear. Boys gain more strength than girls, with girls demonstrating an earlier return to linear increases in strength later in puberty.[108]
- Maximal increase in muscle thickness, as well as increases in muscle fascicle length, occurs about the time of the PHV.[105]
- Preadolescent and adolescents can safely increase strength and power after participating in a well-designed and properly supervised resistance training program.[106,110,111]
- Use of maximal lifts and competitive style weight lifting is not recommended prior to skeletal maturity.[107,110]
- Physiological mismatching is possible between 13 and 17 years of age and may increase the risk of injury

resulting from differences in body size, age, and maturity status. Biological age should be considered as well as chronological age in youth sports and training programs.[108]
- The health benefits from participation in a well-designed and appropriately supervised resistance training program far outweigh the potential risks. Benefits are similar to those reported above for children.

Adults
- Maximal strength is achieved in the 30s and maintained until the 50s.[38]
- Strength training results in improved performance in trained and untrained individuals.
- Strength training needs to be specific to the task, such as speed, power, intensity, and endurance.
- If strengthening is performed throughout middle and older adulthood, age-related strength loss is mitigated but *not* eliminated.[52,112]
- Only 41% of men and 28% of women met the recommendations of the American College of Sports Medicine (ACSM) on physical activity beneficial for health.[113]

Older Adults
- Progressive resistance training is an effective and safe way to increase strength in older adults.[114–117]
- Women may respond differently to strength training.[118–120]
- Frailty and advanced age are not a contraindication to exercise.[116,121] A sedentary lifestyle is far more dangerous than activity in the older adult.
- Participation in a regular progressive resistive exercise can combat the functional declines associated with aging.[114,122–124]
- Training for power may be more important than training for strength because of the carryover to functional activities, such as rising from a chair or climbing stairs.[124–126]
- Gait speed is positively affected by progressive resistance strength training.[127–129] Gait speed is a powerful predictor of health.[130,131]
- Recommendations for strength training in older adults can be found in the position stand of the American College of Sports Medicine[48] and the *Canadian Journal of Public Health*.[132,133]

external resistance. The literature defines several types of strength: static, power, and dynamic.[31] *Static*, or *isometric, strength* is the maximal voluntary force produced against an external resistance without any change in muscle length. It is generally measured in specific muscle groups, such as those in the hand, by grip strength, or isokinetically in the quadriceps or hamstrings. *Power* is explosive strength or the ability of muscles to produce a certain amount of force in the shortest amount of time. It is measured as a function of strength. *Dynamic strength* is the force generated by repetitive contractions of a muscle. Therefore, it is closely linked to muscular endurance. Dynamic strength is also known as functional strength in the physical fitness literature.

Muscle endurance is the ability to repeat or maintain muscular contractions over time. It is believed that the capacity of a muscle to increase in muscular endurance is related to the ability of the muscle to use oxygen, or the *oxidative metabolism* of the muscle. This ability is related to the individual's maximal oxygen uptake, or Vo_{2max}, levels. This is defined as the transport of oxygen from the atmosphere for use by the mitochondria of the muscle and is related to individual cardiovascular efficiency (see Chapter 13). Muscle fatigue is the reduced ability to achieve the same amount of force output. Fatigue is related to endurance but is not the same thing. Although endurance is related to the aerobic capacity of the muscle, fatigue may be the result of a failure of motor unit recruitment or altered excitation-contraction coupling. There are many central and peripheral factors that can be responsible for muscle fatigue.

Muscle fatigue is the loss of force and power, which leads to reduced task performance.[134] It is task specific and manifests differently in men and women.[135,136] Furthermore the response to exercise and production of fatigue may change over the life span. The origin of fatigue is multifactorial as are the different domains of fatigue.[137] Some of the same factors implicated in the causation and progression of sarcopenia have been identified as contributing to fatigue, such as the decline in mitochondrial function, oxidative stress, and inflammation. The time to task failure, or the inability to continue a task because of fatigue, is different between young and old and women and men as seen in Fig. 6.12. Factors affecting fatigue include the muscle groups involved, the type and intensity of the contraction, whether the limb is supported, and the environment in which the task is performed.[135]

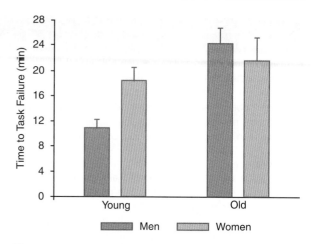

Fig. 6.12 Time to task failure for a sustained isometric fatiguing contraction performed with elbow flexor muscles with young and old men and women. The time to failure was longer for the young women compared with the young men but similar for older men and women. (From Hunter SK, Critchlow A, Enoka RM. Influence of aging on sex differences in muscle fatigability. *J Appl Physiol* 2004;97:1723–1732.)

Decreased muscle strength and increased muscle fatigue hasten the loss of independence for older adults. Functional implications of decreased muscular performance can lead to decreased mobility performance (i.e., stairs, sit-to-stand, walking, and balance), limited ADL and IADL function, postural changes that can lead to greater levels of pain, and risk for falls and fractures (Fig. 6.13).

Childhood and Adolescence

Through childhood and adolescence, increases are seen in muscle mass, cross-sectional area, volume, and thickness. The tendons also increase in cross-sectional area and stiffness. Muscle fascicle length increases especially in adolescence, possibly stimulated by limb growth, and pennation angle of muscle fibers increases. Many of these changes contribute to increases in force production.[105] It is clear that muscular strength increases gradually during early infancy and early childhood. Muscle strength increases linearly through childhood and is fairly equivalent in boys and girls.[34,108] Longitudinal studies show that the adolescent growth spurt in isometric strength occurs within a year before the age at PHV and may coincide with peak weight velocity.[37] In girls, there is improvement in strength through about 15 years of age.[23] Boys

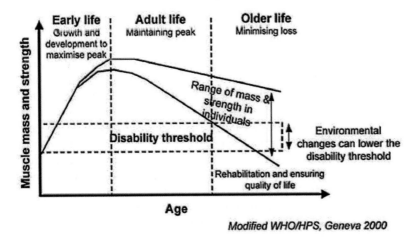

Fig. 6.13 Relating strength changes to disability threshold with aging.

experience a longer growing period of almost 2 years, which along with a sharper acceleration of growth accounts for the gender difference in growth during puberty.[108] Strength, body size, and muscle mass are related. Power as measured by the ability to perform a vertical jump or a standing long jump shows increases in boys and girls from 6 to 12 or 13 years old. After 13, boys continue to improve while girls' scores level off. This age-related trend is seen in the development of strength, aerobic power, and motor performance.[23] Muscular endurance improves linearly with age from 5 to 13 or 14 years in boys, followed by a spurt similar to that for static muscular strength. Muscular endurance also increases with age in girls, but there is no clear evidence of a spurt like that seen in boys.[23]

Children should be encouraged to engage in active play and physical activity from a young age to optimize muscle strength and mass.[138] Children depend on aerobic metabolism during play and can only participate in short bursts of highly intense activity. During short intense bouts of exercise, children have a lesser ability to generate mechanical energy from chemical energy sources.[139] These exercise needs can more easily be met by anaerobic energy production. Genetics, fiber-type differentiation, hormonal influences, and improved coordination all contribute to the development of anaerobic muscle function.[139,140]

Strength can be increased in children before puberty through the use of resistance training. However, the increase in muscle strength occurs without much increase in muscle size.[141] Strength gains are related to nervous system maturation and functions. Increased recruitment of motor units, myelination, and firing frequency of motor units facilitate strength increases.[105,108,110] During puberty, muscle strength and growth continue to be influenced by nervous system development, as well as hormonal influences (testosterone, growth hormone, and IGF). Cross-sectional area, pennation angle of fibers, and continued motor unit differentiation to include type II muscle fibers contribute to increased force production.[108]

Strength Training in Children and Adolescents

Toddlers and young children are physically active, which supports development of muscle strength as they run, climb, push, and pull in play. Once children are old enough to follow directions and begin participating in sports activities (as early as 5–6 years old), they can safely begin participation in well-supervised and well-designed resistance training/strength training programs.[106] Strength training programs for children have been shown to improve muscle strength (30%–50% in 8- to 20-week resistance training programs) and motor skill performance.[107,108] Once children are in school and in community programs, strength training should be incorporated into physical education to build muscle strength and reduce the risk of injury with sport participation through childhood and adolescence.[106]

Strength training will also increase bone strength, as well as tendon thickness and stiffness in children/adolescents.[105] Improvements in body composition (fat-free mass), lipid profiles, insulin sensitivity (in obese children), cardiovascular fitness, and self-esteem have also been reported.[106-108] It is well established that well-supervised, well-designed resistance training programs are safe for children and adolescents and do not put them at risk for epiphyseal injury or other injuries from weight lifting.[107,110]

Resistance training programs for youth can include several forms of resistance, such as body weight resistance, free weights (age-appropriate size), resistance tubing, medicine balls, and weight machines (if size appropriate for youth).[106-108] Other recommendations are to include 5–10 minutes of warmup and cool down; perform exercises through a full range of motion; focus on major muscle groups, both flexor and extensor muscles, upper and lower extremities; use submaximal load to help a child learn correct form and technique and then increase load slowly as the child progresses. Resistance training should be done 2–3 times/week on nonconsecutive days. Most importantly, supervision, education of children and parents about form and safety, and age-appropriate design of the program for each child are critical.[106-108] Use of maximal lifts and power lifting is not recommended for children and adolescents, until skeletal maturity is attained.[110]

There is consensus that resistance training is beneficial to children and adolescents because it can lead to improved muscular function and health benefits.[106,108-110,142] Participation in resistance training also builds motor competence in youth and can contribute to a physically active lifestyle across the life span.

Adulthood and Aging

As stated earlier in this chapter, beginning by age 40 adults lose muscle mass as they age. But, adults have the ability to improve strength by resistance training.[143] Exercise and training need to be guided specifically for how the muscle is expected to function in order to see desired improvements. Examples include static exercise for holding a muscle contraction, plyometrics for power, and endurance training to improve cardiopulmonary function. Training needs to be specific to the type of task being performed and intensity must be challenging for the individual. Once a strength base is established, specific power or endurance training can follow. The variability of motor

performance between young and old adults appears to be the result of muscle force production fluctuations.[144] Fluctuations in muscle force production during a voluntary contraction are influenced by the architecture or shape of the muscle, the type of contraction the muscle is undergoing, the intensity of the contraction, and the properties of the motor units involved. The rate at which a muscle develops force (acceleration) during a slow concentric or eccentric contraction can fluctuate around a mean. Healthy older adults were found to demonstrate greater force fluctuations during submaximal contractions than younger adults. Depending on the muscle group involved, these fluctuations could be decreased by either increased physical activity or strengthening.[144] The motor unit discharge rate to both the agonist and antagonist muscles was most likely responsible for the difference seen between young and older adults.

Loss of muscle strength is associated with a loss of function in older adults. Strength changes in older adulthood are discussed in Table 7-1. The strength-function relationship is curvilinear. There appears to be a minimum amount of strength required for a given task; this threshold may vary from task to task. Strong correlations between strength and function may exist only in individuals who have less than the "threshold" amount of strength. The amount of strength and the mode of muscle contraction—isometric, concentric, or eccentric—are specific to the task to be performed. For example, isometric hip abductor strength may be more representative of the force that needs to be generated during a single limb stance than a concentric contraction of the same muscle group. By using the best measure of strength for a particular task, Chandler and co-workers[145] were able to predict the relative strength of the correlations between muscle strength and certain functional activities.

The strength of the quadriceps has been specifically studied as it relates to falls and steadiness in standing. Sarcopenia can result in force generation fluctuations that might hinder the prevention of falling. Lower limb muscle strengthening seems to be an effective intervention for preventing falls.[146,147] After 16 weeks of resistance training, older adults improved in their use of tripping reactions.[148] Maximum push-off force improved in the trained group. Faller and nonfallers were distinguished by increased unsteadiness during eccentric quadriceps contractions.[149] Symons and associates[122] found that after a 12-week strength training program, older adults improved their performance in stair ascent and descent.

Muscle power also relates to the ability to perform functional skills, and loss of muscle power with aging may have a greater impact on the functional ability of older adults than muscle strength.[99] As stated earlier, power diminishes with age; in fact, power declines faster than strength.[99,104] Puthoff and Nielsen[123] studied the relationships between impairments in strength and power of the lower extremities and function in older adults. Their regression analysis showed that power had a stronger indirect effect on function than strength. Peak power measurements explained more of the variance in functional activities than strength measurements. The researchers concluded that older adults would benefit from velocity-specific resistance training, that is, work at both low and high velocities in addition to strength training.

Endurance is related to the "use it or lose it" concept and can be assessed by looking at muscle fatigue. As previously defined, muscle fatigue "develops gradually soon after the onset of sustained physical activity.[135]" Baudry and associates[150] demonstrated more fatigability in older adults than younger adults with maximal concentric and eccentric contractions of the dorsiflexor muscles. They attributed the fatigue in older adults to impaired neuromuscular propagation and to changes in the control of excitation-contraction coupling by Ca^{2+}. The latter change in excitation-contraction coupling was given as a reason for the fatigue in young adults.

Endurance exercises may help normalize mitochondrial function in older individuals.[151] In a cross-sectional study, researchers measured insulin sensitivity and mitochondrial function in two groups of endurance-trained and sedentary young and older adults. Endurance training ameliorated the age-related decline in mitochondrial oxidative capacity in older adults. Both the older and younger adults who underwent endurance training had higher levels of insulin sensitivity than the sedentary adults, but the amount of difference did not reach statistical significance.

Muscle Strength, Endurance, and Power Training in Older Adults

Older adults can improve muscular strength and endurance and substantially increase their functional capacity. Strength training helps offset the loss of muscle and the decline in strength seen with normal aging, according to the American College of Sports Medicine's position stand.[48] Older adults should participate in aerobic activities, strength training, and exercises for postural stability and flexibility. Vandervoort[152] states that the benefits and guidelines for strength training in older individuals can be summed up by, again, the old adage "use it or lose it."

Exercise is efficacious even in the oldest old. Physical frailty can be delayed by increasing the activity level of the older adult. Resistance exercise training and aerobic exercise training have been found to increase muscle strength and aerobic capacity by at least 20%–30% in older adults.[48] In a Cochrane review,[114] progressive resistive training was shown to produce functional improvements in mobility and performance. Older adults were able to improve in activities such as getting up from a chair and stair climbing. These improvements were generally greater than improvements in walking speed, a very powerful predictor of health. Interestingly, the older adults were also able to improve their performance of more complex activities, such as preparing a meal and taking a bath, with progressive strength training.

Strength training in older adults increases muscle strength by increasing muscle mass and by improving the recruitment of motor units, and increasing their firing rate.[153] Muscle mass can be increased through training at an intensity corresponding to 60%–85% of the individual maximum voluntary strength. Improving the rate of force development requires training at a higher intensity (above 85%), in the elderly just as in younger persons.[153] The recommendation from this study is that healthy older people should train 3 or 4 times weekly for the best results. Even people starting from a deconditioned state can benefit from muscle strengthening. Studies in which resistance training was performed either alone or as part of multicomponent exercise programs revealed greater strength gains in older adults with physical frailty or severe functional declines.[132] The side effects are rare for this training. Progressive strength training in the elderly is efficient, even with higher intensities, to reduce sarcopenia, and to retain motor function.

Eccentric loading of muscles is recommended for older adults so that they take advantage of their relatively higher eccentric strength.[50] Eccentric exercise with older adults is more effective in decreasing muscle atrophy and facilitates higher velocity contraction and force production than other resistance exercise. It may also stimulate a greater satellite cell response then concentric contraction.[154] Eccentric training can start with repetitive submaximal exercise, which will increase muscle strength and mobility in older adults. When higher intensity or greater volume of eccentric exercise can be tolerated, increases in the cross-sectional area of type II muscle fibers and a greater number of type II phenotypes may be seen[154] Although eccentric exercise has been found to improve strength,[155] concentric training demonstrated the greatest gains when compared with isometric or eccentric training.[122] Eighteen men and 12 women with mean age of 73 participated in a 12-week training program using a Biodex. They were divided into three groups: isometric, concentric, and eccentric. All three exhibited increases in strength: peak isometric, isokinetic concentric, and eccentric of the knee extensors. The strength improvement manifested as functional improvement in stair climbing.

Resistance training has been shown to increase muscle mass and strength, increase cross-sectional area, increase neuromuscular system function, and increase type II satellite cell function in older adults.[78] The use of progressive strength training for older adults has become a vital part of evidence-based practice for preventive and rehabilitative care. Exercise is undoubtedly one of the pillars of healthy aging.[156,157]

Progressive resistive exercise is the most common type of exercise used with older adults and has been shown to be very effective in increasing their strength.[127] In a meta-analysis, Steib et al.[125] concluded that there was strong evidence for training at high intensities for maximizing strength adaptations compared with moderate to lower intensities. However, the ability to maximize strength does not necessarily carry over to functional improvement.[158] In fact, low to moderate exercise intensity was shown to have considerable positive effects on the function and strength measures of older adults. Specific exercises related to ADL are seen as a promising strategy for enhancing function in older adults. Interestingly, studies using power training showed improved chair rising and stair climbing but did not provide an advantage to performing a timed up-and-go test or positively impact walking speed.[99] More research is recommended to establish appropriate recommendations for resistive training in older adults.

Aerobic training has been shown to increase muscle cross-sectional area, number of muscle fibers, muscle hypertrophy, improve mitochondrial function, and decrease inflammation in older adults.[78] Aerobic exercise and endurance training can increase Vo_{2max}, which typically declines with age. Aerobic exercise improves the ability of the muscle to use oxygen. Endurance training increases Vo_{2max} by increasing cardiac output or by widening the arterial-to-venous oxygen difference.[159] For example, the maximum amount of oxygen available to a 75-year-old master athlete may be 85 mL/min/kg compared with 15 mL/min/kg for a debilitated 75-year-old person. If 12 mL/min/kg is required to walk at 3 miles/h, walking would "cost" the athlete 14% of Vo_{2max} compared with 80% for the debilitated older adult. However, Aagaard and colleagues[52] recommended long-term strength training over aerobic training to counter the age-related loss of muscle mass and subsequent strength with increasing age, reinforcing the ACSM guidelines, which include multiple forms of exercise for older adults to maximize function. Ideally, muscles need to produce force at all contraction velocities (eccentric and concentric). The optimal contraction velocity needs to be correlated with the functional demands of the task. If loads are varied, it may improve functional performance. Traditional resistance training does not improve eccentric force production, which is important for fall prevention and for many ADL activities.[144,149] (For additional discussion on cardiovascular changes with aging and fitness issues, see Chapters 7 and 13.)

In 2000, Kraemer and Newton[160] recommended velocity-specific resistance training for improvement in power. Traditional resistance training and power training have both been shown to increase muscle strength and muscle power.[102] High-velocity power training has been shown to be more effective than traditional resistance training in increasing the function of older adults.[99,103,161]

Power training has been found to be safe and effective for older adults, including the frail elderly, especially if progressed slowly.[99,103,162] It has been recommended that the power training program should be preceded by a 2-week muscle strength and endurance conditioning program, to best prepare the older adult for power training.[103] Low load (30%–35% 1 RM) power training has been found to be most effective at improving functional skills in older adults. A power training program at 30% 1 RM has also been found to best improve balance in older adults, aiding in fall prevention.[101] The fast speed with low loads is more reflective of the requirements of daily tasks (such as standing from a chair, climbing stairs, and crossing a crosswalk) and improves older adults' safety within their community.[103,161] Recommendations for power training programs for older adults include two to three sessions per week (even one session per week can be effective); using a resistance load between 34 and 75 1RM; performing one to three sets of exercises at 6–10 repetitions each. If necessary, only 3–5 repetitions can be used so that velocity can be maximized.[103] If the older adult cannot participate in a supervised program with free weights and/or exercise machines, use of weighted vests, TheraBand®, aquatic resistance exercise, or performing functional activities (i.e., sit-to-stand from a chair) at high speed are also effective for power training.[99,103]

SUMMARY

Many factors can influence muscle development both before and after birth, including genetics, nutrition, and activity levels. Muscle maturation occurs in childhood, and the rate of that maturation may limit the speed and dexterity with which a child can perform motor tasks. Strength development in childhood and adolescence increases with age.[32,37] Anaerobic function also improves during the same time period.[139] Strength gains increase with age to maturity and then begin to decline in middle adulthood. By optimizing muscle strength gain and development in childhood and adolescence, greater muscle strength and function are carried into adulthood. Through adulthood, especially prior to age 50 years, strength training programs are important to minimize strength loss and functional declines in older adulthood.[41] Power training is also an important consideration for older adults to maintain and improve functional abilities, such as rising from a chair, stair climbing, and walking, for older adults.

After the age of 50, the loss of muscle mass, known as sarcopenia, can affect strength and functional abilities. As we age, maintaining functional independence has a great deal to do with remaining physically active. During the last decades, key research has been published on the effects of strength and power training in older adults. Knowledge of how and why weakness occurs is far more abundant than in previous decades. Age-related changes in muscle cannot be stopped, but they can be slowed. The only known way to slow them is to maintain a healthy nutritional status and exercise on a regular basis. Exercise needs to be resistive in nature and include power training, eccentric loading, and functional activities. The human muscle remains responsive to these factors throughout the life span. Even aged muscle is trainable with the appropriate endurance and resistance goals. As part of our role as advocates for healthy aging, we refer you to the National Institutes of Health website http://nihseniorhealth.gov/exerciseforolderadults/toc.html, which is designed to motivate older adults to exercise.

REFERENCES

1. Motohashi N, Asakura A. Muscle satellite cell heterogeneity and self-renewal. *Front Cell Dev.* 2014:2. https://doi.org/10.3389/fcell.2014.00001.
2. Kumar K, Radhakrishnan R, 2022. What are the five main functions of the muscular system. Medicinenet.com/what-are-the-5-finctions-of-the-muscular-system/article.htm. Accessed April 30, 2022.
3. Lieber RL, Friden J. Functional and clinical significance of skeletal muscle architecture. *Muscle Nerve.* 2000;23:1647–1666.
4. Lieber RL. *Skeletal Muscle Structure, Function, and Plasticity.* Philadelphia: Wolters Kluwer/Lippincott Williams & Wilkins; 2010.
5. Mukund K, Subramaniam S. Skeletal muscle: a review of molecular structure and function in health and disease. *Wiley Interdiscip Rev Syst Biol Med.* 2020;12(1):e1462. https://doi.org/10.1002/wsbm.1462.
6. Leiber RL, Roberts TH, Blemker SS, Lee SSM, Herzog W. Skeletal muscle mechanics, energetics and plasticity. *J Neuroeng Rehabil.* 2017;14:108. https://doi.org/10.1186/s12984-017-0318y.
7. Rossi D, Pierantozzi E, Osamwonuyi A, Buonocores The sarcoplasmic reticulum of skeletal muscle cells: a labyrinth of membrane contact sites. *Biomolecules.* 2022;12:488. https://doi.org/10.3390/biom12040488.
8. McArdle WD, Katch FI, Katch VL. *Exercise Physiology: Energy, Nutrition and Human Performance.* 7th ed. Philadelphia: Wolter Kluwer/Lippincott Williams & Wilkins; 2010.
9. Murga M, Nogara L, Baraldo M, Reggiani C, Mann M, Shiaffino S. Protein profile of fiber types in human skeletal muscle: a single-fiber proteomics study. *Skeletal*

Muscle, 11. 2021;24. https://doi.org/10.1186/s13395-021-00279-0.

10. Talbot J, Maves L. Skeletal muscle fiber type: using insights from muscle developmental biology to dissect targets for susceptibility and resistance to muscle disease. *Wiley Interdiscip Rev Dev Biol.* 2016;5(4):518–534. https://doi.org/10.1002/wdev.230.

11. Vikne H, Strom V, Pripp AH, Gjovaag T. Human skeletal muscle fiber type percentage and area after reduced muscle use: a systematic review and meta-analysis. *Scand J Med Sci Sports.* 2020;30:1298–1317. https://doi.org/10.1111/sms.13675.

12. Moore KL, Torchia MG. Muscular System. In. Moore KL, Persaud TVN, Torchia MG, eds. *The Developing Human; Clinically Oriented Embryology.* 11th ed. Philadelphia: Elsevier; 2020:33-339e.1.

13. Carlson BM. *Human Embryology and Developmental Biology.* 4th ed. St Louis: Mosby; 2009.

14. Abofil M, Azab AE, Alsheban A. Skeletal muscle: insights into embryonic development, satellite cells, histology, ultrastructure, innervation, contraction and relaxation, causes, pathophysiology and treatment of volumetric muscle injury. *J Biotech and Bioprocessing.* 2021;2(4). https://doi.org/10.31579/2766-2314/038.

15. Hagiwara N. Developmental organization of skeletal muscle fiber types and the motor unit. *Trends in Devel Biology.* 2014;8:55–64. 83-91.

16. Almeida CF, Fernandes SA, Ribeiro AF, Okamoto OK, Vainzof M. Muscle satellite cells: exploring the basic biology to rule them. *Stem Cell International.* 2016:Article ID 1078686. DOI: 10.1155/2016/1078686.

17. Le Grand F, Rudnicki M. Satellite and stem cells in muscle growth and repair. *Development.* 2007;134:3953–3957.

18. Dumont NA, Wang YX, Rudnicki MA. Intrinsic and extrinsic mechanisms regulating satellite cell function. *Development.* 2016;142:1572–1581. https://doi.org/10.1242/dev.11.

19. Yan X, Zhu MJ, Dodson MV, Du M. Developmental programming of fetal skeletal muscle and adipose tissue. *Journal of Genomics.* 2013;1:29–38. https://doi.org/10.7150/jgen.3930.

20. Racca AW, Beck AE, Rao VS, Flint GV, et al. Contractility and kinetics of human fetal and human adult skeletal muscle. *J Physiol.* 2013;59(12):3049–3061. https://doi.org/10.1113/jphysiol.2013.252650.

21. Schiaffino S, Rossi AC, Smerdu V, Leinwald LA, Reggiani C. Developmental myosins: expression patterns and functional significance. *Skeletal Muscle.* 2015;5:22. https://doi.org/10.1186/s13395-015-0046-6.

22. Hesselmans LF, Jennekens FG, Van Den Oord CJ, et al. Development of innervation of skeletal muscle fibers in man: relation to acetylcholine receptors. *Anat Rec.* 1993;236:553–562.

23. Malina RM, Bouchard C, Bar-Or O. *Growth, Maturation and Physical Activity.* 2nd ed. Champaign, IL: Human Kinetics; 2004.

24. Plotkin DL, Robers MD, Haun CT, Schoenfeld BJ. Muscle fiber type transitions with exercise training: shifting perspectives. *Sports.* 2021;9:127. https://doi.org/10.3390/sports9090127.

25. Lexell J, Sjostrom M, Nordlund A, et al. Growth and development of human muscle: a quantitative morphological study of whole vastus lateralis from childhood to adult age. *Muscle Nerve.* 1992;15:4040–4049.

26. Elder GC, Kakulas BA. Histochemical and contractile property changes during human muscle development. *Muscle Nerve.* 1993;16:1246–1253.

27. Lin JP, Brown JK, Walsh EG. Physiological maturation of muscles in childhood. *Lancet.* 1994;343:1386–1389.

28. Lin JP, Brown JK, Walsh EG. The maturation of motor dexterity, or why Johnny can't go any faster. *Dev Med Child Neurol.* 1996;38:244–254.

29. Malina RM. Growth of muscle and muscle mass. In: Faulkner R, Tanner JM, eds. *Human Growth: A Comprehensive Treatise.* vol. 2. New York: *Postnatal Growth* Plenum Press; 1986:77–99.

30. Fiorotto ML, Davis TA. Critical windows for the programming effects of early-life nutrition on skeletal muscle mass. In: Colombo J, Koletzko B, Lampl M, eds. *Recent Research in Nutrition and Growth.* vol 89. Nestlé Nutr Inst Workshop Ser; 2018:25–35.

31. Beunen G, Thomis M. Muscular strength development in children and adolescents. *Pediatr Exerc Sci.* 2000;12:174–197.

32. Tonson A, Ratel S, Le Fur Y, et al. Effect of maturation on the relationship between muscle size and force production. *Med Sci Sports Exerc.* 2008;40(5):918–925.

33. Xu Y, Wen Z, Deng K, Li R, Yu Q, Xiao SM. Relationships of sex hormones with muscle mass and muscle strength in male adolescents at different stages of puberty. *PlosONE.* 2021; 16(12) e0260521. doi: 10.1371/journal.pone. 0260521.

34. Jones DA, Round JM. Muscle development during childhood and adolescence. In: Hebestreit H, Bar-Or O, eds. *The Young Athlete.* Oxford UK: Blackwell Publishing; 2008:18–26.

35. Wiggin M, Wilkinson K, Habetz S, et al. Percentile values of isokinetic peak torque in children six through thirteen years old. *Pediatr Phys Ther.* 2006;18:3–18.

36. Sinclair D, Dangerfield P. *Human Growth After Birth.* 6th ed. Oxford, UK: Oxford University Press; 1998.

37. De Ste Croix M. Advances in paediatric strength assessment: changing our perspective on strength development. *J Sport Sci Med.* 2007;6:292–304.

38. Vandervoort AA. Aging of the human neuromuscular system. *Muscle Nerve*. 2002;25:17–25.

39. Suominen H. Physical activity and health: musculoskeletal issues. *Adv Physiother*. 2007;9:65–75.

40. Connelly DM. Resisted exercise training of institutionalized older adults for improved strength and functional mobility: a review. *Top Geriatr Rehabil*. 2000;15:6–28.

41. Wiedmer P, Jung T, Castro JP, Pomatto LCD, et al. Sarcopenia: Molecular mechanisms and open questions. *Aging Research Reviews*. 2021;65:101200. https://doi.org/10.1016/jarr.2020/101200.

42. Wilkinson DJ, Piasecki M, Atherton PJ. Age-related loss of muscle mass and function: measurement and physiology of muscle fibre atrophy and muscle fibre loss in humans. *Ageing Research Review*. 2018;47:123–132. https://doi.org/10.1016/jar.2018.07.005.

43. Lexell J. Human aging, muscle mass, and fiber type composition. *J Gerontol*. 1995;50A(special issue):11–16.

44. Power GA, Rice CL, Vandervoort AA. Increased residual force enhancement in older adults is associated with maintenance of eccentric strength. *PLosOne*. 2012;7(10):e48044. https://doi.org/10.1371/journal.pone.0048044.

45. Roig M, MacIntyre DL, Eng JJ, Narici MV, et al. Preservation of eccentric strength in older adults: evidence, mechanisms and implications for training and rehabilitation. *Exp. Gerontol*. 2010;45(6):400–409. https://doi.org/10.1016/j.exger.2010.03.008.

46. Wu R, Ditrillo M, Delahunt E, DeVito G. Age related changes in motor function (II). Decline in motor performance outcomes. *Int J Sports Med*. 2021;43:215–226. https://doi.org/10.1055/a-1265-7073.

47. Goodpaster BH, Park SW, Harris TB, et al. The loss of skeletal muscle strength, mass, and quality in older adults: the health, aging and body composition study. *J Gerontol A Biol Sci Med Sci*. 2006;61A:1059–1064.

48. American College of Sports Medicine Position stand: exercise and physical activity for older adults. *Med Sci Sports Exerc*. 2009;41(7):1510–1530.

49. Phillips BA, Lo SK, Mastaglia FL. Muscle force measured using "break" testing with a hand-held myometer in normal subjects aged 20–69 years. *Arch Phys Med Rehabil*. 2000;81:653–661.

50. Krishnathasan D, Vandervoort AA. Eccentric strength training prescription for older adults. *Top Geriatr Rehabil*. 2000;15:29–40.

51. Rozand V, Sundberg CW, Hunter SK, Smith AE. Age-related deficits in voluntary activation: a systematic review and meta-analysis. *Med Sci Sports Exerc*. 2020;52(3):549–560. https://doi.org/10.1249/MSS.0000000000002179.

52. Aagaard P, Magnusson PS, Larsson B, et al. Mechanical muscle function, morphology, and fiber type in lifelong trained elderly. *Med Sci Sports Exerc*. 2007;39(11):1989–1996.

53. Cruz-Jentoft AJ, Bahat G, Bauer J, Boirie Y, et al. Sarcopenia: revised European consensus on definition and diagnosis. *Age Ageing*. 2019;48(1):16–31.

54. Steffl M, Bohannon RW, Sontakova L, et al. Relationship between sarcopenia and physical activity in older people: a systematic review and meta-analysis. *Clin Interv Aging*. 2017;12:835–845.

55. Iannuzzi-Sucich M, Prestwood KM, Kenny AM. Prevalence of sarcopenia and predictors of skeletal muscle mass in healthy, older men and women. *J Gerontol A Biol Sci Med Sci*. 2002;57AM772M777.

56. Santilli V, Bernetti A, Mangone M, Paoloni M. Clinical definition of sarcopenia. *Clin Cases Miner Bone Metab*. 2014 Sep;11(3):177–180.

57. Janssen I, Heymsfield SB, Wang AM, et al. Skeletal muscle mass and distribution in 468 men and women ages 18–88 yr. *J Appl Physiol*. 2000;89:81–88.

58. Morley JE, Abbatecola AM, Argiles JM, et al. Sarcopenia with limited mobility: an international consensus. *J Am Med Dir Assoc*. 2011;12:403–409.

59. Bischoff-Ferrari HA, Orav JE, Kanis JA, et al. Comparative performance of current definitions of sarcopenia against the prospective incidence of falls among community-dwelling seniors age 65 and older. *Osteoporos Int*. 2015;26:2793–2802.

60. Schaap LA, van Schoor NM, Lips P, et al. Associations of sarcopenia definitions, and their components, with the incidence of recurrent falling and fractures: the longitudinal aging study Amsterdam. *J Gerontol A Biol Sci Med Sci*. 2018;73:1199–1204.

61. Malmsrom TK, Miller DK, Simonsick EM, et al. SARC-F: a symptom score to predict persons with sarcopenia at risk for poor functional outcomes. *J Cachexia Sarcopenia Muscle*. 2016;7:28–36.

62. Bahat G, Ilhan B. Sarcopenia and the cardiometabolic syndrome: a narrative review. *Eur Geriatr Med*. 2016;6:220–223.

63. Bone AE, Hepgul N, Kon S, et al. Sarcopenia and frailty in chronic respiratory disease. *Chron Respir Dis*. 2017;14:85–99.

64. Chang KV, Hsu TH, Wu WT, et al. Association between sarcopenia and cognitive impairment: a systematic review and meta-analysis. *J Am Med Dir Assoc*. 2016;171164.e7-1164.e15.

65. Beaudart C, Biver E, Reginster JY, et al. Validation of the SarQoL(R), a specific health-related quality of life questionnaire for Sarcopenia. *J Cachexia Sarcopenia Muscle*. 2017;8:238–244.

66. Akune T, Muraki S, Oka H, et al. Incidence of certified need of care in the long-term care insurance system

and its risk factors in the elderly of Japanese population-based cohorts: the ROAD study. *Geriatr Gerontol Int*. 2014;14:695–701.

67. Baumgartner RN, Koehler KM, Gallagher D, et al. Epidemiology of sarcopenia among the elderly in New Mexico. *Am J Epidemiol*. 1998;147:755–763.

68. Janssen I, Heymsfield SB, Ross R. Low relative skeletal muscle mass (sarcopenia) in older persons is associated with functional impairment and physical disability. *J Am Geriatr Soc*. 2002;50:889–896.

69. McGregor RA, Cameron-Smith D, Poppitt SD. It is not just muscle mass: a review of muscle quality, composition and metabolism during ageing as determinants of muscle function and mobility in later life. *Longev Healthspan*. 2014;3:9.

70. Jones TE, Stephenson KW, King JG, et al. Sarcopenia – mechanisms and treatments. *J Geriatr Phys Ther*. 2009;32:39–45.

71. Di Orio A, Abate M, Di Renzo D, et al. Sarcopenia: age-related skeletal muscle changes form determinants to physical disability. *Int J Immunopathol Pharmacol*. 2006;19(4):703–719.

72. Doherty TJ. Invited review: aging and sarcopenia. *J Appl Physiol*. 2003;95:1717–1727.

73. Marcel TJ. Sarcopenia: causes, consequences, and prevention. *J Gerontol A Biol Sci Med Sci*. 2003;58A(10): 911–916.

74. Eynon N, Yamin C, Ben-Sira D. Optimal health and function among the elderly: lessening severity of ADL disability. *Eur Rev Aging Phys Act*. 2009;6:55–61.

75. Thompson LV. Age-related muscle dysfunction. *Exp Gerontol*. 2009;44(1-2):106–111.

76. Gomes MJ, Martinez PF, Pagan LU, et al. Skeletal muscle aging: influence of oxidative stress and physical exercise. *Oncotarget*. 2017;8(12):20428–20440. https://doi.org/10.18632/oncotarget.14670.

77. Baumann CW, Kwak D, Liu HM, Thompson LV. Age-induced oxidative stress: how does it influence skeletal muscle quantity and quality. *J Appl Physiol (1985)*. 2016 Nov 1;121(5):1047–1052. https://doi.org/10.1152/japplphysiol.00321.2016.

78. McCormick R, Vasilaki A. Age-related changes in skeletal muscle: changes to life-style as a therapy. *Biogerontology*. 2018;19(6):519–536. https://doi.org/10.1007/s10522-018-9775-3.

79. Woods JA, Wilund KR, Martin SA, Kistler BM. Exercise inflammation and aging. *Aging Dis*. 2012;3(1):130–140.

80. Powers SK, Jackson MJ. Exercise-induced oxidative stress: cellular mechanisms and impact on muscle force production. *Physiol Rev*. 2008;88:1243–1276.

81. Monteiro ER, Vingren JL, Corrêa Neto VG, Neves EB, Steele J, Novaes JS. Effects of different between test rest intervals in reproducibility of the 10-repetition maximum load test: a pilot study with recreationally resistance trained men. *Int J Exerc Sci*. 2019;12(4):932–940.

82. Schaap LA, Saskia MF, Deeg DJH, et al. Inflammatory markers and loss of muscle mass (sarcopenia) and strength. *Am J Med*. 2009;119:526.e9–526.e17.

83. Roth SM, Metter EJ, Ling S, et al. Inflammatory factors in age-related muscle wasting. *Curr Opin Rheumatol*. 2006;18(6):625–630.

84. Tuttle CSL, Thang LAN, Maier AB. Markers of inflammation and their association with muscle strength and mass: a systematic review and meta-analysis. *Aging Research Reviews*. 2020;64:101185. https://doi.org/10.1016/jar.2020.101185.

85. Roos MR, Rice CL, Vandervoort AA. Age-related change in motor unit function. *Muscle Nerve*. 1997;20:679–690.

86. Lexell J. Evidence for nervous system degeneration with advancing age. *J Nutr*. 1997;1271011Sendash1013S.

87. Wu R, DeVito G, Delahunt E, Ditroilo M. Age-related changes in motor function (1): Mechanical and Neuromuscular factors. *Int J Sports Med*. 2020;41:709–719. https://doi.org/10.1055/a-1144-3408.

88. Hortobagyi T, Zheng DH, Weidner M, et al. The influence of aging on muscle strength and muscle fiber characteristics with special reference to eccentric strength. *J Gerontol A Biol Sci Med Sci*. 1995;50:B399B406.

89. Gokhin DS, Fowler VM. The sarcoplasmic reticulum: actin and tropomodulin hit the links. *Bioarchitecture*. 2011;1(4):175–179. https://doi.org/10.4161/bioa.1.4.17533.

90. Seo DY, Lee SR, Nari Kim N, et al. Age-related changes in skeletal muscle mitochondria: the role of exercise. *Integrative Med Res*. 2016;5(3):182–186.

91. Sun N, Youle RJ, Finkel T. The mitochondrial basis of aging. *Mol Cell*. 2016 Mar 3;61(5):654–666.

92. Chistiakov DA, Sobenin IA, Revin VV, Orekhov AN, Bobryshev YV. Mitochondrial aging and age-related dysfunction of mitochondria. *Biomed Res Int*. 2014;2014:238463. https://doi.org/10.1155/2014/238463.

93. Marzetti E, Calvani R, Bernabei R, Leeuwenburgh C. Apoptosis in skeletal myocytes: a potential target for interventions against sarcopenia and physical frailty—a mini-review. *Gerontology*. 2012;58:99–106.

94. Snijders T, Nederveen JP, McKay BR, Joanisse S, et al. Satellite cells in human skeletal muscle plasticity. *Fronteirs in Physiology*. 2015;6:283. https://doi.org/10.3389/fphys.2015.00283.

95. Nair KS. Aging muscle. *Am J Clin Nutr*. 2005;81:953–963.

96. Kumar V, Selby A, Rankin D, et al. Age-related differences in the dose-response relationship of muscle protein synthesis to resistance exercise in young and old men.

J Physiol. 2009;587(1):211–217. https://doi.org/10.1113/jphysiol.2008.164483.

97. Evans WJ. Protein nutrition, exercise and aging. J Am Coll Nutr. 2004;23(6):601Sendash609S.

98. Boire Y. Physiopathological mechanism of sarcopenia. J Nutr Health Aging. 2009;13(8):717–723.

99. Reid KF, Fielding RA. Skeletal muscle power: a critical determinant of physical functioning in older adults. Exerc Sport Sci *Rev.* 2012;40(1):4–12. https://doi.org/10.1097/JES.0b013e31823b5f13.

100. Miljkovic N, Lim JY, Miljkovic I, Frontera WR. Aging of skeletal muscle fibers. *Ann Rehabil Med.* 2015;39(2):155–162. https://doi.org/10.5535/arm.2015.39.2.155.

101. Orr R, deVos NJ, Singh NA, et al. Power training improves balance in healthy older adults. *Journal of Gerontology, MEDICAL SCIENCES.* 2006;61A(1):78–85.

102. Henwood RE, Reik S, Taaffe DR. Strength versus muscle power-specific resistance training in community-dwelling older adults. *Journal of Gerontology, MEDICAL SCIENCES.* 2008;63A(1).

103. Rice J, Keough JWL. Power training: can it improve functional performance in older adults? A systematic review. Int J Exer Sci. 2009;9(2):131–151.

104. Raz IS, Bird SR, Shield AJ. Aging and the force-velocity relationship of muscles. *Exp Gerontol.* 2010;45:81–90.

105. Kumar NTA, Oliver JL, Lloyd RS, Pedley JS, Radnor JM. The influence of growth, maturation and resistance training on muscle-tendon and neuromuscular adaptations: a narrative review. *Sports.* 2021;9:59. https://doi.org/10.3390/sports9050059.

106. Stricker PR, Faigenbaum AD, McCambridge TM. Resistance training for children and adolescents. *Pediatrics.* 2020;145(6):e20201011. https://doi.org/10.1542/peds.2020-1011.

107. Dahab KS, McCambridge TM. Strength training in children and adolescents: raising the bar for young athletes. *Sports Health.* 2009;1(3):223–227. https://doi.org/10.1177/1941738109334215.

108. Lloyd RS, Faigenbaum AD, Stone MH, et al. Position statement on youth resistance training: the 2014 international consensus. *Br J Sports Med.* 2013;0:1–12. https://doi.org/10.1136/bjsports-2013-09.2952.

109. Behm DF, Faigenbaum AD, Falk B, et al. Canadian society for exercise physiology position paper: resistance training in children and adolescents. *Appl Physiol Nutr Metab.* 2008;33:547–561.

110. Myers AM, Beam NW, Fakhoury JD. Resistance training for children and adolescents. *Transl Pediatr.* 2017;6(3):137–141. https://doi.org/10.21037/tp.2017.04.01.

111. Faigenbaum AD, Kraemer WJ, Blimkie CJR, et al. Youth resistance training: updated position statement paper from the National Strength and Conditioning Association. *J Strength Cond Res.* 2009;23(Suppl 5):S60S80.

112. Deschenes MR. Effects of aging on muscle fibre type and size. *Sports Med.* 2004;34(12):809–824.

113. Mynarski W, Rozpara M, Nawrocka A, et al. Physical activity of middle-age adults aged 50–65 years in view of health recommendations. *Eur Rev Aging Phys Act.* 2014;11:141–147. https://doi.org/10.1007/s11556-014-0138-z.

114. Lui CJ, Latham NK. Progressive resistance strength training for improving physical function in older adults. *Cochrane Database Syst Rev.* 2009;3:CD002759.

115. Hunter GR, McCarthy FP, Bamman MM. Effects of resistance training on older adults. *Sports Med.* 2004;34(5):329–348.

116. Seynnes O, Fiatarone Singh MA, Hue O, et al. Physiological and functional responses to low-moderate versus high-intensity progressive resistance training in frail elders. *J Gerontol A Biol Sci Med Sci.* 2004;59(5):503–509.

117. Papa EV, Dong X, Hassan M. Resistance training for activity limitations in older adults with skeletal muscle function deficits: a systematic review. *Clin Interv Aging.* 2017;12:955–961. https://doi.org/10.2147/CIA.S104674. Published 2017 Jun 13.

118. Hakkinen K, Pakarinen A, Kraemer WJ, et al. Selective muscle hypertrophy, changes in EMG and force, and serum hormones during strength training in older women. *J Appl Physiol.* 2001;91:569–580.

119. Mueller M, Breil FA, Vogt M, et al. Different response to eccentric and concentric training in older men and women. *Eur J Appl Physiol.* 2009;107:145–153.

120. Ansdell P, Thomas K, Hicks KM, et al. Physiological sex differences affect the integrative response to exercise: acute and chronic implications. *Exp Physiol.* 2020;105(12):2007–2021.

121. Yoo SZ, No MH, Heo JW, et al. Role of exercise in age-related sarcopenia. *J Exerc Rehabil.* 2018;14(4):551–558. https://doi.org/10.12965/jer.1836268.134. Published 2018 Aug 24.

122. Symons TB, Vandervoort AA, Rice CL, et al. Effects of maximal isometric and isokinetic resistance training on strength and functional mobility in older adults. *J Gerontol A Biol Sci Med Sci.* 2005;60A(6):777–781.

123. Puthoff ML, Nielsen DH. Relationships among impairments in lower-extremity strength and poser, functional limitations, and disability in older adults. *Phys Ther.* 2007;87:1334–1347.

124. Henwood TR, Riek S, Taaffe DR. Strength versus muscle power-specific resistance training in community-dwelling older adults. *J Gerontol A Biol Sci Med Sci.* 2008;63A(1):83–91.

125. Steib S, Schoene D, Pfeifer K. Dose-response relationship of resistance training in older adults: a meta-analysis. *Med Sci Sports Exerc*. 2010;42(5):902–914.

126. Alcazar J, Losa-Reyna J, Rodriguez-Lopez C, et al. The sit-to-stand muscle power test: An easy, inexpensive and portable procedure to assess muscle power in older people. *Exp Gerontol*. 2018 Oct 2;112:38–43. https://doi.org/10.1016/j.exger.2018.08.006. Epub 2018 Sep 1. PMID: 30179662.

127. Latham NK, Anderson C, Bennett D, et al. Progressive resistance strength training for physical disability in older people. *Cochrane Database Syst Rev*. 2003;2:CD002759.

128. Barry BK, Carson RG. Transfer of resistance training to enhance rapid coordinated force production by older adults. *Exp Brain Res*. 2004;159(2):225–238.

129. Van Abbema R, De Greef M, Crajé C, et al. What type, or combination of exercise can improve preferred gait speed in older adults? A meta-analysis. *BMC Geriatr*. 2015;15:72. https://doi.org/10.1186/s12877-015-0061-9.

130. Cesari M, Pahor M, Lauretani F, et al. Skeletal muscle and mortality results from the InCHIANTI study. *J Gerontol A Biol Sci Med Sci*. 2009;64A(3):377–384.

131. Middleton A, Fritz SL, Lusardi M. Walking speed: the functional vital sign. *J Aging Phys Act*. 2015;23(2):314–322. https://doi.org/10.1123/japa.2013-0236.

132. Fragala MS, Cadore EL, Dorgo S, et al. Resistance training for older adults: position statement from the National Strength and Conditioning Association. *J Strength Conditioning Res*. 2019;33(8):2019–2052. https://doi.org/10.1519/JSC.0000000000003230.

133. Paterson DH, Jones GR, Rice CL. Ageing and physical activity: evidence to develop exercise recommendations for older adults. *Can J Public Health*. 2007;98(Suppl 2): S69S108.

134. Fitts RH. Mechanisms of muscular fatigue. In: Poortmans JR, ed. *Principles of Exercise Biochemistry*. 3rd ed. New York: Karger; 2004:279–300.

135. Enoka RM, Duchateau J. Muscle fatigue: what, why and how it influences muscle function. *J Physiol*. 2008;586:11–23.

136. Hunter SK. Sex differences and mechanisms of task-specific muscle fatigue. *Exerc Sport Sci Rev*. 2009;37(3): 113–122.

137. Alexander NB, Taffet GE, Horne FM, et al. Bedside-to-Bench conference: research agenda for idiopathic fatigue and aging. *J Am Geriatr Soc*. 2010;58:967–975.

138. Ito T, Suguria H, Ito Y, Noritake K, Ochi N. Relationship between skeletal muscle mass index and physical activity of Japanese children: A cross-sectional, observational study. *PlusONE*. 2021;16(5):e0251025. https://doi.org/10.1371/journal.pone.0251025.

139. Van Praagh E. Anaerobic fitness tests: what are we measuring? *Med Sport Sci*. 2007;50:26 45.

140. Van Praagh E. Development of anaerobic function during childhood and adolescence. *Pediatr Exerc Sci*. 2000;12:150–173.

141. Rowland TW. *Children's Exercise Physiology*. 2nd ed. Champaign, IL: Human Kinetics; 2005.

142. Faigenbaum AD. Resistance training for children and adolescents: are there health outcomes? *Am J Lifestyle Med*. 2007;1:190–200.

143. Lowndes J, Carpenter RL, Zoeller RF, et al. Association of age with muscle size and strength before and after short-term resistance training in young adults. *J Strength Cond Res*. 2009;234(7):1915–1920.

144. Enoka RM, Christou EA, Hunter SK, et al. Mechanisms that contribute to differences in motor performance between young and old adults. *J Electromyogr Kinesiol*. 2003;13:1–12.

145. Chandler JM, Duncan PW, Kochersberger G, et al. Is lower extremity strength gain associated with improvement in physical performance and disability in frail, community-dwelling elders? *Arch Phys Med Rehabil*. 1998;79:24–30.

146. Ishigaki EY, Ramos LG, Carvalho ES, Lunardi AC. Effectiveness of muscle strengthening and description of protocols for preventing falls in the elderly: a systematic review. *Braz J Phys Ther*. 2014;18(2):111–118. https://doi.org/10.1590/s1413-35552012005000148.

147. Padula CA, Disano C, Ruggiero C, Carpentier M, Reppucci M, Forloney B, Hughes C. Impact of lower extremity strengthening exercises and mobility on fall rates in hospitalized adults. *J Nurs Care Qual*. 2011 Jul-Sep;26(3):279–285. https://doi.org/10.1097/NCQ.0b013e318207decb. PMID: 21209594.

148. Pijnappels M, Reeves ND, Maganaris CN, et al. Tripping without falling: lower limb strength, a limitation for balance recovery and a target for training in the elderly. *J Electromyogr Kinesiol*. 2008;18:188–196.

149. Carville SF, Perry MC, Rutherford OM, et al. Steadiness of quadriceps contractions in young and older adults with and without a history of falling. *Eur J Appl Physiol*. 2007;100:527–533.

150. Baudry S, Klass M, Pasquet B, et al. Age-related fatigability of the ankle dorsiflexor muscles during concentric and eccentric contractions. *Eur J Appl Physiol*. 2007;100:515–526.

151. Lanza IR, Short DK, Raghavakaimal S, et al. Endurance exercise as a countermeasure for aging. *Diabetes*. 2008;57(11):2933–2943.

152. Vandervoort AA. *Introduction. Top Geriatr Rehabil.* 15. viendashviii; 2000.

153. Mayer F, Schrage-Rosenberger F, Carlsohn A, Cassel M, Müller S, Scharhag J. The intensity and effects of strength training in the elderly. *Dtsch Arztebl Int.* 2011;108(21):359–364. https://doi.org/10.3238/arztebl.2011.0359.

154. Kim DY, Oh SL, Lim JY. Applications of eccentric exercise to improve muscle and mobility function of older adults. *Annals of Geriatric Medicine and Research.* 2022;26(1):4–15. https://doi.org/10.4235/agmr.21.0138.

155. Hortobagyi T, DeVita P. Favorable neuromuscular and cardiovascular responses to 7 days of exercise with an eccentric overload in elderly women. *J Gerontol A Biol Sci Med Sci.* 2000;55(8):B401B410.

156. Peterson MD, Gordon PM. Resistance exercise for the aging adult: clinical implications and prescription guidelines. *Am J Med.* 2011;124(3):194–198.

157. Bjorkgren M, Borg F, Tan K, et al. Introducing progressive strength training programs in Singapore's elder care settings. Front Med. 2021;8:515898. https://doi.org/10.3389/fmed.2021.515898.

158. Liu CJ, Shiroy DM, Jones LY, et al. Systematic review of functional training on muscle strength, physical functioning, and activities of daily living in older adults. *Eur Rev Aging Phys Act.* 2014;11:95–106. https://doi.org/10.1007/s11556-014-0144-1.

159. Thompson LV. Physiological changes associated with aging. In: Guccione AA, ed. *Geriatric Physical Therapy.* 2nd ed. St Louis: Mosby; 2000:28–55.

160. Kraemer WJ, Newton RU. Training for muscular power. *Phys Med Rehabil Clin N Am.* 2000;11:341–368.

161. Sayers SP, Gibson K. High-speed power training in older adults: a shift of external resistance at which peak power is produced. *J Strength Cond Res.* 2014;28(3):616–621. https://doi.org/10.1519/JSC.0b013e3182a361b8/.

162. Caserotti P, Aagaard P, Buttrup Larsen J, Puggarard L. Explosive heave-resistance training in old and very old adults: changes in rapid muscle force, strength and power. *MedSci Sport.* 2008;18(6):773–782.

7

Cardiovascular and Pulmonary System Changes

OBJECTIVES

After studying this chapter, the reader will be able to:
1. Describe structural and functional characteristics of the cardiovascular and pulmonary systems as they relate to physical functioning.

2. Discuss age-related structural and functional characteristics of the cardiovascular and pulmonary systems.
3. Relate age-related changes in the cardiovascular and pulmonary systems to physical functioning, activity, and participation.

Together, the cardiovascular and pulmonary systems deliver necessary nutrients and oxygen to body tissues, as well as remove waste products. Blood circulating through the vascular system provides the transport system for these substances. Oxygen is delivered to the blood via the pulmonary system. An understanding of the structure, function, and development of these two systems as they relate to how well a person can participate in daily activities is important to assess and promote functional movement and wellness across the life span.

COMPONENTS OF THE CARDIOVASCULAR AND PULMONARY SYSTEMS

Cardiovascular System

Components

The cardiovascular system is made up of the heart and the vascular network. Its purpose is to pump blood and to deliver it throughout the body. The blood is pumped from the heart through a high-pressure arterial system to the target organs. There, nutrients and waste products are exchanged between capillaries and tissues. The low-pressure venous system then returns blood to the heart. *Heart rate* refers to the number of times the heart

beats per minute (bpm); *stroke volume* refers to the amount of blood that is pumped from the ventricle with each heartbeat. By multiplying heart rate by stroke volume, one can determine the amount of blood pumped from the ventricles in 1 minute, which is referred to as *cardiac output.*

The heart. The heart is made up of four chambers and acts as the pump of the cardiovascular system. The cardiovascular pump works very differently before and after birth. Fig. 7.1 depicts the prenatal circulation that permits most of the oxygenated blood to bypass the liver and lungs via three shunts: (1) ductus venosus, (2) foramen ovale, and (3) ductus arteriosus. Poorly oxygenated blood returns to the placenta for oxygen and nutrients from the umbilical arteries.[1] Dramatic changes occur in the cardiovascular and pulmonary systems at birth when the infant's lungs fill with air. The shunts are no longer needed and immediately start to close. Fig. 7.2 illustrates postnatal circulation of blood through the heart, lungs, and periphery. After birth, the atria move blood into the ventricles, which then pump with sufficient force to deliver blood to the lungs and the periphery. The chambers of the right side of the heart receive blood from the periphery and pump it to the lungs to be oxygenated. The chambers on the left side of the heart then receive the oxygenated blood and pump it through the aorta to

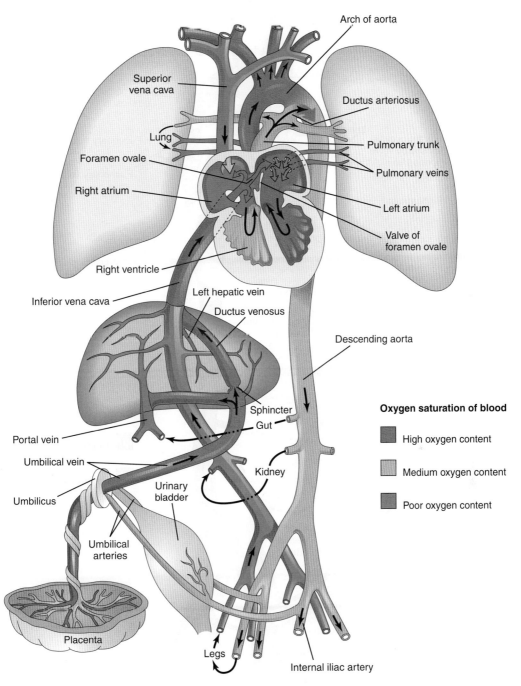

Fig. 7.1 Schematic of fetal circulation. The shades of blue (dark to light) indicate the oxygen saturation of the blood, and the *arrows* show the course of the blood from the placenta to the heart. The organs are not drawn to scale. Three shunts—(1) ductus venosus, (2) foramen ovale, and (3) ductus arteriosus—permit most of the blood to bypass the liver and lungs. The poorly oxygenated blood returns to the placenta for oxygen and nutrients through the umbilical arteries. (From Moore KL, Persaud TVN, Torchia, MG. Ch 13: Cardiovascular System. In: Moore KL, Persaud TVN, Torchia MG. eds. *The Developing Human.* 11th ed. Philadelphia: Elsevier; 2020. Figure 13.46.)

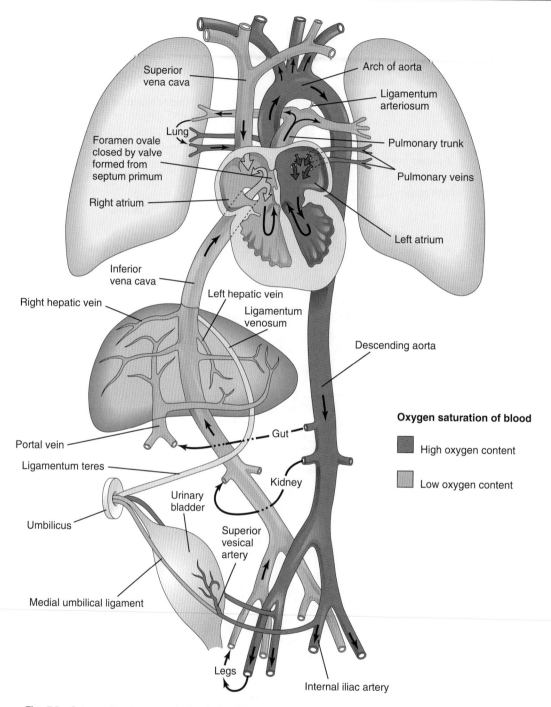

Fig. 7.2 Schematic of neonatal circulation. The adult *derivatives* of the fetal vessels and structures that become nonfunctional at birth are also shown. The arrows indicate the course of the blood in the infant. The organs are not drawn to scale. After birth, the *three shunts* that short-circuited the blood during fetal life cease to function, and the pulmonary and systemic circulations *separate*. (From Moore KL, Persaud TVN, Torchia, MG. Ch 13: Cardiovascular System. In: Moore KL, Persaud TVN, Torchia MG, eds. *The Developing Human*. 11th ed. Philadelphia: Elsevier; 2020. Figure 13.47.)

the systemic circulation. Valves in the heart ensure unidirectional blood flow. The tricuspid and mitral valves, found between the atria and ventricles, prevent blood from flowing back into the atria during ventricular contraction. The aortic and pulmonary valves, also called the *semilunar valves*, prevent blood from flowing back into the ventricles from the aorta and pulmonary artery.

Structurally, the heart is made up of three layers, which are also called *tunics* (Fig. 7.3). The inner layer, the *endocardium*, is made up of a single layer of squamous endothelial cells and a layer of connective tissue. The connective tissue contains blood vessels, nerves, and branches of the conducting system of the heart. The middle layer, the *myocardium*, is the thick muscular layer of the heart and is richly supplied with capillaries. Cardiac muscle cells in the myocardium are able to conduct electricity, but they also have a long refractory period, allowing them to maintain rhythmic heart contraction. The outer layer, the *epicardium*, is made up of loose connective tissue and fat that is covered by simple squamous epithelium. Large blood vessels, such as the coronary arteries, and nerves that supply the heart are found in the epicardium.

Contraction of the heart muscle is controlled by the cardiac conducting system, which consists of the sinoatrial node, atrioventricular node, and atrioventricular bundle of His (Fig. 7.4).[2] The conduction system contains specialized cardiac muscle cells that carry impulses faster than other myocardial cells. The stimulus for cardiac contraction originates in the sinoatrial node, the pacemaker of the heart. Autonomic nerve and ganglion cells are also found near and in the node. These cells influence the circulatory and nervous system and help regulate heart rate and contractility. The atrioventricular node receives the impulse from the sinoatrial node and delays it slightly, allowing the atria time to

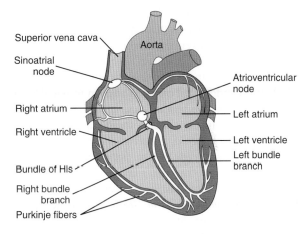

Fig. 7.4 The conducting system of the heart. (From Gartner LP. *Textbook of Histology*, 5th ed. Chapter 11: Circulatory System; Elsevier, 2021: 249-270. Figure 11.24)

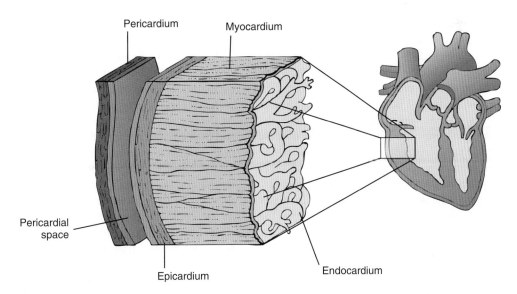

Fig. 7.3 Layers of the heart. (Hall JE, Hall ME. *Guyton and Hall Textbook of Medical Physiology*. 14th ed. Chapter 9: Cardiac Muscle; The Heart as a Pump and Function of the Heart Valves; WB Saunders, 2021;113–126.)

empty before the ventricles contract. The atrioventricular bundle of His and its branches then carry the stimulus to the ventricles. From there, the contractile stimulus is transmitted from one cardiac muscle fiber to another, resulting in a wave of cardiac contractions. The conduction system of the heart is a coordinating system. Each part of it can conduct or initiate an impulse on its own, but the rhythm is controlled because the sinoatrial node fires first. When the sinoatrial node is not functioning properly, cardiac arrhythmias occur.

The vascular system. Three main types of vessels make up the vascular system: *arteries*, *capillaries*, and *veins*. Arteries and veins are structurally similar to the heart in that they are made up of three concentric layers (Fig. 7.5). The inner layer, *tunica intima*, is made up of a layer of endothelial cells and a subendothelial layer of elastic connective tissue. Some smooth muscle cells are also found in the subendothelial layer. The middle layer, *tunica media*, consists of concentric layers of smooth muscle cells, elastic fibers, collagen fibers, and proteoglycans. The outer layer, *tunica adventitia*, is made up of fibroelastic connective tissue. Small blood vessels, *vasa vasorum*, are found in the media and adventitia layers of large vessels. They nourish the thicker layers of the vessel, where sufficient nutrition cannot be supplied by diffusion from the circulating blood.

Arteries carry blood from the heart to the rest of the body and minimize fluctuations in pressure caused by the heartbeat. For instance, when the ventricles contract, the arteries are stretched, decreasing pressure. When the ventricles relax, the arteries return to their original size and maintain the level of pressure.

Arteries can be divided into three groups. The large elastic arteries, called *conducting arteries*, include the aorta and its main branches. The tunica media of these vessels is made up of layers of elastic membrane, which makes them efficient at absorbing the pressure changes that accompany each heartbeat. Almost no elastin layers are present in the aorta at birth, but this increases to 40 to 70 layers in the adult.[3] The second category, the *muscular*, or *distributing arteries*, are branches of the large elastic arteries that supply blood to the organs and extremities. The tunica media of the distributing arteries is made of up to 40 layers of smooth muscle cells that regulate blood flow in response to nervous system or hormonal input. Connective tissues, including elastic and collagen fibers, can be found between the muscular

layers. The third category of arteries, the *arterioles*, are small vessels that deliver blood to the capillaries. The tunica intima of the arteriole consists of a layer of endothelium and an internal elastic membrane. The tunica media is made of one to two layers of smooth muscle cells and a few elastic fibers.[2] Vasoconstriction and vasodilation of the arterioles control the systemic blood pressure so that only a slow, steady stream of blood enters the capillaries. The arterioles are innervated by the autonomic nervous system and can quickly react to functional needs of the tissue.

Capillaries provide a site for the exchange of nutrients and waste products between the blood and the tissue, connect the arterial and venous systems, and contain a large volume of the blood in the body. The capillary itself is a small vessel, made up of a single layer of endothelial cells surrounded by a thin layer of collagen fibers. Areas of the body with high metabolic needs, such as the lungs, liver, kidneys, cardiac muscle, and skeletal muscle, have large capillary networks.

Veins are responsible for carrying deoxygenated blood back to the heart and for the transport of waste products from the tissue. Two exceptions are the pulmonary vein, which takes oxygenated blood from the lungs to the heart, and the umbilical vein, which also supplies oxygenated blood to the fetal circulation. Veins have larger diameters and thinner walls than do arteries. Because of their size and the large number of veins that make up the venous system, blood flows back to the heart slowly and at low pressure.

Veins can be divided into three major categories by size. *Venules*, the smallest veins, receive blood from the capillaries. The diameter of the venule is greater than that of the capillary and serves to slow the rate of blood flow. As the venule size increases, layers of connective tissue and then smooth muscle cells are added. When the size of the venule is approximately 50 µm, elastic fibers and smooth muscle fibers can be found between the tunica intima and the tunica adventitia. The next category of *small- to medium-sized* veins includes most named veins in the body and their branches. These veins contain valves that maintain unidirectional flow of blood. The tunica intima and tunica media are thin, whereas the tunica adventitia is thick. The *large veins* make up the third category of veins and include the superior vena cava, inferior vena cava, portal vein, pulmonary veins, abdominal veins, and main tributaries. The tunica adventitia is the thickest and most developed component of

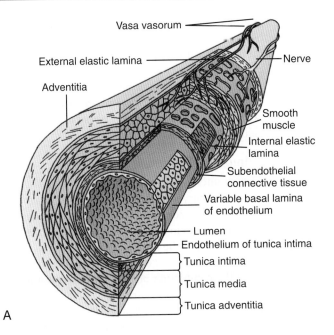

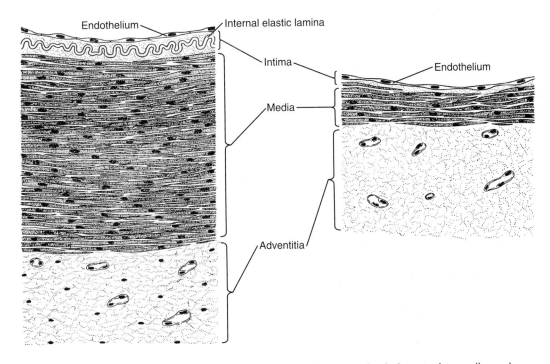

Fig. 7.5 (**A**) Diagram of a typical artery showing the three layers: tunica intima, tunica media, and tunica adventitia. (**B**) Comparison of muscular artery *(left)* and accompanying vein *(right)*. (**A**, From Gartner LP, Hiatt JL. *Color Textbook of Histology*. Philadelphia: WB Saunders; 1997:213; **B**, from Junqueira LC, Carneiro J, Kelley RO. *Basic Histology*. 10th ed. Large Medical Books McGraw-Hill. Medical Pub Division, 2003.)

these veins, containing longitudinal bundles of smooth muscle fibers. These muscle cells strengthen the venous wall and help to prevent distention.

Control

Regulation of heart rate and dilation/constriction of the vessels of the vascular system are influenced by the autonomic nervous system and by the presence of chemicals in the circulation. Nervous system control originates in the medulla and is carried via the sympathetic and parasympathetic branches of the autonomic nervous system.

Autonomic fibers are found within the cardiac conducting system. Sympathetic input to the heart increases the rate and strength of cardiac contraction via the release of catecholamines (epinephrine and norepinephrine). Sympathetic innervation of smooth muscle cells in the tunica media of the arteries and the tunica media and tunica adventitia of the veins stimulates vasoconstriction. Parasympathetic input to the heart is received via the vagus nerve and slows the heart rate by releasing acetylcholine. Skeletal muscle arteries also dilate in response to parasympathetic input.

The vascular system relates sensory information to the nervous system through the stretch-sensitive *baroreceptors*, found in the aorta and carotid sinus, and the *chemoreceptors*, found in the carotid and aortic bodies. These receptors react to changes in blood pressure, levels of oxygen and carbon dioxide in the circulating blood, and acidity (pH) of the blood.

Mechanics of Circulation

Blood flow is regulated by pressures exerted by the various structures in the system. Within the heart, *preload* is the amount of pressure necessary to stretch the ventricles during cardiac filling. *Afterload* is the amount of pressure that must be exerted by the ventricles to overcome aortic pressure, open the aortic valve, and push the blood out toward the periphery. The vessels continue to control blood flow, not only because of the neural and chemical influences but also because of their physical properties. Length and diameter of the vessels help to determine peripheral vascular resistance and to influence the speed of blood flow. Blood pressure is the pressure exerted by the blood on the vessels as it flows through them.

For efficient mechanical control of blood flow, the blood pressure must be sufficient for blood to flow through the system and must stretch the ventricles during preload. It must likewise not be so high that

afterload is increased, making the ventricles work harder to overcome aortic pressure and to empty. In individuals with *hypertension* (high blood pressure), the chronic increased aortic pressure eventually leads to left ventricular hypertrophy because the left ventricle has been working so hard to maintain adequate stroke volume. This can eventually contribute to congestive heart failure.

Pulmonary System

Components

The pulmonary system consists of the lungs and the structures that connect the lungs to the external environment. It is a closed system, open to the external environment only at the nose and mouth.

The system can be divided into two major structural parts: the conducting portion and the respiratory portion (Fig. 7.6). The respiratory system does more than just control gaseous exchange. It also regulates blood pH, assists with blood pressure control, and provides nonspecific mechanical immune defense mechanisms. Functionally, the pulmonary system can be divided into the ventilatory pump (air in and out) and the respiratory component (gas exchange).

Conducting portion. When considering the structural components of the pulmonary system, the conducting portion of the pulmonary system provides a pathway for air to travel between the environment and the lungs. In this portion, no gas exchange takes place, but the air is cleaned, moistened, and warmed. The conducting portion of the pulmonary system includes the nose, pharynx, larynx, and trachea and portions of the bronchial tree in the lungs. The conducting portion of the bronchial tree includes the two main bronchi, bronchi to the main lobes and to the segments of the lungs, and bronchioles. The diameter of these conducting tubes decreases with each successive branching, helping to regulate the flow of air during inspiration and expiration. The *bronchi* are made up of hyaline cartilage and smooth muscle cells. The muscle cells are arranged in spirals and increase in number closer to the respiratory portion of the pulmonary system. The *bronchioles* are made up of smooth muscle cells and elastic fibers. Sympathetic nervous system input via the vagus nerve influences contraction of the smooth muscle cells, which can change the length and diameter of the conducting vessels in the bronchial tree.

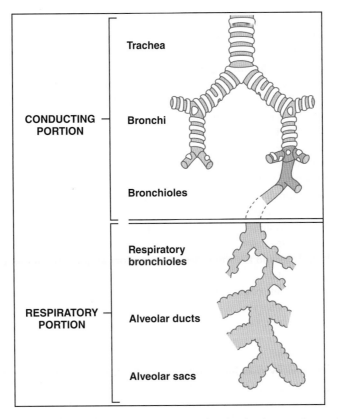

Fig. 7.6 The main divisions of the pulmonary system: the conducting portion and the respiratory portion. (From Costanzo LS: *Physiology.* Philadelphia: WB Saunders; 1998:164.)

Respiratory portion. The respiratory portion of the pulmonary system includes the remaining branches of the bronchial tree, alveolar ducts, alveolar sacs, and alveoli. As air is moved through these structures, gas exchange takes place. Respiratory bronchioles differ from conducting bronchioles because they have alveoli along their walls. At the alveolar level, only a very thin barrier is found between the air and the circulating blood. Alveoli are not only found in the respiratory bronchioles; large numbers of alveoli branch off from the alveolar ducts and alveolar sacs. *Alveolar sacs* (clusters of alveoli) and alveoli branch off from alveolar ducts, which contain smooth muscle cells, elastic fibers, and collagen fibers. Elastic and reticular fibers are found where the alveoli arise from the respiratory bronchioles, alveolar ducts, or alveolar sacs. The elastic fibers help to open the alveoli during inspiration and allow recoil during exhalation. Reticular fibers help maintain the shape of the alveoli.

Alveolar epithelium is made up of two types of cells. *Type I* alveolar cells are flat and thin respiratory epithelial cells, providing a large surface area for gas exchange. *Type II* cells are responsible for the production of *surfactant*, the detergent-like substance that mixes with water to decrease the alveolar surface tension. The decreased surface tension allows the alveoli to open more easily during respiration. Without *surfactant*, alveolar collapse can occur. This is especially important for the newborn. Lack of *surfactant* in the premature infant results in respiratory distress. Surfactant is constantly produced and turned over throughout life.

Air can also move from one part of the respiratory system to another via collateral ventilation mechanisms. Two mechanisms of collateral ventilation are pores of Kohn and Lambert canals. *Pores of Kohn* are gaps in the alveolar walls that provide an opening from one alveolus and its neighbor. *Lambert canals*, or *channels*, are small pathways from the respiratory bronchi to nearby alveoli.[4] The pores of Kohn also help with distribution of surfactant over the alveolar surface, which helps maintain the surface tension and prevent atelectasis.[5]

Functional components of the pulmonary system. The pulmonary system can also be divided into two functional components: the ventilatory pump and the respiratory component. Changes in elements of these functional components across the life span can influence function of the pulmonary system. The ventilatory pump component controls the flow of air. It is made up of three groups of respiratory muscles: the diaphragm, rib cage muscles, and the abdominal muscles.[6] "Each group acts on the chest wall and its compartments, that is lung-apposed rib cage, the diaphragm-apposed rib cage, and the abdomen."[6] The rib cage muscles consist of the intercostals, parasternals, scalene, and neck muscles. They are both inspiratory and expiratory.

The respiratory component is the site of gas exchange and consists of the lungs, intrapulmonary airways, and intrapulmonary vessels.

Control Mechanisms and Regulation

Control of ventilation is achieved by two interacting systems: the nervous system and chemoreceptors. Both systems are automatic but can be overridden by the need to talk, swallow, or perform other desired tasks like swimming underwater. The neural and chemical systems act on the muscular contraction of the diaphragm and intercostal muscles that are involved in the inspiratory phase of ventilation.

Neural System

The pulmonary system is innervated by the parasympathetic and sympathetic branches of the autonomic nervous system. Parasympathetic input results in bronchial constriction, whereas sympathetic input results in bronchodilation. Sensory and motor nerve fibers are found in the lung to the level of the terminal bronchioles.

At least three brain stem centers coordinate the rhythmic ventilatory cycle and maintain depth of ventilation. These sites are located in the medulla and pons of the brain stem. The inspiratory neurons in the medulla provide the stimulus to fire the muscles of breathing. One center in the pons modulates the medullary inspiratory neurons, which regulates the depth of ventilation. Another center in the pons is active during the transition between inspiration and expiration.

Chemical System

The chemical system regulates alveolar ventilation and monitors blood gases. Chemoreceptors detect changes in the blood levels of oxygen and carbon dioxide, as well as the pH of the blood, stimulating appropriate respiratory changes. Chemoreceptors located in the medulla respond to the hydrogen ion concentration in the extracellular fluid of the brain. Carbon dioxide in the extracellular fluid reacts with water to form hydrogen ions. A rise in arterial P_{CO_2} causes an increase in hydrogen ion concentration and consequently an increase in ventilation.

Ventilation can also be stimulated by a large decrease in arterial P_{O_2}. This mechanism uses the peripheral chemoreceptors: the aortic and carotid bodies. The chemoreceptors are directly influenced by the oxygen content of circulating arterial blood. A decrease in oxygen content excites the receptors to cause an increase in the depth and rate of breathing. Peripheral receptors provide an accessory mechanism for controlling breathing activity. The central receptors account for the majority of increased ventilation due to chemical change.

Breathing patterns can also be modified by sensory input from the lungs and chest wall. For example, proprioceptive input from stretch receptors in the lungs also stimulates ventilation.

Mechanics of Ventilation

The lungs, thorax, intercostal muscles, and diaphragm provide a pumping action that transports gas between the environment and the alveoli. During inspiration, the intercostal muscles contract to elevate the rib cage. The diaphragm also contracts, increasing the diameter of the thoracic cavity. This muscle activity expands the pleural cavity and results in increased negative pressure in the thoracic cavity. Atmospheric air rushes in, and the lungs expand. Bronchi and bronchioles increase in diameter. The expansion of the lungs activates stretch receptors, inhibiting inspiration. Exhalation occurs passively, with muscle relaxation and elastic recoil of the chest wall. Inhibitory input to inspiration is decreased, once again activating inspiration.

The ability of the musculoskeletal pump to transport inspiratory and expiratory gases is influenced by the compliance and resistance of the chest wall and lungs. Flexibility of the joints of the thoracic cavity contributes to achieving optimal expansion of the space. Resistance and elasticity of the pulmonary tissues must be overcome by contraction of the respiratory muscles, diaphragm, intercostal muscles, and accessory muscles of respiration. Resistance of the conducting airways also affects the amount of work necessary to deliver air to the respiratory system.

The amount of air contained in the lungs is defined by various functional volumes (Fig. 7.7). The maximal amount of air that can be contained in the lungs is referred to as the total lung capacity. The amount of air moved during resting inspiration and exhalation is referred to as the tidal volume (TV). The additional inspired air that can be taken into the lungs with a deep breath is called the inspiratory reserve volume (IRV); the additional air that can be pushed out of the lungs with forced exhalation is called the expiratory reserve volume (ERV). The sum of these three volumes is called the vital capacity (VC). The residual volume (RV) is the amount of air that is left in the lungs after exhalation. Minute ventilation (MV) is the total amount of air exchanged by the pulmonary system in 1 minute. Forced expiratory volume (FEV) can also be measured, and the amount of gas expired in the first second of a forced VC test is referred to as FEV_1. The FEV_1 is used to measure airway resistance.

Resistance and compliance factors, the breathing rate (number of breaths/minute), and the amount of air being moved with each breath determine the energy cost of breathing. The pulmonary system itself requires oxygen to fuel the work of breathing. The source of that oxygen is the bronchial arteries, which deliver blood from the aorta to the lung tissue. Blood is then returned to the heart via the pulmonary and bronchial veins.

DEVELOPMENT OF THE CARDIOVASCULAR AND PULMONARY SYSTEMS ACROSS THE LIFE SPAN

Prenatal Period
Cardiovascular System

The cardiovascular system is the earliest system of the body to function in the developing embryo, with blood circulation starting in the third week of gestation. Functionally, this circulation is necessary because the embryo has grown, and simple diffusion of nutrients and waste products across cell membranes can no longer meet nutritional demands.[1]

By the end of the third week of gestation, a primitive heart tube has been formed from clusters of mesoderm cells and neural crest cells. A heartbeat can be heard at approximately 22 days gestation.[1] As this tube elongates, a series of dilations and constrictions differentiate the vessel into an atrium, a ventricle, the truncus arteriosus, and the sinus venosus. The sinus venosus functions early as the pacemaker of the conducting system of the heart and is the precursor to the sinoatrial node, atrioventricular node, and bundle of His. At approximately 4 weeks of gestation, areas of swelling form on the walls

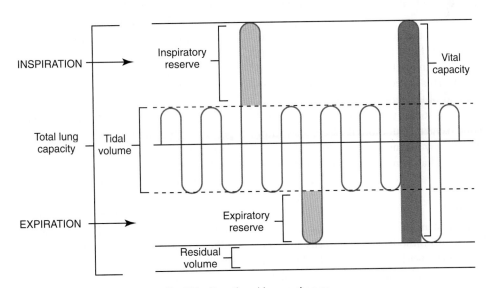

Fig. 7.7 Functional lung volumes.

of the atrioventricular canal. These swellings, called *endocardial cushions*, grow together during the fifth week of gestation and begin to divide the heart into left and right chambers. The primitive atrium is also divided into two chambers by the formation of the septum primum and the septum secundum at approximately 5 weeks gestation.[7] An oval opening left between the interatrial septae, called the *foramen ovale*, is important for fetal circulation, allowing blood to flow from the right to left atria. Near the end of the fourth week of gestation, contractions of the heart coordinate unidirectional flow of blood. By the seventh week, the heart tube has become a four-chambered vessel.[1]

The embryo's primitive heart tube establishes links with its blood vessels and with the placenta as early as 13–15 days of gestation. Circulation is then established between the mother and the embryo, ensuring the exchange of nutrients and removal of waste products. Maternal nutrients and oxygen are transported to the fetus via the umbilical vein; waste products and carbon dioxide are removed via the umbilical artery. By the fifth week of development, embryonic vessel formation is under way.

Vascular development begins with the differentiation of mesodermal cells into vessels, which then form larger vascular networks in organs such as the liver and endocardium of the heart. Further development of the vessels occurs as branches are formed from existing vessels. This process is called *angiogenesis* and can occur in embryonic development, as well as throughout the life span.[7]

The fetus receives all necessary oxygen from the mother; little blood flow is necessary through the lungs. Fetal hemoglobin levels are higher than postnatal hemoglobin levels. This is necessary because the oxygen saturation of blood of the fetus from the umbilical circulation is only 50%–60% in the fetus compared with an arterial blood oxygen saturation of 90%–95% within minutes after birth.[8] By having an increased fetal hemoglobin level, the fetus has a greater capacity to carry oxygen to the tissues.

Pulmonary System

The pulmonary system of the embryo arises from both endodermal and mesodermal germ cells and first appears in the fourth week of gestation. Endodermal cells from the primitive pharynx form the epithelial lining of the trachea, larynx, bronchi, and lungs. Mesoderm surrounding the developing lung buds contributes to the development of smooth muscle, connective tissue, and cartilage within these structures.

Early development of the fetal pulmonary system is shown in Fig. 7.8. At 28 days of gestation, *bronchial buds* have developed at the end of the laryngotracheal tube and have divided into the right and left lung buds. At 35 days, secondary bronchi have appeared. By 42 days, all of the branches of the conducting airways have been formed. Between 42 and 56 days of gestation, branching has continued to the level of at least two respiratory bronchioles. By the end of the embryonic period, the two lungs, major airways, and pleural cavity are formed.[9,10] Formation of the pulmonary arterial tree accompanies the branching of the respiratory tree.

Early in the fetal period, the bronchial tree continues to form and smooth muscle begins to develop at the proximal segments of the airways.[10] By 12–26 weeks of gestation, distal airways begin to form and conducting and respiratory airways are differentiated. Type I and Type II epithelial cells appear.[10] Type I cells are responsible for gas exchange and Type II cells produce surfactant.[11] The bronchial epithelium thins and flattens, increasing the diameter of the bronchi and terminal bronchioles. Capillaries also appear in the epithelium. From 24 weeks of gestation until birth, development of the *terminal respiratory units* continues. These may also be referred to as *terminal sacs* or *primitive alveoli*. Type II epithelial cells appear in the lining of the primitive alveoli and begin to secrete surfactant, which allows the alveoli to expand. Primitive alveoli continue to multiply in the last few weeks of the normal gestational period.

Type II epithelial cells begin producing surfactant as early as 20–22 weeks of gestation.[11] Surfactant is necessary for maximum lung expansion after birth, maintaining expansion of the alveoli. Once surfactant is produced, the amniotic fluid begins to contain lecithin, a phospholipid. The ratio of two types of phospholipids, lecithin and sphingomyelin (L/S ratio), is used as an index of lung maturity. A ratio of 2:1 or greater indicates that the lungs are mature and that the risk of development of respiratory distress syndrome in the fetus is minimal.[12] By 26–28 weeks of gestation, the fetus has sufficient vascularized terminal sacs and surfactant to survive if born prematurely.[11]

The intrauterine lung is not responsible for gas exchange. Weak attempts at fetal breathing appear to

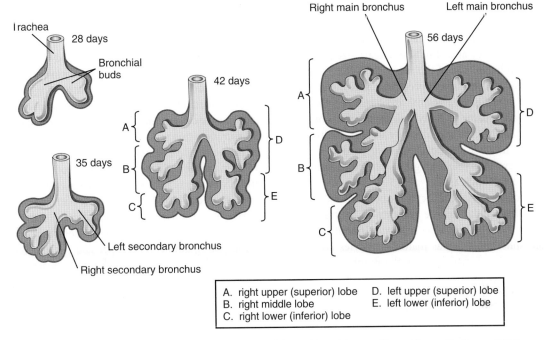

A. right upper (superior) lobe   D. left upper (superior) lobe
B. right middle lobe   E. left lower (inferior) lobe
C. right lower (inferior) lobe

Fig. 7.8 **Successive stages in the development of bronchi and lungs.** (From Moore KL, Persaud TVN, Torchia MG. Ch 10: Respiratory System. In: Moore KL, Persaud TVN, Torchia MG, eds. *The Developing Human.* 11th ed. Philadelphia: Elsevier; 2020, Figure 10.9.)

be present in preparation for respiration after birth. Instead, the lung tissue secretes liquid that is swallowed or added to amniotic fluid. This fluid production slows shortly before birth so that the lungs are only 50% filled with fluid at birth. This fluid has to be removed as the lungs inflate after birth. Like the cardiovascular system, the pulmonary system undergoes dramatic change in the moments after birth.

Infancy and Young Childhood

Cardiovascular and Pulmonary Adjustments at Birth

Immediately after birth, blood must be circulated to the lung tissue, and the lungs must inflate. Much of the fluid that fills the lungs is pushed out through the nose and mouth during labor; remaining fluid can be drained by the pulmonary vasculature and lymphatic system as the newborn begins spontaneous breathing and aeration of the lungs occurs.[13] With each of the first breaths, more and more air is retained in the lungs, building up the newborn's functional residual capacity (RV plus ERV). With inspiration, alveolar expansion occurs, delivering oxygenated air to the alveoli.

After birth, blood must be shunted into the pulmonary circulation to receive oxygen from the alveoli. As the lungs expand, pulmonary vascular resistance decreases, and blood flow to the lungs increases. With the occlusion of the umbilical cord, the ductus venosus, which had delivered blood from the umbilical vein to the inferior vena cava, closes. This results in decreased pressure in the inferior vena cava and right atrium. As left atrial pressure becomes greater than right atrial pressure, the foramen ovale closes. Another circulatory change occurs as increased systemic and aortic pressures pump the blood toward the pulmonary artery, reversing the direction of blood flow through the ductus arteriosus. The ductus arteriosus constricts and eventually closes (see Figs. 8.1 and 8.2), with the infant transitioning fully to adult circulation by 4–8 weeks of age.[11,13,14]

Cardiovascular System

The newborn heart lies horizontally in the chest cavity, but a more vertical position is assumed as the lungs expand and the chest cavity grows. Irregularity in the electrocardiogram of the newborn is not unusual because stabilization of the autonomic nervous system, conductivity of cardiac muscle fibers, heart position, and hemodynamics are not yet completed.[15]

Through infancy and childhood, heart size increases at a rate similar to that of the increase in fat-free body weight. Heart volumes are approximately 40 mL at birth, 80 mL at 6 months, and 160 mL by 2 years of age. The ratio of heart volume to body weight remains constant at approximately 10 mL/kg of body weight.[15] Although there is no increase in the number of cardiac muscle fibers (myocytes) as the heart grows, the cross-sectional area of the fibers increases.

Several changes in the myocyte are noted during development, allowing the mature myocyte to contract with more force than the immature myocyte. Immature myocytes are spherical, whereas mature myocytes are more rectangular. As myocytes mature, the number of myofibrils per cross-sectional area increases, and with increased myofibrils, the contractile properties of the myocyte increase. The length of the myofibril also increases which also contributes to increased contractile force. Increased size and number of mitochondria in the mature cardiomyocyte also increase the potential for ATP production.[16] As myocytes mature, the myofibrils assume a parallel orientation and increase their force-generating potential.[16,17]

The vascularization of the heart muscle increases from one vessel for six muscle fibers in the newborn to one vessel for each muscle fiber, as seen in the adult. At birth, the thicknesses of the right and left ventricle walls are equal, but as the left ventricle starts pumping against increased pressure, the left ventricular wall increases in size and becomes approximately twice as thick as the right ventricular wall by adulthood.[18]

Arteries and veins also increase in size as body weight and height increase. The thickness of the vessel wall increases as increased functional demands are placed on the vessels. Development of smooth muscle within the walls of the vessels occurs more slowly. No muscle cells are present at birth in the alveolar blood vessels. Muscle cells can be seen in pulmonary vasculature at the level of the respiratory bronchiole by 4 months of age and at the alveolar ducts by 3 years of age. Some alveolar arteries have muscle cells in their walls at 10 years, but others do not complete this process until 19 years of age.[19]

The heart rate and stroke volume of infants and young children are very different from those of adults. Because stroke volume is related to heart size, the smaller the heart, the less blood that can be pumped with each heartbeat. At birth, stroke volume is only 3–4 mL, whereas it may be 40 mL in the preadolescent and 60 mL in the young adult. To compensate for smaller stroke volumes, children demonstrate higher heart rates than adults (Table 7.1). Boys and girls younger than 10 years have similar heart rates, but after puberty, girls' heart rates are 3–5 bpm higher than those of boys.[15]

Blood pressure also changes from infancy through childhood. These changes are related to ongoing development of (1) the autonomic nervous system, (2) peripheral vascular resistance, and (3) body mass. Blood pressure increases in children are strongly related to increases in height and weight. Over the past decade, population-based increases have been seen in both population norms of blood pressure in children and in incidence of hypertension.[20–22] Pediatric hypertension is discussed in more detail in Clinical Implications Box 7.1.

Blood volume also increases with body size; the total blood volume of the newborn is 300–400 mL, whereas the adolescent or young adult has approximately 5 L of blood. Hemoglobin levels in the blood vary with age, affecting the oxygen-carrying capacity of the blood. In

TABLE 7.1   Normal Vital Sign Values by Age

Age Group	Respiratory Rate (Per Minute)	Pulse (Per Minute)	Blood Pressure (mm Hg)
Neonate		80–180	60/30
Infant	20–40	80–160	96/60
Toddler	20–30	50–150	98/64
School-aged child	16–24	75–110	106/68
Adolescent	12–20	50–100	114/74
Adult	12–18	60–100	120/80

From Higuet A, Idrissi SH, Wateleet JB, 2016. MedlinePlus Medical Encyclopedia, Vital Signs. https://medlineplus.gov/ency/article/002341.htm. Accessed 10-2-2022.

CLINICAL IMPLICATIONS BOX 7.1
Hypertension: An Issue for Children and Adults

Hypertension (HTN) has long been identified as a serious health problem for adults, increasing the risk for development of heart disease, stroke, renal disease, etc. Globally, HTN is the leading cause of preventable, premature death in adults,[23] and HTN rates doubled in adults from 1990 to 2019.[24] However, it is estimated that less than 50% of cases are diagnosed and less then 25% of cases of HTN are adequately controlled.[24,25] A study of prevalence and incidence of HTN from 1995 to 2005 estimated that the global prevalence of hypertension would increase by at least 25% by 2025, but some population-based studies indicated that the increase would be even greater.[26] Over the past 20 years, improvements have been seen in prevalence of HTN in high-income countries, but HTN is a greater problem in low- and middle-income countries,[24] and more than 1 billion people are reported to have HTN globally.[23] In the past decade, increased attention has been paid to the prevalence of hypertension in children and its related outcomes. Pediatric HTN is reported to related to adult hypertension, increased risk of cardiac disease, renal disease, and mortality.[25,27]

Hypertension in Adults

Blood pressure does appear to increase with age and has also been linked to obesity, reduced levels of physical activity, elevated sodium intake, and other dietary choices.[28,29] Other medical conditions, such as renal disease, diabetes mellitus, sleep apnea, and thyroid disease, can also contribute to development of hypertension. In older adults, vascular stiffness, age-related changes in sympathetic nervous system control of the vasculature,[30] and increased salt sensitivity (especially in women) contribute to prevalence of HTN in 60% of individuals between 60 and 69 years of age and greater than 75% of individuals over 80 years of age.[28,31] Globally, several guidelines are published related to the diagnosis and management of hypertension in adults. Information provided in this Clinical Implication Box is based upon the clinical practice guideline developed in the United States.[29]

Diagnosis is based on the values of systolic and diastolic blood pressure as normal, elevated, hypertension stage 1, or hypertension stage 2. A diagnosis of HTN is based upon an average of at least two blood pressure readings/visits, over two separate visits (Table 7.1A).[32]

Risks/Outcomes of HTN in Adults

- Stroke
- Cardiovascular disease/mortality
- Kidney damage
- Cognitive changes

Intervention for HTN in Adults

Intervention to control hypertension in adulthood focuses on lifestyle modifications that will support weight loss, increase level of physical activity, and dietary changes. A diet that includes fresh fruits and vegetables, low-fat foods, and low salt is recommended (see Table 7.1B). Medications are also used to control factors contributing to HTN. Several categories of medications have been demonstrated to effectively control hypertension. Pharmaceutical management of hypertension is complex and managed by the patient's physician.

Hypertension in Children

Hypertension in children has become a global health concern. Prevalence of hypertension in children has increased over the past decades in several countries. From 2000 to 2015, a 75%–79% increase in global prevalence was identified for individuals from 6 to 19 years of age.[33] The global estimate of children and adolescents with hypertension is 4%, and almost 10% of this population demonstrated elevated blood pressure in the prehypertension range.[25,33] The problem of childhood and adolescent hypertension is greater in low- and middle-income countries, with a recent study in Africa reporting over 7% prevalence of hypertension and over 11% of prehypertension.[34] In India, the prevalence of hypertension in 5- to 15-year-old children was reported at greater than 20%, and in China greater than 18%.[23] Global prevalence of hypertension in 6–19-year-olds increases to almost 5% in individuals who are overweight and greater than 15% in those who are obese.[33] This increased prevalence with overweight and obese children is also reported in Africa, where obesity has become a significant problem over the past decades.[34] Hypertension related to obesity can be seen in children younger than 5 years of age.[25] In addition to obesity and physical inactivity, dyslipidemia and hyperglycemia are also risk factors for pediatric and adolescent HTN.[35]

Both primary and secondary hypertension are seen in children. Primary hypertension is associated with prevalence of obesity in children, dietary sodium levels, and sedentary lifestyle. Socioeconomic factors, ethnic

TABLE 7.1A Diagnostic Table

	Systolic Blood Pressure	Diastolic Blood Pressure
Normal	<120 mm Hg	<80 mm Hg
Elevated	120–129 mm Hg	<80 mm Hg
HTN stage 1	130–139 mm Hg	80–89 mm Hg
HTN stage 2	≥140 mm Hg	≥90 mm Hg

CLINICAL IMPLICATIONS BOX 7.1
Hypertension: An Issue for Children and Adults

TABLE 7.1B   Lifestyle Modifications to Prevent and Manage Hypertension[a]

Modification	Recommendation	Approximate SBP Reduction (Range)[b]
Weight reduction	Maintain normal body weight (body mass index 18.5–24.9 kg/m²)	5–20 mmHg/10 kg
Adopt DASH eating plan	Consume a diet rich in fruits, vegetables, and low-fat dairy products with a reduced content of saturated and total fat	8–14 mmHg
Dietary sodium reduction	Reduce dietary sodium intake to no more than 100 mmol per day (2.4 g sodium or 6 g sodium chloride)	2–8 mmHg
Physical activity	Engage in regular aerobic physical activity such as brisk walking (at least 30 min per day, most days of the week)	4–9 mmHg
Moderation of alcohol consumption	Limit consumption to no more than 2 drinks (e.g., 24 oz beer, 10 oz wine, or 3 oz 80-proof whiskey) per day in most men, and to no more than 1 drink per day in women and lighter weight persons	2–4 mmHg

[a]For overall cardiovascular risk reduction stop smoking.
[b]The effects of implementing these modifications are dose- and time-dependent, and could be greater for some individuals.
DASH, Dietary approaches to stop hypertension; SBP, systolic blood pressure
From National Heart, Lung, Blood Institute, US Department of Health and Human Services. The Seventh Report of the Joint Natitonal Committee on Prevention, Detection, evaluation, and Treatment of High Blood Pressure, 2004. https://www.nhlbi.nih.gov/files/docs/guidelines/jnc7full.pdf

differences, and family history are other factors that may contribute to the development of primary hypertension in children and adolescents. Perinatal factors such as low birth weight, prematurity, and maternal factors (pre-eclampsia, hypertension, body mass index, and age) also influence development of hypertension in children.[25] Rates of primary hypertension are increasing rapidly in children and adolescents. Secondary hypertension, resulting from other conditions such as renal, heart, and endocrine disease or use of medications or nutritional supplements, is more common in children than adults, especially infants and young children. As incidence of primary hypertension has increased in children, only about 10% of childhood hypertension is identified as secondary hypertension.[35]

HTN. The European,[36] Canadian,[37] and American Academy of Pediatrics[38] guidelines are summarized in Table 7.1C.

Risks/Outcomes of HTN in Children and Adolescents

Children and adolescents with HTN have an increased prevalence of:
- Cardiac changes such as left ventricular hypertrophy, thickening of the carotid artery intima, and arterial stiffness.[25,27]
- Cognitive changes resulting in lower performance on neurocognitive testing and cognitive impairment earlier in life.[35] Increased incidence of learning disability in children with HTN has also been reported.[38]

Diagnosis

It is recommended that children over the age of 3 years have routine screening of blood pressure, using a blood pressure cuff appropriate for child size. It is recommended that readings of increased blood pressure be confirmed on three consecutive visits before a diagnosis or HTN or pre-HTN is made. If blood pressure is above the 90th percentile or 95th percentile on three separate clinic visits, a diagnosis of prehypertension or hypertension is made. Guidelines are available from several groups regarding diagnostic criteria for pediatric and adolescent

Intervention

Intervention to control hypertension in children focuses on lifestyle modifications that support weight loss, increase level of physical activity, reduced sodium intake, and dietary changes. A diet that includes fresh fruits and vegetables, low-fat foods, reduced sugar, and low salt is recommended.[25,35] If lifestyle modifications do not adequately correct pediatric and adolescent HTN, medications may also be prescribed.[35] Diagnostic and intervention information related to children and adolescence is summarized in Table 7.1D.

Continued

CLINICAL IMPLICATIONS BOX 7.1
Hypertension: An Issue for Children and Adults

TABLE 7.1C Classification of Office-Based BP in Children and Adolescents by the American Academy of Pediatrics 2017, European Society of Hypertension 2016, and Hypertension Canada 2020 Guidelines

Guidelines	American Academy of Pediatrics (2017)[38]	European Society of Hypertension (2016)[36]	Hypertension Canada (2020)[37]
BP screening end measurement	– Annual BP measurement in children ≥3 years of age, or at every visit if risk factors for hypertension – Oscillometric methods can be used for screening, but must be confirmed by auscultatory method – Elevated BP should be confirmed on three separate clinic visits—ABPM recommended	– BP measurement should be performed in children ≥3 years of age, and can repeat every 2 years if BP normal – Auscultatory method preferred – Elevated BP should be confirmed on three separate clinic visits – ABPM recommended	– BP should be regularly measured in children ≥3 years of age. No recommendation on screening, frequency – Oscillometric methods can be used for screening, but must be conferred by auscultatory method – Elevated BP should be confirmed on three separate clinic visits – ABPM should be considered
Hypertension threshold	≥95th percentile (<13 years) Or ≥130/80 (≥13 years)	≥95th percentile (<16 years) Or ≥140/90 mm Hg (≥16 years)	-95th percentile Or >120/80 mm Hg (6–11 years) Or >130/85 mm Hg (≥12 years)
Target BP (general pediatric population)	90th percentile (<13 years) Or <130/80 (≥13 years)	<95th percentile recommended <90th percentile should be considered	<95th percentile <90th percentile (for patients with risk factors or target organ damage)
Target BP (pediatric CKD)	24-h MAP (by ABPM) of <50th percentile	<75th percentile (nonproteinuric CKD) <50th percentile (proteinuric CKD)	<90th percentile

ABPM, Ambulatory blood pressure monitoring; BP, blood pressure; CKD, chronic kidney disease; MAP, mean arterial pressure.
Robinson CH, Chanchlani R High blood pressure in children and adolescents: Current perspectives and strategies to improve future kidney and cardiovascular health. Kidney Int Rep. 2022;7:954–970.

TABLE 7.1D Lifestyle Modifications to Prevent and Manage Hypertension in Children and Adolescents

Modification	Recommendation	Variation by Source
Physical activity	40–60 min of moderate to vigorous aerobic activity at least 3–5 days/week. Resistance exercise 2–3 times/week	AAP 2017 recommends 40 min/day. European guidelines recommend 60 min/day and resistance exercise.
Limit sedentary activity	Limit time in sedentary activity to no more than 2 h/day	

CLINICAL IMPLICATIONS BOX 7.1
Hypertension: An Issue for Children and Adults

TABLE 7.1D Lifestyle Modifications to Prevent and Manage Hypertension in Children and Adolescents—cont'd

Modification	Recommendation	Variation by Source
Diet	Follow DASH diet—increase fruits, vegetables, whole grains; low-fat dairy; fish, poultry, lean red meat/limit sugar and sodium Sodium intake <2300 mg/day	European guidelines specify sodium intake guideline
Weight loss	Weight loss for overweight and obese children	
Limit exposure to smoke	Smoke-free environment	Listed in European guidelines
Parental and family involvement in lifestyle modifications	Parent and family participation in lifestyle modification program	Listed in European guidelines

Based upon recommendations of the American Academy of Pediatrics[38] and the European Society of Hypertension.[36]

the newborn, hemoglobin levels are high (20 g/100 mL), but they fall to 10 g/100 mL by 3–6 months of age. Hemoglobin values then slowly increase with age to adult levels of 16 g/100 mL for men and 14 g/100 mL for women.[15]

Pulmonary System

Ventilatory pump development. From a mechanical point of view, the shape of the chest wall and limitations in posture and movement affect the infant's breathing efficiency. At birth, the infant maintains a posture of shoulder elevation, limiting the cervical dimensions of the thorax. The ribs are made up primarily of cartilage and are in a horizontal position, giving the lower thorax a circular dimension (Fig. 7.9). This results in a relatively flexible thorax and affects the alignment of the diaphragm. The diaphragm and other ventilatory muscles of the newborn are made up of more type IIa muscle fibers than type I muscle fibers, affecting muscle strength and endurance.[14] The structural immaturity of the thorax, combined with a lack of development and control of the ventilatory muscles, prevents the infant from stabilizing the rib cage and effectively using the diaphragm to breathe. The compliancy of the infant's thorax both minimizes inspiratory forces of the rib cage and makes the infant susceptible to paradoxical movement during inspiration.[39] Because of the inefficiency of the respiratory muscles, horizontal rib cage alignment, and airway resistance, the infant experiences a high workload with breathing, and respiratory fatigue can occur.[14]

As the infant learns to move the head and upper body against gravity and to reach in the first 3–6 months, muscular development allows increased expansion and use of the upper chest in breathing. In the second half of the first year, the infant learns to sit, stand, and walk, systematically overcoming the force of gravity. As the upright sitting position is assumed, the force of gravity and forces from developing abdominal musculature will pull the ribs downward into a more angular position. This not only expands the thoracic cavity but also increases spacing between the ribs, allowing the intercostal muscles to work more efficiently. Throughout childhood, the rib cage becomes more rigid as osteophytes are laid down to replace cartilage. With growth, the diaphragm is pulled into a dome shape that improves the length-tension relationship of the muscle and improves function. Active use of the abdominal muscles stabilizes the rib cage within the more rigid thorax, providing a stable base for diaphragmatic action.[39,40]

The depth and rate of ventilation change in relationship to the activity or work to be performed. The diaphragm is the major muscle of inspiration until around 5–7 years of age, after which the thoracic muscles play a larger role. By age 4 years, the chest wall has elongated and takes up more than half the trunk.[40] The intercostal muscles connecting all the ribs are fully developed. Four

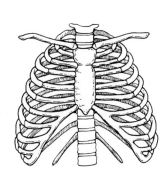 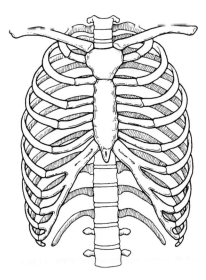

Fig. 7.9 Comparison of the infant thorax *(left)* with the mature thorax *(right)*. A major difference between the infant and mature adult thorax, other than the size, is the orientation of the ribs. The ribs are oriented horizontally in the infant thorax but are angled downward in the adult.

structures can contribute to breathing: the diaphragm, the chest wall, the neck, and abdominals. The usual breathing pattern consists of using a combination of diaphragm and chest wall movements. The relationship among work capacity, ventilation, and oxygen consumption in the child continues to mature into adolescence.

Respiratory system development. Only a small percentage of the total number of alveoli to be developed are present at birth. From birth to 3 years of age, some of the nonrespiratory bronchioles in the conducting airway system that were formed prenatally are converted to respiratory bronchioles. This increases the gas exchange capacity of the lungs. It has been considered that new alveoli develop rapidly in the first 2–3 years of life and continue to develop until approximately 8 years of age, when the adult number of 300 million alveoli is attained.[11,15,41] Current studies using advanced assessment methods demonstrate that alveolar development (alveolarization), although most robust in the first 2–3 years of life, continues until adolescence or early adulthood when growth of the lungs is complete.[10,42] With the advanced assessment methods, it is also hypothesized that the adult has 300–700 million alveoli.[42] The size and complexity of the alveoli increase throughout infancy and childhood, significantly increasing the available surface area for gas exchange. Alveolar diameter has been shown to increase through 22 years

of age.[41] The growth of the alveolar surface appears to be related to the increased oxygen demand of working tissue. The pulmonary arterial and venous vasculature develops concurrently with the development of alveoli. Capillarization of the alveoli develops in parallel to the alveolarization.[10,43]

The conducting and respiratory airways increase in length and diameter until growth of the thoracic cavity is complete. Children under 5 years of age have a large number of small airways that are less than 2 mm in diameter. Small airways can be problematic in two ways. First, they offer increased resistance to airflow, thereby increasing the work of breathing. Second, they are very easily obstructed by foreign objects.[14] Conducting airway volume increases through young adulthood and correlates with increases in height.[41]

The bronchioles and alveoli of infants and young children are weaker and less efficient than those of adults. Smooth muscle in the walls of the bronchioles does not develop until the child is 3–4 years old. As a result, the airway is more susceptible to collapse, thus trapping air. The development of elastic tissue in the alveoli may be incomplete until after adolescence; this means decreased lung compliance and distensibility for infants and young children. This makes it harder for the infant and small child to fully inflate their lungs and maintain lung volume. In children younger than 7 years, decreased elastic recoil causes the airways to close at a greater lung volume than in older children and adults. When combined with small airway size, this relative lack of recoil places young children more at risk for complications from respiratory diseases.

One other structural difference between the pulmonary systems of children and adults is the absence of collateral ventilation mechanisms in children. This decreased collateral circulation may increase the risk of respiratory infection and atelectasis in children. Pores of Kohn have not been seen in children younger than 4 years of age, and continue to develop during childhood. Lambert canals also develop during childhood.[4,14,44]

In summary, the development of the lungs into their adult form continues well into adolescence and young adulthood. Lung volume increases proportionally with increases in body size and increases as the number of alveoli increases.[15] VC values are related to height. Size of the conducting airways is related to stature, and the total number of alveoli an individual develops is proportional to height, which reinforces the relationship between lung volume and body size.[19,41] In the first year of life, the infant has little pulmonary reserve and must increase breathing frequency to meet demands for increased oxygen. IRV and ERV sufficient to meet increased needs are evident at about 1 year of age.

Differences between a child's and an adult's pulmonary function are seen in breathing pattern and in breathing frequency. The newborn infant undergoes dramatic changes in intrathoracic pressure, lung inflation, and pulmonary circulation. It is not unusual to observe irregular breathing patterns, including periods of apnea, during this time. Small airway size, together with the limited number of developed alveoli, leave the young infant with a small lung volume. As a result, the newborn's respiratory rate is higher than at any other time in the life span (Table 7.1).

Adolescence

Growth and functional changes of the cardiovascular and pulmonary systems continue through childhood and into adolescence. During the adolescent growth spurt, gender differences in cardiovascular and pulmonary function become apparent. Left ventricular mass increases in parallel with body mass equally for boys and girls until 9–12 years of age. In adolescence, the left ventricular mass of boys is greater than that of girls. Adolescents who participate in endurance-type sports also have a greater left ventricular mass than their peers who do not participate in this type of activity.[15] By adolescence, blood volume of boys is also greater than that of girls.

The amount of muscle in the heart increases, resulting in increased blood pressure and decreased heart rate.[18] Increased blood pressure is primarily related to increased body weight. In girls, blood pressure increases during their prepubertal growth spurt and then levels off. In boys, blood pressure gradually increases with lean body mass through 18 years of age. By the end of adolescence, systolic blood pressures of boys become slightly greater than those of girls, while no gender difference is seen for diastolic blood pressure.[15] It should be noted that more recently, increases in blood pressure for both boys and girls have been linked to body weight and increasing levels of obesity (see Clinical Implications Box 7.1). Gender differences in heart rate are also reported: the basal heart rate of girls is 3–5 bpm faster than that of boys. Stroke volume also increases but does not appear to be related only to heart size.

In the year preceding the peak height velocity, stroke volume changes appear to be related to an increased arterial-venous oxygen difference. This implies that more oxygen is being extracted by the tissues, which may be due to age-related changes in muscle mass, muscle enzyme profusion, and the ratio of capillaries to muscle fiber. In the year after peak height velocity, increased stroke volume may be related to an increased cardiac preload condition with increased venous return.[45]

The adolescent growth spurt is also reflected in lung size and lung volume. Lung and thoracic development continues through puberty in males, but is almost complete in females at the time of menarche. In males, the thoracic volume index correlates best with lung volumes, while in females height correlates with lung volume. Changes in lung volumes after maximal height is attained are thought to be related to muscle strength. Muscle strength increases in males through puberty, but plateaus in females at approximately age 15.[46] Ventilation increases between 11 and 17 years in boys and only between 11 and 13 years in girls, based on a study by Zhou and associates.[47] Peak ventilation and tidal volume increase almost linearly with age, body mass, stature, and free-fat mass in both sexes.[48]

Proximal airways and vasculature increase in size. Alveoli become larger, and greater amounts of elastic fiber can be found in the alveolar wall. The capillaries in the alveolar region also become larger, supporting increased gas exchange. By age 19, muscle is developed in the walls of the arteries found at the alveoli, increasing the efficient control of blood flow by vasodilation and vasoconstriction.[49]

Adulthood and Aging

Normal function of the cardiovascular and pulmonary systems in early and middle adulthood is described in the beginning of this chapter. Heart size and weight may continue to increase in adulthood, primarily because of fat deposition.[18,50] Some gender differences in function of the cardiovascular and pulmonary systems do exist. During submaximal exercise, the cardiac output of women is 5%–10% greater than that of men. This may be related to stroke volume differences and the fact that women have slightly less hemoglobin (14 g/100 mL blood) than men (15–16 g/100 mL blood).[5] Age-related changes in mean heart weight are not readily demonstrated in men, but in women, the mean heart weight increases between the fourth and seventh decades of life.[51] Women may also experience greater aortic stiffening after menopause.[52]

With increasing age, anatomical and physiological changes are seen in the cardiovascular and pulmonary systems. At least initially, these age-related changes do not seem to significantly interfere with function. Functional losses are more evident beginning in the seventh decade of life.[53] It is also difficult to differentiate cardiovascular and pulmonary changes related purely to aging from those caused by asymptomatic disease or deconditioning. As discussed in Chapter 13, it is thought that physically active adults can minimize the impact of aging on cardiovascular and pulmonary function.

Age is a major risk factor for cardiovascular disease. More than 50% of all heart failure patients and 90% of deaths occur in people over the age of 70.[54] Changes in cardiovascular structure and function seen with aging can increase the presence of cardiovascular risk factors.[55,56] Cardiovascular disease is a leading cause of death across the globe, with the incidence increasing with age.[55,56]

Cardiovascular System

The heart. Structural changes are seen in the heart and cardiac cells with aging. In general, the number of myocytes (muscle cells) decreases, whereas their size increases.[55,56] In the myocardium, increasing amounts of elastic tissue, fat, and collagen contribute to increased stiffness and decreased compliance of the ventricles. Cross-linkage of collagen in the myocardium also contributes to increased stiffness. Accumulation of lipofuscin, a waste product associated with oxidative damage, is also seen in the cardiac muscle cells, resulting in a darkening of the myocardium. Lipofuscin deposits interfere with mitochondrial turnover in the cardiac myocyte and contribute to cellular aging and cell death.[57-59]

A slight increase in the size of the heart, especially the left ventricle, occurs in some people, but there is an actual loss of muscle mass. The hypertrophy is primarily due to the thickening of the intraventricular septum. The heart wall thickens, so the amount of blood that the chamber can hold may actually decrease despite the increased overall heart size. Thicker walls also become stiffer, which does not allow the chambers to fill with as much blood before each ventricle pumps. The age-related stiffening of the heart walls causes the left ventricle to not fill as well and can sometimes lead to heart failure.[60]

Thickening of the left ventricular wall is seen in both men and women and may be related to the loss of myocytes, with increased size of remaining myocytes and increased amount of connective tissue. The thickening of the left ventricular wall seems to be related to age, but independent of body mass index (BMI), valve disease, coronary artery disease, and hypertension.[56] Increases are greater in women than men, especially when estrogen levels decrease. Over a 10-year period, men demonstrated a 15% increased risk for left ventricular hypertrophy, whereas women demonstrated a 67% increase in risk.[61] Some of this thickening may be related to hypertrophy of the remaining myocytes secondary to the increased demand on the heart necessary to pump blood through a less-compliant vascular system. As the walls of the arteries and arterioles become thicker, the space within the arteries expands slightly. Elastic tissue within the walls of the arteries and arterioles is lost. Together, these changes make the vessels stiffer and less resilient.[54] As a result, blood pressure increases in older adults when the heart contracts (systole). The decreased compliance in the vasculature contributes to systolic hypertension, which predominates in older adulthood, raising the pulse pressure and therefore the work of the left ventricle.[52,54,62] Since the arteries and arterioles are less elastic, blood pressure cannot adjust quickly when people stand, making older people at risk for orthostatic hypotension when they stand up suddenly. Additionally, these blood vessels cannot relax as quickly during the rhythmic pumping of the heart, which keeps blood pressure higher during rest. A decreased sensitivity of the baroreceptors can also lead to postural hypotension in response to stress and can lead to variable blood pressure changes during the day. This diminished response also makes it difficult to maintain blood pressure with blood loss. The belief is that the age-related thickening of the blood vessels interferes with the baroreceptors' ability to accurately determine the need to alter blood pressure, increasing the risk of postural hypotension with resultant risk for falls and injury.[60]

The volume of the left ventricle is slightly decreased, and the left atrium is slightly dilated.[56] In the endocardium, thickened areas of elastic and collagen fibers can be noted, especially in the atria. Fragmentation and disorganization of elastic, collagen, and muscle fibers also occur.[57] Increased fat is found within the epicardium, especially over the right ventricle and in the atrioventricular groove.[51,63]

With aging, changes are also seen in the heart valves and in the conduction system. The valves inside the heart (aortic semilunar valve, semilunar valve, bicuspid valve, tricuspid valve), which control the direction of blood flow, thicken, calcify, and become stiffer.[56] A heart murmur caused by valve stiffness is fairly common in older adults.[54] Collagen and lipid accumulation, as well as calcification, within the aortic and mitral valves impairs the ability of the valves to completely close. Collagen and fat are also laid down in the left bundle branches of the conduction system. By age 60, the number of pacemaker cell in the sinoatrial node decreases by 50%–75% of the amount seen in younger person.[59] By age 75, less than 10% of the number of sinoatrial node cells found in the adult heart are seen.[54,64] Decreased pacemaker cells in the sinoatrial node can lead to slightly slower heart rates.[59] Cellular loss is also noted in the atrioventricular node and bundle of His. These changes in the conduction system may contribute to the increased incidence of premature ventricular complexes and differences seen on the older adult's electrocardiogram. The QRS wave shifts to the left, and ST segment depression is seen.

The vasculature. The vasculature undergoes change throughout life, with vessels becoming thicker, more rigid, and more dilated. In general, the vascular course becomes more tortuous. Changes attributed to aging are initially seen in the coronary arteries at approximately 20 years of age and in the remainder of the arterial system after 40 years of age. Dilation occurs in proximal arteries such as the aorta, whereas thickening of the arterial wall predominates in the peripheral arteries. Larger arteries have a high elastin content in young adults.[60] Elastic arteries change more than muscular arteries, with irregular thickening of elastic tissue, fragmenting of elastic fibers, lipid infiltration, and calcification. These changes are seen earliest in the proximal portions of the large arteries.[54] The tunica media of the artery is made up of smooth muscle cells and is controlled by the vasomotor center of the medulla. This center plays an important role in regulating blood pressure by controlling vasodilatation and vasoconstriction. This control becomes more difficult with increased vessel rigidity as one ages.[60] The older vessel is thickened and less elastic, which results in less compliance. Arteriosclerosis refers to decreased compliance of the arteries, which is a normal consequence of age-related changes in the arterial walls.[54,55] This is contrasted to atherosclerosis, a pathological deposition of fatty plaques on the inner layer of the vessel, which also results in increased resistance to blood flow through the vessel. The cholesterol ratio changes with age with a decrease in HDL (good cholesterol) and an increase in LDL (bad cholesterol). The endothelium of the blood vessel can become injured with age and lead to atherosclerosis.[60] Research has shown that regular aerobic, endurance exercise can minimize the age-related changes in central arterial compliance. This possibly reflects the mechanism by which exercise decreases the risk of cardiovascular disease in older adults.[62,65,66]

Functional changes. The changes in the cardiovascular system associated with aging functionally affect the heart rate, blood pressure, stroke volume, and adaptability of the system to stress. The structural changes of the left ventricular wall reduce the ability of the ventricle to fill and contract. These changes do not have much effect on an individual at rest or during light exercise, but maximal exercise capacity decreases. In a resting person, the cardiac output measured as the amount of blood pumped through the heart in a minute averages 4–6 L, regardless of age in the absence of disease. An older adult cannot, however, keep up with a younger person during vigorous exercise. Maximal cardiac output (the maximal amount of blood the heart can pump in 1 min) decreases with aging by 25% and maximal oxygen uptake (VO_2 max) decreases by as much as 50%

between the ages of 20 and 80 years.[54] Even master athletes will experience decreases in VO_2 max with aging, inactivity can accelerate the loss, and sedentary individuals may experience VO_2 max loss by 10% each decade after age 25.[54]

The sensitivity of regulatory mechanisms, such as the baroreceptors, is diminished in the older individual, affecting the adaptability of the cardiovascular system to stressful situations such as cough, the Valsalva maneuver, and orthostasis. In older adults, the effectiveness of the sympathetic nervous system response to drops in blood pressure appears to be reduced due to stiffening of the vascular system.[67] This may help explain why older adults more often experience orthostatic hypotension than younger adults.[30,68] Increased plasma catecholamine levels and decreased end-organ responsiveness to adrenergic stimulation also affect the ability of the system to increase heart rate, contractility of the heart, and vasodilation of the vessels in response to stress. Because of decreased adaptability, the heart takes longer to reach a steady state or to recover from exercise. Older adults who are physically active appear to have improvements of the baroreflex control of heart rate than their sedentary peers, reflecting the role of exercise in improving vagal control of the heart.[68]

The resting heart rate changes minimally with aging, but maximum heart rate decreases. Mean heart rate has been shown to decrease slightly with age, but the change reportedly has minimal statistical significance.[69] Because heart rate varies with several factors, including the level of fitness, a wide range of resting heart rates is within normal limits for the older adult. The decrease in the maximum heart rate may be related to (1) decreased activity of the cardiac pacemaker, (2) decreased sensitivity to catecholamines, and (3) increased ventricular filling time. Increased ventricular filling time results from decreased ventricular compliance. Contraction time and diastole may also be increased because of slowed calcium uptake in the sarcoplasmic reticulum of the cardiac cells. Because of poor calcium transport and storage, the heart muscle will take longer to reach peak tension and to relax. Decreased venous tone, slowed relaxation of the ventricles, thickening of the mitral valve, and left ventricular stiffness may result in a decreased left ventricular filling time.[56] In older adults, the heart fills with blood more slowly than younger individuals, resulting in a lower proportion of total diastolic filling occurring during this passive, early diastolic phase, which is primarily due to an increase in the isovolumic relaxation time.

Stiffening of the aorta and major arteries increases systemic blood pressure, and poor perfusion of the skeletal muscle contributes to an increase in afterload.[31,62,70]

At rest and during exercise, blood pressure increases through adulthood and older adulthood. Blood pressure remains significantly related to adiposity through adulthood.[71] Systolic blood pressure rises in older adults, while diastolic blood pressure may decrease after the sixth decade.[31] The widening difference between systolic and diastolic blood pressure results in an increased pulse pressure, which can stress the heart and vasculature. The increase in systolic blood pressure is related to reduced loss of smooth muscle cells in the arterial wall, increased collagen content and cross-linkage within the vessels, thinning of the arterial wall, and calcium deposition in the vessel. These changes lead to increased stiffness in the vessels.[31] Moderate-intensity aerobic exercise appears to lower resting systolic blood pressure.[62] Low-intensity aerobic training in older adult hypertensive patients has also been shown to lower blood pressure, with these patients returning to a pretraining level of blood pressure when exercise was discontinued.[72] This finding seems to reflect that lifestyle factors also play a role in determining the blood pressure of the older adult. Even with attention to lifestyle choices that maintain appropriate body weight and regular physical activity, it appears that aging of the cardiovascular system leaves the older adult susceptible to development of hypertension (see Clinical Implications Box 7.1).

Delivery of oxygen to the peripheral tissues is altered with aging. The efficiency of oxygen extraction from the blood at the tissue level decreases with age, narrowing the arterial-venous oxygen difference. Loss of muscle strength, decreased muscle enzyme levels, and diminished size of the capillary network that perfuse muscle limit oxygen extraction from the circulating blood. Other vascular changes with aging, obstruction of major vessels, and decreased levels of hemoglobin are also factors. With increasing age, increased obesity, and decreased efficiency of sweating, blood is shunted away from the muscles and to the skin, assisting in body cooling. This also reduces blood flow to the tissues and contributes to the decreased efficiency of oxygen extraction.[73-75]

Age-related cardiovascular risk can also be caused by an imbalance of the autonomic nervous system (ANS) with increased sympathetic and decreased parasympathetic input, in addition to previously mentioned pathologies. The renin/angiotensin system which helps regulate blood pressure is controlled by the ANS. Impaired autonomic control contributes to loss of general function.[76,77]

In summary, there are decreases in maximal aerobic capacity, maximal heart rate, maximum cardiac output, peak heart rate and oxygen consumption, endothelial reactivity, maximal skeletal blood flow, and arterial distensibility. Increases in left ventricular mass with thickening of walls, loss of valvular flexibility, epicardial fat, peripheral vascular resistance, and total and LDL cholesterol are seen in aging adults.

Pulmonary System

Both the ventilatory pump and respiratory system are affected by aging. Because of this, older adults are at increased risk for respiratory failure because of changes in the lungs. Risk of ventilatory failure also increases because of changes in the ventilatory pump.[60,78]

Ventilatory pump changes. Structural changes occur with aging and create a stiffer, bony thorax, which increases the work of breathing. The thorax becomes shortened vertically and larger in the anterior-posterior dimension. Thoracic kyphosis and decreased mobility of the joints allow rib rotation. Increased calcification of the rib cartilage, and changes in the articulation between the ribs and vertebrae may also contribute to increased stiffness. Elasticity of cartilage and collagen in the annulus fibrosus decreases, and loss of fluid from the nucleus pulposus results in a flattened, less-resilient disk. Because of the resting position of the thorax, the intrathoracic pressure at end-expiration is higher, again increasing airway resistance and effort during breathing. Functionally, these changes result in decreased chest wall expansion during breathing. In a young adult, a 40% change in lung volume is noted with thoracic expansion, but only a 30% change is seen in older adults.[78,79]

The presence of osteoporosis and/or poor postural habits, may lead to structural deficits such as kyphosis and reduce the height of the thoracic cage due to loss of disc height and/or compression fractures. This reduces the ability of the chest wall to expand with inhalation. This decreased chest wall compliance results in an increase in the amount of work to inhale air. A kyphotic posture also puts the diaphragm at a mechanical disadvantage and reduces the efficiency of the contraction.

The intervertebral disc can gradually lose water and shrink, making them more compressed. Overall, these changes can lead to a decreased respiratory reserve for the entire system.[50]

Elasticity and compliance are also decreased within the lung because of changes in collagen and elastin. Cross-linkage of collagen is seen, and there is a loss of elastin in the airways and blood vessels. This results in decreased recoil of the lung and premature closure of small airways, especially at higher lung volumes.[78,80] This can result in air-trapping and an inability to completely empty the lungs. In the conducting airways, elasticity of bronchial cartilage is diminished. This results in a slightly increased diameter of the large airways. Hyaline cartilage structures in the trachea may become ossified. Bronchial mucous glands increase in number, thickening the mucus layer in the airway and offering more resistance to airflow. The number and thickness of elastic fibers in the walls of smaller airways decrease, again increasing the resistance to airflow and diminishing elastic recoil of the lungs. As elastic recoil of the lungs is diminished, RV increases and VC is reduced. Lungs, alveoli, and alveolar ducts enlarge with age. As a result, more time is needed for inspired air to reach the alveolar area. Decreased elasticity of the alveoli makes them susceptible to collapse on expiration. There is a decrease in the number of cilia in the lungs, making it more difficult to expel phlegm, bacteria, or mucous. This can lead to an increased risk for pneumonia or other respiratory problems.[81] Normally, healthy alveoli maintain a number of macrophages to fight infection, but these decrease in number as one ages.[60]

Respiratory muscles become less efficient with age. Inspiratory muscle strength and endurance appear to decrease, primarily due to loss of muscle mass in the diaphragm and the intercostals.[60,78] Structural changes in the thoracic cavity alter the length-tension relationship of the respiratory muscles, increasing the work of breathing. For example, the resting position of the diaphragm changes as the thoracic height decreases and diameter increases. Increased RV of the aging lung will also affect the resting position of the diaphragm. The abdominal muscles become weaker and less effective at stabilizing the diaphragm. Because of these changes, the older adult has to increase breathing rate rather than tidal volume to increase MV and has a less effective cough. This also increases the work of breathing and the risk for respiratory infections.[60,81]

Respiratory system changes. Many changes are noted in the aging lung. The loss of elastic recoil of the lung, as mentioned earlier, decreases the effectiveness of the ventilatory pump. The alveolar surface area also changes. By the time a person reaches their 90s, they have lost 25% of the alveolar surface area.[60] A loss of surface area results from a decrease in the actual number of alveoli per unit of lung volume; loss of alveolar wall tissue; and increased size of the respiratory bronchioles, alveolar sacs, and alveolar ducts.

The pulmonary vasculature undergoes the same changes within its vascular wall that were discussed earlier. The capillary bed at the alveolar interface becomes smaller, which, when combined with increased alveolar size, limits the diffusing capacity of the system. Pulmonary blood flow and blood volume within the capillary bed decrease. As a result, pulmonary gas exchange is affected. Pulmonary function and aerobic capacity decline by 40% between ages 25 and 80.[82] The alveolar-to-arteriole oxygen gradient increases as the arterial Po_2 decreases. The decrease in PaO_2 with age has been well documented,[19,82] but some references note a decrease in PaO_2 until the age of 70–75 years, after which PaO_2 plateaus.[78,82] Arterial Pco_2 remains constant throughout adulthood.

Functionally, the impact of these changes is reflected in lung volumes and arterial blood gas values at rest and during exercise. Although total lung capacity does not change, VC decreases while functional residual capacity and RV increase. By 70 years of age, VC is reported to decrease to 75% of earlier values, and RV increases by 50%.[19,60] At age 25 in men, VC is about 5 L, declining to 3.9 L by age 65. For women, it decreases from 3.5 L to 2.8 L. These changes are due primarily to the gradual loss of respiratory muscle strength and increase in chest wall rigidity.[60] IRV and ERV also decrease because of the decreased elasticity of the lung. The loss of elasticity causes the airways to close at a higher volume during expiration, which affects the amount of oxygenated air that is distributed to the tissue. The pulmonary system works harder to deliver less oxygen to the tissues in older adults.

In summary, aging causes decreases in VC, maximal airflow rates, strength of respiratory muscles, elasticity of lung fibers, elastic recoil, tidal volume, number of cilia, alveolar surface area, and vascularity. Increases can be seen in stiffness of the chest wall, RV, functional residual capacity, and respiratory rate.

FUNCTIONAL IMPLICATIONS OF CHANGES IN THE CARDIOVASCULAR AND PULMONARY SYSTEMS

Because of anatomical and physiological differences in the cardiovascular and pulmonary systems of the infant, child, adolescent, and adult, function and efficiency differ in each age group. Through childhood, most changes are related to changes in body size. Gender differences become apparent in adolescence. In adulthood and older adulthood, effects of environment and normal aging alter the efficiency and capacity of the cardiovascular and pulmonary systems. Lifestyle habits that affect respiratory system function in older adults include nutrition, smoking habits, and exercise. In the presence of protein malnutrition, muscle atrophy may be seen in the respiratory muscles. Smoking has a negative effect on both the cardiovascular and pulmonary systems.

Efficiency of the cardiovascular and pulmonary systems is reflected in measures such as cardiac output, MV, and maximal aerobic capacity. *Cardiac output* is a measure of the efficiency of the cardiovascular system. *MV*, the volume of air moved into the lungs in 1 minute, is a measure of the efficiency of the pulmonary system. These two measures, when considered with the ability of working tissue to use oxygen for energy production, indicate an individual's *maximal aerobic capacity*, or level of cardiovascular and pulmonary fitness.

Cardiac output varies with an individual's age. The cardiac output of children is less than that of adults both at rest and during exercise. Small heart size limits stroke volume to such a degree that even the increased heart rate of children cannot compensate. Functionally, the lower cardiac output does not affect a child's level of activity because even with less hemoglobin than an adult, the child efficiently extracts oxygen from the blood. In addition, the small body size of children and their ability to easily dissipate heat over their relatively large body surface area enables them to function with a smaller cardiac output. Cardiac output increases as the body grows. In older adults, cardiac output declines because the heart must pump harder to overcome increased stiffness of the vessels, stiffness of the ventricular wall increases, and diastolic filling becomes more difficult.[62] With aging, both maximal heart rate and maximal stroke volume are decreased. Because cardiac output during maximal exercise is the product of these two values, it also decreases with age.[5]

Oxygen transportation to working tissues is another important factor in determining an individual's maximal aerobic capacity. Efficient ventilation carries inspired air to a well-developed and expanded alveolar network. Efficient circulation provides sufficient oxygenated blood to the pulmonary capillary network and to the capillaries of working tissues. Factors such as airway resistance, compliance of the thorax, functioning of the respiratory muscles, and compliance/elasticity of the lung and airways affect efficiency. The functional volumes of air in the lungs, such as the tidal volume, vary with the demands placed on the pulmonary system. As more oxygen is required during light to moderate exercise, tidal volume increases.[19]

Cardiorespiratory fitness in older adults is impacted by changes in cardiac factors and diminished ability of the peripheral tissues to extract oxygen. Beginning at age 30–40 years, declines in peak VO_2 begin to be seen. The decline is 3%–6% per decade initially. Although the rate of decline increases after age 45, the decline accelerates even more after the age of 70 years with a decline of 20% per decade.[83,84] Cardiorespiratory fitness of older men and women decreases to approximately 65% of peak aerobic capacity in young adulthood.[84] Both the decrease in cardiac output and the diminished ability of the peripheral tissues (muscle) to extract oxygen contribute to the decrease in maximal oxygen uptake.[85,86] It appears that the rate of decline in cardiorespiratory fitness is greater in older men than women, but when adjusted for fat-free body mass, the changes in aerobic capacity are similar in men and women.[83] Individuals who have maintained high levels of physical activity through their lifetime and have higher levels of peak oxygen uptake as they enter older adulthood maintain higher cardiorespiratory fitness than their more sedentary peers but still have accelerated decreases in cardiorespiratory fitness with increasing age.[83,84]

Many of the effects of aging on the heart and blood vessels can be reduced by regular exercise. Exercise helps people maintain cardiovascular fitness as well as muscular fitness as they age. Exercise is beneficial regardless of the age at which it is started. Moderate exercise is one of the best things older persons can do to keep their heart, lungs, and the rest of their body healthy. Lifestyle factors such as physical activity and exercise have a significant impact not only on preventing cardiovascular diseases later in life but also attenuating age-related cardiovascular function decline in the absence of disease.

Aging can increase the susceptibility to respiratory infections. Older adults have reduced clearance of particles due to decreased cilia and ciliary action. A reduced cough reflex increases the risk for mucous to collect in airways, and along with reduced elastic recoil can lead to problems. Additionally, older adults have a higher risk for aspiration of food or oropharyngeal secretions.[60]

Changes in the functional lung volumes and decreased efficiency of the respiratory muscles reduce an older individual's ability to increase tidal volume and MV in response to exercise. The pulmonary system is less able to adapt to stress because of (1) the loss of elastic recoil and chest wall compliance, (2) changes in central nervous system control, (3) innervation of respiratory muscles, and (4) impaired perception of carbon dioxide levels. Breathing frequency is increased in an attempt to provide necessary oxygen transport. The inability of the pulmonary system to meet needs is also thought to limit exercise in the older individual.[64,82] These changes are minimized in the healthy, active, nonsmoking older adult, and endurance training is thought to improve inspiratory muscle strength and lung function.[5]

SUMMARY

The cardiovascular and pulmonary systems work closely together to provide the food and fuel necessary for physical function. Changes in these systems over the life span can alter the functional ability of the systems and those of the individual. Some of these changes appear to be the result of normal development, whereas others may be determined by lifestyle choices. Research shows that regular physical activity can have a positive impact on function and health and that exercise at any age is important to maintain these two important systems at maximal efficiency.

Cardiovascular and pulmonary efficiency contributes to an individual's level of physical fitness. Fitness is a measure of a person's functional ability and health. Clinically, cardiovascular disease is a significant problem for adults. Risk factors for cardiovascular disease can sometimes be identified in young children. It is important to consider cardiovascular and pulmonary development and function across the life span as clinicians work with their clients to prevent cardiovascular disease and to minimize the effects of aging on these systems. A more extensive discussion of fitness issues across the life span, including the effects of exercise and training on the body systems, can be found in Chapter 13.

REFERENCES

1. Moore KL, Persaud TVN Torchia MG. Ch 13: Cardiovascular system. In: Moore KL, Persaud TVN, Torchia MG, eds. *The Developing Human.* 11th ed. Philadelphia: Elsevier; 2020:263–313.
2. Gartner LP. *Textbook of Histology.* 5th ed. Philadelphia: Elsevier; 2021:249–270.e2 [chapter 11].
3. Ross MH, Kaye GL, Pawlina W. *Histology: A Text and Atlas.* 4th ed. Baltimore: Lippincott, Williams & Wilkins; 2003.
4. Terry PB, Traystman RJ. The clinical significance of collateral ventilation. *Ann Am Thorac Soc.* 2016;13(12):2251–2257.
5. McArdle WD, Katch FL, Katch VL. *Exercise Physiology: Energy, Nutrition and Human Performance.* 7th ed. Philadelphia: Lippincott, Williams & Wilkins; 2010.
6. Aliverti A. The respiratory muscles during exercise. *Breathe (Sheff).* 2016;12(2):165–168.
7. Carlson BM. Ch 17: Cardiovascular System. In: Carlson BM, ed. *Human Embryology and Developmental Biology.* 6th ed. Philadelphia: Elsevier; 2019:391–434.e2.
8. Lara-Canton I, Badurdeen S, Dekker J, et al. Oxygen saturation and heart rate in healthy term and late preterm infants with delayed cord clamping. *Pediatr res.* 2022. https://doi.org/10.1038/s41390-021-01805-y.
9. Carlson BM. Ch 15: Digestive and Respiratory Systems and Body Cavities. In: Carlson BM, ed. *Human Embryology and Developmental Biology.* 6th ed. Philadelphia: Elsevier; 2019:318–352.e2.
10. Schnittny JC. Development of the lung. *Cell Tissue Res.* 2017;367:427–444. https://doi.org/10.1007/s00441-016-2405-0.
11. Moore KL, Persaud TVN, Torchia MG. Ch 10 Respiratory System. In: Moore KL, Persaud TVN, Torchia MG, eds. *The Developing Human.* 11th edition. Philadelphia: Elsevier; 2020:181–192.e1.
12. Luo G, Norwitz ER. Revisiting amniocenteses for fetal lung maturity after 36 weeks' gestation. *Rev Obstet Gynecol.* 2008;1(2):61–68.
13. Hooper SB, Polglase GM, Roehr CC. Cardiopulmonary changes with aeration of the newborn lung. *PaediatrRespirRev.* 2015;16(3):147–150. https://doi.org/10.1016/jprrv.2015.03.003.
14. Saikia D, Mahanta B. Cardiovascular and respiratory physiology in children. *Indian Journal of Anaesthesia.* 2019;63(9):690–697. https://doi.org/10.4103/IJA_490_19.
15. Malina RM, Bouchard C, Bar-Or O. *Growth, Maturation and Physical Activity.* 2nd ed. Human Kinetics: Champaign, Ill; 2004.
16. Guo and Pu. Cardiomyocyte maturation: new phase in development. *Circulation Research.* 2020;126(8):1086–1106. https://doi.org/10.1161/CIRCRESAHA.119.315862.
17. Anderson PAW. The heart and development. *Semin Perinatol.* 1996;20:482–509.
18. Sinclair D, Dangerfield P. *Human Growth After Birth.* 6th ed. New York: Oxford University Press; 1998.
19. Murray JF. *The Normal Lung.* 2nd ed. Philadelphia: WB Saunders; 1986.
20. Flynn JT. Pediatric hypertension update. *Curr Opin Nephrol Hypertens.* 2010;19:292–297.
21. Feber J, Ahmed M. Hypertension in children: new trends and challenges. *Clin Sci.* 2010;119:151–161.
22. Liang YJ, Xi B, Hu YH, et al. Trends in blood pressure and hypertension among Chinese children and adolescents: China Health and Nutrition Surveys 1991–2004. *Blood Press.* 2010;20(1):45–53.
23. Ashraf M, Irshad M, Parry NA. Pediatric hypertension: an updated review. *Clinical Hypertension.* 2020;26:22. https://doi.org/10.1186/x40885-020-00156-W.
24. Zhou B, Perel P, Menaxah GA, Ezzati M. Global epidemiology, health burden and effective interventions for elevated blood pressure and hypertension. *Nature Reviews Cardiology.* 2021;18:785–802.
25. Robinson CH, Chanchlani R. High blood pressure in children and adolescents: Current perspectives and strategies to improve future kidney and cardiovascular health. *Kidney Int Rep.* 2022;7:954–970.
26. Tu K, Chen Z, Lipscombe LL. Prevalence and incidence of hypertension from 1995 to 2005: a population-based study. *CMAJ.* 2008;178(11):1429–1435.
27. Yang L, Magnussen CG, Yang L, Bovet P, Xi B. Elevated blood pressure in childhood or adolescence and cardiovascular outcomes in adulthood: a systematic review. *Hypertension.* 2020;75 https://doi.org/10.1161/HYPERTENSIONAHA.119.14168.2020:948-955. 7.
28. National Institutes of Health (NIH), 2004 The 7th report of the Joint National Committee on Prevention, Detec-

tion, Evaluation and Treatment of High Blood Pressure. NIH Publication No. 04-5230, August US Department of Health and Human Services:

29. Whelton P, Carey R, Aronow W, et al. 2017 ACC/AHA/AAPA/ABC/ACPM/AGS/APhA/ASH/ASPC/NMA/PCNA Guideline for the Prevention, Detection, Evaluation, and Management of High Blood Pressure in Adults. *J Am Coll Cardiol*. 2018;71(19):e127–e248. https://doi.org/10.1016/j.jacc.2017.11.006.

30. Studinger P, Goldstein R, Taylor JA. Age- and fitness-related alterations in vascular sympathetic control. *J Physiol*. 2009;587:2049–2057.

31. Acelajado MC, Oparil S. Hypertension in the elderly. *Clin Geriatr Med*. 2009;25:391–412.

32. Flack JM, Adekola B. Blood pressure and the new ACC/AHA hypertension guidelines. *Trends Cardiovasc Med*. 2020;30:160–164.

33. Song P, Zhang Y, Yu J, et al. Global prevalence of hypertension in children: a systematic review and meta-analysis. *JAMA Pediatr*. 2019;173(12):1154–1163.

34. Crouch SH, Soepnel LM, Kolkenbeck-Ruh A, et al. Paediatric hypertension in Africa: a systematic review and meta-analysis. *EClinicalMedicine*. 2021;43:101229.

35. de Simone G, Mancusi C, Hanssen H, et al. Hypertension in children and adolescents. *Eur Heart J*. 2022;43(35):3290–3301.

36. Lurbe E, Agabiti-Rosei E, Cruickshank JK, et al. 2016 European Society of Hypertension guidelines for the management of high blood pressure in children and adolescents. *J Hypertens*. 2016;34:1887–1920.

37. Rabi DM, McBrien KA, Sapir-Pichhadze R, et al. Hypertension Canada's 2020 comprehensive guidelines for the prevention, diagnosis, risk assessment, and treatment of hypertension in adults and children. *Can J Cardiol*. 2020;36:596–624.

38. Flynn JT, Kaelber DC, Baker-Smith CM, et al. Clinical practice guideline for screening and management of high blood pressure in children and adolescents. *Pediatrics*. 2017;140:e20171904. https://doi.org/10.1542/peds.2017-1904.

39. Reilly KJ, Moore CA. Respiratory movement patterns during vocalizations at 7 and 11 months of age. *J Speech Lang Hear Res*. 2009;52:223–239.

40. Massery M. Multisystem clinical implications of impaired breathing mechanics and postural control. In: Frownfelter D, Dean E, eds. *Cardiovascular and Pulmonary Physical Therapy Evidence and Practice*. 5th ed. St Louis: MO/ Mosby/Elsevier Health Science; 2012:633–653.

41. Zeeman KL, Bennett WD. Airways and alveoli from childhood to the adult lung measured by aerosol-derived airway morphometry. *Journal of Applied Physiology*.

2006;100:965–971. https://doi.org/10.1152/japplphysiol.00409.2005.

42. Herring MJ, Putney LF, Wyatt G, Finkbeiner WE, Hyde DM. Growth of alveoli during postnatal development in humans based on steriological estimation. *Am J of Physiol Lung Cell Mol Physiol*. 2014;307(4): https://doi.org/10.1152/ajplung.00094.2014.LK338-L344.

43. Mullassery D, Smith NP. Lung development. *Seminars in Pediatric Surgery*. 2015;24:152–155. https://doi.org/10.1053/j.sempedsurg.2015.01.011.

44. Omran HI Al. Unilateral double round pneumonia in a child: a case report and literature review. *Radiology Case Reports*. 2021;16(11):3266–3269. https://doi.org/10.1016/jradcr.2021.07.

45. Cunningham DA, Paterson DH, Blimke CJR. The development of the cardiorespiratory system with growth and physical activity. In: Boileau RA, ed. *Advances in Pediatric Sport Science, Vol 1*: Biological Issues. Champaign, IL: Human Kinetics; 1984:85–116.

46. Neve V, Girard F, Flahault A, Boule M. Lung and thorax development during adolescence: relationship with pubertal status. Europ. *Respiratory Journal*. 2002;20:1292–1298. https://doi.org/10.1183/09031936.02.00208102.

47. Zhou F, Yin X, Phillipe K, Houssein A, Gastinger S, Prioux J. Ventilatory responses at submaximal exercise intensities in healthy children and adolescents during the growth spurt period: a semi-longitudinal study. *Eur J Appl Physiol*. 2021;121:3211–3223. https://doi.org/10.1007/s00421-021-04776-4.

48. Armstrong N, Welsman J. Influence of sex-specific concurrent changes in age, maturity status, and morphological covariates on the development of peak ventilatory variables in 10-17-year-olds. *Eur J Appl Physiol*. 2021;121:783–792. https://doi.org/10.1007/s00421-020-04569-1.

49. Davis JA, Dobbings J. *Scientific Foundations of Pediatrics*. Baltimore: University Park Press; 1981.

50. Chester JG, Rudolph JL. Vital signs in older patients: age-related changes. *J Am Med Directors Assoc*. 2011;12(5):337–343.

51. Kitzman DW, Edwards WD. Minireview: age-related changes in the anatomy of the normal human heart. *J Geriatr Med Sci*. 1990;45:33–39.

52. Lee HY, Oh BH. Aging and arterial stiffness. *Circ J*. 2010;71:2257–2262.

53. Cunningham DA, Paterson DH. Discussion: exercise, fitness and aging. In: Bouchard C, Shephard RJ, Stephens T, eds. *Exercise, Fitness and Health: A Consensus of Current Knowledge*. Champaign, IL: Human Kinetics; 1990: 699–704.

54. Strait JB, Lakatta EG. Aging-associated cardiovascular changes and their relationship to heart failure. *Heart Failure Clinics*. 2012;8(1):143–164.

55. Baron-Castaneda A. Geriatric Cardiology: a challenge for the twenty first century. *Rev Colomb Cardiol*. 2019;26(6):308–309.

56. Agrawal T, Nagueh SF. Changes in cardiac structure and function with aging. *J CardiovascAging*. 2022;2:13. https://doi.org/10.20517/jca.2021.40.

57. Terman A, Gustafsson B, Brunk UT. Autophage, organelles and ageing. *J Pathol*. 2007;211(2):124–143.

58. Terman A, Kurz T, Gustafsson B, et al. The involvement of lysosomes in myocardial aging and disease. *Curr Cardiol Rev*. 2008;4(2):107–115.

59. North BJ, Sinclair DA. The intersection between aging and cardiovascular disease. *Circulation Res*. 2012;110:1097–1108.

60. Knight J, Nigam Y. Anatomy and physiology in ageing 1: the cardiovascular system. *Nursing Times* [online]. 2017;113(2):22–24.

61. Lieb W, Xanthakis V, Sullivan LM, et al. Longitudinal tracking of left ventricular mass over the adult life course: clinical correlates of short- and long-term change in the Framingham offspring study. *Circulation*. 2009;119(240):3085–3092.

62. Sattelmair JR, Pertman JH, Forman DE. Effects of physical activity on cardiovascular and noncardiovascular outcomes in older adults. *Clin Geriatr Med*. 2009;25: 677–702.

63. Bertaso AG, Bertol D, Duncan BB, Foppa M. Epicardial fat: definition, measurements and systematic review of main outcomes. *Arq Bras Cardiol*. 2013 Jul;101(1):e18–e28. https://doi.org/10.5935/abc.20130138.PMID: 23917514; PMCID: PMC3998169.

64. Tecklin JS. Cardiopulmonary changes with aging. In: Irwin S, Tecklin, eds. Cardiopulmonary Physical Therapy: A Guide to Practice. St. Louis: Mosby; 2004:102–120. 4th ed.

65. Tanaka H, Dinenno FA, Monahan KD, et al. Aging, habitual exercise and dynamic arterial compliance. *Circulation*. 2000;102:1270–1275.

66. Grässler B, Thielmann B, Böckelmann I, Hökelmann A. Effects of different exercise interventions on heart rate variability and cardiovascular health factors in older adults: a systemic review. *Eur Rev Aging Phys Act*. 2021;18(1):24.

67. Hart EC, Joyner MJ, Wallin BG, et al. Age-related differences in the sympathetic-hemodynamic balance in men. *Hypertension*. 2009;54(1):127–133.

68. Shi X, Schaller FA, Tierney N, et al. Physically active lifestyle enhances vagal-cardiac function but not central autonomic neural interaction in elderly humans. *Exp Biol Med*. 2008;233:209–218.

69. Santos MA, Sousa AC, Reis FP, Santos TR, Lima SO, Barreto-Filho JA. Does the aging process significantly modify the Mean Heart Rate? *Arq Bras Cardiol*. 2013 Nov;101(5):388–398. https://doi.org/10.5935/abc.20130188. Epub 2013 Sep 13. PMID: 24029962; PMCID: PMC4081162.

70. Shephard RJ. The cardiovascular benefits of exercise in the elderly. *Top Geriatr Rehabil*. 1985;1:1–10.

71. Gerber LM, Stern PM. Relationship of body size to blood pressure: sex-specific and developmental influences. *Hum Biol*. 1999;71(4):505–528.

72. Motoyama M, Sunami Y, Kinoshita F, et al. Blood pressure lowering effect of low-intensity aerobic training in elderly hypertensive patients. *Med Sci Sports Exerc*. 1998;30:818–823.

73. Fiogbé E, de Vassimon-Barroso V, de Medeiros Takahashi AC. Exercise training in older adults, what effects on muscle oxygenation? A systematic review. *Arch Gerontol Geriatr*. 2017 July;71:89–98. https://doi.org/10.1016/j.archger.2017.03.001. Epub 2017 Mar 20. PMID: 2841050.

74. Sagiv M, Goldhammer E, Ben-Sira D, et al. Factors defining oxygen uptake at peak exercise in aged people. *Eur Rev Aging Phys Act*. 2010;7:1–2. https://doi.org/10.1007/s11556-010-0061-x.

75. Montero D, Díaz-Cañestro C. Endurance training and maximal oxygen consumption with ageing: role of maximal cardiac output and oxygen extraction. *European Journal of Prevent Cardiol*. May 2016;23(7):33–743. https://doi.org/10.1177/2047487315617118.

76. Miller AJ, Arnold AC. The renin-angiotensin system and cardiovascular autonomic control in aging. *Peptides*. 2022 Apr;150:170733. https://doi.org/10.1016/j.peptides.2021.170733.

77. Miller AJ, Arnold AC. The renin-angiotensin system in cardiovascular autonomic control: recent developments and clinical implications. *Clin Auton Res*. 2019 Apr;29(2):231–243. https://doi.org/10.1007/s10286-018-0572-5.

78. Rossi A, Ganassini A, Tantacci C, et al. Aging and the respiratory system. *Aging Clin Exp Res*. 1996;8:143–161.

79. Lee SH, Yim SJ, Kim HC. Aging of the respiratory system. *Kosin Med J*. 2016;31(1):11–18. https://doi.org/10.7180/kmj.2016.31.1.11.

80. Sharm G, Goodwin J. Effects of aging on respiratory system physiology and immunology. *Clin Interv Aging*. 2006;1(3):253–260.

81. Freitas FS, Ibianpina CC, Alvim CG, et al. Relationship between cough strength and functional level in elderly. *Braz J Phys Ther*. 2010;14(6):470–476.

82. Roman MA, Rossiter HB, Casaburi R. Exercise, ageing and the lung. *Eur Respir J*. 2016;48:1471–1486.

83. Fleg JL, Morrell CH, Bos AG, et al. Accelerated longitudinal decline of aerobic capacity in healthy older adults. *Circulation*. 2005;112:674–682.

84. Jackson AS, Sui X, Hebert JR, et al. Role of lifestyle and aging on longitudinal change in cardiorespiratory fitness. *Arch Intern Med.* 2009;169(19):1781–1787.

85. McGuire DK, Levine BD, Williamson JW, et al. A 30-year follow-up of the Dallas bed rest and training study: I. Effect of age on the cardiovascular response to exercise. *Circulation.* 2001;104:1350–1357.

86. McGavock JM, Hastings JL, Snell PG, et al. A forty-year follow-up of the Dallas bed rest and training study: the effect of age on the cardiovascular response to exercise in men. *J Gerontol A Biol Sci Med Sci.* 2009;64A(2): 293–299.

8

Nervous System Changes

OBJECTIVES

After studying this chapter, the reader will be able to:

1. Describe the role and functions of the nervous system.
2. Discuss unique structural and functional changes of the nervous system in the developing fetus, infant, child, adolescent, adult, and older adult.
3. Relate nervous system changes over time to functional differences in movement, memory, and cognition.
4. Incorporate issues of life span development of the nervous system into patient examination and intervention.
5. Discuss clinical implications of alcohol use across the life span.

The nervous system is frequently referred to as the *command center for human function*. It not only receives information but also integrates all incoming messages to orchestrate fluid, appropriate responses. The nervous system truly oversees all other body systems as they cooperate to perform day-to-day activities and control the major functions of moving, thinking, and feeling.

Movement is controlled when the nervous system functions as an initiator, a modulator, and a comparator, activating the muscular and skeletal systems. Movement is not the product of any one system, nor does one system act in isolation from the others to produce movement. Attention is necessary for motor function. Abnormal movement might result from a problem in the skeletal, muscular, cardiopulmonary, or nervous system. For example, in either muscle disease (e.g., muscular dystrophy) or peripheral nerve injury, the end result is movement dysfunction.

A unique role of the nervous system is thought processing, that is, cognition and intelligence. Psychological theorists such as Erikson[1] have little to say about how the brain "thinks." Physiologists believe that the ability of the brain to form memories is a mechanism for intelligence. Memory formation is contingent on an individual's level of alertness and ability to focus attention. Memory formation occurs in an area of the brain called the *hippocampus*.[2] The frontal area of the brain has been linked to abstract thought and personality. Its protracted development in adolescence is what finally allows a teenager to become a thinking adult. After head trauma, a patient's sensory, motor, and cognitive deficits can be attributed to damage to a specific area of the brain. In other areas of the brain, called *association areas*, sensory input is connected to meaning. For example, in the visual association areas, visual input is connected with the memory and names of shapes.

Another important aspect of nervous system control is its role in motivation and emotions. One of the oldest parts of the brain, called the *limbic system*, is responsible for attending to sensory and motor cues; monitoring basic drives for food, water, and sexual gratification; and attaching emotional meaning to actions. The limbic system aids in memory formation as it attaches emotional meaning to memory. The ability of the nervous system to react to these cues is not well understood. Emotions can provide powerful motivation for movement. The affective component of movement dysfunction is often the most difficult to deal with, as when trying to motivate a person to perform better physically.

The nervous system exhibits a great deal of plasticity throughout the life span. The brain is constantly changing and adapting to experience: those experiences that are expected and those that are unique to the individual. "Neuroplasticity refers to the inherently dynamic biological capacity of the central nervous system (CNS) to undergo maturation, change structurally and functionally in response to experience and to adapt following injury. This malleability is achieved by modulating subsets of genetic, molecular, and cellular mechanisms that influence the dynamics of synaptic connections and neural circuitry formation culminating in gain or loss of behavior or function."[3] There have been monumental conceptual advances in neuroplasticity over the last 60 years.[4] Neuroplasticity has become a theoretical base for rehabilitation interventions.

COMPONENTS OF THE NERVOUS SYSTEM

At the cellular level, the nervous system is made up of two different types of cells: neurons and glial cells. Both cell types are derived from embryonic ectoderm. *Neurons* and their processes allow the nervous system to communicate and direct movement activities. *Neuroglia* provide guidance, support, and protection for neurons. On a larger scale, structures such as the brain, spinal cord, cranial and peripheral nerves make up the functional infrastructure of the nervous system.

Neurons

Neurons are complex structures that form the major communication system of the body. A typical neuron is composed of a cell body, an axon that carries impulses to other neurons, and multiple dendrites that receive incoming stimuli from other neurons. Neurons communicate via electrical impulse conduction down axons and across synapses to other neurons, muscles, or glands. Neurons vary in size and shape according to their function. For example, pyramidal neurons found in the cerebral cortex and Purkinje cells in the cerebellum (Fig. 8.1) are the major output cells for their respective areas. Dendrites are branched to receive multiple inputs from other neurons. The pattern of branching indicates

the purpose of the neuron. The Purkinje cells in the cerebellum have elaborate branching allowing them to integrate many inputs and allow for motor learning.[5] Pyramidal cell axons make up projection, association, and commissural fibers. They travel to the spinal cord, to other areas of the brain, and from one hemisphere to the other. Purkinje cells send information from the cerebellum to the cerebellar nuclei and vestibular nuclei. The structure of the neuron often reflects its role in the communications network of the nervous system.

The neuron communicates by initiating a signal, called an *action potential*. The potential travels down the axon by *saltatory conduction*. The electrical signal leaps from one gap in the myelin to another. These gaps are called *Nodes of Ranvier*, or simply nodes. The axon or nerve fiber terminates in an end bulb that synapses with a target cell. Many axons can converge on a single target. Axons can also branch to transmit signals to more than one target cell or more than one location on a target cell. Information from one source, such as the visual system, can be conveyed to many different sites through divergence. These convergent or divergent impulses can be summated in time or space to either make it easier or more difficult to generate an action potential. An axon can generate up to 1000 action potentials per second.

Myelin is a lipid/protein substance that covers axons. In the CNS, myelin is produced by neuroglial cells called *oligodendrocytes*; in the peripheral nervous system (PNS), myelin is produced by Schwann cells. Schwann cells are also neuroglia and the only support cells for the PNS. Myelin makes action potential conduction more efficient by increasing the speed of nerve impulse conduction and decreasing the metabolic cost of the action potential. How fast impulses can be conducted depends on whether the nerve is myelinated or unmyelinated and on the diameter of the nerve fiber. The larger the diameter of the nerve, the faster the conduction of the action potential. The thicker the myelin surrounding the axon, the greater the conduction of the action potential. Because there are fewer ion channels in the myelin, less adenosine triphosphate (ATP) is needed to support the generation of an action potential.

Neuroglia

Neuroglia cells provide guidance, support, nutrition, and protection to neurons. As nonneuronal cells, they can be thought of as the connective tissue of the nervous system. Four types of neuroglial cells have been identified in the

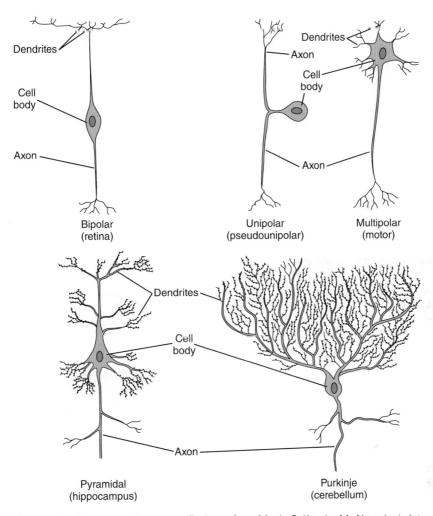

Fig. 8.1 Diagram of various types of neurons. (Redrawn from Martin S, Kessler M. *Neurologic Interventions for Physical Therapy.* 2nd ed. St. Louis: Saunders; 2007:9; Lundy-Ekman L. *Neuroscience Fundamentals for Rehabilitation.* 3rd ed. St. Louis: Saunders; 2007:437; Gartner LP, Hiatt JL. *Color Textbook of Histology.* 2nd ed. Philadelphia: WB Saunders; 2001:187.)

CNS: astrocytes, oligodendrocytes, microglia, and ependymal cells (Fig. 8.2). Astrocytes provide a vascular link via footlike projections between blood vessels and neurons in the brain and the spinal cord. Astrocytes regulate the concentration of sodium and potassium ions and neurotransmitters as well as create a glial scar in response to injury to the brain or spinal cord. In the brain, astrocytes are part of the blood-brain barrier (BBB), which regulate the influx of vital nutrients and keep out harmful substances. The "foot processes" surround the outside of capillary endothelial cells and may assist in the formation and maintenance of the BBB. In preterm infants, this barrier has not been

formed. Therefore, foreign matter such as meconium, the first stool, may be deposited in brain structures and cause movement dysfunction.[6] *Oligodendrocytes* produce the myelin that covers the neural processes of the CNS. The large number of this type of neuroglial cell is a hallmark of the increasing evolutionary complexity of the nervous system. *Microglia* are derived from mesenchyme and can be found scattered throughout the CNS. These small cells develop late in the fetal period after the CNS has been supplied by blood vessels. They are the phagocytes of the CNS. As major scavenger cells, they migrate to any area of injury to remove cellular debris, regardless of whether the damage

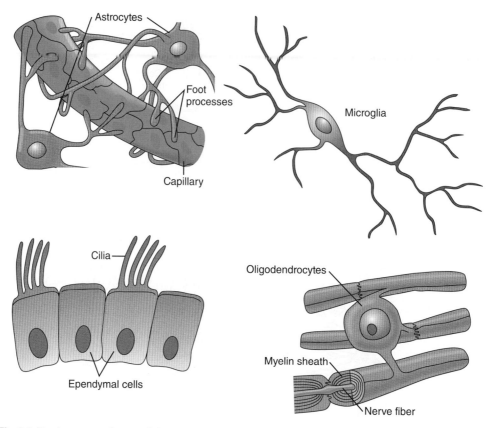

Fig. 8.2 The four types of neuroglial cells: astrocytes, microglia, oligodendrocytes, and ependymal cells. (From Copstead LEC, Banasik JL. *Pathophysiology: Biological and Behavioral Perspectives.* 2nd ed. Philadelphia: WB Saunders; 2000:987.)

is in the spinal cord or in the brain. *Ependymal cells* line the interior wall of the ventricals, the central canal of the spinal cord, and produce and circulate cerebrospinal fluid (CSF).[7] Use of ependymal stem cells is being explored as a treatment for spinal cord injury.[8]

Central Nervous System

The brain, brainstem, and spinal cord are collectively referred to as the CNS. The brain consists of two cerebral hemispheres, or cortices, the *brain stem* and the *cerebellum*. Each hemisphere of the cortex is divided into four lobes—frontal, parietal, temporal, and occipital, which are responsible for unique functions (Fig. 8.3, Table 8.1). The limbic system is described after the functions of each individual lobe. Its structures are deep within the brain and involve association areas located in more than one lobe of the brain. The areas that are directly related to processing sensory and motor information or coordinating movement are

known as primary and association sensory (or motor) areas (Fig. 8.4).

Cerebral Cortex

The surface of the cortex has an average thickness of 2.5 mm[9] and is composed of gray matter. The inner surface is made up of white matter fiber tracts. As seen in Fig. 8.3, the surface consists of ridges (*gyri*) and depressions (*sulci*). This folded architecture allows for an increase in surface area without increasing the size of the brain. There is increased space for cortical neurons. The thickness of the cortex and its surface area constitute what is measured as brain volume.

Lobes of the Cerebral Cortex
Frontal Lobe

The *frontal lobe* contains the primary motor cortex. The frontal lobe is responsible for the voluntary control of

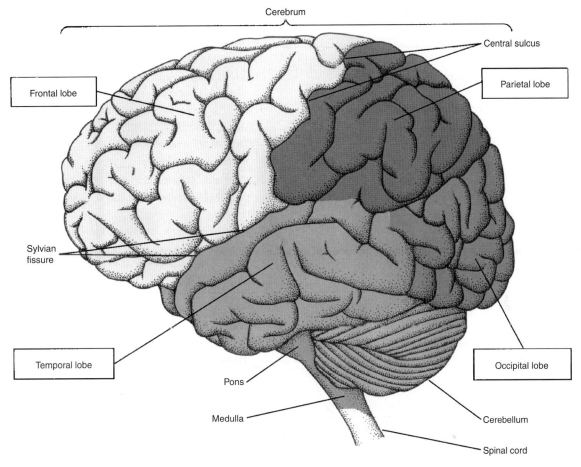

Fig. 8.3 Lobes of the brain. (From Guyton AC: Basic neuroscience: anatomy and physiology, ed 2, Philadelphia: WB Saunders; 1991.)

complex motor activities. It also exhibits a strong influence over cognitive functions including judgment, attention, awareness, and abstract thinking. Broca's area, the main motor area for speech, is located within the frontal lobe near the primary motor regions that control the lips, tongue, and larynx. Speech production is supported by a *dorsal* stream that extends from the parietal cortex to the frontal cortex of the left hemisphere and ends with "speech signals being 'mapped' onto cortical areas specific for articulation, resulting in fluent speech."[10] Damage to Broca's area results in expressive aphasia. The same area in the right hemisphere is involved in nonverbal communication. See Table 8.2 for functions of the additional motor areas in the frontal lobe.

Temporal Lobe

The *temporal lobe* contains the primary auditory cortex. It decodes the pitch and volume of sounds. Attaching meaning to sounds occurs via an associative auditory pathway. The *ventral stream* involves the lateral temporal lobes, inferior frontal lobe, and inferior parietal lobe to make sense of auditory information.[10] Wernicke's area in the temporal lobe is part of the pathway and ascribes meaning to words. When this area is damaged, it results in receptive aphasia. The amygdala and hippocampus also reside in the temporal lobe. These structures are crucial for acquiring factual memory, which is a function of declarative memory.

TABLE 8.1   **Functions of the Lobes of the Cortex of the Brain**

Lobe	Structure	Function
Frontal	Primary motor cortex	Voluntary controlled movements
	Premotor area	Control of trunk and girdle muscles; anticipatory postural adjustments
	Supplementary area	Initiation of movement; orientation of eyes and head; bilateral, sequential movement
	Broca area in left hemisphere	Motor programming of speech
	Same area in right hemisphere	Nonverbal communication
Temporal	Primary auditory cortex	Discriminates loudness and pitch of sounds
	Wernicke area	Hears and comprehends spoken language; intelligence
Parietal	Primary somatosensory cortex	Discriminates texture, shape, and size of objects
	Primary vestibular cortex	Distinguishes head movements and head positions
Occipital	Primary visual cortex	Differentiates intensity of light, shape, size, and location of objects

Data from Lundy-Ekman L. *Neuroscience: Fundamentals for Rehabilitation*. 5th ed. St. Louis: Elsevier; 2018.

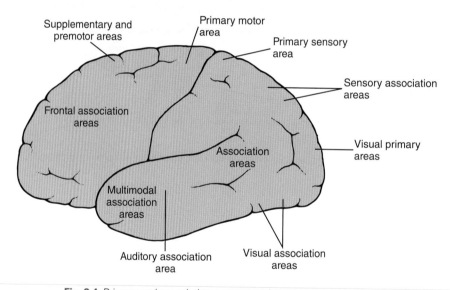

Fig. 8.4 Primary and association sensory and motor areas of the brain.

Parietal Lobe

The *parietal lobe* contains the primary somatosensory cortex. Incoming sensory information is processed and allows for discrimination of texture, shape, and size of objects. Perception is the process of attaching meaning to sensation and requires interaction between the mind, body, and environment.[11] Perceptual learning requires having a functioning parietal lobe.[5] The primary vestibular cortex is involved in distinguishing head movements and head positions. Right-handed individuals have a right vestibular dominance and left-handed individuals have a left vestibular dominance. This explains why a right-handed person who has a right-hemispheric stroke may present with hemispatial neglect of one side of the body, since it involves the vestibular system.[12]

TABLE 8.2 Functions of Motor Areas of the Cortex	
Motor Area	Function
Primary motor cortex	Voluntary controlled movements
Premotor area	Control of the trunk and girdle muscles, anticipatory postural adjustments
Supplemental motor area	Initiation of movement, orientation planning, bimanual and sequential movements

Data from Lundy-Ekman L. *Neuroscience: Fundamentals for Rehabilitation*. 5th ed. St. Louis: Elsevier; 2018.

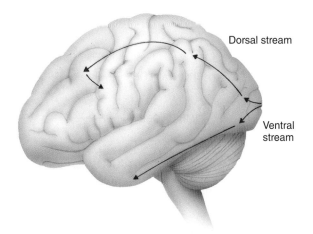

Fig. 8.5 Use of visual information by the cerebral cortex: the dorsal action stream and the ventral perceptual stream. They are also known as the "where" and "what" streams, respectively. (Source: Lundy-Ekman L. *Neuroscience: Fundamentals for Rehabilitation*. 5th ed. St. Louis: Elsevier; 2018: 429. Figure 21.4.)

Occipital Lobe

The *occipital lobe* contains the primary visual cortex. The eye takes in information from the visual field and transmits it from the retina to the primary visual cortex via the thalamus. Neurons in the primary visual cortex discriminate texture, shape, and size of objects while the secondary visual cortex detects color and motion.[11] "The visual association cortex is extensive and is located throughout the cerebral hemispheres along two main streams"[5] that project forward from the primary visual cortex (see Fig. 8.5). "The dorsal stream includes regions in the parietal lobes and determines object location. The ventral stream includes regions in the temporal lobes and determines object identity."[5]

Limbic System

The *limbic system* is very complex. It consists of a group of interconnected deep brain structures (Fig. 8.6), including the amygdala, hippocampus, cingulate gyrus, and thalamic and hypothalamic nuclei (not depicted). It is not an anatomical lobe of the brain as such but a functional classification.[10] The cingulate cortex and its connections play important roles in emotion, action, and memory.[13] Memories are stronger when attached to emotions. The limbic system regulates visceral and hormonal functions, such as eating, drinking, and reproduction. It appears to control memory, affection, fear, pain, pleasure, sorrow, rage, and sexual interest. The role of the limbic system in memory is discussed at the end of this chapter.

Association Cortices

Association cortices are those areas of the cortex not directly involved with sensation or movement. The medial prefrontal cortex (PFC) has verbal and auditory connections in order to identify the emotional content of spoken or heard language and respond appropriately. Awareness of one's own and others' emotions is located in this area. The dorsolateral PFC (DLPFC) is active in all learning and goal-directed behavior (also called executive function [EF]); self-awareness; and elaboration of thought. The DLPFC and the temporoparietal association cortex provide the neural substrate for working memory (WM). The last of the frontal association areas, the orbitofrontal cortex, is also involved in emotion and reward-related processing. The parietoinsular vestibular cortex receives tactile and visual information in addition to vestibular information. This vestibular association cortex constructs our sense of balance based on input from all three sensory systems. Auditory and visual association areas as previously described provide meaning to what we hear and see.

Hemispheric Specialization

The concept that each side of the brain is specialized to perform certain functions has been widely accepted. This sidedness is called hemispheric specialization or lateralization. Although the two cerebral hemispheres appear to be mirror images of each other, gross anatomical differences have been demonstrated. Research has established that the processing and production of

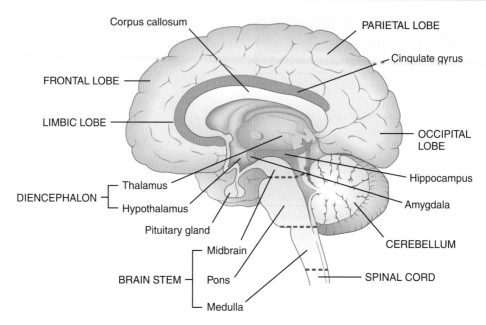

Fig. 8.6 Schematic midsagittal view of the brain shows the relationship between the cerebral cortex, cerebellum, spinal cord, and brainstem and the subcortical structures involved in the limbic system.

language are localized in the left hemisphere and spatial abilities are localized in the right. The hemisphere that is responsible for language is considered the dominant hemisphere. The differences are likely to be related to handedness because 96% of the population, including all right-handed people, are left hemisphere, dominant. Even in people who are strongly left-hand dominant, only 27% have a right hemisphere language dominance. A small percentage (15%) of ambidextrous individuals also have a right hemisphere language dominance.[10] The asymmetry of the two hemispheres is present even in infants. Table 8.3 outlines the respective functions of the dominant and nondominant cerebral hemispheres.

The nervous system is somatotopically organized to relay signals throughout the body. Somatotopic arrangement of neurons in pathways allows for the localization of somatosensory stimulation. These topographic maps allow specialized axons from one part of the body to be in proximity to axons carrying related signals from adjacent parts of the body. This is true in both the motor and sensory cortices, where the parts of the body are represented. The size of the part is directly related to the functional importance of the part. For example, the sensory homunculus seen in Fig. 8.7 depicts a caricature of a human being with oversized lips and thumb. The

same type of organizational relationship is present in the visual cortex as a visuotopic map and in the auditory cortex as a tonotopic map. This type of mapping occurs at every level of the nervous system.

Subcortical Structures

Thalamic complex. The thalamus and the hypothalamus (Fig. 8.6) lie deep within the cortex and make up a thalamic complex. It is composed of the thalamus, epithalamus, subthalamus, and hypothalamus. All sensory systems, except for the olfactory, relay information through the thalamus to the cortex. The thalamus sends sensory information to the appropriate primary and association areas of the cortex for interpretation. Association nuclei integrate touch and visual information, in addition to processing emotional and memory information. Motor output from the basal ganglia and the cerebellum is also processed in the thalamus and sent on to the cortex to influence motor behavior. Nonspecific nuclei in the thalamus are important for regulating consciousness, arousal, and attention.[11]

The hypothalamus is situated underneath the thalamus, at the base of the brain. It is responsible for maintaining balance of the internal environment, or homeostasis. This structure is involved in the regulation

TABLE 8.3 Behaviors Attributed to the Dominant and Nondominant Brain Hemispheres

Behavior	Dominant Hemisphere	Nondominant Hemisphere
Cognitive style/intellect	Processing information in a sequential, linear manner	Processing information in a simultaneous, holistic, or gestalt manner
	Observing and analyzing details	Grasping overall organization or pattern
Perception/cognition	Processing and producing language, processing verbal cues and instructions	Processing nonverbal stimuli (environmental sounds, speech intonations, complex shapes, designs)
		Visual-spatial perception
		Drawing inferences, synthesizing information
Academic skills	Reading: sound-symbol relationships, word recognition, reading comprehension	Mathematical reasoning and judgment Alignment of numerals in calculations
	Performing mathematical calculations	
Motor and task performance	Planning and sequencing movements	Sustaining a movement or posture, consistency in movement performance
	Performing movements and gestures to command	
Behavior and emotions	Organization, expressing positive emotions	Ability to self-correct, judgment, awareness of disability, and safety concerns
		Expressing negative emotions and perceiving emotion

Modified from O'Sullivan SB, Schmitz TJ. *Physical Rehabilitation: Assessment and Treatment*. 4th ed. Philadelphia: FA Davis; 2001:536 and O'Sullivan SB. Stroke. In: O'Sullivan SB, Schmitz TJ, Fulk GD, eds. *Physical Rehabilitation: Assessment and Treatment*. 6th ed. Philadelphia: FA Davis; 2014.

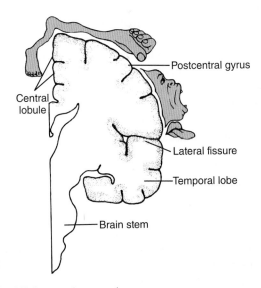

Fig. 8.7 Sensory homunculus.

of automatic functions such as thirst, hunger, digestion, blood pressure, body temperature, sexual activity, and sleep-wake cycles. The hypothalamus integrates the functions of the endocrine and autonomic nervous system by regulating the pituitary gland and its release of hormones. Hormones are chemicals produced by endocrine glands which travel via the blood stream to target receptors and produce biochemical reactions (see Chapter 10).[14]

Basal ganglia. The *basal ganglia* are another group of nuclei found at the base of the cerebrum. This subcortical structure is, in reality, a group of structures composed of the caudate, putamen, globus pallidus, nucleus accumbens, substantia nigra, and subthalamic nuclei. The basal ganglia regulate posture, muscle tone, and force production and are involved in cognitive functions related to movement. These related functions include motivation, memory for location of objects, changing behavior based on task demands, and awareness of body position in space. Four circuits have been identified that involve the basal ganglia: "(1) A motor loop, concerned with voluntary and learned movements. (2) A cognitive loop, concerned with motor planning and movement intentions. (3) A limbic loop, concerned with the emotional aspects of movements. (4) An oculomotor loop, concerned with voluntary saccadic eye movements."[10] The basal ganglia do not normally initiate movement but are involved in all movements. The basal ganglia use the brain's reward system to facilitate learning action sequences by trial-and-error learning.[15] The basal ganglia and more specifically the striatal circuitry (caudate nucleus, putamen, and nucleus accumbens) are involved not only in motor learning but also in cognitive skill learning and emotion-related action patterns.[15] When basal ganglia function is compromised because of a loss of the neurotransmitter dopamine, as happens in Parkinson disease, planning and programming of movement is impaired.

Cerebellum. The *cerebellum* is also made up of two hemispheres connected by a vermis. The hemispheres control the limbs and allow us to produce smooth, complex, multi-joint movements. The vermis controls the trunk and central area of the body thereby assisting in posture and balance of the core. The cerebellum is involved in the initiation and timing of movements and in monitoring postural tone. By receiving sensory input from the vestibular, auditory, and visual systems, as well as from the spinal cord, the cerebellum compares actual movement with anticipated motor performance, thereby functioning as a comparator. The cerebellum receives input from the cerebral cortex via nuclei in the pons, part of the brainstem. The cerebellum influences nuclei in the thalamus and brainstem to control movement, and its circuits are modified during motor learning. The cerebellum is all about timing, the timing of motor actions, and the perceptual processing, which requires exact representation of temporal information. Smooth movement requires regulation of initiation, timing, sequencing, and force generation of agonist and antagonist muscle contractions.[5] The cerebellum is responsible for sensorimotor learning based on the detection of errors in task performance.[16]

Brainstem. The brainstem represents a transition between the brain and the spinal cord (see Fig. 8.6). Its structures include the midbrain, pons, and medulla; each section is responsible for specific functions. The *midbrain* connects the diencephalon to the *pons* and is a relay station for tracts passing between the pons and the cerebellum or

spinal cord. Reflex centers for visual, auditory, and tactile responses are also found in the midbrain. The red nucleus, located in the midbrain, receives information from the cerebellum and the cerebral cortex and connects to the spinal cord via the rubrospinal tract. Activity in this tract contributes to upper limb flexion. The *pons* consists of bundles of axons that travel between the cerebellum and the rest of the CNS and assist the medulla to regulate the rate of breathing. Reflex centers in the pons assist with orientation of the head in response to auditory and vestibular stimulation. Postural muscle activity is controlled partially by tracts arising from vestibular nuclei located at the junction of the pons and medulla and connecting to the spinal cord. Cranial nerves (CN) V through VIII are located in the pons, which carry sensory and motor information to and from the face. The *medulla* houses nuclei that control and coordinate cardiovascular responses, breathing, and swallowing. The medulla contributes to the control of eye and head movements, which may be observed when head turning in an infant produces extension of the face arm (the arm toward which the face is turned) and flexion of the skull arm. This asymmetrical tonic neck reflex (ATNR) requires circuits in the medulla.[11] The eyes also turn toward the extended arm, allowing the infant to regard the hand.

Loosely arranged groups of neurons within the core of the brainstem are responsible for keeping us alert to novel stimuli or for picking up information pertinent to movement safety. This group of neurons is called the *reticular formation* (RF). This system regulates the level of consciousness and the daily cycle of arousal, which includes periods of sleep and waking. Consciousness is governed by the ascending reticular activating system (ARAS). It is a complicated network that connects part of the RF to the cortex, nonspecific thalamic nuclei, the basal forebrain (anterior to the hypothalamus), and the hypothalamus. These latter structures constitute the cerebral part of the consciousness system.[11] Research has focused on using the functional connectivity of the ARAS to predict recovery of consciousness in people with traumatic brain injury.[17] The brainstem produces generalized arousal and integrates all sensory information and cortical input. A part of the reticular formation contains autonomic nuclei, which interact with the parasympathetic and sympathetic portions of the autonomic nervous system to assist the regulation of functions critical for life. Another part of the RF regulates the flow of information regarding pain, level of awareness, and somatic motor activity. The brainstem acts to filter sensory input, such as pain, to the cortex.

Spinal Cord. The spinal cord is a continuation of the brainstem and consists of groups of axons, called *tracts* that ascend or descend within its structure to relay input to and from CNS structures. Ascending tracts carry sensory information, and descending tracts direct movement. The two primary ascending tracts are the *dorsal column* and the *anterolateral/spinothalamic* tract. The dorsal columns carry information about position sense (proprioception), two-point discrimination, deep touch, and vibration. The anterolateral/spinothalamic tract carries pain and temperature sensations to the thalamus for awareness. Light touch and pressure are carried in the ventral spinothalamic tract.

The major descending tract located within the spinal cord originates in the frontal lobe from the primary motor cortex, the supplementary and premotor areas (see Fig. 8.4). This efferent or motor tract is the corticospinal tract. The descending corticospinal tract carries impulses from the cortex, cerebellum, and basal ganglia down the spinal tract that synapse on cell bodies of motor neurons to control distal muscle movement in the arms, fingers, legs, and feet. The corticospinal tract is essential for planning, initiating, and coordinating voluntary movement.

Two additional descending motor tracts are the *reticulospinal* and *vestibulospinal tracts*, which travel from the reticular formation and the vestibular nucleus, respectively, to the spinal cord. The reticular formation is involved in providing feedforward control of posture as it anticipates a change in body posture and acts to ready posture for movement such as in gait. The vestibular nucleus provides information about movements generated in response to sensory signals of a postural disturbance and is part of a feedback mechanism for postural control. Gross motor movements can be controlled by these two brainstem pathways, but the motor cortex connections to the alpha motor neuron via the corticospinal tract are necessary for fine, fractionated extremity movements.

Peripheral Nervous System

The PNS consists of cranial and spinal nerves and their accompanying nerve nuclei and ganglia. Groups of cell bodies within the CNS are called *nuclei*, while groups of neuron cell bodies in the PNS are *ganglia*. Cranial and spinal nerves extend from the CNS to muscles and glands. Cranial nerves are located in the brainstem and can be either sensory nerves or motor nerves, or mixed.

Spinal nerves exit the spinal cord and combine into peripheral nerves. All 31 pairs of spinal nerves are part of the PNS and have sensory and motor components. The PNS is divided into a sensory or afferent division (discussed in Chapter 9) and an efferent or motor division. The motor division is further divided into the somatic nervous system and the autonomic nervous system. The *somatic nervous system* conducts impulses to skeletal muscle; the *autonomic nervous system* (ANS) conducts impulses to smooth muscle, cardiac muscle, and glands. Both the somatic and the autonomic systems produce muscular contractions and change the rate of those contractions, but only the ANS causes the secretion of hormones. The ANS is primarily responsible for maintaining an internal balance of visceral functions related to the heart, smooth muscle, and glands. It consists of three divisions: sympathetic, parasympathetic, and enteric. The sympathetic and parasympathetic divisions of the ANS use acetylcholine as a neurotransmitter at the preganglionic synapse, as diagrammed in Fig. 8.8. The parasympathetic division also uses acetylcholine at postganglionic synapses, whereas the sympathetic division uses norepinephrine to transmit nerve impulses to effector organs. Some effects of ANS activity are outlined in Table 8.4. The third division of the ANS, the enteric nervous system (ENS), consists of two major plexuses: the myenteric and the submucosal. The ENS is contained within the walls of the gastrointestinal (GI) tract and controls digestive function. Microbiota in the gut play an important role in the development of the ENS and CNS.[18] Although the GI tract receives both sympathetic and parasympathetic input, the ENS is neither part of either division of the ANS. It is the most complex and largest unit of the PNS with a built-in neural network, allowing it to act independently to some degree. The ENS and CNS communicate bidirectionally.[19]

COMMUNICATION WITHIN THE NERVOUS SYSTEM

The nervous system is connected via synapses. The axon of a neuron contacts the cell body or dendrite of another neuron to make a synapse. The axon is the output cell of the neuron, while dendrites are the input cells of the neuron. As the system matures, more and more connections are made, both axonal and dendritic. A labyrinth of relay stations with an infinite number of ways to take

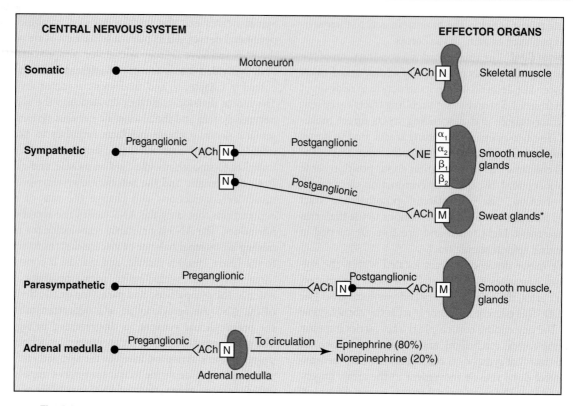

Fig. 8.8 Organization of the autonomic nervous system. (From Costanzo LS. *Physiology*. Philadelphia: WB Saunders; 1998:40.)

in, disseminate, and combine information is formed (Fig. 8.9). Dendritic spines are highly specialized subcellular structures that can change shape in a matter of seconds.[20] The increasing density and complexity of dendrites, the input cells, are a mark of advanced communication seen in phylogenetically higher animals. Dendritic branching increases the synaptic potential of the nervous system. Developmentally, branching occurs after initial pathways are formed with changes in spine morphology supporting changes in synaptic strength. The dynamic nature of change in dendritic spines provides a mechanism for correct information processing and storage in neural networks. Synaptic remodeling occurs throughout the life span in response to experience.[4,20,21]

Synapses

Neuron-to-neuron transmission of nerve impulses occurs at an interneuronal junction called a *synapse*. There are two basic types of synapses: chemical and electrical. Electrical synapses, referred to as *gap junctions*,

occur between dendrites and somas of adjacent neurons. Only a few gap junctions are present in the adult human nervous system. One example is found in the medulla where they function to produce a synchronous action such as inspiration. A second example involves saccadic eye movements.[10] The human nervous system uses predominantly chemical synapses that are activated by substances called *neurotransmitters*.

More than 60 different chemical substances have been classified as neurotransmitters.[22] Neurotransmitters are chemicals released by neurons to signal target cells. A few of the best known are acetylcholine, norepinephrine, serotonin (5-HT), glutamate, gamma-aminobutyric acid (GABA), and dopamine. Dopamine, norepinephrine, and 5-HT are slow-acting. Dopamine is involved in the reward system and is known as the "pleasure chemical."[22] Norepinephrine is both a hormone and a neurotransmitter and is responsible for the "fight or flight response." 5-HT modulates mood by producing a calming effect. Glutamate is the major

TABLE 8.4 Selected Effects of Autonomic Nervous System Activity

Organ	Effect of Sympathetic Stimulation	Effect of Parasympathetic Stimulation
Eye		
Pupil	Decrease dilation	Decrease constriction
Heart		
SA node	Increase heart rate	Decrease heart rate
Muscle	Increase rate and force	Decrease rate and force
Arterioles	Constriction	Dilation
Veins	Constriction	None
Lungs		
Bronchi	Dilation	Constriction
Gut		
Lumen	Decrease peristalsis	Increase peristalsis
Sphincter	Increase tone (usually)	Relax tone (usually)
Liver	Release glucose	Slight glucose synthesis
Kidney	Decrease output and renin secretion	None
Bladder	Relax detrusor muscle	Contract detrusor muscle
Contract trigone muscle	Relax trigone muscle	
Glands		
Lacrimal	None/slight secretion	Copious secretion
Sweat	Copious sweat	Sweaty palms of hands
Basal metabolism	Increase	None

excitatory neurotransmitter that promotes learning and memory. GABA is the major inhibitory neurotransmitter that acts to block neural signaling. It is important in constructing brain circuits during early development. Both are fast-acting. Transmission time for neurotransmitters ranges from milliseconds to minutes.[11] When an action potential reaches the end of an axon, it triggers the release of a neurotransmitter from synaptic vesicles. Sodium ions facilitate the depolarization of the presynaptic membrane, and calcium ions facilitate the release of the neurotransmitter. The transmitter diffuses across the space between the two neurons and binds to receptors on the postsynaptic neuron membrane.

Neuromodulators are chemical substances that are released at extrasynaptic sites, often into the extracellular space. They adjust the function of many neurons by opening ion channels, altering metabolism, or changing gene expression.[11] The same chemical can act as a neurotransmitter in one instance (acting at a synapse) and act as a neuromodulator in another place such as the hypothalamus. Neuromodulators act more slowly and farther away from the synaptic cleft.

Neurons can synapse on other neurons called *interneurons*, or they can synapse on muscle or glands. Interneurons are a major source of synaptic input to motor neurons. Interneurons are the links between motor neurons that form functional networks. Interneurons in the spinal cord receive sensory input that provides reflexive coordination between muscle groups. In addition, signals received from interneurons can facilitate or inhibit the firing of motor neurons.

Cortical Connections

Communication within the cerebrum is by way of subcortical white matter fibers deep into the cortex. The subcortical white fibers are classified in three ways

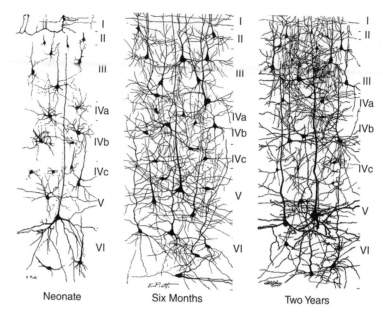

Neonate   Six Months   Two Years

Fig. 8.9 Dendritic growth in the visual cortex of an infant. (Reprinted with permission Corel JL. *The Postnatal Development of the Human Cerebral Cortex.* Vols. I-VIII. Cambridge, MA: Harvard University Press; 1975 [originally published in 1939].)

according to what they connect: association fibers, commissural fibers, and projection fibers.

Association Fibers

Association fibers connect cortical association areas within a given region and a single hemisphere. Short association fibers connect adjacent gyri and longer fibers connect specific combinations of various lobes, all within a single hemisphere.

Commissural Fibers

Commissural fibers are those that connect structures with the same relative position. The major and largest group of commissural fibers is the *corpus callosum* (Fig. 8.6), which transmits information between similar areas of the two sides of the brain. For example, the anterior part of the corpus callosum transmits from the anterior cortex of one hemisphere to the anterior cortex of the opposite hemisphere. The anterior and posterior commissures connect the right and left temporal lobes, respectively.

Projection Fibers

Projection fibers share information vertically. Information goes from the cerebral cortex to the spinal cord, brainstem, basal ganglia, and thalamus and comes to the

cerebral cortex from subcortical structures. Afferent fibers bring sensory input into the spinal cord via the posterior spinal root and connect with or continue as ascending tracts that carry information to various parts of the brain. Efferent fibers carry out commands from the motor cortex and PFC, which travel in descending tracts to the anterior horn of the spinal cord. Tracts are named for where they start and where they end.

ADAPTATION OF THE NERVOUS SYSTEM

Neural Plasticity

Neural plasticity is the ability of the nervous system to change. Five patterns of neural plasticity have been identified: developmental plasticity, adaptive plasticity, reactive plasticity, excessive plasticity, and plasticity that induces brain vulnerability.[3] Normal developmental plasticity is what builds the brain from neurons to networks. Impaired developmental plasticity hinders brain development and is exemplified by genetic disorders and autism spectrum disorders. Adaptive plasticity reorganizes and promotes adaptive function. Examples of this type of plasticity are experience-dependent and activity-dependent plasticity as seen in motor training. Reactive plasticity can occur following a pre- and postnatal injury or sensory deprivation. Two examples of sensory deprivation include infants born with congenital deafness and children with amblyopia (see Chapter 9). Excessive plasticity can lead to brain circuits that are unable to adapt to changes in connectivity such as in seizure generation. Another example of excessive plasticity is seen when someone, often a musician, develops focal dystonia as a consequence of excessive practice.[23] Hypoxic ischemic encephalopathy is the major example of plasticity that induces neuron vulnerability. A premature infant is still developing brain networks and exhibits developmental plasticity but that same plasticity may also make the brain more vulnerable to damage if the infant sustains hypoxia, which results in ischemic encephalopathy.[3]

In the course of typical prenatal and postnatal development, the infant is expected to be exposed to sufficient environmental stimuli at appropriate times. This type of *experience-expectant* neural plasticity is exemplified in the sensory systems that are ready to function at birth but require experience with light and sound to complete maturation. *Experience-dependent* neural plasticity allows the nervous system to incorporate other types of information from environmental experiences that are relatively unpredictable and idiosyncratic. These experiences are unique to the individual and depend on the context in which development occurs, such as the physical, social, and cultural environment. Climate, social expectations, and child-rearing practices can alter movement experiences. What each child learns depends on the unique physical challenges encountered. Motor learning, as part of motor development, is an example of *activity-dependent neural plasticity*. Experiences of infants in different cultures may result in alterations in the acquisition of motor abilities. *Activity-dependent plasticity* drives changes in synapses or neuronal circuits as a result of experience or learning (Fig. 8.10).

Activity-dependent changes in neural circuitry occur in response to experience. Learning and behavior modulate neurogenesis throughout life. Synaptic plasticity is the ability of neurons to modify the strength of their connections.[24] Persistent changes in dendritic spine morphology are seen when synaptic strength increases.[20] The size of the dendritic spine is correlated with the strength of the synapse it forms. Postnatal experience plays a major role in further inducing developmental changes in synaptic strength by axon and dendritic

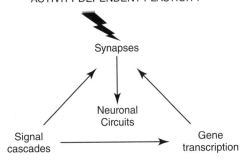

ACTIVITY-DEPENDENT PLASTICITY

Fig. 8.10 Activity-dependent plasticity and refinement of synaptic connections are mediated through modulation of activity at synapses, which activate signaling cascades and gene transcription. Environmental sensory and behavioral conditions, drugs, toxins, nutritional disturbances, and genetic mutations affect the final formation of neuronal networks in the developing brain at multiple levels in this process. (From Johnson MV. Clinical disorders of brain plasticity. *Brain Dev.* 2004;26:73–80.)

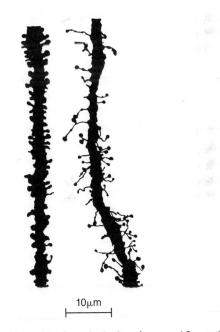

10μm

Fig. 8.11 Dendritic spines from the brains of a normal 6-month-old child *(left)* and a severely cognitively impaired 10-month-old child *(right)*. (From Purpura D. Dendritic spine "dysgenesis" and mental retardation, *Science* 1974;186:1126–1128.)

pruning (see later).[4] Some types of intellectual disability and cognitive disorders have been linked to dendritic spine density abnormalities (Fig. 8.11).[20] The changes in structure and function of the building blocks of the nervous system are prime examples of neural plasticity.

Physical activity (PA) and exercise promote brain plasticity throughout the life span.[25,26] PA provides environmental enrichment for the brain[27] as evidenced by improvement in EF, global cognition, and attention. Higher-order cognitive functions such as decision-making and spatial and language learning have been found to depend on neural plasticity mechanisms such as long-term potentiation (LTP).[4] LTP is the term to describe the strengthening of synapses based on recent patterns of activity. LTP results in a stronger response of a postsynaptic nerve cell to stimulation. LTP is a mechanism for activity-dependent neural plasticity. Movement experiences develop not only motor skills but also cognitive abilities such as learning language and solving problems.

Neuron Cell Death

Neuron cell death occurs via necrosis, apoptosis, or autophagy.[28] Necrosis is uncontrolled cell death following a severe injury such as hypoxia or inflammation. The cell cannot function. It responds by swelling and is unable to maintain homeostasis with its surrounding environment (see "Response to Injury"). Necrosis causes a loss of cell contents into the surrounding tissues and results in damage to those tissues. Apoptosis is controlled cell death that results in clearing the cells from the body with little damage to surrounding tissues. Autophagy is a mechanism that can either protect or kill stressed cells.

Developmentally, neuron cell death is an important occurrence in the nervous system because it initially overproduces neurons. This overproduction ensures a sufficient number of neurons to complete the "wiring" of the organism and to support optimal function. Two regressive processes mold the developing nervous system. One is *developmental apoptosis* and the other is *axon* and *dendritic pruning*.[29] The metabolic state of the extracellular environment appears to strongly influence this process. Those neurons deprived of trophic support, that is, those not nourished, degenerate, and die. The trimming of extraneous axon or dendritic connections occurs without harm to the cell of origin and allows for refinement of neural circuits and sculpting of the nervous system. This developmental process is regulated by interaction between neurons and glial cells. Pruning of axons is accompanied by apoptosis. Disruption of these mechanisms can result in abnormal pruning, which has been associated with brain dysfunction such as Down syndrome (DS). Developmentally appropriate removal of exuberant neural connections is a way to develop efficient and functional movement in keeping with the neuronal group selection theory of Edelman. Axonal and synaptic pruning occurs in two waves, one during the first 2 years of life and the second in adolescence. The later developmental period is when symptoms of psychiatric disorders such as schizophrenia and anxiety may manifest.[30]

Autophagy is an evolutionary process that protects healthy cells during times of metabolic stress[28] and plays a role in maintaining neuronal homeostasis.[31] It is often used to recycle cellular components such as amino acids.[32] A lack of or deficiency in autophagy over the life span leads to an accumulation of protein aggregates, which are associated with neurodegenerative diseases such as Alzheimer disease (AD) and Parkinson disease.[33] Cellular and molecular changes due to aging render neurons vulnerable to damage. A major cause of age-related damage to neurons is oxidative stress. Other causes of cell death include mitochondrial dysfunction, impaired "waste disposal" mechanism, dysregulation of neuronal Ca^{2+} homeostasis, and inflammation.[34] Aging results in a decline in the number of synapses and abnormal synaptic transmission in many brain regions, especially those involved in memory, cognition, and movement.[35]

Response to Injury
Peripheral Nerve

The response of a peripheral nerve to injury is different than that in the CNS. Myelin in the PNS is less dense than CNS myelin. This difference contributes to the ability of peripheral nerve axons to regrow in response to damage. Schwann cells can produce myelin after injury. Depending on the severity of the peripheral nerve injury, the nerve regenerates, and muscle function returns. When peripheral nerve damage is severe enough to disrupt the myelin sheath and the axon, the axon degenerates back to the node of Ranvier, which is most proximal to the injury. This is called Wallerian degeneration. After a time, the axon regrows and tries to reestablish contact with the postsynaptic target and restore function. In a young healthy person, a peripheral nerve may grow a millimeter a day or an inch a month, given ideal circumstances.[36] The path of nerve growth can be followed by the Tinel sign (a tingling when the nerve is tapped) as the severed nerve grows and reestablishes contact with its receptor. In the most severe type of peripheral nerve injury, surgical intervention is required to reestablish the connection.

Central Nervous System

Adaptability within the CNS is functionally limited to reorganization because in most cases regeneration does not occur. Typically, when a neuron dies, it is replaced by neuroglial cells. When the brain is damaged by ischemia, some neurons die immediately, and others are at risk of dying if the blood supply is not reestablished. The latter is programmed cell death or apoptosis that is triggered by an environmental event that sets in motion a cascade of events resulting in cell death. *Excitotoxicity* happens when excessive intracellular calcium causes leakage of mitochondrial components into the cytoplasm.[5] Calcium is not typically toxic to neurons as its usual function is to trigger the release of neurotransmitters. Excess secretion of the excitatory neurotransmitter glutamate can cause destruction and death of previously injured neurons in two ways, calcium-induced *apoptosis*, as described earlier, and *osmotic necrosis*.[5] Water comes into the neuron, producing swelling, eventual rupture, and an inflammatory response. Adjacent neurons, not directly injured, may become inhibited from functioning. Blood flow changes can occur in areas remote from the original damage such that some areas of the cortex become less excitable.[37]

Recovery from neural injury involves resolution of edema, reperfusion of the damaged area, and mechanisms of neural plasticity. The initial inhibition of function occurs because of edema, shock, decreased blood flow, and underutilization of glucose. Spinal shock is an example of the inhibition of function following an acute spinal cord injury. Synaptic effectiveness is altered following neural injury. *Denervation hypersensitivity* contributes to a decline in synaptic effectiveness when presynaptic neurons are destroyed, thereby depriving postsynaptic neurons of sufficient amounts of neurotransmitters. When local edema resolves, synaptic effectiveness improves and the extent of the spinal cord injury can be evaluated.

The same process that is involved in the development of brain networks is involved in reorganizing the brain networks after damage.[24] Through neural plasticity, existing synaptic connections are strengthened, which can modify neural networks and allow brain regions to become more or less responsive to other parts of the brain or the body. A second way neural plasticity adds to recovery is by producing new synaptic connections (*reactive synaptogenesis*) to denervated body parts. Physical therapy interventions aimed at functional tasks such as the use of a treadmill for locomotor training take advantage of activity-dependent neural plasticity to reorganize the brain.[38–40]

SUMMARY OF STRUCTURE AND FUNCTION

Neurons are the means by which the nervous system communicates. All information is received by specialized receptors and transmitted along several distinct pathways to various regions of the brain, where it is interpreted, acted on, stored, or ignored. Structurally, neurons are produced to match their functions within the nervous system. Neurons increase their ability to communicate by the branching of dendrites and making new synaptic connections. The nervous system exhibits a great deal of plasticity throughout the life span. The brain is constantly changing and adapting to experience: those experiences that are expected and those that are unique to the individual. Research continues to explore the ontogeny of memory and learning; analyze the structural and functional responses of the nervous system when it is damaged and delineate ways to utilize neural plasticity to improve a person's potential for recovery.

LIFE SPAN CHANGES

Prenatal Period

The CNS develops from specialized ectoderm at 3 weeks of gestation when the neural tube is formed. The brain is created from the cranial two-thirds, and the spinal cord from the caudal one-third, of the neural tube by the end of the fourth week of gestation—1 month before the mother feels the fetus move.[41] When this process is disturbed, severe brain and spinal cord anomalies may result, including anencephaly and myelomeningocele. During the fourth week of gestation, the embryo develops head and tail folds because of the rapid growth of the cranial region and spinal cord. The head continues to enlarge during the succeeding weeks, with the brain being folded back onto itself. By 8 weeks, the head of the embryo is half the size of the body. At the end of the eighth week, the fetus looks definitely human and has completed the most critical period of CNS development.

Development of the nervous system is a complicated process. Via cytogenesis or cell production, the maximum number of neurons and glia are produced.

Neurons of the spinal cord and brainstem are generated by the tenth week. The neurons of the forebrain, including the cerebral hemispheres, are produced by 20 weeks. During histogenesis, or tissue formation, the structures of the brain and spinal cord are formed. Neurons move or migrate to their correct location within the nervous system, where they differentiate into different nerve cell types, form synaptic connections, and enlarge. Neuronal targets produce trophic substances that guide neuronal connections. Neuronal connections need to have the correct number of axons so that axons innervate the correct number of target cells.[42] Initially, there is polyneuronal innervation of prenatal muscle fibers compared with the 1:1 relationship seen in postnatal life.[11]

Nerve cell types are genetically determined. Therefore, the size and shape of the nerve cell, the pattern of axon or dendrite branching, and even the type of neurotransmitter a neuron will use are innately determined. The cerebral cortex begins as one layer only a few cells thick, known as the *germinal zone*.[43] Cell generation order and cell position in the cortex have an inside-out relationship because of the mechanism of cell migration. The cells formed earliest occupy the deepest layer of the cortex; the cells formed later occupy progressively more superficial layers. These cells migrate using a system of guides, the radial glial fibers, which extend from the surface of the ventricles to the surface of the cortex. Structurally, the six layers of the cortex are completed during the last months of gestation and the first postnatal months of life.[43]

The first endocrine gland, the thyroid, develops at 24 days.[41] By the 11th week, it begins to secrete thyroxin, a hormone necessary for proper brain growth. This hormone triggers the cessation of nerve cell proliferation and initiates nerve cell migration.[44] Without the thyroid hormone, axons are poorly myelinated and neurons do not completely branch. Too little hormone produces *cretinism*, a condition in which there is arrested mental and physical development.

Neuroglia form from the neuroepithelium as early as 3 weeks, although proliferation does not start until later in gestation. Microglia are derived from mesenchymal cells late in the fetal period after blood vessels have established their connections. Microglia are the innate immune cells of the CNS and influence neural development and function. Radial glial cells (specialized microglia) provide a kind of road map for migrating Purkinje cells to complete the development of the structure of the cerebellum and its connections.[45] Migration is facilitated by a chemical affinity between neuronal and glial surfaces, at least in the cerebellum.

Internal brain structures such as the thalamus and hypothalamus are present at 7 weeks of gestation. The internal structure of the spinal cord is achieved in 10 weeks. During the next 5–15 weeks, general structural features—sulci and gyri, cervical and lumbar enlargements of the spinal cord—are attained.[41] The 12 pairs of cranial nerves emerge during the fifth and sixth weeks of gestation.

In addition to giving rise to the neural tube, the neural plate gives rise to neural crest cells, which are the precursors of the PNS. The PNS begins as paired masses of neural crest cells, one on each side of the neural tube, that differentiate into the sensory ganglia of the spinal nerves. The neural crest cells in the brain region migrate to form sensory ganglia for cranial nerves V, VII, VIII, IX, and X.[41] Other structures also are produced from the neural crest cells: Schwann cells, meninges (the connective tissue covering of the brain), and many musculoskeletal components of the head.

Motor nerve fibers begin to appear in the spinal cord at the end of the fourth week of gestation, forming the spinal nerves. Next, the dorsal nerve root (consisting of sensory fibers) appears. It is made up of the axons of neural crest cells that have migrated to the dorsolateral part of the spinal cord, forming a spinal ganglion. The spinal nerves exit between the vertebrae, elongate, and grow into the limb buds, where they supply muscles that are differentiated from *mesenchyme*. The muscles innervated by segments of the spinal nerve are referred to as *myotomes*. Skin innervation occurs in the same segmental fashion, resulting in *dermatomes*.

Synapse formation occurs relatively late in the development of the nervous system, just before 6–7 weeks. Synapse formation is highly variable in pattern and distribution. The development of connections between the sensory neurons and the motor neurons is critical to laying the framework for spinal reflexes and for the pairing of sensory and motor information. A spinal reflex is the pairing of a sensory neuron and a motor neuron so that incoming stimuli produce a motor response. Once established, spinal reflexes are permanent and considered "hard-wired." Reflexes can be monosynaptic or polysynaptic; that is, they can involve one or more than one synapse. The establishment of reflex connections provides the fetus and eventually the infant with survival reflexes, such as suck-swallow, rooting, and gag. Fetal movement begins in utero at about 6–7 weeks of gestation. Reflex movements in response to touch have been chronicled as early as 7–8 weeks of gestation. Reflex connections are established in utero in a cephalocaudal direction; arm withdrawal occurs earlier than leg withdrawal.

As another late-stage phenomenon of neural development, myelination starts after neuron formation (8–16 weeks of gestation) and overlaps with neuron migration (12–20 weeks of gestation). Myelination occurs first in those areas of the nervous system that will be used first. Myelin is initially laid down in the cervical part of the spinal medulla and in the cranial nerves related to sucking and swallowing, abilities needed for survival. The first axons to be myelinated are the anterior (motor) roots of the spinal cord at about 4 months of gestation. One month later, the posterior, or sensory, roots begin the process. Myelin is deposited as a sheath or covering in the spinal cord at the same time that functional connections (i.e., synapses) are being formed.[46] The vestibulocochlear system (cranial nerve VIII) is myelinated at the end of the fifth month of gestation[47] and is related to awareness of the head and body position in space.

Rapid periods of growth such as those seen in the fetal period are critical periods when the nervous system is most vulnerable to damage. The nervous system requires adequate nutrition for cell formation and myelination to occur.[48] For example, lipids in the form of fatty acids must be transported through the BBB because there are no endogenous fats in the brain.

Fetuses are exposed to metabolites from the mother's microbiota in utero before developing their own microbiota. Microbiota is the term used to describe the collection of microbes that inhabit the body. Infants are colonized by microorganisms at birth.[18] Gut microbiota affect ENS and CNS development pre- and postnatally.[18,19,49] The composition of the microbiota of the infant reflects the mode of delivery, the feeding method, and the mother's microbial composition. There appears to be a critical period when the gut microbiota can cause lasting effects on the development of the CNS and ENS. Animal studies have shown gut microbiota can modulate critical process such as myelination, glial cell function, synaptic pruning, and permeability of the BBB.[18]

Birth occurs before CNS development is complete because the fetus outgrows the space, and the metabolic demand of the developing brain mass cannot be met by the mother's placenta.[50] Malnutrition or trauma can have dramatic effects on the developing system. A lack of prenatal and postnatal nutrition results in a decrease in the number of synapses formed and in the amount of dendritic branching and myelination.[51] Incomplete or disrupted development of the ENS can result in long-term GI problems.[19]

Infancy and Early Childhood

At birth, the brain is one-fourth the weight of the adult brain, whereas the head is already 70% of its adult size. Critical periods for brain growth occur between 3 and 10 months and between 15 and 24 months of age.[52] Brain weight doubles by 6 months of age and is half the weight of the adult brain. Malnutrition is a deficiency that can include overnutrition or undernutrition. Growth in children during the first 1000 days (from conception to 24 months of age) is crucial for their cognitive and physical development.[53] Malnutrition during the first 2 years of life reduces the number of glial cells formed,[54] which may result in poorer vascular support for nervous system function. The relationship between brain weight and brain growth is depicted in Fig. 8.12. Inadequate nutrition can lead to inadequate linear growth, which can result in wasting (low weight for height), stunting (low height for age), or underweight (low weight for age). Stunting has been thought to be irreversible after 2 years of age[55] but the debate continues.[56]

Brain metabolism changes with CNS maturation during infancy. Tracking glucose metabolism in the brain postnatally provides another means to document functional maturation. The pattern of activity, that is, where glucose is being used, corresponds to the areas of the brain that are maturing. In the newborn, the highest activity is found in the primary motor and sensory cortex, thalamus, brainstem, and midline of the cerebellum. By 2–3 months, increases in glucose use are evident in the parietal, temporal, and primary visual cortex; basal ganglia; and cerebellar hemispheres. The frontal cortex is the last area to demonstrate increased glucose use. The increase begins between 6 and 8 months, and by 8–12 months, use is widespread in the frontal lobes.[57] The increase in glucose use in the frontal lobes also corresponds to the expansion of dendritic branching and capillary networks in the frontal lobe.

At birth, the regional cerebral rates of glucose use demonstrate a two-fold increase compared to the adult brain until around 4–5 years of age. Fig. 8.13 depicts the

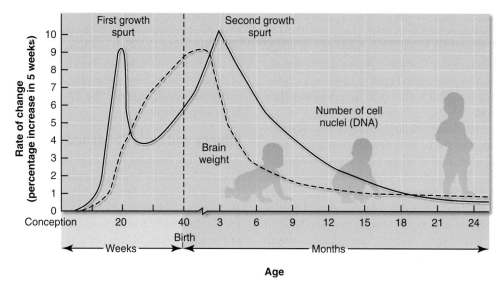

Fig. 8.12 Relationship of brain weight *(dotted line)* and growth *(solid line)*. The DNA curve has two peaks: one reflecting neuron multiplication, and the other reflecting glial multiplication. (Data from Dobbing J. Undernutrition and the developing brain. *Am J Dis Child.* 1970;120:411–415.)

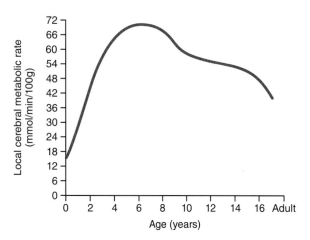

Fig. 8.13 Brain metabolism rate of glucose utilization. (Adapted from Chugani HT. A critical period of brain development: studies of cerebral glucose utilization with PET. *Prev Med.* 1998;27:184–188.)

changes that occur in the metabolic rate of glucose use in the brain over time. The rate plateaus and then starts to decline to the adult rate by 16–18 years of age.[57] These changes partially mirror the time course for synaptogenesis. Synaptic proliferation occurs in the period between birth and 4 years of age. The typical 2-year-old has twice as many cerebral cortex synapses as an adult.[58] Between the ages of 2 and 3, the brain contains about 15,000 synapses per neuron. Pruning of excess synapses begins early in childhood, continues through adolescence, and stabilizes during early adulthood.[59] The decline in the rate of glucose use for brain metabolism during adolescence is due to synaptic elimination that occurs in the cortex with a further diminishment of energy requirement to adulthood.[60]

Myelination of the PNS is largely complete at birth,[61] allowing the newborn immediate access to information about the environment through touch, motion, smell, and taste. The infant uses these sensory cues to carry out vital functions of eating, breathing, sleeping, and excreting. All cranial nerves (with the exception of the optic nerve) are completely myelinated at birth.

Although the PNS is ready to function at birth, myelination has only been occurring for 2 months in the brain (assuming that the infant is born at term, 40 weeks of gestation). Myelination occurs rapidly across the first 2–3 years of life. The primary motor cortex develops ahead of the primary sensory cortex. Fig. 8.14 shows when some major structures undergo myelination. "In general, … brain development progresses from posterior to anterior and from inferior to superior.[59]" The cerebellum and the brainstem myelinate before the cerebral

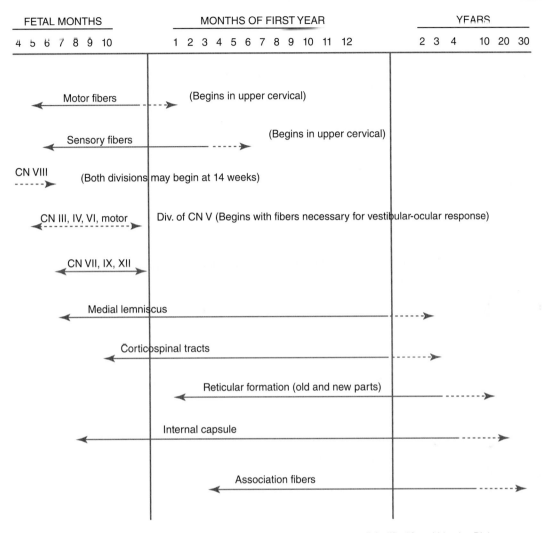

Fig. 8.14 Timetable of myelination of selected nervous system structures. (Modified from Yakovlev PI, Lecours AR. The myelogenetic cycles of regional maturation of the brain. In Minkowski A, ed. *Regional Development of the Brain in Early Life.* Oxford, UK: Blackwell; 1967.)

hemispheres.[62] The midbrain and spinal cord are the most advanced portions at birth in terms of myelination. Early myelination of the brainstem supports the many vital functions controlled there and accounts for the fact that the newborn sleeps most of the time and is totally dependent on caregivers.

The first 2 months after birth are considered a period of CNS organization. During this time, the infant establishes physiological control of sleep and wakefulness as evidenced by the relationship between sleep states and electroencephalographic patterns, and by increasing

the number and duration of periods of alertness. Social behavior begins around 2 months of age with the advent of the social smile. Circadian rhythm, or the 24-hour biological cycle, is established between 2 and 4 months of age without regard for night and day.[63] In other words, this is a time when infants can get their days and nights mixed up.

ANS changes occur during the first year of life as the newborn responds more via the sympathetic nervous system to ever-changing stressors such as light, gravity, and air. As internal body processes such as GI motility stabilize, behavioral responses gradually become more characteristic of the parasympathetic nervous system, which maintains the status quo or steady state.

Nerve conduction velocity increases over time in both skin and muscle fibers because of the change to saltatory conduction and the increase in nerve fiber diameter with age. Values for nerve conduction speed change remarkably quickly after birth. For example, ulnar nerve conduction in infants and young children increases from 30 to 50 m/second from birth to 9 months of age and reaches adult values (60 m/second) by 3 years of age.[64]

Brain structures are ready to support the development of function during the first year of life. The major efferent (motor) tract, the corticospinal tract, begins myelination 1 month before birth and completes the process by 1 year. The corticospinal tract in the newborn has not yet innervated the anterior horn, so during the first 6 months of life the infant demonstrates a Babinski sign.[11] Stroking the foot from the heel along the lateral border of the foot and then under the toes results in extension of the great toe. Although the presence of this sign in individuals older than 6 months is indicative of corticospinal tract damage, in a young infant it is a sign of immaturity. There appears to be a correlation between late corticospinal tract development and late motor development.[65] Furthermore, the fact that the pattern of terminations of the corticospinal tract axons changes over the course of postnatal development is an example of *activity-dependent plasticity*. The structure of the corticospinal axon terminals reflects sensory-motor cortex activity.[66] Atypical somatosensory feedback can lead to maladaptive plasticity.[67] The sensory area of the brain catches up to the motor area by the age of 2. During the second year of life, the increasing speed and complexity of movement are probably related to myelination. The process slows after 2 years and is mostly complete by 10 years of age.

The richness of the experiences that a child is exposed to during the first 3 years of life can be critical to cognitive and language development.[68] Brain growth during childhood is thought to coincide with the stages of cognitive development as described by Piaget[69] and the development of language.[70] The infant's brain weight at 1 year is 60% of its adult weight, a gain of 10% in 6 months. During the next year, growth continues until 75% of adult brain weight is reached by age 2. The relationship of brain weight, age, and language acquisition is shown in Table 8.5. Myelination of structures that support speech development, such as the tectum, an integration center for auditory information, and the striatum, an integration center for language, occurs within the first year of life. Myelination of the striatum by 1 year of age coincides with the child's first spoken word. The pattern and density of dendritic branching have also been linked to language development, especially the specialization of the left hemisphere as the language center in the majority of individuals.[70] A 2-year-old child can put together two-word combinations and by age 3 can speak in phrases and short sentences.

Childhood and Adolescence

Myelination advances quickly in early childhood, the first 5 years of life.[71] During this time, children develop fundamental motor and language skills. The developmental process of myelination is highly influenced by neural activity. Motor and cognitive skills become refined as ongoing myelination of the nervous system continues to increase the speed of conduction of nerve impulses and motor control becomes more automatic. Total brain volume has reached 90% of adult values by 6 years of age, with additional increments continuing during the rest of childhood and early adolescence.[72] A 6-year-old is able to speak in five- to six-word sentences.

TABLE 8.5 Relationship of Age, Brain Weight, and Language Acquisition		
Age	**Brain Weight (% of Adult Weight)**	**Language Level**
Birth	25	Crying; no words
1 year	60	Average age of first spoken word
18 mo to 2 years	75	Two-word combinations
3 years	80	Phrases and short sentences
6 years	90	Five- to six-word sentences
Puberty	100	Abstract language concepts

Despite the fact that children exhibit a partially mature corticospinal tract between 6 and 9 years of age, the ability to conduct nervous impulses at adultlike speeds is not sufficient for proficient motor performance. A group of young school-age children could not perform a motor task as well as adults.[73] The corticospinal tract becomes morphologically mature by 10 years of age but not electrophysiologically mature until age 13.[73,74] In other words, the structure of the tract is adultlike in its connections and anatomical configuration before the tract is able to exhibit adult levels of neurotransmission.

Myelination during adolescence includes secondary association areas important in sensorimotor processing and associative learning. The last areas to be myelinated are the association cortices in the frontal, parietal, and temporal lobes, along with other association fibers. Dendritic branching in the areas of the cortex involved with speech and language reaches adult levels of complexity between 12 and 16 years of age.[70] Additionally, low-frequency electroencephalographic rhythms change to adult high-frequency rhythms by 10–13 years of age.[75] The adolescent may continue to improve motor skills with practice. Females demonstrate performance increases earlier than males, but males' motor performance peaks during late adolescence. Further change in motor performance after adolescence is highly variable and depends more on the amount of practice, instruction, motivation, and innate ability.

Cortical gray matter (neurons and glial cells) volume has previously been reported to peak around the onset of puberty but it actually is highest in childhood and decreases through adolescence.[72] Whole brain volume increases until sometime between 10 and 15 years of age.[76] Puberty is a group of endocrine processes that occurs to mark adolescence. Puberty is initiated by the hypothalamic-pituitary-gonadal (HPG) axis that releases hormones to produce internal and external changes to primary and secondary sexual characteristics allowing for reproduction.[77] These changes include, but are not limited to, development of the primary and secondary sexual characteristics, changes in body composition, growth in height and weight, and the onset of menses (see Chapter 10).

Adulthood

The majority of structures in the CNS are myelinated by the third decade.[78] However, myelination continues into the fifth decade of adulthood[71] in those areas responsible for integrating information for purposeful action, the association areas of the brain. White matter consists of myelinated axon fibers. Loss of myelinated fibers occurs in adulthood, but myelin can be repaired. White matter volume peaks in the fourth decade.[79] Myelin changes are possible during adulthood due to neural plasticity. These can be subtle structural changes such as thickness of the myelin, its distribution along an axon, to generation of new *oligondrocytes*, the myelinating cells in the CNS.[80] Research in myelin plasticity is focused on its relationship to memory and learning as well as age-related cognitive decline. Gray matter is stable during early adulthood. Whole brain volume continues to decrease from adolescence to around age 20 when it stabilizes prior to a decline around age 40.[81]

Different regions of the brain grow at different rates across the first three decades of life. Mills and colleagues studied structural brain development from late childhood (8 years) to early adulthood (~25 years) using anatomical magnetic resonance imaging (MRI) data to track changes in total gray matter volume, cortex volume, mean cortical thickness, and white matter surface area. All of these measures decreased in mid-adolescence and remained stable in early adulthood (20s). In this study, cerebral white matter increases during the transition to adolescence and begins to stabilize in mid-to-late-adolescence continuing into early adulthood.[76] The age at which brain structures stabilize is a measure of maturity. The greatest variability in brain development is seen in adolescence and early adulthood.[76] A total of about 15% of brain weight and volume is lost throughout the life span, beginning in middle adulthood. Knowledge of individual variability may allow the identification of individuals with atypical neural development.

Microstructural changes in brain white matter have been studied using diffusion tensor imaging (DTI). Changes in fractional anisotrophy (FA) and mean diffusivity (MD) are used to describe changes in white matter fibers with age. Tian and Ma[82] studied a group of individuals from early to middle adulthood (18–55 years of age). The pattern of the changes in the above two measures was able to predict the subjects' brain age. In early development FA ↑ and MD ↓ while with aging the reverse is seen FA ↓ and MD ↑. These changes represent mild demyelination and loss of myelinated axons in the corticospinal tract, which contribute to decreased perceptual speed. Another study of young to middle-aged adults focused on age-related decline in dopamine (DA) systems and functional connectivity.[83] Decline in the amount of DA starts in the third decade with a 10% loss with each successive decade.[84] A decline in DA is inversely related to cognitive measures. This exploratory study demonstrated that men had age-related changes in connectivity between the main DA-producing nuclei in the midbrain and cerebellar and cortical regions but women did not. There is considerable interindividual variability in the patterns of brain changes.[85]

The speed with which sensory nerves conduct impulses begins to decline after 30 years of age.[86] Motor nerve conduction velocity, according to Schaumburg and colleagues,[87] decreases by 1 m/second per decade after 15–24 years of age. Motor and sensory nerve conduction velocity of the median, peroneal, and tibial nerves all declined after age 40 in a study by Palve and Palve.[88]

The basal ganglia, which implement movement programs, maintain stability during adulthood.[89] As stated earlier, research has shown that new neurons are produced in the hippocampus in adulthood.[90] In fact, exercise has been found to increase adult hippocampal neurogenesis and plasticity.[91] In a randomized controlled trial with 120 older adults, aerobic exercise training was found to increase the size of the hippocampus and improve memory.[92] The nervous system changes that result from aging begin at age 20. Brain weight and thickness of the cortex decline, whereas the relative number of glial cells increases. Whether the number of neurons increases, decreases, or stays the same with reduced neuron size is still being debated. Despite all of these occurrences, a few overall changes in the structure of the brain and nervous system exceed 25% of the total area through adulthood, except in disease states and only during the last few months of life.[93] The built-in redundancy of the nervous system by way of synaptic plasticity is such that even if neurons are lost in one place, other connections may be gained. Most areas of the brainstem that deal with vital functions are stable throughout adulthood and show minimal change with aging.

Older Adulthood

Brain volume declines in older adults. The PFC and hippocampus shrink at roughly 1%–2% annually in individuals over the age of 55,[94] with higher rates of atrophy seen in individuals beginning to experience cognitive impairment.[95] Although the rate and trajectory of decline varies from region to region, the general finding is that regions that support memory and EFs show earlier and more rapid decline. The effects of aging on the brain and cognition are widespread and have multiple etiologies. Aging has effects on the molecules, cells, hormones, neurotransmitters, and vasculature structure, all of which may affect brain functions including cognition. With aging, the brain shrinks in volume, particularly in the frontal cortex. Age-related differences were generally small prior to age 50, but declined significantly and continuously after age 50 with the actual rate of decline increasing with age, particularly over age 70, and progressing into the 90 s. Frontal lobe volumes showed the greatest decline with age (approximately 12%), and smaller differences were found for the temporal lobes (approximately 9%).[96] Age-related differences in occipital and parietal lobes were modest. Age-related gender differences were generally small, except for the frontal lobe, where men had significantly smaller lobar brain volumes throughout the age range studied. A previous study also showed an association between increasing age, a reduction in prefrontal cortical volume, increased subcortical white matter lesions, and a decrease in EF.[97]

Interestingly, the loss of brain volume is mirrored by age-related changes in cognitive function with the most significant losses occurring when performing memory and executive tasks.[98] Yet, it is these cognitive domains and brain areas that appear the most sensitive to PA training.[99] Age-related cortical atrophy is considered usual aging and is often associated with cognitive decline in older adults who do not have dementia.[100] The primary determinant of cortical volume reductions is cortical thinning.[101] While cortical thinning occurs throughout the life span,[102] the thinning that occurs in older adults is more likely due to neuronal shrinkage and reduction of dendritic spines and synapses than synaptic pruning that happens during development. A major problem with identifying primary aging changes in the nervous system is that it is impossible to know with any degree of certainty if these are signs of preclinical pathology. The potential that both intrinsic and extrinsic environmental factors can produce changes with aging further compounds the problem of identifying what are primary aging changes. Some degree of brain volume and neuron loss is probably inevitable, but it is not possible to state unequivocally what is "normal" or "typical" because universal or primary aging changes are difficult to separate from those that are harbingers

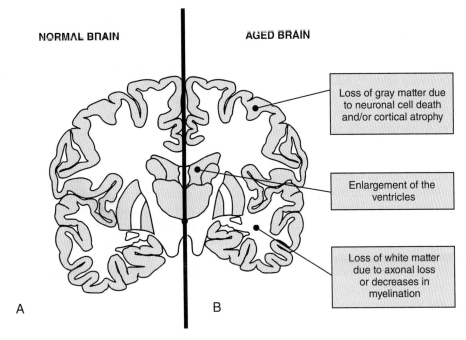

NORMAL BRAIN   AGED BRAIN

Loss of gray matter due
to neuronal cell death
and/or cortical atrophy

Enlargement of the
ventricles

Loss of white matter
due to axonal loss
or decreases in
myelination

A   B

Fig. 8.15 Comparison of a normal and an aged brain. (**A**) A normal hemisection of the human cortex. (**B**) Aged human cortex. Researchers have observed several age-related gross anatomical changes, including a loss or atrophy of cortical neurons, a decrease in white matter (due to axonal or myelin loss), and an enlargement of the ventricles. (From Fox CM, Alder RN. Neural mechanisms of aging. In Cohen H, ed. *Neuroscience for Rehabilitation.* 2nd ed. Philadelphia: Lippincott Williams & Wilkins; 1999:401–418.)

of pathology. A cross-sectional comparison of a normal brain and an aging brain is shown in Fig. 8.15.

Age-related decline in brain weight and volume is accompanied by neuronal atrophy, cell death, and ventricular enlargement. Resnick and colleagues[103] documented on average a 1.4 cm³ increase in ventricular volume per year in healthy older adults. Gyral atrophy includes the loss of gray and white matter, whereas white matter loss includes the loss of myelin. The volume of CSF remains constant until age 40, then increases with another rise after age 60.[104] Significant differences in brain volume are seen between young-old, middle-old, and oldest-old subjects.[105] Volume loss is seen to be minimal after age 65 with decline progressing at small constant rates from young-old to middle-old to oldest-old. The rate of loss is small and constant in healthy older adults.

Minor to moderate neuron loss and the loss of the ability of dendrites to produce new spines (sprouting) have been reported in many parts of the brain, but the link to a decline in function is far from apparent.

Structural losses may be a result of an age-dependent decline in use because dendrites continue to grow into old age. Synaptic remodeling and growth also occur late in adulthood. Synaptic plasticity can be assessed using positron emission tomography as a measure of cognitive reserve capacity. Dendritic complexity in older individuals who are cognitively intact supports the idea that the nervous system is still able to adapt well into the 70 s.[106]

White matter is the CNS structure that declines the most with advanced age. After reaching a maximum in middle age, myelin declines in older age. The process of myelin repair is unable to keep up with age-related myelin breakdown in older age. Commissures, major bundles of white matter that provide interhemispheric communication, are essential to human memory. Loss of myelinated nerve fibers in the frontal lobes and association areas with older age could explain the decline in cognitive processing speed seen in the elderly.[107] White matter loss is more accelerated in people in their 70 s and 80 s compared to those in their 50 s and 60 s. Resnick and associates[103] used MRI to longitudinally study the shrinking brain in adults aged 59–85 years at baseline. They found substantial declines in both gray and white matter. Minor changes in electroencephalographic patterns, such as a slowing of the alpha waves, have been reported with aging.[108] Additional evidence, however, suggests that no significant changes in pattern occur with age.[109] In fact, the temporal wave slowing, so often attributed to normal aging, has been linked to pathological brain changes.[110]

The structural and functional integrity of the cerebellum predicts motor control and cognitive performance in an older population.[111,112] Decreased cerebellar gray matter volume in older adults is associated with poorer cognitive and sensorimotor task performance.[113,114] Volume reduction is also associated with memory decline.[114] Disruption of cortico-cerebellar and cerebellar-hippocampus connectivity is documented in older adultsand linked to cognitive and memory decline.[114,115] The cerebellum also exhibits age-related changes that are associated with declines in posture, balance, and gait seen in the older adult.[116,117]

Glucose metabolism and aerobic glycolysis decline with aging.[118–120] Cerebral glucose metabolic rates are higher in women than in men.[121,122] In a study by Feng and colleagues,[123] glucose metabolism decline began at age 60 in both men and women. The decline involved the frontal and temporal lobes bilaterally as well as the inferior cingulate gyrus. Metabolic differences were documented in the caudate nucleus in men and in the occipital lobe for women. Aging trends differed between genders. In a longitudinal study by Beason-Held and associates,[124] cerebral blood flow was shown to decrease with age in areas of the frontal, temporal, and occipital lobes. Structures such as the thalamus and caudate that border the lateral ventricles also showed a decrease in blood flow, which may reflect age-associated increases in ventricular volume.[103] Areas of the brain that showed an increase in blood flow included the hippocampus, cerebellum, and the prefrontal white matter. It has been postulated that these areas may represent preserved function in the brain relative to the global decline in blood flow seen with advanced age.[124]

The hippocampus exhibits a number of neurofibrillary tangles (NFTs) within the neuron cell body as a result of aging.[125] Although the incidence of NFTs increases with age in the healthy brain, an even greater incidence is seen in patients with dementia.[106] Neuritic or senile plaques and lipofuscin accumulation are additional cellular hallmarks of aging. A *senile plaque* is a thickened mass of degenerating *neurites* (small axons, some dendrites, astrocytes) with an *amyloid* (starchy glycoprotein) deposit in the center.

The role of lipofuscin in normal aging and as a risk factor for AD has been studied and reviewed.[126] Lipofuscin, a byproduct of cell metabolism, is a pigment associated with aging. It accumulates in all cells of the brain. It is also deposited in other tissues of the body such as the heart and gut. Lipofuscin is found within postmitotic cells and is a main marker of brain vulnerability, oxidative stress, and dementia-related pathologies. At first, it was considered a harmless hallmark of aging; however, its presence has now been found to be detrimental as it continually accumulates in cells. The latest evidence shows that lipofuscin accumulation strongly correlates with the excessive production of reactive oxygen, which prevents lipofuscin from being removed by the normal biological recycling mechanisms. This generates a cascade of negative events at a subcellular level. The negative effects are exerted at the DNA level, which culminate in a dysregulation of the cell's normal function. The internal function of the cells is interrupted and causes abnormal gene expression. Mitochondria also incur structural alterations, which lead to a reduction in ATP synthesis, which generates an increase in free radicals.[127]

On a biochemical level, the loss of enzymes involved in neurotransmitter synthesis has been documented along with a moderate loss of receptor sites for certain neurotransmitters in both the CNS and the PNS.[128] A decline in motor system performance has been linked to a steady decrease in dopamine uptake sites because of an age-related loss of axons in basal ganglia pathways.[129] Loss of serotonin receptors in the cortex has been postulated to predispose older individuals to depression and cognitive impairment.[130] Specifically, the muscarinic type of cholinergic receptors decreases by 50%–60% in the caudate, putamen, hippocampus, and frontal cortex between the ages of 4 and 93 years.[131] The declines in the serotonergic and cholinergic systems play a role in cognitive decline associated with pathological aging.

Modest declines in dopamine content of the basal ganglia have been measured after midlife.[131] This 25% loss is in sharp contrast to the losses exhibited with severe lesions involving the basal ganglia or in Parkinson disease. The age-related alterations in the basal ganglia resemble those that occur in Parkinson disease, but the cell dropout is not as severe. Despite the similarity of brain cell degeneration, the causes for the changes are likely to be different.[132]

Aging changes in the ANS can be linked to changes in the sensitivity of sympathetic receptors to circulating neurotransmitters. *Aging* has been described as a hyper-adrenergic state (high adrenaline) because of the more intense cardiac and vascular sympathetic responses seen in older adults.[133,134] In a review by Seals and Esler,[135] an age-related increase in total body sympathetic nervous system activity was reaffirmed. This increase is region specific and includes the gut, skeletal muscle vasculature, heart, and liver as targets but not the kidneys.[136] Less epinephrine (adrenaline) is released from the adrenal medulla in older adults at rest and in response to stress.[137] Plasma levels of noradrenaline (norepinephrine) increase 10%–15% per decade over the adult age range.[137]

Peripherally, over age 60, the loss of motor neurons and myelinated anterior root fibers contributes significantly to the gradual loss of muscle mass and strength seen with aging.[138] Decreased awareness of touch and vibration are two documented peripheral changes that occur after the age of 60.[139,140] Sensory changes are discussed more thoroughly in Chapter 9. The concept of "use it or lose it" cannot be overlooked when assessing the competence of any body system to adapt over time. It is especially true for the nervous system. As we age, lifestyles and habits formed early in life will be what motivate, inspire, and provide an impetus to move. If exercise, fitness, and health are valued and the individual stays physically fit and actively participates in life, how will the outcome differ?

FUNCTIONAL IMPLICATIONS

Two aspects of nervous system function—reaction time and cognition—are used to illustrate the relationship between nervous system development and acquisition of function. Reaction time is a measure of nervous system efficiency during movement. *Cognition* is the function of our brain that enables interaction with the environment. It is a complex brain function, whereas *reaction time* is a simple function. Both aspects of nervous system function—cognition and reaction time—change over time.

Reaction Time

The batter sees the ball, swings, and hits the ball. *Reaction time* is defined as the amount of time between the presentation of a stimulus and the motor response. Reaction time consists of three parts: (1) sensory transmission of input, (2) motor execution time, and (3) central processing.[141] The latter component makes up 80% of the total reaction time. Reaction time requires attention because attention is a prerequisite for sensory information to get into WM, a concept that is discussed under cognition. Investigators using electromyography separate premotor time from motor time. *Premotor time* (PMT) is the time between the stimulus and electromyographic activity and reflects the neural components of reaction time. PMT represents components 1 and 3. *Motor time* (MT) is defined as the time between the electromyographic activity and the movement and therefore reflects the muscular component of reaction time.

As would be expected, the reaction time of children is slower than that of adults. Reaction time improves throughout childhood and into adolescence.[142] There is a substantial decrease in reaction time until the age of 9–10 years with a more gradual reduction beyond that time. In a recent study of motor and nonmotor processes, researchers[143] found that the components of reaction time (PMT and MT) develop at the same rate throughout childhood and adolescence. Physical maturation affects information processing speed in 9- and 10-year-olds, with early maturers being faster than late maturers.[144] Processing speed relative to cognitive tasks also increases in childhood with significant gain seen between 9 and 10 years and 11 and 12 years.[142] Reaction time peaks in young adulthood at age 24[145] and then declines.[146]

Both premotor and motor times are related to chronological age. PMT (the neural component) is slower in all older individuals regardless of the task. MT (the motor component) depends more on the type of task, especially the amount of muscular force required. Simple tasks such as hand movement show more age-related effects on the premotor time;[147] jumping[148] and movement against resistance[149] show more age-related effects on the motor time. The more complicated the task, the more likely it is to be influenced by age-related change. In general, the more complicated the decision or task, the bigger is the difference seen in the reaction time of young and older adults.[150]

Complex or choice reaction time studies involve a choice between two responses. Light and Spirduso[151] confirmed that as the task becomes more complex, reaction time increases with the increasing age of the individual. In a complex task such as trying to recover balance, an individual's risk of falling increases with age. After the age of 60, reaction time variability increases relative to that of younger individuals. When Fozard and colleagues[152] compared simple and choice reaction times in a group of men and women ranging in age from 20 to 90 years, however, they found only a slight slowing of simple reaction time but a more dramatic slowing in choice reaction time. Ebiad and associates[153] found that the decline in cognitive processing speed across the life span was not completely explained by a decline in motor reaction time.

Health and exercise may modify age-related changes in reaction time.[154] When the level of PA of the individual is considered, active older subjects have been found to have faster reaction times than sedentary older subjects.[155] Also, variability within older subjects increases such that on a day-to-day basis, responses are not as consistent as they are in younger individuals. The rate of slowing depends a great deal on the task. Thus, results involving reaction time in the elderly must be regarded cautiously.

Fitness training has positive benefits on both peripheral and central aspects of reaction time. Response times are faster for those individuals who had engaged in exercise for long periods of their lives. Those who exercised performed better than those who did not exercise on reasoning and WM tasks. Training improved the performance of older adults engaged in multiple tasks. These improvements were retained for several months.[156] The aging brain generates new neurons in response to physical exercise, and it is thought that learning selectively enhances synaptogenesis well into adulthood.[25,157] PA also enhances the vascular response of the brain.[25]

Cognition

Cognition is the process of knowing and the application of that knowledge is intelligence. Cognitive processes include selective attention, learning, and memory. The ability to change the structure of the nervous system in response to experience is the basis for learning and memory.[2,158] EFs performed by the brain involve goal-directed, conscious decision-making, and strategy selection. These functions require attention to select features on which to make decisions, to resolve conflicts, and to plan new actions.

Selective Attention/Self-Control

Selective or focal attention is related to a person's ability to assess the many conflicting details of the environment and self and then make choices that influence cognitive and emotional function. The attention network includes the frontal, parietal, and cingulate cortex.[10] Posner and Rothbart[159] posited that the ability to attend develops during the first year of life and is initially demonstrated by the infant's self-regulation of her own distress. Infants can consistently self-calm at 3–4 months when their attention is distracted. They further hypothesized that the mechanism used by infants to cope with feelings of distress, or self-regulate, is transferred and applied to the control of cognition during later infancy and childhood.[159]

The development of self-control begins in infancy with the regulation of distress and involves interaction between areas in the frontal lobe, specifically the cingulate and the amygdala. For example, an 18-month-old shows context-sensitive learning when visually attending to surroundings. Spatial locations are learned when the frontal areas of the brain develop a functional visual field. Self-control is needed for attention, and attention is needed for learning. Executive attention undergoes a dramatic change around 30 months of age. Patterns of response change, with older children becoming more accurate. Casey and co-workers[160] showed a significant correlation between the ability to perform tasks that relied on attentional control and the size of the right anterior cingulate in children aged 5.3–16 years. Further refinement of the attentional system occurs in adulthood. The development of self-control progresses slowly in early life, continues throughout adolescence, and becomes inconsistent during adulthood.[159]

Memory

Memory is necessary for learning and plays a pivotal role in information processing and therefore cognition. Memories can be categorized by what is remembered and how long the memory lasts. The three major types of memories are *procedural memory*, *declarative memory*, and *working memory* (see Table 8.6). The first two types are also known by the terms implicit and explicit. *Procedural memory* is the memory of doing and does not usually require conscious attention. *Declarative memory* involves memory for facts and events and requires conscious effort, that is attention, to be recalled. Memories can be considered *immediate*, *short-term*, or *long-term* depending on

TABLE 8.6 Types of Memory			
Type of Memory	Procedural/Implicit	Declarative/Explicit	Working
Information	Skilled movements and habits	Facts, general knowledge, events, concepts, and location	Goal-relevant information
Neural substrate	Frontal cortex, thalamus, basal ganglia	Lateral prefrontal cortex and medial temporal lobe	Prefrontal and temporoparietal association cortex
Development	Begins first few months of life	Begins at 8–12 months	Begins at 8–12 months and increases to 6–24 years
Examples	Priming Associative learning-conditioning	Event sequence Novelty preference	Relate past events to present

Data from Nelson CA. The ontogeny of human memory: a cognitive neuroscience perspective, *Dev Psychol.* 1995;31:723–738; Purves D, Nelson CA. The nature of early memory. *Prev Med.* 1998;27:172–179; Lundy-Ekman L. *Neuroscience: Fundamentals for Rehabilitation.* 5th ed. St. Louis: Elsevier; 2018; and Camina E, Güell F. The neuroanatomical, neurophysiological and psychological basis of memory: current models and their origins. *Front Pharmacol.* 2017;8:438.

their duration. Immediate memories last for only a few seconds or a few minutes. Short-term memories can last for days or weeks but will eventually be lost if they are not converted to long-term memory. *Working memory* is a type of short-term memory. Long-term memory can be recalled years later and is the result of structural changes at the level of the synapses that influence signal conduction.[161]

Development of Memory

The development of memory occurs throughout life (Table 8.6). Before 6 months of age, there is no conscious memory, only a learned adaptive response. After 6 months of age, an infant learns object permanence, so the infant knows that an object does not disappear when it is out of sight. Conscious, declarative memory is demonstrated as early as 7 months, but verbal recall of events is minimal until a child is about 3 years of age. Place learning, which is dependent on the hippocampus, has been demonstrated in toddlers after the age of 20 months but not before that age.[162] The volume of the hippocampus formation increases sharply to age 2 and increases slowly thereafter until the age of 12. Between 5 and 7 years of age, the child begins to relate past and present memories and to reason more efficiently.[163] Children no longer just monitor perceptual information, such as size, shape, and color, but correlate perceptual information (e.g., "all round objects made of rubber bounce, whereas round stones do not"). They continue to pick up and reflect on salient perceptual cues to solve increasingly complex problems or to perform tasks after the age of 6 or 7 years.[164]

Children's learning capabilities change with age. Memories increase between the ages of 6 and 12 years.[165] Conscious memory is related to the linguistic ability of the child. Verbal comprehension, a measure of semantic memory, is associated with school performance in children 8–10 years of age.[166] WM improves steadily until around 11 years and then levels off according to one study.[165] However, a systematic review concluded that WM ability continues to mature through puberty and into early adulthood.[167] Around the age of 9 or 10 years, children begin to direct their thinking. They can evaluate, plan, and refine their own thinking about how best to solve a problem. Being able to think about thinking is called *metacognition*, a term that subsumes elaborate EFs. The ability to think about remembering is called *metamemory*. We practice metacognition when encountering a patient with an undefined movement dysfunction and thinking of ways to approach the patient's problem. We practice metamemory when planning for a test by reviewing what one does and does not know. Children at 10–12 have recall abilities comparable to adults.[168]

With aging, there is a decrease in complex cognitive skills involving memory. A linear decline in episodic memory occurs with age.[169,170] Furthermore, women scored higher than their male counterparts up to the age of 70.[169] Remembering details of events such as a birthday party or lunch with a friend is often poorer in older adults. Event perception and memory may be changed based on prior familiarity with the event, which leads to poorer encoding of the event memory (Wahlheim and Zacks 2019)[171]. Older adults do not always detect changes that occur from one episode to the next.

A relatively constant performance in semantic and perceptual representation memory tasks with increasing age has been reported.[169] However, another study showed sematic memory declines later in life.[172] Prospective memory such as remembering to take medicine before going to bed declines with age.[173] As procedural memory is motor memory, the inconsistencies may be related to the tasks used to test this type of memory. If the tasks involve aspects of short-term memory, there might be a decline with age. If the task used in testing is purely procedural, it would only require activation of the primary motor cortex, which is relatively well preserved in older adults.[170]

WM is most affected by aging because information must not only be retained but also be manipulated or changed to be retrieved. New information can be registered and retrieved, but new information is forgotten more quickly. The speed with which information is processed slows with age and is a fundamental cause of age-related decline in memory.[85] This activity requires that information storage occurs at the same time as acquisition of new data, something that is difficult for the older learner. Older adults appear to have to redistribute resources from storage to allocation to keep up. The decline of both verbal and visual-spatial WM occurs in older adults. Pliatsikas and colleagues[174] found these changes were modulated by educational level and gender. With increasing age, males show a sharper decline in WM than females, but with increasing education females display greater gains in WM than males.

Intelligence

Cognition is functionally reflected in intelligence and development of EF. Horn and Donaldson[175] described two types of intellectual ability: fluid intelligence and crystallized intelligence Fig. 8.16 *Fluid intelligence* is the ability to form novel associations, to reason logically, and to solve problems. It can be measured by looking at reaction time and memory. Fluid intelligence peaks in the early 20s and declines throughout adulthood. WM is strongly correlated to fluid intelligence.[176] *Crystallized intelligence* is experiential learning, education, and stored information. It is the ability to use judgment to decide on a course of action. This type of intelligence incorporates a lifetime of decision-making and is postulated to improve with age.[175]

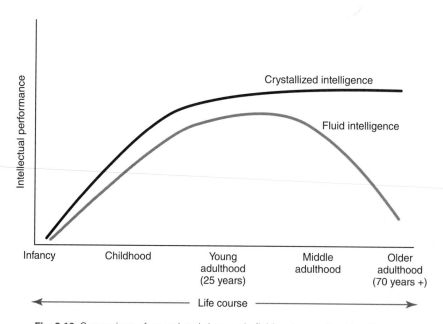

Fig. 8.16 Comparison of age-related changes in fluid and crystallized intelligence.

According to measures of intelligence, intellectual ability peaks between ages 20 and 30 and is maintained until around the age of 60[177] or 70[178] years of age. Despite all we do know about the aging changes related to cognition or intelligence, we do not understand why some older individuals remain alert, sharp, and active participants in the world around them and others lose touch, disengage, or show signs of dementia. Mild intellectual changes seen in later life that are considered "normal" include (1) slowing of reaction time or cognitive processing speed, (2) decline in fluid intelligence, and (3) impairment in some aspects of short-term memory.[153,170]

There are incredible differences in cognitive aging due to the heterogeneity in older adults. In an update of the Betula study, Nyberg and colleagues[85] identified mechanisms that could explain the individual differences seen in cognitive aging among older adults. One mechanism, cognitive reserve, is discussed in Chapter 2. Average onset of cognitive changes occurs around the age of 60 with episodic long-term memory being more sensitive to decline than other types of long-term memory.[83] With aging, the epigenetic regulation of memory becomes dysfunctional and the risk of memory decline increases (Creighton et al., 2020).[179,238] The neuronal epigenome is crucial for the formation of long-lasting memories. The exact mechanisms for these epigenetic changes have not been fully elucidated.

Gazzaley and colleagues[180] looked at the effect of high memory load and distraction on older adults' ability to perform a delayed recognition and recall task. Results showed that as the memory load increases, the older adult makes more errors in recognition. The frontal lobes are affected early by aging, and the PFC is involved with preserving memories in the face of distractions.[181] Changes in memory abilities need to be considered when giving verbal direction to older patients with movement dysfunction. Written instructions that parallel the verbal instructions are often critical to provide adequate carryover in a home program.

Executive Function

Looking at the development of EF and its components will provide an overview of the changes that occur in the brain over the life span. Diamond[176] identified the core triad of components of EF (Fig. 8.17). The components are WM, inhibitory control, and cognitive flexibility. WM and its subcomponents (verbal memory and visual spatial memory) and inhibitory control and its subcomponents (self-control and interference) were discussed previously. Cognitive flexibility is sometimes described

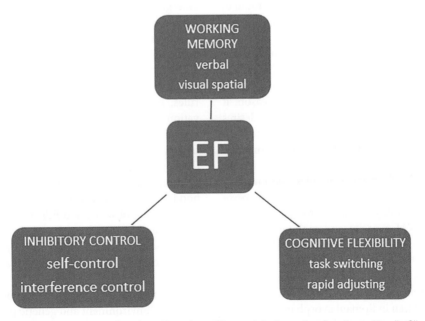

Fig. 8.17 A model of executive function. (Data from Diamond A. Executive functions. *Handb Clin Neurol.* 2020;173:225–240.)

TABLE 8.7   **Development of Executive Function**

Age Period	Working Memory	Inhibitory Control	Cognitive Flexibility
Infancy 0–2	3½- to 5-month-old infants can maintain representations of hidden objects	Evidence seen in reaching behavior in second half of the first year of life	Means and behavior indicates planning in 8- to 12-month-old infants
Preschool 2–3 years 3–5 years	Rigid Sorting by shape or color	Rigid in task performance Impulse control improves up to 6 years	Inflexible thinking Can change perspective (Theory of Mind)
Middle childhood 6–11 years	Continued and marked improvement	Speed and accuracy changes during task performance. 9-year-olds can monitor and regulate own actions	Increased scores on Wisconsin Card Sorting Test Rapidly developing organizational skills between 7 and 10 years of age
Adolescence 12–18/20 years	Continued gradual improvement	Continued improvement	Not at adult level at 13 years
Adulthood 20 years	Continues to mature into early adulthood	Adult level achieved	Adult level achieved

From Anderson P. Assessment and development of executive function (EF) during childhood. *Child Neuropsychol*. 2002;8(2): 71–82; Davidson MC, Amso D, Anderson LC, et al. Development of cognitive control and executive functions from 4 to 13 years: evidence from manipulations of memory, inhibition, and task switching. *Neuropsychologia* 2006;44:2037–2078; Andre J, Picchioni M, Zhang R, Toulopoulou T. Working memory circuit as a function of increasing age in healthy adolescence: a systematic review and meta-analyses. *Neuroimage Clin*. 2016;12:940–948; and Diamond A. Executive functions. *Handb Clin Neurol*. 2020;173:225–240.

as mental flexibility. Its subcomponents are switching between different tasks or mindsets and quickly adjusting to a change of topics or finding an alternate route to a goal. See Table 8.7 for a brief developmental overview of the three components of EF.

"The development of the brain throughout infancy, childhood and adolescence is paralleled by the growth and maturation of the mind."[182] Theory of mind refers to the ability of a person to understand and reason. It implies that the person can appreciate how the desires and intentions of others are the same or different from her own. Children below the age of 4 do not demonstrate this ability. EF can be positively impacted enrichment experiences. For example, being exposed to speaking two languages in the home during infancy leads to an increase in EF.[183] Musical training is more strongly associated with heightened WM capacity and maintenance than enhanced WM updating, especially in late childhood and early adolescence.[184] Conversely, stress early in life can produce EF deficits in children, adolescents, and adults.[158] A frequently used example of this is the negative effects of neglect seen in children in Romanian orphanages.[185]

Davidson and associates[186] looked at cognitive flexibility in children from 4 to 13 years of age. The ability to switch responses requires inhibition of previously learned responses and WM. This ability begins to emerge between 3 and 4 years of age.[187] The child can handle more complicated tasks between 7 and 9 years, with gains continuing into early adolescence but not achieving adult levels.[186]

Puberty is a critical period for development of social cognition. Social cognition is the knowledge of social rules, norms, or behaviors usually learned by observation of others. Social cognition and EF both have extended developmental trajectories along with the frontal neural networks that support their continued development. EF is needed as the adolescent transitions to more independence and autonomy in early adulthood. Taylor and colleagues[188] assessed the longitudinal development of social and EFs in a group of older adolescents and young adults. Social cognition was found to be relatively stable by 17 years and beyond while EF continued to improve in the areas of planning, inhibition, and rule detection. Remodeling of the cortex during adolescence has functional implications for adult development. "Environment and genetic programming interact to regulate synaptic organization during the critical period resulting in a mature cortex."[189] Behaviorally, a teen's performance on tasks involving decision-making, WM, processing speed, and inhibitory control improves during adolescence.[190,191] These tasks represent different facets of EF and reflect pruning of synapses, network reorganization, and myelination. Optimal function of the PFC supports the interaction of the limbic system and the executive network in the dorsolateral PFC. The interplay of the two promotes emotional regulation, using past experience to understand new situations, and making rational decisions.

The PFC is sensitive to environmental influences such as early initiation of drinking and binge drinking.[192] These two patterns of alcohol use increase the adolescent's vulnerability to later alcohol abuse. Functional imaging studies have shown that binge drinking disrupts WM and EF, and triggers impulsive behavior.[193,194] Fig. 8.18 is a model of the effect that alcohol abuse has on adolescent and adult development. This is different from those adolescents exposed to alcohol during fetal development and who have a fetal alcohol spectrum disorder (FASD). This model suggests that interventions to reduce adolescent drinking will improve abilities and reduce the likelihood of addiction.

Adult EF appears to depend on a set of interrelated cortical and cerebellar regions that are also involved in early motor skill acquisition. "The cerebellum and prefrontal cortex participate as critical parts of a neural circuit that is important when (1) a cognitive task is difficult as opposed to easy, (2) a cognitive task is new as opposed to familiar and practiced, (3) conditions of the cognitive task change, as opposed to when they remain stable and predictable, (4) a quick response is required, as opposed to longer response latencies being acceptable, and (5) one must concentrate instead of being able to operate on 'automatic pilot.'[195] Ridler and co-workers[196] showed that the frontocerebellar system used for EF is anatomically related to systems associated with typical infant motor development. They looked at two groups of adults: one group had schizophrenia and the other were nonpsychotic. The group with earlier motor skill development had superior EF, while the group with delayed motor skill development had impaired EF. The researchers concluded that adult executive systems emerge developmentally by integrating additional cerebellar regions which had previously matured in support of early motor skills.[196]

WM decline has been associated with normal aging in older adults. A decline in WM directly affects EF. The frontal brain structure responsible for this decline is primarily located in the PFC.[197] Neuroimaging studies have shown that when older adults perform WM tasks there tends to be greater bilateral frontal activity than

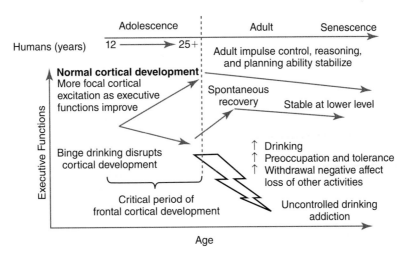

Fig. 8.18 A schematic diagram of how adolescent alcohol abuse disrupts frontal cortical development and maturation of executive function. The upward narrowing arrow emphasizes the normal focusing of cortical excitation during cognitive tasks that occurs during the transition from adolescence to adulthood. The model suggests that interventions to reduce adolescent drinking will improve abilities and reduce addiction. (From Crews F, He J, Hodge C. Adolescent cortical development: a critical period of vulnerability for addition. *Pharmacol Biochem Behav.* 2007;86:189–199.)

in younger adults. Berryhill and Jones[198] found evidence for differential frontal recruitment as a function of strategy when older adults perform WM tasks. Results from Nissim et al.[199] demonstrated an increase in connectivity between the two frontal lobe structures during-active transcranial direct current stimulation (tDCS). Subregions of the frontal lobe have been shown to be essential for manipulation of verbal and spatial knowledge. The prefrontal cortex has exhibited enhanced activity during various cognitive control processes such as selection, maintenance, and retrieval of goal-directed information. The prefrontal cortex has also shown critical involvement during task delay periods and facilitates the ability to keep task-relevant information active, in addition to manipulating that information to accomplish the task. In older adults, both prefrontal cortexes demonstrate enhanced activity in cognitive control processes such as monitoring, manipulating, or processing goal-directed information, all of which are vital to WM. The results of this study demonstrated that acute bilateral frontal tDCS selectively modulates functional brain connectivity in the WM network of older adults, which is not found in younger adults.[199]

Exercise and Cognition

Exercise appears to mediate cognitive changes in the brain that occur from aging. Erickson and colleagues[27] in a review of the 2018 PA guidelines concluded that there was moderate evidence to support the association of moderate-to-vigorous intensity PA with improvements in EF, cognition, processing speed, and memory. There was moderate evidence that PA improves cognitive function in individuals with disorders that impair cognitive function such as a Parkinson disease. Based on observational prospective studies, there was strong evidence for PA being associated with a reduced risk of cognitive decline and dementia, including AD.

Possible protective factors for AD include increased education level, increased mental activity, increased PA/exercise, socialization, intact hearing, nutrition, and conscientiousness.[200–203] There was a 50% drop in risk with individuals who walked 6–9 miles/week. If you have a high level of fitness in your 40s, or maybe even earlier than that, your likelihood of developing AD later on is definitely reduced.[204,205] Exercise and cardiorespiratory fitness are associated with a healthy brain. Exercise increases neurotrophic factor, enhances neuronal survival, increases synaptic development and plasticity, and

may mediate amyloid cascade by decreasing production.[206] Exercise can delay dementia onset and slow the progression of dementia.[206] Starting exercise or PA later in life leads to a reduction in rates of dementia by 37%.[207] Researchers from the Boston University School of Medicine found that people with poor physical fitness in their 40s have significantly lower brain volumes by the time they reach age 60.[208] This decrease in brain volume is a sign of accelerated aging of the brain. The study reviewed exercise data from more than 1200 adults who were around the age of 40, all of whom were part of the larger Framingham Heart Study.[96,209] When these participants were given MRI scans 20 years later, those who were less fit in midlife had much lower levels of brain tissue later on. See Chapter 13 for more information on beneficial effects of exercise.

Atypical Nervous System Development

Typical life span course of the nervous system can be perturbed anywhere along its developmental path. Two examples of disruption of the nervous system are FASDs and AD. These examples provide a marked contrast to typical development in one case and a possible variant of aging in the other case.

Fetal Alcohol Spectrum Disorders

FASDs represent an umbrella designation encompassing the full range of observed outcomes in individuals who experience prenatal alcohol exposure (PAE). PAE is associated with dysfunction of the placenta and higher rates of premature births.[210] Alcohol exposure in any amount during pregnancy is detrimental to neural development.[211,212] Twenty to 30% of pregnant women continue to drink alcohol, with more than 8% reporting frequent or binge drinking.[213] Binge drinking is more detrimental to the fetus than chronic low levels of drinking because it takes the fetus days to detoxify what the mother's liver can dissipate in hours.[214] Lange and colleagues[215] estimated that 1 of every 13 pregnant women who drank alcohol during pregnancy had a child with FASD. Furthermore, the prevalence of FASD is higher than some common birth defects in the United States such as DS and spina bifida. FASD is the result of altered neural plasticity. Development of functional maps of the sensory cortex and the visual cortex, as well as the frontal lobes, is disrupted by alcohol exposure.

The spectrum of FASDs ranges from mild to severe along a continuum. Jones and Smith[216] coined the term FAS in 1973 by describing a triad of signs: facial dysmorphology, prenatal and postnatal growth disturbance, and CNS deficits including intellectual disability. The facial features are shown in Fig. 8.19 and consist of short palpebral fissures, short nose, an elongated midface, wide-set eyes, thin upper lip, and a long, undefined philtrum (area between the nose and upper lip). Children with FAS show decreases in both weight and length/height, characteristically falling below the 10th percentile for age.[217] Neurobehavioral impairments in FAS can range in severity from global intellectual disability to a behavioral impairment without intellectual disability.[217] Higher rates of FAS are seen in high-risk groups: those with lower socioeconomic status; those of racial and ethnic minority populations such as Native American; and children in foster care.[215] FAS and FASDs are the most common nonheritable causes of intellectual disability[218] and are a major public health problem.[219,220] It should be noted that FAS is a diagnosis of exclusion.[221] Despite an update in diagnostic clinical guidelines for FASD,[217] it has been difficult to definitively diagnose FASD before the age 5. Earlier diagnosis is crucial for being able to initiate

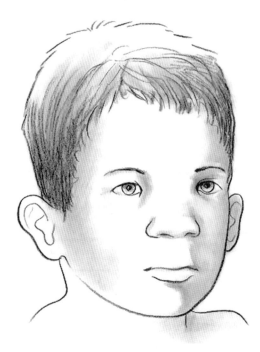

Fig. 8.19 Characteristic facial features of a child with fetal alcohol syndrome. (From Ratliffe KT. *Clinical Pediatric Physical Therapy*. St. Louis: Mosby; 1998:331.)

early intervention for those with FASD. PAE results in problems during middle childhood and adolescence, especially in the areas of EF and social interaction. Six to 13-year-olds with PAE performed poorly on tests of interpersonal skills, use of play and leisure time, and coping skills compared to non-exposed children with similar IQs.[222] Rockhold and associates[223] studied the relationship between EF and social function (SF) deficits in a group of preschool and adolescent children with PAE. They found that the relationship between deficits in SF and EF was present in the adolescent group with PAE but not present in the adolescent control group nor in the preschool PAE group. At the 4-year follow-up, preschool participants were found to display this relationship. See the Clinical Implications Box 8.1 for further information regarding how alcohol can affect development across the life span.

Mild Cognitive Impairment and Alzheimer Disease

A major reason that memory loss is so feared by the elderly is because of the association between memory loss and AD. Mild cognitive impairment (MCI) lies somewhere between normal aging and dementia and affects 15% of the nondemented population.[228] Some older adults with MCI have more memory or other cognitive problems than other people of the same age. Both normal aging and MCI are associated with everyday functional memory problems. People with MCI can usually take care of themselves and perform their normal activities.[229] Both groups may have difficulty learning new names, recalling events that happened in the previous day or two, retrieving the name of an old acquaintance, coming up with a specific word in conversation, remembering why one walked into a room, and/or remembering to take medications on time.[230] The main qualitative difference in memory patterns for normal aging and MCI is that the latter show relatively rapid forgetting of newly learned information or decreased retention rates over time. By definition, individuals with MCI have greater memory impairments than same-aged individuals with normal cognitive changes; on average, the memory deficit in MCI is about one to two standard deviations below the mean for age. Memory patterns in MCI more closely resemble those of patients with Alzheimer dementia than those of normal aging.[231] MCI may be an early sign of AD, but not everyone with MCI will develop AD.

CLINICAL IMPLICATIONS BOX 8.1
Alcohol and Development

Use and abuse of alcohol take a huge toll on the health of individuals across the life span. Alcohol is a teratogen and therefore can cause birth defects if ingested during pregnancy. "Alcohol use disorders are the most prevalent substance use disorders in the United States." Alcohol abuse is a public health problem of gargantuan proportions. This clinical box highlights some of the issues related to alcohol use from a developmental perspective.[192,211,212,224]

Prenatal
- Fetal alcohol syndrome is the most severe of the four disorders that comprise fetal alcohol spectrum disorders.
- Prenatal exposure to alcohol puts the developing fetus at risk for developmental disabilities.
- Prenatal exposure puts the individual at risk for alcohol abuse later in life.
- Fetal alcohol spectrum disorders are totally preventable.

Infancy
- Babies can be exposed to alcohol when breastfed.
- Contrary to popular belief, use of alcohol by a lactating mother decreases milk production and disrupts important hormones involved in supporting lactation.
- Prenatal and postnatal exposure to flavors and odors, including alcohol, can predispose to behaviors and preferences during infancy and childhood.

Childhood/Adolescence
- The onset of drinking occurs in middle school.
- Half of adolescents are active drinkers.
- Adolescents are less sensitive to the sedative effects of alcohol but more sensitive to the memory disruptions caused by alcohol ingestion.
- Being insensitive to the intoxicating effects of alcohol has been shown to predict later problems with alcohol, as well as being a characteristic of persons at genetic risk for alcoholism.
- Binge drinking may lead to long-term changes in executive function because of the disruption of the neuromaturation of numerous brain regions, such as the hippocampus, prefrontal cortex, and the limbic system.

- Alcohol is involved in 1519 deaths in college-age students.[225]
- Nine percent of college students meet the criteria for having an alcohol use disorder according to a 2019 national survey.[226]
- A college-age student's brain is still developing and at risk for further damage from over-imbibing.

Adults
- Twenty to 30% of pregnant women used alcohol, and more than 8% engaged in binge drinking according to a survey by the Substance Abuse and Mental Health Services Administration.[213]
- More than half of the women of childbearing age did not use birth control and used alcohol, and 8% reported binge drinking.
- Prenatal alcohol use is one of the leading preventable causes of developmental disabilities.

Older Adults
- Alcohol misuse in older adults increases the likelihood of physical and mental problems.
- The Dietary Guidelines for Americans 2020–2050 state that moderate drinking is two drinks a day or less for men and one drink or less a day for women. The National Institute on Alcohol Abuse and Alcoholism recommends that persons over 65 years of age limit themselves to only one drink a day.[227]
- Twenty percent of older adults (60–64) and 11% of those over age 65 surveyed nationally reported being "binge drinkers," which is drinking five or more drinks on one occasion at least 12 times in the previous year.
- Alcohol use in the elderly is a public health issue.
- Hazardous drinking is a pattern of alcohol consumption that carries a risk of harmful consequences to the drinker or others.
- Harmful drinking is a pattern of drinking that causes physical or mental damage to the drinker's health but without being dependent.

Alzheimer Disease

AD is a progressive neurodegenerative disease marked by deficits in episodic memory, WM, and EF. Examples of executive dysfunction include poor selective and divided attention, failed inhibition of interfering stimuli, and poor math and verbal skills. AD is the most common form of dementia, accounting for up to 50%–70% of all forms of dementia.[232] Over 6 million people have been diagnosed with AD.[232] The number of individuals with AD is expected to rise to 14–16 million by 2050. Prevalence of AD doubles with each decade after the age of 65. A positive family history significantly increases the risk of developing AD. One first-degree relative increases the risk by 4 times, two or more increase the risk by 40 times. Five to 10% of cases of AD have a positive family history. AD is more common in African Americans and Hispanics (0.5% develop AD at the age of 60, 10%–13% at age 70, and 10%–30% at age 80).[232] Incidence may be as high as 50% at age 85. AD is 2.8 times more prevalent in females, possibly due to their longer life span. AD is progressive and irreversible.[232] Over 50% of skilled nursing facility (SNF) residents have AD and two-thirds of SNF residents have cognitive impairments. Life expectancy is decreased by 3 years with a diagnosis of AD. Diabetes mellitus is linked to a 65% increased risk of developing AD.[233]

Females have an increased risk of developing AD. After menopause, the drop in estrogen negatively influences brain processes that increase the risk of developing AD.[234] Estrogen supplementation decreases the prevalence of AD, but may be unsafe for cardiovascular health.[235] There may be a critical period when estrogen replacement alone may be beneficial for cognitive function in women. "Estrogen levels affect spine density on pyramidal neurons in the prefrontal cortex; these neurons may provide many of the same circuits implicated in AAMI [age-associated memory impairment]."[236] Therefore there appears to be an interaction between reproductive and neural senescence.

Clinical features of AD include progressive cognitive decline, short-term memory loss, delayed free recall and cognition, decreased EF, difficulty following simple commands, and increased distractibility. Other clinical features are decreased judgment, insight, and empathy. Language problems include aphasia, anomia, reading, and comprehension. Many patients deny they have any problems at all. Individuals with AD retain their social skills early on, but later experience physical and personality changes such as lack of inhibition and paranoia.[232] Prognosis for individuals with AD disease is poor. Medication can only slow progression, not reverse it. The cause of death is usually due to complications. The time of onset to the time of death usually spans 7–11 years. AD is listed as the sixth cause of death in the United States, and fifth overall in individuals over the age of 65. The younger the diagnosis, the faster the disease progresses.[232]

Age and genetics are two risk factors for the development of AD. With increased age comes an increased risk of AD; the prevalence goes up with each decade. Aging contributes to an increased potential for neuronal injury. The presence of neurofibrillary (tau) tangles (NFT) inside the neurons and of amyloid plaques outside the neurons are hallmarks of AD neuropathology. The genes associated with the amyloid precursor protein on chromosome 21 and presenilin-1 and presenilin-2 are involved in only a small percentage of cases of AD but are common in Trisomy 21 or DS. These individuals have an earlier onset of AD, before the age of 60. About 30% of people with DS who are in their 50s have AD. About 50% of people with DS in their 60s have AD.[237]

AD is associated with the loss of synaptic connection, neuronal death and atrophy of cerebral cortex, and acetylcholine depletion. On autopsy, amyloid plaques and NFT are evident. The amyloid plaques disrupt communications between nerve cells, cause death, and reduce the amount of acetylcholine available. Severity of cognitive decline correlates more closely to NFTs rather than the amount of amyloid. The area of the brain affected may differ, but the hippocampus is usually affected first (memories). Parietal and frontal lobe degeneration cause impaired judgment, and the parietal and limbic regions cause psychiatric symptoms. Motor problems can occur if the hypothalamus and cortex are affected. The 10 warning signs of AD are contrasted with typical age-related functional changes in Clinical Implications Box 8.2.

CLINICAL IMPLICATIONS BOX 8.2
Alzheimer Disease: Ten Early Signs

Alzheimer disease (AD) is the most common form of progressive degenerative dementia. There are presently 6.5 million people living with AD in the United States, and it is the sixth leading cause of death in adults.[232] Diagnosis is based on a history of progressive deterioration in at least two aspects of cognition, one of which is typically memory. The 10 early warning signs of AD are listed below and contrasted with typically age-related functional changes.[232]

Early Warning Signs

1. Memory loss that disrupts daily life
2. Challenges in planning or solving problems
3. Difficulty completing familiar tasks
4. Confusion with time or place
5. Trouble understanding visual images and spatial relationships
6. New problems with words in speaking or writing
7. Misplacing things and losing the ability to retrace steps
8. Decreased or poor judgment
9. Withdrawal from work or social activities
10. Changes in mood and personality

Typical Age-Related Changes[232]

- Sometimes forgetting names or appointments, but remembering them later.
- Making occasional errors when managing finances or household bills.
- Occasionally needing help to record a TV show or use microwave settings.
- Getting confused about the day of the week, but figuring it out later.
- Vision changes related to cataracts.
- Sometimes having trouble finding the right word.
- Misplacing things from time to time and retracing steps to find them.
- Making a bad decision once in a while, like neglecting to change the oil in the car.
- Sometimes feeling uninterested in family or social obligations.
- Developing very specific ways of doing things and becoming irritable when a routine is disrupted.

In summary, there is no clear line regarding normal cognitive aging. As people age, subtle changes in memory occur naturally as part of the aging process. However, sometimes these changes occur sooner than anticipated or faster than expected. These changes often go unnoticed, but at other times can be disturbing to ourselves or others. Changes are usually mild and affect visual and verbal memory. Normal cognitive aging affects more immediate memory and the ability to name objects. Age-associated memory impairments involve benign senescent forgetfulness, slower cognitive processing, minimum decline in executive functioning and memory, and ability to remember later.

SUMMARY

When looking at the function of the nervous system, we must understand that it is constantly changing in response to environmental demands, both from within and from without. The degree of adaptation and accommodation varies from one person to another. Movement, language, and cognitive changes that occur across the life span are based on the interaction between the structure and function of the nervous system that is mediated by epigenetic modification. Experience can produce structural changes within the nervous system. How and why we learn to move, talk, and think depends on the integrity of our nervous system. Our ability to learn about and to adapt to the environment reflects the neural plasticity of each individual's unique experiences and the impact that those experiences have on gene expression across the life span. Enriched environments have the potential to enhance development while physical or psychological stress can result in maladaptive development. Our ability to fully participate in life continues as long as our systems' reserves are maintained and not compromised by disease.

REFERENCES

1. Erikson EH. *Identity, Youth, and Crisis.* New York: WW Norton; 1968.
2. Donato F, Alberini CM, Amso D, Dragoi G, Dranovsky A, Newcombe NS. The ontogeny of hippocampus-dependent memories. *J Neurosci.* 2021;41:920–926.
3. Ismail FY, Fatemi A, Johnston MV. Cerebral plasticity: windows of opportunity in the developing brain. *Eur J Paediatr Neurol.* 2017;21:23–48.
4. Sweatt JD. Neural plasticity and behavior—sixty years of conceptual advances. *J Neurochem.* 2016;139(Suppl 2): 179–199.
5. Kessler M, Pitt J. Neuroanatomy. In: Kessler M, Martin S, eds. *Neurologic Interventions for Physical Therapy.* 4th ed. Philadelphia: Elsevier; 2021:12–40.
6. Volpe JJ. *Neurology of the Newborn.* 3rd ed. Philadelphia, PA: WB Saunders; 1995.
7. Sheikh AA, Mohamed A. Ependymal proliferation: a conduit for tricking the central nervous system into bio-engineering itself. *Biomed Sci Instrum.* 2015;51:309–314.
8. Gazdic M, Volarevic V, Harrell CR, et al. Stem cells therapy for spinal cord injury. *Int J Mol Sci.* 2018;19:1039. https://doi.org/10.3390/ijms19041039.
9. Fischl B, Dale AM. Measuring the thickness of the human cerebral cortex from magnetic resonance images. *Proc Natl Acad Sci U S A.* 2000;97:11050–11055. https://doi.org/10.1073/pnas.200033797.
10. Mtui E, Gruener G, Dockery P. *Fitzgerald's Clinical Neuroanatomy and Neuroscience.* 8th ed. Poland: Elsevier Limited; 2021.
11. Lundy-Ekman L. *Neuroscience: Fundamentals for Rehabilitation.* 5th ed. St. Louis, MO: Elsevier; 2018.
12. Dieterich M, Brandt T. The parietal lobe and the vestibular system. *Handb Clin Neurol.* 2018;151:119–140. https://doi.org/10.1016/B978-0-444-63622-5.00006-1.
13. Rolls ET. The cingulate cortex and limbic systems for emotion, action, and memory. *Brain Struct Funct.* 2019;224:3001–3018. https://doi.org/10.1007/s00429-019-01945-2.
14. Hiller-Sturmhöfel S, Bartke A. The endocrine system: an overview. *Alcohol Health Res World.* 1998;22:153–164.
15. Graybiel AM, Grafton ST. The striatum: where skills and habits meet. *Cold Spring Harb Perspect Biol.* 2015;7: a021691. https://doi.org/10.1101/cshperspect.a021691.
16. Tseng YW, Diedrichsen J, Krakauer JW, Shadmehr R, Bastian AJ. Sensory prediction errors drive cerebellum-dependent adaptation of reaching. *J Neurophysiol.* 2007;8:54–62. https://doi.org/10.1152/jn.00266.2007.
17. Jang SH, Kwon YH. Recovery of the ascending reticular activating system and consciousness following compre-hensive management in a patient with traumatic brain injury. *Yeungnam Univ J Med.* 2022;39(4):332–335.
18. Heiss CN, Olofsson LE. The role of gut microbiota in development, function and disorders of the central nervous system. *J Endocrinol.* 2019;31:e12684. https://doi.org/10.1111/jne.12684.
19. Rao M, Gershon MD. Enteric nervous system development: what could possibly go wrong? *Nat Rev Neurosci.* 2018;19:552–565.
20. Carlisle HJ, Kennedy MB. Spine architecture and synaptic plasticity. *Trends Neurosci.* 2005;28(4):182–187.
21. Lippman J, Dunaevsky A. Dendritic spine morphogenesis and plasticity. *J Neurobiol.* 2005;64(1):47–57.
22. Sukel K. Neurotransmission: Neurotransmitters. https://www.dana.org/wp-content/uploads/2019/05/fact-sheet-neurotransmission-neurotransmitters-baw-2020.pdf Accessed December 28, 2021.
23. Schmidt A, Jabusch H, Altenmüller E, et al. Etiology of musician's dystonia familial or environmental? *Neurology.* 2009;72:1248–1254. https://doi.org/10.1212/01.wnl.0000345670.63363.d1.
24. Bassi MS, Iezzi E, Gilio L, Centonze D, Buttari F. Synaptic plasticity shapes brain connectivity: implications for network topology. *In J Mol Sci.* 2019;20:6193. https://doi.org/10.3390/ijms20246193.
25. Anish EJ. Exercise and its effects on the central nervous system. *Curr Sports Med Rep.* 2005;4:18–23. https://doi.org/10.1097/01.csmr.0000306066.14026.77.
26. Carson Smith J, Erickson KI, Rao SM. Introduction to the JINS special issue: physical activity and brain plasticity. *J Int Neuropsychol Soc.* 2015;21:743–744. https://doi.org/10.1017/S1355617715001149.
27. Erickson KI, Hillman C, Stillman CM, et al. Physical activity, cognition, and brain outcomes: a review of the 2018 Physical Activity Guidelines. *Med Sci Sports Exerc.* 2019;51:1242–1251. https://doi.org/10.1249/MSS.0000000000001936.
28. D'Arcy MS. Cell death: a review of the major forms of apoptosis, necrosis and autophagy. *Cell Biol Int.* 2019;43: 582–592. https://doi.org/10.1002/cbin.11137.
29. Riccomagno MM, Kolodkin AL. Sculpting neural circuits by axon and dendrite pruning. *Annu Rev Cell Dev Biol.* 2015;31:779–805. https://doi.org/10.1146/annurev-cellbio-100913-013038.
30. Casey BJ, Jones RM, Hare TA. The adolescent brain. *Ann N Y Acad Sci.* 2008;1124:111–126.
31. Stavoe AKH, Holzbaur ELF. Autophagy in neurons. *Annu Rev Cell Dev Biol.* 2019;35:477–500. https://doi.org/10.1146/annurev-cellbio-100818-125242.
32. Mizushima N, Levine B, Cuervo AM, Klionsky DJ. Autophagy fights disease through cellular self-digestion. *Nature.* 2008;2008(451):1069–1075.

33. Valencia M, Kim SR, Jang Y, Lee SH. Neuronal autophagy: characteristic features and roles in neuronal pathophysiology. *Biomol Ther*. 2021;29:605–614.

34. Mattson MP, Arumugam TV. Hallmarks of brain aging: adaptive and pathological modification by metabolic states. *Cell Metab*. 2018;27:1176–1199. https://doi.org/10.1016/j.cmet.2018.05.011.

35. Sikora E, Bielak-Zmijewska A, Dudkowska M, et al. Cellular senescence in brain aging. *Front Aging Neurosci*. 2021;13:646924. https://doi.org/10.3389/fnagi.2021.646924.

36. Dvorak L, Mansfield PJ. *Essentials of Neuroanatomy for Rehabilitation*. Boston: Pearson; 2013.

37. Landers M. Treatment-induced neuroplasticity following focal injury to the motor cortex. *Int J Rehabil Res*. 2004;27:1–5.

38. Knikou M. Neural control of locomotion and training-induced plasticity after spinal and cerebral lesions. *Clin Neurophysiol*. 2010;121:1655–1668. https://doi.org/10.1016/j.clinph.2010.01.039.

39. Knikou M. Plasticity of corticospinal neural control after locomotor training in human spinal cord injury. *Neural Plast*. 2012;2012:254948. https://doi.org/10.1155/2012/254948.

40. Clos P, Lepers R, Garnier YM. Locomotor activities as a way of inducing neuroplasticity: insights from conventional approaches and perspectives on eccentric exercises. *Eur J Appl Physiol*. 2021;121:697–706. https://doi.org/10.1007/s00421-020-04575-3.

41. Moore KL, Persaud TVN, Torchia MG. *The Developing Human*. 11th ed. Philadelphia: Elsevier; 2020.

42. Purves D, Augustine GJ, Fitzpatrick LC, et al.*Neuroscience*. Sunderland, MA: Sinauer Associates; 1997.

43. Green E. Developmental neurology. In: Stokes M, ed. *Neurological Physiotherapy*. St. Louis: Mosby; 1998:215–228.

44. Bernal J. Thyroid hormones in brain development and function. In: Feingold KR, Anawalt B, Boyce A, eds. *Endotext*. South Dartmouth, MA: MDText.com, Inc.; 2000.

45. Stoessel MB, Majewska AK. Little cells of the little brain: microglia in cerebellar development and function. *Trends Neurosci*. 2021;44(7):564–578. https://doi.org/10.1016/j.tins.2021.04.001.

46. Martinez M. Biochemical changes during early myelination of the human brain. In: Evrard P, Minkowski A, eds. *Developmental Neurobiology*. Vol. 12. New York: Raven Press; 1989:185–200.

47. Almli CR, Moore NM. Normal sequential behavior and physiological changes throughout the developmental arc. In: Umphred DA, ed. *Neurological rehabilitation*. 3rd ed. St. Louis: CV Mosby; 1995:33–65.

48. Matonti L, Blasetti A, Chiarelli F. Nutrition and growth in children. *Minerva Pediatr*. 2020;72(6):462–471. https://doi.org/10.23736/S0026-4946.20.05981-2.

49. De Vadder F, Grasset E, Holm LM, et al. Gut microbiota regulates maturation of the adult enteric nervous system via enteric serotonin networks. *Proc Natl Acad Sci U S A*. 2018;115:6458–6463. https://doi.org/10.1073/pnas.1720017115.

50. Meo SA, Hassain A. Metabolic physiology in pregnancy. *J Pak Med Assoc*. 2016;66(9 Suppl 1):S8–S10. PMID: 27582161.

51. Deoni S, Dean D 3rd, Joelson S, O'Regan J, Schneider N. Early nutrition influences developmental myelination and cognition in infants and young children. *Neuroimage*. 2018;178:649–659. https://doi.org/10.1016/j.neuroimage.2017.12.056.

52. Rabinowicz T, De Courten-Myers G, McDonald-Comber Petetot J, et al. Human cortex development: estimates of neuronal numbers indicate major loss late in gestation. *J Neuropathol Exp Neurol*. 1996;55:320–328.

53. Dattilo AM, Saavedra JM. Nutrition Education: Application of Theory and Strategies during the First 1,000 Days for Healthy Growth. *Nestle Nutr Inst Workshop Ser*. 2019;92:1–18. https://doi.org/10.1159/000499544.

54. Dobbing J. Infant nutrition and later achievement. *Nutr Rev*. 1984;42:1–7.

55. Crookston BT, Schott W, Cueto S, Dearden KA, Engle P, Georgiadis A, Lundeen EA, Penny ME, Stein AD, Behrman JR. Postinfancy growth, schooling, and cognitive achievement: young lives. *Am J Clin Nutrition*. 2013;98:1555–1563.

56. Alderman H, Behrman JR, Glewwe P, Fernald L, Walker S. Evidence of impact of interventions on growth and development during early and middle childhood. In: Bundy DAP, Silva ND, Horton S, Jamison DT, Patton GC, eds. *Child and Adolescent Health and Development*. 3rd ed. Washington (DC): The International Bank for Reconstruction and Development / The World Bank; 2017. Chapter 7.

57. Chugani HT. A critical period of brain development: studies of cerebral glucose utilization with PET. *Prev Med*. 1998;27:184–188.

58. Johnston MV. Clinical disorders of brain plasticity. *Brain Dev*. 2004;26:73–80.

59. Gothelf D, Furfaro JA, Penniman LC, et al. The contribution of novel brain imaging techniques to understanding the neurobiology of mental retardation and developmental disabilities. *Ment Retard Dev Disabil Res Rev*. 2005;11:331–339.

60. Chugani HT. Development of regional brain glucose metabolism in relation to behavior and plasticity. In:

Dawson G, Fischer KW, eds. *Human Behavior and the Developing Brain*. New York: Guilford; 1994:153–175.

61. Bishop B, Craik RL. *Neural Plasticity*. Washington, D.C: American Physical Therapy Association; 1982.

62. Sowell ER, Thompson PM, Toga AW. Mapping changes in the human cortex throughout the span of life. *Neuroscientist*. 2004;10(4):372–392.

63. Stratton P. Rhythmic functions in the newborn. In: Stratton P, ed. *Psychobiology of the Human Newborn*. New York: J Wiley & Sons; 1982:119–145.

64. Thomas JE, Lambert EH. Ulnar nerve conduction velocity and H-reflex in infants and children. *J Appl Physiol*. 1960;15:1–9.

65. Martin JH. The corticospinal system: from development to motor control. *Neuroscientist*. 2005;11(2):161–173.

66. Friel KM, Martin JH. Role of sensory-motor cortex activity in postnatal development of corticospinal axon terminals in the cat. *J Comp Neurol*. 2005;485(1):43–56.

67. Delcour M, Russier M, Castets F, et al. Early movement restriction leads to maladaptive plasticity in the sensorimotor cortex and to movement disorders. *Sci Rep*. 2018;8:16328. https://doi.org/10.1038/s41598-018-34312-y.

68. Miguel PM, Pereira LO, Silveira PP, Meaney MJ. Early environmental influences on the development of children's brain structure and function. *Dev Med Child Neurol*. 2019;61:1127–1133. https://doi.org/10.1111/dmcn.14182.

69. Piaget J. *Origins of Intelligence*. New York: WW Norton; 1952.

70. Hallett T, Proctor A. Maturation of the central nervous system as related to communication and cognitive development. *Infant Young Child*. 1996;8:1–15.

71. Lebel C, Deoni S. The development of brain white matter microstructure. *Neuroimage*. 2018;182:207–218. https://doi.org/10.1016/j.neuroimage.2017.12.097.

72. Mills KL, Goddings A-L, Herting MM, et al. Structural brain development between childhood and adulthood: convergence across four longitudinal samples. *Neuroimage*. 2016;141:273–281. https://doi.org/10.1016/jneuroimage.2016.07.044.

73. Heinen F, Fietek UM, Berweck S, et al. Fast corticospinal system and motor performance in children: conduction precedes skill. *Pediatr Neurol*. 1998;19:217–221.

74. Nezu A, Kimura S, Uehara S, et al. Magnetic stimulation of motor cortex in children: maturity of corticospinal pathway and problem of clinical application. *Brain Dev*. 1997;19:176–180.

75. Valadian I, Porter D. *Physical Growth and Development from Conception to Maturity*. Boston: Little, Brown; 1977.

76. Mills KL, Siegmund KD, Tamnes CK, et al. Inter-individual variability in structural brain development from late childhood to young adulthood. *Neuroimage*. 2021;242:118450. http://doi.org/10.1016/j.neuroimage.2021.

77. Herting MM, Sowell ER. Puberty and structural brain development in humans. *Front Neuroendocrinol*. 2017;44:122–137. https://doi.org/10.1016/j.yfrne.2016.12.003.

78. Yakovlev PI, Lecours A-R. The myelogenetic cycles of regional maturation of the brain. In: Minkowski A, ed. *Regional Development of the Brain Early in Life*. Boston: Blackwell Scientific Publications Inc.; 1967:3–70.

79. Lebel C, Gee M, Camicioli R, Wieler M, Martin W, Beaulieu C. Diffusion tensor imaging of white matter tract evolution over the lifespan. *Neuroimage*. 2012;60:340–352. https://doi.org/10.1016/j.neuroimage.2011.11.094.

80. Chapman TW, Hill RA. Myelin plasticity in adulthood and aging. *Neurosci Lett*. 2020;715:134645. https://doi.org/10.1016/j.neulet.2019.134645.

81. Hedman AM, van Haren NEM, Schnack HG, Kahn RS, Hulshoff Pol HE. Human brain changes across the life span: a review of 56 longitudinal magnetic resonance imaging studies 2012. *Hum. Brain Mapp*. 2012;33:1987–2002. https://doi.org/10.1002/hbm.21334.

82. Tian L, Ma L. Microstructural changes of the human brain from early to mid-adulthood. *Front Human Neurosci*. 2017;11:393. https://doi.org/10.4489/fnhum.2017.00393.

83. Peterson AC, Zhang S, Hu S, Chao HH, Li CR. The effects of age, from young to middle adulthood, and gender on resting state functional connectivity of the dopaminergic midbrain. *Front Hum Neurosci*. 2017;11:52. https://doi.org/10.3389/fnhum.2017.00052.

84. Reeves S, Bench C, Howard R. Ageing and the nigrostriatal dopaminergic system. *Int. J. Geriatr. Psychiatry*. 2002;17:359–370. https://doi.org/10.1002/gps.606.

85. Nyberg L, Boraxbekk CJ, Sörman DE, et al. Biological and environmental predictors of heterogeneity in neurocognitive ageing: evidence from Betula and other longitudinal studies. *Ageing Res Rev*. 2020;64:101184. https://doi.org/10.1016/j.arr.2020.101184.

86. Buchtal F, Rosenfalck A, Behse F. Sensory potentials of normal and diseased nerves. In: Dyck PJ, Thomas PK, Griffin JW, eds. *Peripheral neuropathy*. 2nd ed. Philadelphia: WB Saunders; 1984:442–464.

87. Schaumburg HH, Spencer PS, Ochoa J. The aging human peripheral nervous system. In: Katzman R, Terry RD, eds. *The Neurology of Aging*. Philadelphia: FA Davis; 1983:111–122.

88. Palve SS, Palve SB. Impact of aging on nerve conduction velocities and late responses in healthy individuals. *J Neurosci Rural Pract*. 2018;9:112–116.

89. Whitbourne SK. *The Aging Individual: Physical and Psychological Perspectives*. New York: Springer; 1996.

90. Bruel-Jungerman E, Rampon C, Laroche S. Adult hippocampal neurogenesis, synaptic plasticity and memory: facts and hypotheses. *Rev Neurosci*. 2007;18 .93=114.

91. Micheli L, Ceccarelli M, D'Andrea G, Tirone F. Depression and adult neurogenesis: positive effects of the antidepressant fluoxetine and of physical exercise. *Brain Res Bull*. 2018;143:181–193. https://doi.org/10.1016/j.brainresbull.2018.09.002.

92. Erickson KI, Voss MW, Prakash RS, Basak C, Szabo A, Chaddock L, Kim JS, Heo S, Alves H, White SM, Wojcicki TR, Mailey E, Vieira VJ, Martin SA, Pence BD, Woods JA, McAuley E, Kramer AF. Exercise training increases size of hippocampus and improves memory. *Proc Natl Acad Sci U S A*. 2011;108:3017–3022. https://doi.org/10.1073/pnas.1015950108.

93. Cotman CW, Holets VR. Structural changes at synapses with age: plasticity and regeneration. In: Finch CE, Schneider EL, eds. *Handbook of the Biology of Aging*. New York: Van Nostrand Reinhold; 1985:617–644.

94. Raz N, Lindenberger U, Rodrigue KM, et al. Regional brain changes in aging healthy adults: general trends, individual differences and modifiers. *Cereb Cortex*. 2005;15:1676–1689. https://doi.org/10.1093/cercor/bhi044.

95. Jack Jr CR, Wiste HJ, Vemuri P, et al. Alzheimer's Disease Neuroimaging Initiative. Brain beta-amyloid measures and magnetic resonance imaging atrophy both predict time-to-progression from mild cognitive impairment to Alzheimer's disease. *Brain*. 2010;133: 3336–3348. https://doi.org/10.1093/brain/awq277.

96. DeCarli C, Massaro J, Harvey D, et al. Measures of brain morphology and infarction in the Framingham Heart Study: establishing what is normal. *Neurobiol Aging*. 2005;26:491–510.

97. Gunning-Dixon FM, Raz N. Neuroanatomical correlates of selected executive functions in middle-aged and older adults: a prospective MRI study. *Neuropsychologia*. 2003;41(14):1929–1941.

98. Reuter-Lorenz PA, Park DC. Human neuroscience and the aging mind: a new look at old problems. *J Gerontol B Psychol Sci Soc Sci*. 2010;65:405–415. https://doi.org/10.1093/geronb/gbq035.

99. Erickson KI, Gildengers AG, Butters MA. Physical activity and brain plasticity in late adulthood. *Dialogues Clin Neurosci*. 2013;15:99–108. https://doi.org/10.31887/DCNS.2013.15.1/kerickson.

100. Fleischman DA, Leurgans S, Arfanakis K, et al. Gray-matter macrostructure in cognitively healthy older persons: associations with age and cognition. *Brain Struct Funct*. 2014;219:2029–2049. https://doi.org/10.1007/s00429-013-0622-7.

101. Storsve AB, Fjell AM, Tamnes CK, et al. Differential longitudinal changes in cortical thickness, surface area and volume across the adult life span: regions of accelerating and decelerating change. *J Neurosci*. 2014;34:8488–8498. https://doi.org/10.1523/JNEUROSCI.0391-14.2014.

102. Fjell AM, Grydeland H, Krogsrud SK, et al. Development and aging of cortical thickness correspond to genetic organization patterns. *Proc Natl Acad Sci U S A*. 2015;112 https://doi.org/10.1073/pnas.1508831112. 15462-1547.

103. Resnick SM, Pham DL, Kraut MA, et al. Longitudinal magnetic resonance imaging studies of older adults: a shrinking brain. *J Neurosci*. 2003;23(8):3295–3301.

104. Bondareff W. Brain & Central Nervous System. ed 2. In: Birren JE, ed. *Encyclopedia of Gerontology*. Vol 1. Boston: Academic Press; 2007:187–190.

105. Mueller EA, Moore MM, Kerr DC, et al. Brain volume preserved in healthy elderly through the eleventh decade. *Neurology*. 1998;51:1555–1562.

106. Mrak RE, Griffin ST, Graham DI. Aging-associated changes in human brain. *J Neuropathol Exp Neurol*. 1997;56:1269–1275.

107. Bartzokis G, Lu PH, Tingus K, et al. Lifespan trajectory of myelin integrity and maximum motor speed. *Neurobiol Aging*. 2010;31:1554–1562. https://doi.org/10.1016/j.neurobiolaging.2008.08.015.

108. Friedlander WJ. Electroencephalographic alpha rate in adults as a function of age. *Geriatrics*. 1958;13: 29–31.

109. Shigeta M, Julin P, Almkvist O, et al. EEG in successful aging: a 5-year follow-up study from the eighth to the ninth decade of life. *Electroencephalogr Clin Neurophysiol*. 1995;95:77–83.

110. Keefover RW. Aging and cognition. *Neurol Clin*. 1998; 16:625–648.

111. Emch M, von Bastian CC, Koch K. Neural correlates of verbal working memory: an fMRI meta-analysis. *Front Hum Neurosci*. 2019;13:180.

112. Kim T, Lee KH, Oh H, et al. Cerebellar structural abnormalities associated with cognitive function in patients with first-episode psychosis. *Front Psychiatry*. 2018;9:286. https://doi.org/10.3389/fpsyt.2018.00286.

113. Bernard JA, Seidler RD. Relationships between regional cerebellar volume and sensorimotor and cognitive function in young and older adults. *Cerebellum*. 2013:12. https://doi.org/10.1007/s12311-013-0481-z.

114. Cui D, Ahand L, Zheng F, et al. Volumetric reduction of cerebellar lobules associated with memory decline across the adult lifespan. *Quant Imaging Med Surg*. 2020;10:148–159. https://doi.org/10.21037/qims.2019.10.19.

115. Uwisengeyimana JD, Nguchu BA, Wang Y, et al. Cognitive function and cerebellar morphometric changes relate to abnormal intra-cerebellar and cerebro-cerebellum functional connectivity in old adults. *Exp Gerontol.* 2020;140:111060. https://doi.org/10.1016/j.exger.2020.111060.

116. Cavallari M, Moscufo N, Skudlarski P, et al. Mobility impairment is associated with reduced microstructural integrity of the inferior and superior cerebellar peduncles in elderly with no clinical signs of cerebellar dysfunction. *NeuroImage Clin.* 2013;2:332–340. https://doi.org/10.1016/j.nicl.2013.02.003.

117. Kafri M, Sasson E, Assaf Y, et al. High-level gait disorder: associations with specific white matter changes observed on advanced diffusion imaging. *J Neuroimaging.* 2013;23:39–46.

118. DeSanti S, de Leon MJ, Convit A, et al. Age-related changes in brain: II. Positron emission tomography of frontal and temporal lobe glucose metabolism in normal subjects. *Psychiatr Q.* 1995;66:357–370.

119. Aanerud J, Borghammer P, Rodell A, Jónsdottir KY, Gjedde A. Sex differences of human cortical blood flow and energy metabolism. *J Cereb Blood Flow Metab.* 2017;37:2433–2440. https://doi.org/10.1177/0271678X16668536.

120. Goyal MS, Vlassenko AG, Blazey TM, Su Y, Couture LE, Durbin TJ, Bateman RJ, Benzinger TL, Morris JC, Raichle ME. Loss of brain aerobic glycolysis in normal human aging. *Cell Metab.* 2017;26(353-360):e3. https://doi.org/10.1016/j.cmet.2017.07.010.

121. Andreason PJ, Zametkin AJ, Guo AC, Baldwin P, Cohen RM. Gender-related differences in regional cerebral glucose metabolism in normal volunteers. *Psychiatry Res.* 1994;51:175–183. https://doi.org/10.1016/0165-1781(94)90037-x.

122. Thompson PM, Jahanshad N, Ching CRK, et al. ENIGMA and global neuroscience: a decade of large-scale studies of the brain in health and disease across more than 40 countries. *Transl Psychiatry.* 2020;10:100. https://doi.org/10.1038/s41398-020-0705-1.

123. Feng B, Cao J, Yu Y, et al. Gender-related differences in regional cerebral glucose metabolism in normal aging brain. *Front Aging Neurosci.* 2022;14:809767. https://doi.org/10.3389/fnagi.2022.809767.

124. Beason-Held LL, Kraut MA, Resnick SM. I. Longitudinal changes in aging brain function. *Neurobiol Aging.* 2006;29:483–496.

125. Bell MA, Ball MJ. Neuritic plaques and vessels of visual cortex in aging and Alzheimer's dementia. *Neurobiol Aging.* 1990;11:359–370.

126. Keller JN. Age-related neuropathology, cognitive decline, and Alzheimer's disease. *Ageing Res Rev.* 2006;5:1–13.

127. Illie OD, Ciobica A, Riga S, et al. Mini-review on lipofuscin and aging. focusing on the molecular interface, the biological recycling mechanism, oxidative stress, and the gut-brain axis functionality. *Medicina (Kaunas).* 2020;56:626. https://doi.org/10.3390/medicina56110626.

128. Anyanwu EC. Neurochemical changes in the aging process: implications in medication in the elderly. *ScientificWorldJournal.* 2007;7:1603–1610. https://doi.org/10.1100/tsw.2007.112.

129. Volkow ND, Gur RC, Wang GJ, et al. Association between decline in brain dopamine activity with age and cognitive and motor impairment in healthy individuals. *Am J Psychiatry.* 1998;155:344–349.

130. Seyedabadi M, Fakhfouri G, Ramezani V, Mehr SE, Rahimian R. The role of serotonin in memory: interactions with neurotransmitters and downstream signaling. *Exp Brain Res.* 2014 Mar;232(3):723–738. https://doi.org/10.1007/s00221-013-3818-4.

131. DeKosky ST, Palmer AM. Neurochemistry of aging. In: Albert ML, Knoefel JE, eds. *Clinical Neurology of Aging.* 2nd ed. New York: Oxford University Press; 1994:79–101.

132. Hubble JP. Aging and the basal ganglia. *Neurol Clin.* 1998;16.649–657.

133. Milne B, Hong M. Increasing longevity by decreasing sympathetic stress-early beta receptor blockade pharmacotherapy. *Med Hypotheses.* 2004;62(5):755–758. https://doi.org/10.1016/j.mehy.2003.10.027.

134. Balasubramanian P, Hall D, Subramanian M. Sympathetic nervous system as a target for aging and obesity-related cardiovascular diseases. *Geroscience.* 2019 Feb;41(1):13–24. https://doi.org/10.1007/s11357-018-0048-5.

135. Seals DR, Esler MD. Human ageing and sympathoadrenal system. *J Physiol.* 2000;528:407–417.

136. Esler M, Lambert G, Kaye D, et al. Influence of ageing on the sympathetic nervous system and adrenal medulla at rest and during stress. *Biogerontology.* 2002;3:45–49.

137. Ziegler MG, Lake CR, Kopin IJ. Plasma noradrenaline increases with age. *Nature.* 1976;261:333–335. https://doi.org/10.1038/261333a0.

138. Lexell J. Evidence for nervous system degeneration with advancing age. *J Nutr.* 1997;127 1011Sendash1013S.

139. McIntyre S, Nagi SS, McGlone F, Olausson H. The effects of ageing on tactile function in humans. *Neurosci.* 2021;464:53–58.

140. Cavazzana A, Röhrborn A, Garthus-Niegel S, et al. Sensory-specific impairment among older people. An investigation using both sensory thresholds and subjective measures across the five senses. *PLoS One.* 2018;13 (8):e0202969.

141. Dmochowski JP, Norcia AM. Cortical components of reaction-time during perceptual decisions in humans.

PLoS One. 2015;10:e0143339. https://doi.org/10.1371/journal.pone.0143339.

142. Kail R. Developmental change in speed of processing during childhood and adolescence. *Psychol Bull.* 1991;109:490–501. https://doi.org/10.1037/0033-2909.109.3.490.

143. Śmigasiewicz K, Servant M, Ambrosi S, Blaye A, Burle B. Speeding-up while growing-up: synchronous functional development of motor and non-motor processes across childhood and adolescence. *PLoS One.* 2021;16:e0255892. https://doi.org/10.1371/journal.pone.0255892.

144. Eaton WO, Ritchot KIM. Physical maturation and information-processing speed in middle childhood. *Dev Psychol.* 1995;31:967–972.

145. Thompson JJ, Blair MR, Henrey AJ. Over the hill at 24: persistent age-related cognitive-motor decline in reaction times in an ecologically valid video game task begins in early adulthood. *PLoS One.* 2014;9:e94215. https://doi.org/10.1371/journal.pone.0094215.

146. Tam HM, Lam CL, Huang H, Wang B, Lee TM. Age-related difference in relationships between cognitive processing speed and general cognitive status. *Appl Neuropsychol Adult.* 2015;22:94–99. https://doi.org/10.1080/23279095.2013.860602.

147. Welford AT. Between bodily changes and performance; some possible reasons for slowing with age. *Exp Aging Res.* 1984;10:73–88.

148. Onishi N. Changes of the jumping reaction time in relation to age. *J Sci Labour.* 1966;42:5–16.

149. Singleton WT. The change of movement timing with age. *Br J Psychol.* 1954;45:166–172.

150. Spirduso WW, Francis KL, MacRae PG. *Physical Dimensions of Aging.* Champaign, IL: Human Kinetics; 2005.

151. Light KE, Spirduso WW. Effects of adult aging on the movement complexity factor of response programming. *J Gerontol.* 1990;45 P107P109.

152. Fozard JL, Vercruyssen M, Reynolds SL, et al. Age differences and changes in reaction time: the Baltimore longitudinal study of aging. *J Gerontol B Psychol Sci Soc Sci.* 1994;49:179–189.

153. Ebaid D, Crewther SG, MacCalman K, Brown A, Crewther DP. Cognitive processing speed across the lifespan: beyond the influence of motor speed. *Front Aging Neurosci.* 2017;9:62. https://doi.org/10.3389/fnagi.2017.00062.

154. Emery CF, Huppert FA, Schein RL. Relationships among age, exercise, health, and cognitive function in a British sample. *Gerontologist.* 1995;35:378–385.

155. Spirduso WW. Physical fitness, aging and psychomotor speed: a review. *J Gerontol.* 1980;35:850–865.

156. Churchill JD, Galvez R, Colcombe S, et al. Exercise, experience and the aging brain. *Neurobiol Aging.* 2002;23:941–955.

157. Fabel K, Kempermann G. Physical activity and the regulation of neurogenesis in the adult and aging brain. *Neuromolecular Med.* 2008;10(2):59–66.

158. Kolb B, Harker A, Gibb R. Principles of plasticity in the developing brain. *Dev Med Child Neurol.* 2017;59:1218–1223. https://doi.org/10.1111/dmcn.13546.

159. Posner MI, Rothbart MK. Attention, self-regulation and consciousness. *Philos Trans R Soc Lond B Biol Sci.* 1998;353:1915–1927.

160. Casey BJ, Trainor R, Giedd J, et al. The role of the anterior cingulate in automatic and controlled processes: a developmental neuroanatomical study. *Dev Psychobiol.* 1997;3:61–69.

161. Camina E, Güell F. The neuroanatomical, neurophysiological and psychological basis of memory: current models and their origins. *Front Pharmacol.* 2017;8:438. https://doi.org/10.3389/fphar.2017.00438.

162. Newcombe NS, Balcomb F, Ferrara K, Hansen M, Koski J. Two rooms, two representations? Episodic-like memory in toddlers and preschoolers. *Dev Sci.* 2014;17:743–756.

163. Mussen PH, Conger JJ, Kagan J, eds. *Child Development and Personality.* 4th ed. New York: Harper & Row; 1974.

164. Paris SC, Lindauer BK. The development of cognitive skills during childhood. In: Wolman BB, ed.*Handbook of Developmental Psychology.* Englewood Cliffs, NJ: Prentice-Hall; 1982:333–349.

165. Thaler NS, Goldstein G, Pettegrew JW, Luther JF, Reynolds CR, Allen DN. Developmental aspects of working and associative memory. *Arch Clin Neuropsychol.* 2013;28:348–355. https://doi.org/10.1093/arclin/acs114.

166. Varga NL, Esposito AG, Bauer PJ. Cognitive correlates of memory integration across development: explaining variability in an educationally relevant phenomenon. *J Exp Psychol Gen.* 2019;148:739–762. https://doi.org/10.1037/xge0000581.

167. Andre J, Picchioni M, Zhang R, Toulopoulou T. Working memory circuit as a function of increasing age in healthy adolescence: a systematic review and meta-analyses. *Neuroimage Clin.* 2016;12:940–948. https://doi.org/10.1016/j.nicl.2015.12.002.

168. Czernochowski D, Mecklinger A, Johansson M. Age-related changes in the control of episodic retrieval: an ERP study of recognition memory in children and adults. *Dev Sci.* 2009;12:1026–1040. https://doi.org/10.1111/j.1467-7687.2009.00841.x.

169. Nilsson LG. Memory function in normal aging. *Acta Neurol Scand Suppl.* 2003;179:7–13.

170. Harada CN, Natelson Love MC, Triebel K. Normal cognitive aging. *Clin Geriatr Med.* 2013;29:737–752. https://doi.org/10.1016/j.cger.2013.07.002.

171. Wahlheim CN, Zacks JM. Memory guides the processing of event changes for older and younger adults. *J Exp Psychol Gen.* 2019;148:30–50.

172. Rönnlund M, Nyberg L, Bäckman L, Nilsson LG. Stability, growth, and decline in adult life span development of declarative memory: cross-sectional and longitudinal data from a population-based study. *Psychol Aging.* 2005;20:3–18. https://doi.org/10.1037/0882-7974.20.1.3.

173. Schnitzspahn KM, Stahl C, Zeintl M, Kaller CP, Kliegel M. The role of shifting, updating, and inhibition in prospective memory performance in young and older adults. *Dev Psychol.* 2013;49:1544–1553. https://doi.org/10.1037/a0030579.

174. Pliatsikas C, Veríssimo J, Babcock L, et al. Working memory in older adults declines with age, but is modulated by sex and education. *Q J Exp Psychol (Hove).* 2019;72:1308–1327. https://doi.org/10.1177/1747021818791994.

175. Horn JL, Donaldson G. Cognitive development in adulthood. In: Brim OG, Kagan J, eds.*Constancy and Change in Human Development.* Cambridge, MA: Harvard University Press; 1980:445–529.

176. Diamond A. Executive functions. *Handb Clin Neurol.* 2020;173:225–240. https://doi.org/10.1016/B978-0-444-64150-2.00020-4.

177. Plassman BL, Welsh KA, Helms M, Brandt J, Page WF, Breitner JCS. Intelligence and education as predictors of cognitive state in late life: a 50-year follow-up. *Neurology.* 1995;45:1446–1450.

178. Aartsen MJ, Smiths CHM, van Tilburg T, Knopscheer KCPM, Deeg DJH. Activity in older adults: cause or consequence of cognitive functioning? A longitudinal study on everyday activities and cognitive performance in older adults. *J Gerontol: Psychological Science.* 2002;57B:P153–P162.

179. Creighton SD, Stefanelli G, Reda AN, Zovkic IB. Epigenetic mechanisms of learning and memory: implications for aging. *Int J Mol Sci.* 2020;21:6918.

180. Gazzaley A, Sheridan MA, Cooney JW, et al. Age-related deficits in component processes of working memory. *Neuropsychology.* 2007;21(5):532–539.

181. Sakai K, Rowe JB, Passingham RE. Active maintenance in prefrontal area 46 creates distractor-resistant memory. *Nat Neurosci.* 2002;5:479–485.

182. Ito M. Nurturing the brain as an emerging research field involving child neurology. *Brain Dev.* 2004;26:429–433.

183. Kovács AM, Mehler J. Cognitive gains in 7-month-old bilingual infants. *Proc Natl Acad Sci U S A.* 2009;106:6556–6560. https://doi.org/10.1073/pnas.0811323106.

184. Saarikivi KA, Huotilainen M, Tervaniemi M, Putkinen V. Selectively enhanced development of working memory in musically trained children and adolescents. *Front Integr Neurosci.* 2019;13:62. https://doi.org/10.3389/fnint.2019.00062.

185. Hostinar CE, Stellern SA, Schaefer C, Carlson SM, Gunnar MR. Associations between early life adversity and executive function in children adopted internationally from orphanages. *Proc Natl Acad Sci U S A.* 2012;109(Suppl 2):17208–17212. https://doi.org/10.1073/pnas.1121246109.

186. Davidson MC, Amso D, Anderson LC, et al. Development of cognitive control and executive functions from 4 to 13 years: evidence from manipulations of memory, inhibition, and task switching. *Neuropsychologia.* 2006;44:2037–2078.

187. Espy K. The shape school: assessing executive function in preschool children. *Dev Neuropsychol.* 1997;13:495–499.

188. Taylor SJ, Barker LA, Heavey L, McHale S. The longitudinal development of social and executive functions in late adolescence and early adulthood. *Front. Behav Neurosci.* 2015;9:252. https://doi.org/10.3389/fnbeh.2015.00252.

189. Crews F, He J, Hodge C. Adolescent cortical development: a critical period of vulnerability for addition. *Pharmacol Biochem Behav.* 2007;86:189–199.

190. Luciana M, Conklin HM, Hooper CJ, et al. The development of nonverbal working memory and executive control processes in adolescents. *Child Dev.* 2005;76(3):697–712.

191. Luna B, Garver KE, Urban TA, et al. Maturation of cognitive processes from late childhood to adulthood. *Child Dev.* 2004;75(5):1357–1372.

192. Jadhav KS, Boutrel B. Prefrontal cortex development and emergence of self-regulatory competence: the two cardinal features of adolescence disrupted in context of alcohol abuse. *Eur J Neurosci.* 2019;50:2274–2281. https://doi.org/10.1111/ejn.14316.

193. Carbia C, Cadaveira F, Lopez-Caneda E, et al. Working memory over a six-year period in young binge drinkers. *Alcohol.* 2017;61:17–23.

194. Gil-Hernandez S, Garcia-Moreno LM. Executive performance and dysexecutive symptoms in binge drinking adolescents. *Alcohol.* 2016;51:79–87.

195. Diamond A. Close interrelation of motor development and cognitive development and of the cerebellum and prefrontal cortex. *Child Dev.* 2000;71(1):44–56.

196. Ridler K, Veijola JM, Tanskanen P, et al. Fronto-cerebellar systems are associated with infant motor and adult executive functions in healthy adults but not in schizophrenia. *Proc Natl Acad Sci U S A.* 2006;103(42):15651–15665.

197. Indahlastari A, Albizu A, Kraft JN, et al. Individualized tDCS modeling predicts functional connectivity changes within the working memory network in older adults. *Brain Stimulation*. 2021;5:1205–1215.

198. Berryhill ME, Jones KT. tDCS selectively improves working memory in older adults with more education. *Neurosci Letters*. 2012;521:148–151.

199. Nissim NR, O'Shea A, Indahlastari A, et al. Effects of in-scanner bilateral frontal tDCS on functional connectivity of the working memory network in older adults. *Front Aging Neurosci*. 2019;11:51. https://doi.org/10.3389/fnagi.2019.00051.

200. Silva MVF, Loures CdMG, Alves LCV, et al. Alzheimer's disease: risk factors and potentially protective measures. *J Biomed Sci*. 2019;26:33. https://doi.org/10.1186/s12929-019-0524-y.

201. Beydoun MA, Beydoun HA, Fanelli-Kuczmarski MT, et al. Association of serum antioxidant vitamins and carotenoids with incident Alzheimer disease and all-cause dementia among US adults. *Neurology*. 2022. https://doi.org/10.1212/WNL.0000000000200289.

202. Larson EB, et al. Exercise is associated with reduced risk for incident dementia among persons 65 years of age and older. *An Intern Med*. 2006;144:73–81.

203. Laurin D, et al. Physical activity and risk of cognitive impairment and dementia in elderly persons. *Arch Neurol*. 2001;38:498–504.

204. Intlekofer KA, Cotman CW. Exercise counteracts declining hippocampal function in aging and Alzheimer's disease. *Neurobiol Dis*. 2013;57:47–55. https://doi.org/10.1016/j.nbd.2012.06.011.

205. Torre JC. Exercise plays a preventive role against Alzheimer's disease. *J Alzheimer Dis*. 2010;20:773–783.

206. Meng Q, Lin MS, Tzeng IS. Relationship between exercise and Alzheimer's disease: a narrative literature review. *Front Neurosci*. 2020;14:131.

207. Buchman AS, Yu L, Wilson RS, et al. Physical activity, common brain pathologies, and cognition in community-dwelling older adults. *Neurology*. 2019;92(8):e811–e822. https://doi.org/10.1212/WNL.0000000000006954.

208. Spartano NL, Himali JJ, Beiser AS, et al. Midlife exercise blood pressure, heart rate, and fitness relate to brain volume 2 decades later. *Neurol*. 2016;86(14):1313–1319. https://doi.org/10.1212/WNL.0000000000002415.

209. Jefferson AL, Himali JJ, Beiser AS, et al. Cardiac index is associated with brain aging. The Framingham Heart Study. *Circulation*. 2010;12:690–697.

210. Jańczewska I, Wierzba J, Cichoń-Kotek M, Jańczewska A. Fetal alcohol spectrum disorders—diagnostic difficulties in the neonatal period and new diagnostic approaches. *Dev Period Med*. 2019;23:60–66. https://doi.org/10.34763/devperiodmed.20192301.6066.

211. Sundelin-Wahlsten V, Hallberg G, Helander A. Higher alcohol consumption in early pregnancy or low-to-moderate drinking during pregnancy may affect children's behaviour and development at one year and six months. *Acta Paediatr*. 2017;106:446–453. https://doi.org/10.1111/apa.13664.

212. Römer P, Mathes B, Reinelt T, Stoyanova P, Petermann F, Zierul C. Systematic review showed that low and moderate prenatal alcohol and nicotine exposure affected early child development. *Acta Paediatr*. 2020;109:2491–2501. https://doi.org/10.1111/apa.15453.

213. Substance Abuse and Mental Health Services Administration, Center for Behavioral Statistics and Quality. 2019 National Survey on Drug Use and Health. Table 6.23B—Alcohol Use Disorder in Past Year among Persons Aged 18 to 22, by College Enrollment Status and Demographic Characteristics: Percentages, 2018 and 2019. https://www.samhsa.gov/data/sites/default/files/reports/rpt29394/NSDUHDetailedTabs2019/NSDUHDetTabsSect6pe2019.htm#tab6–23b. Accessed March 28, 2022.

214. Ratliffe KT. *Clinical Pediatric Physical Therapy*. St. Louis: Mosby; 1998.

215. Lange S, Probst C, Gmel G, Rehm J, Burd L, Popova S. Global prevalence of fetal alcohol spectrum disorder among children and youth: a systematic review and meta-analysis. *JAMA Pediatr*. 2017;171:948–956. https://doi.org/10.1001/jamapediatrics.2017.1919.

216. Jones KL, Smith SW. Recognition of the fetal alcohol syndrome in early infancy. *Lancet*. 1973;2:999–1001.

217. Hoyme HE, Kalberg WO, Elliott AJ, et al. Updated clinical guidelines for diagnosing fetal alcohol spectrum disorders. *Pediatrics*. 2016;138:e20154256. https://doi.org/10.1542/peds.2015-4256.

218. Denny L, Coles S, Blitz R. Fetal alcohol syndrome and fetal alcohol spectrum disorders. *Am Fam Physician*. 2017;96:515–522.

219. May PA, Chambers CD, Kalberg WO, et al. Prevalence of fetal alcohol spectrum disorders in 4 US communities. *JAMA*. 2018;319(5):474–482.

220. Kalberg WO, May PA, Buckley D, et al. Early-Life predictors of fetal alcohol spectrum disorders. *Pediatrics*. 2019;144(6):e20182141.

221. Leibson T, Neuman G, Chudley AE, Koren G. The differential diagnosis of fetal alcohol spectrum disorder. *J Popul Ther Clin Pharmacol*. 2014;21:e1–e30.

222. Thomas SE, Kelly SJ, Mattson SN, Riley EP. Comparison of social abilities of children with fetal alcohol syndrome to those of children with similar IQ scores and

normal controls. *Alcohol Clin Exp Res.* 1998;22:528–533. https://doi.org/10.1111/j.1530-0277.1998.tb03684.x.

223. Rockhold MN, Krueger AM, de Water E, et al. Executive and social functioning across development in children and adolescents with prenatal alcohol exposure. *Alcohol Clin Exp Res.* 2021;45:457–469. https://doi.org/10.1111/acer.14538.

224. Vorgias D, Bernstein B.Fetal Alcohol Syndrome. Treasure Island (FL): StatPearls Publishing; 2022. https://www.ncbi.nlm.nih.gov/books/NBK448178/. Acccessed March 15, 2022.

225. Hingson R, Zha W, Smyth D. Magnitude and trends in heavy episodic drinking, alcohol-impaired driving, and alcohol-related mortality and overdose hospitalizations among emerging adults of college ages 18-24 in the United States, 1998–2014. J Stud Alcohol Drugs. 2017; 78:540–548. https://doi.org/10.15288/jsad.2017.78.540.

226. National Institute on Alcohol Abuse and Alcoholism. https://www.niaaa.nih.gov/publications/brochures-and-fact-sheets/college-drinking. Accessed February 10, 2022.

227. National Institute on Alcohol Abuse and Alcoholism. https://www.niaaa.nih.gov/alcohols-effects-health/special-populations-co-occurring-disorders/older-adults. Accessed March 28, 2022.

228. National Institute on Aging. What is mild cognitive impairment. https://www.nia.nih.gov/health/what-mild-cognitive-impairment. Accessed May 10, 2022.

229. Greenaway MC, Lacritz LH, Binegar D, et al. Patterns of verbal memory performance in mild cognitive impairment, Alzheimer disease, and normal aging. Cognitive Behavioral Neurol. 2006;19:79–84.

230. Parikh PK, MA, Troyer AK, Maione AM, Murphy KJ. The impact of memory change on daily life in normal aging and mild cognitive impairment. *Gerontologist.* 2016;56:877–885. https://doi.org/10.1093/geront/gnv030.

231. Albert MS, DeKosky ST, Dickson D, et al. The diagnosis of mild cognitive impairment due to Alzheimer's disease: recommendations from the National Institute on Aging-Alzheimer's Association workgroups on diagnostic guidelines for Alzheimer's disease. *Alzheim Dementia.* 2011;7:270–279.

232. Alzheimer's Association. https://www.alz.org/. Accessed May 10, 2022.

233. Crane PK, Walker R, Hubbard RA, et al. Glucose levels and risk of dementia. *N Engl J Med.* 2013;369:540–548. https://doi.org/10.1056/NEJMoa1215740.

234. Candore G, Balistreri CR, Grimaldi MP, et al. Age-related inflammatory diseases: role of genetics and gender in the pathophysiology of Alzheimer's disease. *Ann N Y Acad Sci.* 2006;1089:472–486.

235. Ratnakumar A, Zimmerman SE, Jordan BA, Mar JC. Estrogen activates Alzheimer's disease genes. *Alzheimers Dement (N Y).* 2019;5:906–917. https://doi.org/10.1016/j.trci.2019.09.004.

236. Morrison JH, Hof PR. Life and death of neurons in the aging cerebral cortex. *Int Rev Neurobiol.* 2007;81:41–57.

237. de Graaf G, Buckley F, Skotko BG. Estimation of the number of people with Down syndrome in the United States. *Genet Med.* 2017;19(4):439–447. https://doi.org/10.1038/gim.2016.127.

238. Harman MF, Martin MG. Epigenetic mechanisms related to cognitive decline during aging. *J Neuro Res.* 2020;98:234–246. https://doi.org/10.1002/jnr.24436.

9

Sensory System Changes

After studying this chapter, the reader will be able to:
1. Describe the role and function of sensory systems.
2. Discuss the role of sensation in perception and movement.
3. Describe age-related sensory system changes across the life span.
4. Correlate sensory system changes with function across the life span.

INTRODUCTION

Our senses provide the only means of communicating with and about the world around us. The psychologist J. J. Gibson[1] introduced the concept of *affordance* to describe the complementary effect of the environment on the developing organism. Sensory input provides information from the external and internal environment. Sensation provides feedback for learning about movement (Chapter 4, Fig. 4.3). Sensation affords interaction between the infant and the environment, as well as interaction between the environment and the infant in such a manner that both are changed. The environment includes the biophysical and sociocultural surroundings that affect movement outcome. These surroundings can also encompass people and objects. No wonder Piaget[2] described the origins of intelligence as the sensorimotor period. An infant's initial foray into the world is guided by sensations that are paired with movement to initiate communication, motor control, and intelligence.

Because the sensory system is part of the nervous system, sensory and motor systems have a common goal—movement production. The role of sensory input in the development and control of posture and movement is well documented.[3-7] Initially, sensory input is paired with motor output, resulting in reflexes such as flexor withdrawal and positive support. Infants learn to maintain their posture and balance in response to sensory input with the development of *postural reactions* that automatically occur to maintain the alignment of the head and trunk in response to a weight shift; these include protective extension of the extremities, righting, and equilibrium reactions of the head and trunk. Automatic postural reactions in response to anteroposterior body sway (postural sway) are governed by somatosensory, vestibular, and visual input (see Chapter 11).

Sensory input aids the process of learning movement by providing feedback for movement accuracy, such as in reaching for or rolling toward a desired object. Once movement is learned, sensation may not be as necessary for the movement to occur. When movement becomes more automatic, however, sensation becomes an anticipatory signal to move; for example, gathering your things when you hear the bell ring at the end of class or changing your walk to a run when you think you may miss your bus. The way a movement feels can be recalled when playing a once-forgotten piano piece or riding a bicycle. Once you learn, you do not forget how, although execution may be impaired through nervous or muscular system deficits.

Sensory systems are important to functional movement. The majority of what we know about the senses comes from research with animals and infants. We also need to understand the age-related changes in sensory function across the life span, including the importance of state and stimulus novelty. The normally expected changes in sensory awareness with advanced age are being distinguished from pathological changes, and our knowledge of the functional implications of age-related sensory decrements for movement is being documented.

CHARACTERISTICS OF SENSORY SYSTEMS

Sensation entails the reception of afferent stimuli from both the internal milieu of the body and the external world. To receive input, the body must be sufficiently aroused. The state of arousal of an infant determines the level of responsivity to sensory stimuli. A person in a coma may respond only to painful stimuli. With recovery, sensory awareness improves. Reception of sensory stimuli does not always imply that the sensation reaches conscious awareness or that the sensation is correctly perceived. Each sensory system has its own unique set of receptors and pathways it travels to reach conscious awareness and to be interpreted/perceived.

The senses monitor internal processes related to maintaining homeostasis and producing arousal in the form of general alerting, sexual responses, and fight-or-flight reactions. The arousal functions are choreographed by various subsystems of the nervous system (central, peripheral, and autonomic) in concert with the brainstem reticular activating, hypothalamic, and limbic systems. The interpretation of sensory stimuli is often determined by the state of the autonomic nervous system. Think of how slowly you respond to the alarm clock in the morning when you have an 8 o'clock class. Your parasympathetic system predominates during vegetative functions such as sleep, but you animatedly respond to cold water when showering, a sympathetic response to a brief cold stimulus.

Sensory input comes in via special receptors, is conveyed by nerve fibers, and is disseminated to appropriate regions of the central nervous system (CNS). For example, your eye picks up a moving image and relays the information to the brain, which identifies a hummingbird. In the meantime, your eye muscles track the bird's movements while you safely continue your forward progression on the nature path. Different sensory receptors have sent a variety of messages to the brain that have been interpreted and have resulted in an adaptive response to allow you to enjoy a pleasurable activity while continuing a motor task. Some pathways relay information from only one type of sensory receptor such as mechanoreceptors; others carry information about pain and temperature. All sensory systems have the ability to transform one type of energy (the stimulus) into an electrical signal, code for specific qualities of the stimulus, be represented topographically on many levels of the nervous system, integrate information between one or more sensory systems, and participate in motor responses both in a preparatory and reactive manner.

The Senses
Somatic Senses

Touch, temperature, pain, and awareness of joint position (proprioception) are conveyed by mechanoreceptors, thermoreceptors, and nociceptors. Touch and proprioception contribute to the development of body scheme and awareness of our relationship to the outside world. Touch defines the limits of the body and provides information about people and objects in the environment. Temperature detection ensures survival and efficient physiological function of the body. Pain protects the body from too much pressure, as from sitting too long in one position, and from overexposure to the sun, snow, or chemicals. Somatic receptors convey pressure, vibration, temperature, pain, and some proprioceptive information about the body.

Free nerve endings are found in the skin, muscle, joints, and viscera. These nociceptors convey noxious stimuli. As such, they can respond to mechanical, thermal, and chemical stimuli, either on the skin or internally at the periosteum, arterial walls, and joint surfaces. Thermoreception also occurs by activating free, unencapsulated nerve endings. Thermoreceptors detect hot and cold by responding to changes in their own metabolic rate relative to actual temperature changes in the ambient air. Extremes of hot or cold can be detected as pain through the stimulation of pain receptors in addition to the temperature receptors.

The majority of *mechanoreceptors* are encapsulated and include *Pacinian corpuscles*, *Meissner corpuscles*, *Merkel cells*, and *Ruffini endings*. Pacinian corpuscles respond to tissue vibration and rapid changes in the mechanical state of the tissues.[8] They are found in the skin and joints. Meissner corpuscles are sensitive to light touch and vibration, whereas Merkel cells respond to pressure. The latter receptor is found in hairy skin, and the former two receptors are found primarily in hairless (glabrous) skin. Ruffini endings convey stretch of the skin and of joints.

Muscle spindles and Golgi tendon organs are not only examples of mechanoreceptors but are also classified as proprioceptors. Proprioceptive receptors detect the position of body parts in space and are found in the vestibular part of the ear as well as in the muscles, tendons, and joints. Muscle spindles are stretch-sensitive and provide information about muscle length and velocity of contraction. The awareness of joint movement or kinesthesia along with joint position sense make up the functions often collectively referred to as "proprioception."[9] A classic definition of proprioception considers it a specialized variation of touch including the sensations of joint movement (kinesthesia) and joint position sense.[10] Joint position receptors relay knowledge of joint angulation, especially at end ranges. More than half of the innervation to a muscle conveys information to and from the muscle spindles, the body's primary source of proprioceptive information.[11] The muscle spindle provides sensory feedback during reflexive and voluntary movement.

The Golgi tendon organ, located in the muscle tendon, detects tension generated by the contraction or stretch of that muscle and safeguards the muscle from overwork by inhibiting or stopping the muscle from contracting. Articular receptors in the joint capsule and ligaments also provide proprioceptive information. The Pacinian corpuscles respond to mechanical stimulation during movement, whereas Ruffini endings become active when the joint is at the extremes of its movement. However, the loss of joint receptors because of surgery or anesthesia does not seem to impair motion detection.[12] Various cutaneous sensory receptors are shown in Fig. 9.1.

Vestibular Sense

The ear is a special part of our anatomy that is crucial to motion sense as well as the sense of hearing. It is, therefore, important to understand its various parts and how they work (Fig. 9.2). The vestibular system relays input about the body's relationship to gravity, head position, and head movement. Although it is considered part of proprioception in some regards, it is discussed separately because of its intimate relationship to movement. Vestibular receptors in the inner ear provide information about head position and head movement in space. Vestibular information is used to update postural tone and equilibrium and to ensure gaze stability during head movements.[13] Gaze stability allows the eyes to fix on an image even though the head is moving. The vestibular system resolves intersensory conflicts about balance. If the proprioceptors think the body is not moving and the eyes think the body is moving, the input of the vestibular system decides what the real situation is and relays information to appropriate motor centers.

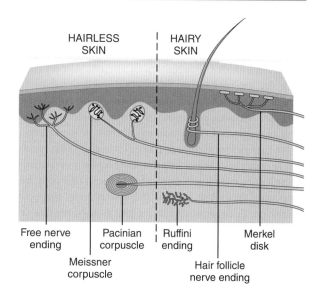

Fig. 9.1 Cutaneous receptors include the free nerve ending, Meissner corpuscle, and Pacinian corpuscle found in hairless skin and the Ruffini ending and Merkel cells in hairy skin. (From Lundy-Ekman L. *Neuroscience Fundamentals for Rehabilitation.* 3rd ed. Philadelphia: WB Saunders; 2007:107.)

The vestibular receptors are located within the membranous labyrinth of the inner ear. The labyrinth is made up of three fluid-filled semicircular ducts and the utricle and saccule (Fig. 9.3). The vestibular receptors are specialized hair cells located in the ampullae of the semicircular ducts and the maculae of the saccule and utricle (Fig. 9.4). The semicircular ducts respond to angular head movement. The saccule and utricle detect gravity; the utricle also monitors the position of the head when one is upright, and the saccule monitors it when one is lying down. Both respond to linear acceleration from the deflection of the hair cells. The three semicircular ducts are oriented at right angles to each other and respond to angular acceleration. When these paired structures are stimulated, the hair cells (receptors) are deformed (bent). They transmit electrical signals via the vestibular part of cranial nerve VIII to the vestibular ganglion and on to the vestibular nuclei in the medulla and vestibulocerebellum. These relay nuclei also communicate with the cervical spinal cord, oculomotor system, cerebellum, vestibular nuclei of the other side of the body, brainstem reticular formation, thalamus, and hypothalamus. Although the vestibular system exerts an influence on all other sensory systems,[13,14] it exerts more influence on the motor systems by contributing to postural tone.

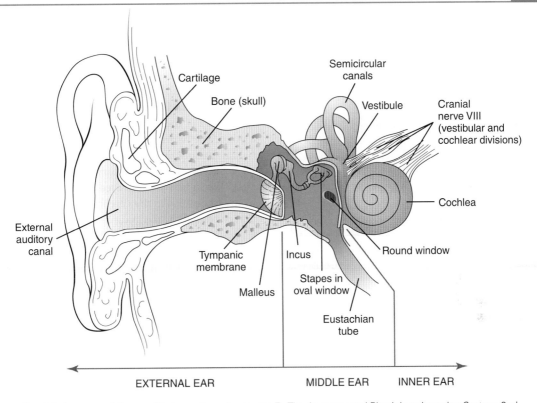

Fig. 9.2 Anatomy of the ear. (Redrawn from Applegate E. *The Anatomy and Physiology Learning System.* 2nd ed. Philadelphia: WB Saunders; 2000:194.)

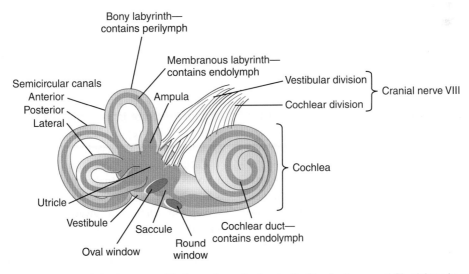

Fig. 9.3 Labyrinths of the inner ear. (Redrawn from Applegate E. *The Anatomy and Physiology Learning System.* 2nd ed. Philadelphia: WB Saunders; 2000:195.)

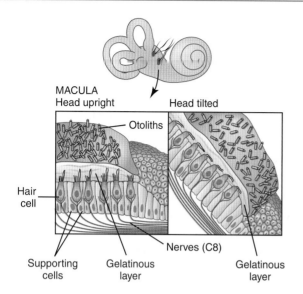

Fig. 9.4 Structure of the macula. (Redrawn from Applegate E. *The Anatomy and Physiology Learning System*. 2nd ed. Philadelphia: WB Saunders; 2000:198.)

Postural tone is sufficient tone in postural muscles to sustain a posture.

Special Senses

Vision, hearing, taste, and smell are considered the traditional special senses and are subserved by specific cranial nerves. Specialized receptors found in the eye, ear, tongue, and nose are specifically and uniquely designed to sense light, sound, taste, and odors. The distance receptors—vision and hearing—have been the most thoroughly studied.

Vision is the most complex special sense. The sharpness of vision (acuity) and the ability to focus on near and far objects (accommodation) are functions of the structure of the eye. The eye is the organ of sight, but the photoreceptors are the rods and cones within the retina of the eye. A very small area of the retina called the macula is capable of detailed and acute vision. The center of this small area, the fovea, consists of only cones. Cranial nerves II, III, IV, and VI are involved in vision. Visual recognition of objects and the interpretation of their meaning involve the occipital cortex and the limbic system.

Hearing is possible because sound waves are transformed into vibration in the ear. Sound is captured by the external ear and funneled to the eardrum, or tympanic membrane. Three small bones form the ossicular chain (the malleus, incus, and stapes) and transmit sound vibration to the cochlea in the inner ear (see Fig. 9.2). Remember that the cochlea is embedded in the temporal bone or bony labyrinth and is a set of fluid-filled coiled tubes. The sound wave travels along the basilar (bottom) membrane of the cochlear duct like a ripple of water on a pond. The hair cells of the organ of Corti lying on the basilar membrane receive the vibration and generate nerve impulses in the auditory division of cranial nerve VIII. The signals are conveyed via complex connections in the brainstem to the cerebral cortex, where sound is perceived and the meaning can be interpreted.

Taste as a sensory modality is involved in the "oral perception of food-derived chemicals that stimulate receptor cells within the taste buds."[15] Taste combines with smell and touch to form flavors. Taste and smell are considered near and far receptors, respectively, and are the only ones that are continually being replaced. Substances in the mouth enter taste pores and interact with the membranes of the taste receptors (buds). The chemical stimulus is transduced into taste sensation. Taste buds are found in special skin structures called *papillae*, which are innervated by the branches of cranial nerves VII, IX, and X. Three distinct types of papillae are present in humans and located on different parts of the tongue, soft palate, and epiglottis (see Fig. 9.5).

Smell is the most primitive special sense. It has a direct connection to the limbic, or emotional, system as well as to the cortex. The olfactory receptor is a remarkably simple structure found in the olfactory mucosa. Olfactory hairs, or cilia, project into the mucus, react to odors, and stimulate the olfactory cells. Many pleasant memories can be triggered by our favorite smells such as baking bread or a pine tree. As a bipolar neuron, the olfactory receptor is the actual cell body of the sensory neuron. The receptor can be replaced if damaged. Its axon forms cranial nerve I.

Perception and integration. Sensory input plays a major role in perceptual development. When meaning is attached to sensory information, sensation becomes perception. Detection, awareness, and localization of sensory information are components of perception. The ability to discriminate comes before interpretation of sensory information. Sensory information is shared between senses to provide for the identification and manipulation of objects and people within the environment.

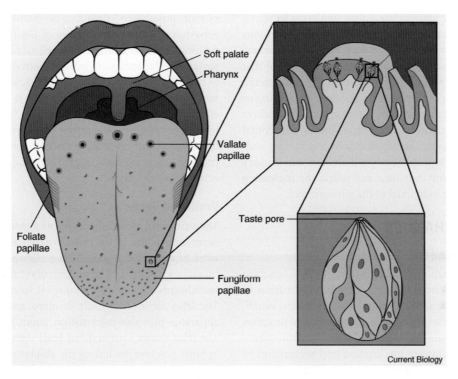

Current Biology

Fig. 9.5 Taste papillae and taste buds. (From Breslin PA. An evolutionary perspective on food and human taste. *Curr Biol.* 2013;23:R409-R418.)

Sensory integration is the ability to use sensory information to move efficiently. *Integration* means putting together many sensory inputs for the purpose of adapting to the task at hand. Integration enhances adaptation by making an individual's response more effective. An individual who has difficulty processing any of the many sensory inputs might exhibit difficulty in planning or executing certain tasks. Perceptual abilities and sensory integration develop over time and reflect the increasing adaptation of the individual to the environment and the tasks encountered within the environment.

There are three types of sensory integration. *Intrasensory* integration occurs when information is shared within the same sensory system. Input from both eyes provides for the perception of depth. *Intersensory* integration occurs when two different sensory systems combine to impart a richer understanding than could be provided by only one sensory dimension. For example, touch and proprioception combine to provide a sense of body scheme. The last type, *sensorimotor* integration, involves the interaction of sensory and motor systems, as with the combining of vision and movement to draw

or write. The combination of head turning, looking, and hearing to localize an auditory cue is another example. The linking of movement awareness and language results in the establishment of directionality or the ability of the child to use spatial cues. Others have called this *spatial cognition.*

The role of *sensation* in perceptual organization was defined by Ayres[14] as being able to make use of sensory information. A later definition explains that the sensory information from within the body and from the environment is processed to allow the individual to move effectively within the environment. Sensory integration is an adaptive phenomenon that takes place within the context of a specific task and environment. It is one thing to maneuver a wheelchair through an obstacle course and quite another to walk on the deck of a rolling ship in a storm.

Cortical and subcortical structures participate in sensory integration. Association cortices, the thalamus, and the brainstem reticular system can process, amplify or dampen, and direct sensory information to other areas of the brain. The thalamus relays the sensory stimulus to the cortex and to the appropriate association areas to plan a response. Recognition and interpretation of the stimulus occur in the primary sensory cortex, such as the realization that you have been touched and the quality of that touch (gentle or rough). The touch is further interpreted in the higher association areas as emotionally pleasing or dangerous. In an open system, interconnected structures regulate and organize sensory input into a conceptual whole to allow us to identify shapes by touch. This ability is called *stereognosis*. Perceptual abilities and sensory integration develop over time and reflect the increasing adaptation of the individual to the environment.

LIFE SPAN CHANGES

Prenatal Period

The senses of touch, smell, and taste are ready to function at birth, as evidenced by the complete myelination of their respective neural pathways. The vestibular, visual, and auditory senses are capable of some level of function at birth but require additional time and environmental experience to complete myelination and maturation of central pathways. The sensory systems develop in utero in the following order: touch, vestibular, smell, hearing, vision, taste, and proprioception.

Somatic Senses

The fetus develops the ability to respond to touch around the mouth as early as 7½ weeks of gestation.[16] The earliest response to touch is avoidance, or turning away. By 17 weeks, cutaneous sensation spreads to the entire body with the exception of the top and back of the head; these areas are subjected to the most sensory input during delivery.

Proprioceptive receptors are well developed by mid–fetal life.[17] Tapping, stretching, or even a change in amniotic fluid pressure can cause a response in the fetus.[18] Muscle spindles are known to differentiate between 11 and 12 weeks.[19] The Golgi tendon organ does not differentiate until 16 weeks of gestation. Pacinian corpuscles are found in the distal parts of limbs at 20 weeks of gestation but are immature.

Sensory nerve endings capable of carrying pain are present throughout the body of the fetus by 20 weeks of gestation. However, the fetus is not aware of the pain because the pathway from the spinal cord to the cortex is incomplete. This pathway connects to the thalamus by 24–26 weeks of gestation, making cortical perception

of pain possible.[20,21] Pain can be transmitted and perceived even before myelination of the nociceptive pain pathway which is completely myelinated by 37 weeks of gestation.[22] Neonates are hypersensitive to pain because of their immature nervous system.[23] Knowing that term and preterm infants feel pain makes it imperative that effective pain management strategies be implemented in this population. According to Perry et al.,[24] efforts to evaluate and alleviate pain in neonates, especially preterm ones, are inconsistent and inadequate despite active research efforts.

Vestibular Sense

The vestibular apparatus begins as a thickening of ectoderm, or placode, in the primitive ear early in the fourth week of gestation. A *placode* is a common precursor of most sensory organs. The semicircular canals, utricle, and saccule are completely formed at 9½ weeks of gestation.[25] The fetus moves constantly in utero, and the vestibular apparatus provides information about that movement. The fetus shows a generalized body response to changes in body position, including the ability to right the head. Movement in utero has been linked to later movement competence.[26] Neural connections link the labyrinths and the oculomotor nuclei in the brainstem between 12 and 24 weeks of gestation, which will be important for establishing gaze stability and spatial orientation. This is the first sensory system to be myelinated and the first to function. However, although it is structurally complete at birth, maturation continues to assist the child to develop postural control, movement, and balance.[27]

Special Senses

Vision. The eyes also develop during the fourth week of gestation from a placode that forms a vesicle. The optic vesicle folds in onto itself to produce a two-layered optic cup, from which the retina is derived. The neural cells of the retina differentiate into 10 layers containing photoreceptors (the rods and cones), cell bodies of bipolar neurons, and ganglion cells. Because of the infolding, the photoreceptors are adjacent to the pigment layer. Therefore light must pass through the retina to reach the receptors.

Neurons in the occipital cortex are organized into their adult layers during the second half of gestation,[28] so they are ready to receive input after birth. Myelination begins at the optic chiasm around 13 weeks of gestation, and the rods and cones differentiate at 16 weeks. Light perception is possible in utero;[29] the fetus exhibits reflexive eye blinking at 6 months of gestation. Thalamic connections begin to myelinate before term and continue until the fifth postnatal month of life. The thalamic connections, those to the lateral geniculate nucleus, are crucial to the development of more sophisticated visual perceptual abilities. Central visual pathways develop postnatally, even though the neurons that constitute these pathways are formed prenatally. These pathways require visual input to complete their development.

Hearing. The ectoderm of the otic placode forms both the membranous labyrinth of the vestibular system and the structures of the inner ear—the cochlear duct and the organ of Corti—during the fourth week of gestation. The hair cells differentiate by 16 weeks of gestation. The remaining structures of the ear, including ligaments and muscles, come from the branchial arches. Hearing in utero is possible as early as 24 weeks of gestation and is consistently present after 28 weeks of gestation.[30,31]

Taste. The tongue is developed from the mandibular arch at 26–31 days of gestation. Formation is completed by the 37th day; the various types of taste buds reach maturity by 13 weeks of gestation.[28] Ingestion of amniotic fluid in utero is thought to contribute to the development of the primitive gut and to the regulation of amniotic fluid volume. Taste is functional in utero in the last third of the pregnancy. The amniotic fluid is rich in chemicals such as sugars, salts, acids, and lactate that can be "tasted" by the fetus.[32,33] This ability is the beginning of gustatory sensory memory that will affect food choices of the future infant and child. The taste buds are initially stimulated by amniotic fluid and later by maternal milk which changes composition based on the mother's diet.

Smell. The olfactory placode also forms during the fourth week of gestation. It is the earliest distance receptor to develop. The fifth cranial nerve innervates the walls of the nose at 5 weeks; the olfactory organ (bulb) is well developed by the fifth and sixth months of gestation. The unmyelinated nerve fibers of cranial nerve I are the olfactory nerve. It is these fibers that end in the olfactory bulb. Olfactory discrimination is possible in preterm infants beyond 29 weeks of gestation.[17]

Infancy and Early Childhood

All sensory systems are capable of functioning at birth because the peripheral nervous system is completely myelinated. However, complete maturation of sensory pathways occurs after birth. Physiological changes occur after birth in all sensory systems, as evidenced by an increase in nerve conduction velocity (time to conduct) with myelination, redistribution of axon branching, and increased synaptic efficiency and efficacy. Functional changes are apparent as the infant interacts more meaningfully with the world. Sensory systems are dependent on sensory experiences to complete their development. This is an example of experience-expectant plasticity.

State and Novelty

Behavioral state and novelty of stimulus play a role in the infant's level of interest in sensory information. A sleeping or overstimulated infant is not able to react to a new stimulus. On the other hand, a quietly alert infant looking at a mobile will generally become attentive to a new toy. Sensory awareness requires that the infant be sufficiently aroused. The concept of state was first described by Prechtl[34] as levels of alertness ranging from sleep to crying. The quiet alert state has been deemed the most appropriate for testing an infant's responses to sensory stimulation. Studies show that an infant's state will affect the level of reflex and motor responsiveness.[35] The ability of the infant to change states smoothly is also an indication of the degree to which the CNS is organized.

Many studies of visual preference in infants have pinpointed the role of novelty in gaining attention and producing motor behavior. The behavior may be looking, reaching, vocalizing, or even quieting, but the common denominator is that the infant responds to a certain level of stimulus novelty. For example, when an infant is shown two pictures, the infant typically attends to the new picture. From the earliest moment that the infant is quietly alert, there is the ability to perceive sensory stimuli and to demonstrate preferences. Novelty and complexity guide infants' exploratory behavior.[36] Learning and adaptation occur much earlier than was once believed. Perceptual abilities once reserved as the province of the older child are consistently being documented in infants. For example, 5-month-old infants use figure/ground perception to develop shape recognition.[37] Sensory perception, that is, the ability to attach meaning to sensory information, occurs from the beginning of extrauterine life.

Self-Perception

Infants develop a sense of self as young as 2–3 months. Hand-to-mouth and hand-to-face behavior is typical in an infant. This cutaneous self-stimulation does not trigger any of the typically observed rooting responses when an external object contacts the same facial location. Rochat and Hespos[38] suggest that the infant can distinguish between self-touch and touch of another person. The self-stimulation would involve proprioceptive stimulation from self-movement as well as touch. When touching their own face, infants experience a unique sensorimotor event that potentially identifies their body as a differentiated body. Rochat categorizes infants' self-exploration of their own bodies as visual-proprioceptive calibration: "infants appear fascinated by the simultaneous experience of seeing and feeling the limbs of their own body moving through space."[39] Three-month-old infants begin to show systematic visual and proprioceptive self-exploration.[40]

During the second year of life, the child develops a sense of "me." Before that time, infants may not distinguish their image from another infant's image in a mirror. In an experiment where a Post-it note is stuck to a child's forehead and the child looks in the mirror and removes the Post-it, the concept of "me" is thought to exist. This action occurs by 21 months but the development of the child's sense of self continues until 4–5 years of age, according to Rochat.[40] The reader is referred to his description of levels of self-awareness and their clinical implications.

Somatic Senses

Touch. The perception of touch and pain is crucial to the newborn's survival. Although the defensive movements to light touch seen in utero fade by birth, the newborn reflexively moves to clear the nose and mouth of any object that obstructs the airway. The first responses to touch are generalized diffuse responses, such as random arm and leg movements. Information from touch is initially used by the infant to locate food. Within a few days after birth, head turning in response to touching the mouth is precisely related to the part of the mouth touched. Although touch and pain are not completely differentiated in the full-term newborn, pain sensitivity has been shown to increase over the first 4 days of life.[41]

Early tactile input plays a role in parent-infant attachment, stress-coping mechanisms, sociability, and cognitive development. The use of tactile input to recognize differences develops gradually; a 1-month-old infant is

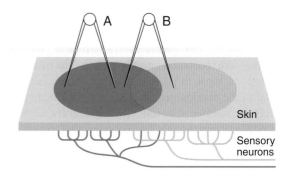

Fig. 9.6 Receptive fields. Areas of skin innervated by each neuron are indicated on the surface of the skin. (A) The caliper points touching the skin would be perceived as one point, because both points are within the receptive field of a single neuron. (B) The caliper points would be perceived as two points, because the points are contacting the receptive fields of two neurons. (From Lundy-Ekman L. *Neuroscience: Fundamentals for Rehabilitation.* 5th ed. Elsevier; 2018:187. Figure 10.3.)

able to distinguish between pacifier shapes.[42] A receptive field is that area in which a sensory stimulus can be perceived as separate from an adjacent field (see Fig. 9.6). The receptive field for touch-mediated reflex responses such as flexor withdrawal becomes more refined or localized with age. Touch to any part of the leg of a newborn causes a reflexive withdrawal. Gradually, the receptive field becomes limited to the sole of the foot.

Touch sensation can be localized generally at 7–9 months; specific localization is demonstrated by 12–16 months of age.[17] General localization is exhibited by the infant's moving the extremity; specific localization involves the infant's touching or looking at the area touched. Toddlers will rub the area or push away the stimulus. Infants at 7 months can touch the place where they were touched.[43] For this to occur, the tactile information of the stimulus must be integrated with proprioceptive or visual information about the current body position in external space.[44,45] The infant then has to use location information about the reaching limb to get to the target. Leed and colleagues[43] found that manual localization improved with age in 7- to 21-month-old infants. Visual localization was also associated with successful reaching. The ability to use touch to identify objects is called *haptic perception.*[1] *Haptic* means "able to lay hold of" and is appropriate because the majority of information about objects comes from manipulation. Nine-month-old infants have been found to possess this ability, as determined by manual exploration.[46] When visual information is combined with touch, infants as young as 6 months can pick out toys that were touched previously without seeing the toy.[47] Infants perceive visual-tactile spatial relationships from at least 6 months of age.[48] "Multisensory interactions between vision and touch may be the developmental mechanism by which infants come to represent the relation[ship] between their body and external space."[49]

Temperature. The newborn must regulate its own body temperature at birth and is sensitive to the temperature of the ambient air. Responses to changes in air temperature are often seen in common body postures assumed by the infant. Infants who are too warm may appear to be "sunbathing," decrease their calorie intake, sleep, and show peripheral vasodilation. Sweating and panting responses mature later. Conversely, the infant will wake and move about if too cool. Discrimination of hot and cold is possible early on and is characterized by more reactivity to cold. Respiratory changes, limb movement, and state changes have been documented for temperatures varying as little as 5°–6°F.

Pain. Pain receptors are equally prevalent in infants and adults,[20] with pain sensitivity appearing to increase in the first month of life.[50] Infants remember pain.[51] Newborn infants and preterm infants may experience pain more acutely because descending inhibition is not present developmentally.[52,53] Management of procedural pain has been studied for over a decade resulting in use of strategies to minimize pain. However, despite recommendations from the American Academy of Pediatrics (AAP) and other experts, neonatal pain continues to be inconsistently assessed and inadequately managed.[54,55] Barriers that lead to suboptimal care such as lack of resources in low- to middle-income countries exist.[56] Therapists should be familiar with pain rating scales for infants and children. Evidence suggests that there may be short- and long-term consequences of not treating pain in infants,[23,52,57] which may include changes in pain sensitivity, poor brain development, diminished social control, poor adaptive behavior, and impulsivity.

Proprioception. Proprioception is the foundation for purposeful movements such as imitation, reaching, and locomotion. It is used for action very early after birth, when the tactile and vestibular systems are functioning. The fact that newborn infants imitate mouth opening and tongue protrusion is interpreted as a pairing of visual and proprioceptive input.[58] In the same way a child handles objects to gain haptic perception,

infants move to gain proprioceptive information. Self-perception in the infant appears to depend on touch and proprioception.[59] Self-touch contributes to the infant's early body representation.[49] When the infant touches the body, tactile and proprioceptive information during and after the movement is combined with knowledge of the body's position in space from the vestibular system. Eventually, visual and auditory information is included in learning about the spatial disposition of the body and limbs within the environment.

Reach and grasp of objects within arm's reach develops at 4–6 months of age.[60] Research has shown that reaching behavior in 5-month-olds depends more on the infant's motor ability and proprioception than on visual control; no difference is seen between reaching in the dark and reaching in the light.[61] Vision becomes more important as the system matures, as evidenced by more successful reaching with vision in the 8- to 9-month-olds who can intercept a moving target.[62]

Achieving and maintaining an upright posture depend on the infant's ability to interpret and respond to information about body sway, which comes from vestibular, visual, and proprioceptive input. Multiple studies have shown that infants use vision proprioceptively in sitting and standing to maintain stable postures.[63–66] When proprioceptive and vestibular input indicated that the body was stable and visual input indicated movement, the majority of subjects made compensatory movements.

Vestibular Sense

The vestibular system defines the body's relationship to gravity and is completely myelinated at birth. Many of the infant's earliest activities are related to achieving and maintaining stable postures against gravity. Preterm infants were initially found to have delayed vestibular responses to movement,[67] especially preterm infants, who are also small for gestational age. This delay in responding is due to immaturity, not pathology,[68] and is related to the difficulty preterm infants have in maintaining alert wakefulness. When alert and awake, even preterm infants can demonstrate vestibular responses.[69] Newborn infants' vestibular function was found to be better when tested in a supine position than in a prone position.[70]

The first postnatal vestibular ocular reflex (VOR) demonstrated by the infant is called the *doll eye phenomenon*. When a typical newborn is held in dorsal suspension and the head is moved horizontally, the eyes appear to move in the opposite direction of the head motion. This eye movement corresponds to the slow component of nystagmus. Persistence of the doll eye phenomenon after the first 2 weeks of life indicates serious brain damage. A normal VOR should be present by 2 months of age[71] and consists of both the slow and fast components of nystagmus being present. Nystagmus is an alternating sequence of fast and slow horizontal eye movements normally seen in response to a series of rotatory movements of the head. The form and amount of nystagmus normally present in infants change between birth and the first year of life.

Saccadic movements of the eye are quick movements, which bring the image onto the fovea of the eye. As the saccadic system matures, the eyes can then demonstrate the fast component of nystagmus, a jerking back to central gaze. Optokinetic nystagmus is nystagmus that results from viewing a rotating drum stimulus. Infants as young as 3–6 months of age can demonstrate optokinetic nystagmus. The saccadic system responsible for the fast component of nystagmus continues to mature up to the age of 2 years.[27,71] A VOR can also generate eye movements to compensate for head motion to maintain a stable retinal image. A lack of this VOR response at 10 months of age is abnormal.[27,72]

Vestibular sensitivity increases from birth to a peak between 6 and 12 months of age. The most striking maturational changes occur in preschool children.[27] After this peak, there is a decline to 2½ years and a more gradual decline to puberty. Before 3 years of age, infants and children engage in repetitive self-stimulation, such as rocking in a rocking chair or spinning themselves around, but this is not a pervasive activity. Infants are more sensitive to vestibular input, and that oversensitivity may explain their relative unsteadiness. The slow maturation of vestibular sensitivity is a result of changes in synaptic strength and connectivity in the brainstem and higher centers.[69] Maturation of the vestibular system contributes to general motor development and postural control.

Special Senses

Vision. Newborns were always thought to have relatively poor, if any, visual abilities at birth. However, as technology for testing has become more sophisticated, so has the understanding of the infant's visual system. Newborns have pattern preference and can maintain attention if a stimulus is novel enough or resembles a face. To obtain visual alerting behavior, newborns need to be approached from the side because they are unable to maintain their heads in the midline until 4 months of age. Visual acuity at birth appears to be about 20/800,[73] and steadily increases with age. Some authors report that adult levels of vision (20/20) are achieved as early as 1 year,[50] but others use 3 years as the age at which adult resolution is possible.[73]

The infant sees initially in black and white. As the cones (the color receptors) mature over the first several months, color vision develops. Two-month-old-infants can see the colors red and yellow. Full-color vision is present by 4 months.

Smooth tracking abilities begin by 2 months of age[60] and progress over an ever-widening arc as the infant matures and head control is achieved. Smooth pursuit is the ability to track a target smoothly without jerking. Myelination of the pathway that subserves smooth pursuit is complete at 5 months.[74] Accommodation is possible at 2 months but improves to adult levels by 6 months. Depth and size perception begin to develop with the ability to use the two eyes together to converge or diverge on near and far objects. This may be aided by the development of head control in the prone position as the infant practices looking down at hands or up at toys.

Vision provides vital information for balance and head control: "perceptual sensitivity to visual information improves rapidly during the first few months after birth."[75] Head control contributes to the ability of the infant to visually fix on objects. Conversely, visual fixation contributes to postural stability of the head and neck. Visual information is used to control posture even before infants can sit. Optical flow is detected peripherally by infants and used as a cue to make a compensatory response. "Optical flow refers to the perceived motion of the visual field that results from an individual's own movement through the environment."[76]

Binocular vision depends on adequate alignment of the eyes. Most infants demonstrate good visual alignment between 3 and 6 months of age. Shimojo and colleagues[77] postulate that the change in binocular function seen at 3 months is related to the separation of the afferent input from the two eyes into columns within the visual cortex. These bands of cells are known as *ocular dominance columns.* If the input from each eye is the same, the columns will be the same size. Two-year-olds exhibit adultlike binocular vision. Table 9.1 provides a list of changes in visual development along with changes in visual-motor behavior during the first two years of life.

Hearing. At birth, the infant physiologically responds to sound by changing respiratory patterns or heart rate. The auditory brainstem response (ABR) is an electrophysiologic measure of function used to test for eighth cranial nerve integrity at 27–28 weeks gestation. It is accurate for detecting sensorineural hearing loss.[78] ABR wave forms change with age. Latencies for all wave forms reach adult values by 18 months.[79] Behaviorally,

the infant may demonstrate facial grimacing, eye blinking, and crying at loud noises. The auditory system is completely myelinated 1 month after birth but the system is not mature until adolescence. Otoacoustic emissions (OAEs) can be recorded at birth using a small sensitive microphone placed in the entrance to the ear canal.[30] OAEs are used to study the maturation of cochlear function. By 3 months of age, head turning to localize sound is well established. In the appropriate state of wakefulness, a newborn may exhibit eye or head turning

TABLE 9.1   Visual Development in First Two Years of Life

Age	Visual Development	Visual-Motor Behavior
Newborn	Focal distance 7–10 in 20/800 acuity	Hands fisted Doll eye Tracks toy to midline Prefers black and white
1 month	Focal distance ≥1–3 ft Frontal visual fields mature	Tracks 180 degrees Prefers face to object Tracks horizontally
2 months	Accommodation develops Depth and size perception developing Dichromatic (red and yellow)	Unilateral hand regard Asymmetrical tonic neck reflex Hands open, manipulates red ring, swipes
3 months	Head turning with eyes Binocular vision begins Improved visual attention	Strong visual inspection of hands at midline Mouths objects
4 months	Sees in full color Well-developed binocular vision Accommodates over wide range of distances	Bilateral reach at midline Hits and shakes objects Instinctive grasp Holds one cube
5 months	Vision directs grasp and manipulation	Turns head to follow vanishing object Raking; holds two cubes
6 months	Adult accommodation 20/40 acuity	Tracks objects in all directions Transfers at midline Palmar grasp
7 months		Transfers hand to hand Radial palmar grasp
8 months	Macula more mature	Anticipates future position of objects in motion Reaches for hidden objects
9 months		Radial digital grasp
10 months		Recognizes object by seeing only part of it Inferior pincer grasp (9–12 months)
12 months	20/20 acuity	Follows rapidly moving objects Visually monitors hand play Neat pincer grasp
2 years	Adult binocular vision	

to sound. New sounds will produce searching behavior in infants older than 4 months and will encourage the infant to babble in vocal play. Vocal imitation follows, with words being produced by the first year.

"The auditory system constructs a perceptual space that takes information from objects and groups, segregates sounds, and provides meaning and access to communication tools such as language."[30] When a moving infant takes or shows an object to a caregiver, the infant is making a moving bid for interaction. The action of initiating shared attention to objects is known to be valuable for language development.[80] Joint attention is needed for motor learning and socialization. Object play has been associated with the emergence of words.[81]

The 2-year-old develops listening skills, which refine the production of speech and facilitate the rapid acquisition of language. Speech is learned by successive approximations of the correct sound. Basic auditory listening skills are mastered by 3 years of age.[17] There is prolonged maturation of auditory development into the teenage years.[30] Changes in attention, cognition, and memory play a role in auditory development. Childrens' exposure to real-world language in the form of adult-child conversation correlates with increased strength of connectivity of language pathways.[82]

Ear infections (otitis media) that result in increased fluid in the ear are a common problem in infants and preschoolers. Because fluid in the middle ear can produce a conductive hearing loss, these infections are now treated aggressively with insertion of tympanostomy tubes based on clinical practice guidelines from the American Academy of Otolaryngology-Head and Neck Surgery Foundation.[83] Two recommendations from the executive summary[84] are noteworthy for therapists. (1) Children should have a hearing evaluation if they have otitis media with effusion for 3 months or longer or prior to surgery for tube insertion. (2) "Clinicians should determine if a child is at risk for speech, language, or learning problems from otitis media because of baseline sensory, physical, cognitive, or behavioral factors."[84] Dynamic balance problems and delays in gross motor development have been reported in children with chronic ear infections.[85]

Taste and smell. These two chemical senses are significant to the newborn. Although obviously linked to feeding, these senses are also involved in parent-infant communication, control of respiration, and cognition.[50] Taste or more specifically flavor assists in modulating oral intake. Flavor is a composite of taste, texture, and smell. Infants discriminate between all five primary taste sensations (sour, salty, sweet, bitter, and umami [savory]) but prefer sweet-tasting solutions to bitter ones.[86,87] Development of flavor preferences begins in utero when flavors ingested by the mother are transmitted to the amniotic fluid. Preferences continue to develop based on the type of formula the infant is fed.[32] A 5-day-old newborn can selectively orient to her mother's breast pad based on odor.[88] Odors such as pine or baby powder can reduce distress and increase attention in 6-month-old infants.[89] Infants may use smell to identify familiar features of the environment, including people, before the visual system is effective in performing this function. Both taste and smell are functional at birth and quickly become connected to feeding reflexes.

Childhood and Adolescence

Sensory changes continue during childhood and adolescence. It is during childhood that the integration of sensation and movement occurs. The perceptual process, although evident in early development, is further refined by the child's increased ability to attend to more than one characteristic of a stimulus, to attach meaning to sensory stimuli, and to plan a motor response. Cognitive and language development is of paramount importance in developing and verbalizing spatial and directional concepts that build on the increased awareness of self and the surroundings.

Somatic Senses

Somatosensation consists of touch registration and perception, proprioception, and haptic ability. Somatosensation increases with age from 2.5 years to 18 years.[90] These improvements are not linear. Individuals exhibit variability in performance. Exploratory procedures used for haptic perception are adultlike by 3 years and haptic perception is fairly well developed by early childhood.[49] Proprioception in the upper extremities improves between 4 and 8 years of age.[29,91] Two-point discrimination is possible by 4 years of age.[92] Children can usually identify familiar objects using only touch at 5 years of age. This type of haptic perception is called stereognosis. Knowledge of where the body is in space and the sequence of movements that must be planned to perform a motor task is based on appropriate interpretation of tactile and proprioceptive input. The ability to motor plan, or praxis, emerges during childhood.

Refinements in proprioceptive input needed for motor output occur from 6 years and continue into adolescence.[93] Values are lowest in childhood (6- to 8-year-olds) and increase to a peak in young adulthood.[94] Tactile and proprioceptive sensation recalibrates the changing adolescent's body scheme and the affective view of the body in response to pubertal growth between 13 and 17 years in males and 11 and 15 years in females.[91]

Self-Perception

The coupling of movement and perception is a central process in perceptual development of self-recognition. Bigelow[95] identified how children use proprioceptive information in visual self-recognition. Children recognized moving images of themselves sooner than they did static pictures, which supports the belief that children move their bodies purposefully to gain proprioceptive information. Thelen[96] believed that individuals perceive in order to move and move in order to perceive. Rochat thinks that the highest level of self-awareness is achieved around the age of 5. This belief is supported by the ability of children to develop representations of objects and people in their mind between the ages of 4 and 5. Infants begin with no awareness of self and as children are able to develop a higher level of self-awareness by age 5. For example, 5-year-olds are very aware of inequity and have learned to capitalize on the ethic of fairness.

Kinesthetic perception is composed of *kinesthetic acuity* and *kinesthetic memory*. *Kinesthetic acuity* is the ability to proprioceptively discriminate differences in location, distance, weight, force, speed, and acceleration of movement. For example, an individual can distinguish objects by weight when held in the hand while blindfolded. Kinesthetic acuity improves with age. Based on research using the Kinesthetic Acuity Test (KAT), Elliot and associates[97] reported that performance in children improves from ages 5 through 12 and sometimes beyond. Livesey and Parks[98] and Livesey and Intilli[99] used the KAT with preschool children and documented that kinesthetic sense can be tested in children as young as 3 years of age. They found that kinesthetic sense improves with age and that boys performed better than girls. However, when visual-spatial cues were reduced in

a follow-up study, the gender differences were no longer present. Kinesthetic acuity improves more quickly than kinesthetic memory. Memory for movement is referred to as *kinesthetic memory*. Examples of movement tasks performed from memory are a dance routine and the sequence of step-hopping that occurs in skipping. Adult levels of kinesthetic acuity are achieved by 8 years of age, whereas kinesthetic memory maturity is not usually achieved until after the age of 12.[100]

Vestibular Sense

Vestibular responses change greatly between preadolescence and adulthood.[68] Children demonstrate a more vigorous nystagmus in response to vestibular stimulation than adults, who respond less intensely as the system matures. Maturation of vestibular nystagmus is thought to be completed by 10 years of age.[68] Charpiot and colleagues[101] studied the VOR and balance maturation in 6- to 12-year-olds. They found that the 10- to 12-year-olds used vestibular input for balance more than the younger children in the study. Previously, Hirabayashi and Iwaski[4] reported that vestibular function relative to postural control did not reach adult levels even at age 15. Goulème and associates[102] found that girls in the most challenging balance situations maintained better postural control than boys by using vestibular input. Sinno and colleagues[103] found that vestibular ratio scores using the sensory organization test for balance increased with age in their subjects who ranged from 3 to 16.8 years. Scores of 15- to 17-year-olds in this study were not significantly different from scores in a control group of adults. See Chapter 11 for a further discussion of sensory organization in postural control.

Special Senses

Vision. Many aspects of visual perception develop in childhood. The child shows refinement of size constancy: the ability to recognize that objects remain the same size even if the distance of the viewer from the object changes. The ability to separate the figure from the background, or *figure-ground perception*, improves with age. By 8 years of age, most children are as good as adults in performing this perceptual task.[104]

Visual perception related to object identification, movement, and task performance seems to follow the same trend. By 5 years of age, children demonstrate *visual closure*, or the ability to discern a shape when seeing only part of it. Between 5 and 10 years of age, children accurately track moving objects, such as a softball.[105] Perceptual judgments regarding the size of various objects at different distances become mature at the age of 11 years.[106] Adult levels of depth perception are achieved at 12 years of age.

Spatial awareness. *Spatial awareness* is the internalization of our own location in space and object localization. The teacher stands in front of the students with the blackboard behind her. Visuospatial processing utilizes two distinct pathways in the brain. The dorsal pathway processes spatial information and the ventral pathway processes form perception.[107] *Space perception* is the ability to perceive direction or distance. Combining visual information with proprioception allows the child to recognize the location and orientation of objects within the environment. By age 3–4 years, most children have conceptualized the spatial dichotomies of over/under, top/bottom, front/back, and in/out. The sequence of acquisition of these spatial directions is vertical to horizontal, then diagonal or oblique.[100] Knowledge of the spatial environment is necessary to construct effective motor programs. Objects are first related to the child and later related to other objects. Space perception and spatial awareness are needed for successful execution of a motor program when accommodating to changing environmental demands.

Most 5-year-old children know the right side of the body from the left side. This concept of *laterality* is a conscious internal awareness of the two sides of the body. However, it is not until children are 8 years of age that they consistently and accurately answer questions about right-left discrimination.[100] It is also at this age that children can begin to relay information in directional terms such as "the playground is on the right."

Directionality, the motor expression of laterality and spatial orientation, develops between 4 and 12 years of age.[100] Four-year-olds understand spatial dichotomies such as up/down, in/out, and top/bottom. Directionality is initially demonstrated when children mirror imitate the movements of the person in front of them. At 7 years of age, the child uses the body as a directional reference: "The ball is in front of me." Next, the child can reference objects objectively, such as, "The water fountain is on the left." By 10 years of age, children can identify the right and left of the person in front of them. The child no longer mirrors movements but will move the right arm when the other person moves the right arm. At 12 years

of age, children can use a natural frame of reference to describe that the sun sets in the west.

Adulthood and Aging

Sensory abilities present in adolescence continue to guide motor activities. Information from different sensory systems continues to be combined during adulthood. This *intersensory integration* allows the adult mover to use visual and auditory cues to provide increased perception of the task at hand. Many combinations of sensory inputs are possible. The response time in a motor task can be shortened when a person attends to a combination of sensory inputs rather than to a single sensory input.[108,109] Despite the development of intersensory associations and the maintenance of a steady functional state of sensory receptors up to middle age, a decline in sensory function does begin in adulthood and progresses with advanced age. Peripheral and central changes are documented in many of the sensory systems, although these changes are not always directly related to a decline in function, nor are they universal.

Somatic Senses

Some older adults show a diminished ability to detect touch, vibration, proprioception, temperature, and pain.[110] Structural changes in the skin such as loss of dermal thickness, decline in nutrient transfer, and loss of collagen and elastin fibers contribute to a decline in the functions of the skin. Wrinkles and loss of skin firmness can contribute to a decline in touch discrimination (See Chapter 10).[111] The sense of touch is needed to handle objects and detect stimuli. Loss of touch sensitivity and acuity can significantly affect the quality of life. Physiologically, the growth rate, healing response, sensory perception, and thermoregulation of the skin decline.[111]

Touch. The skin receptors responsible for the perception of pressure and light touch, *Pacinian* and *Meissner corpuscles*, decline in number with age.[9] By the ninth decade, they are only one-third of their original densit. Both of these receptors also undergo morphological or structural changes. Decreased vibrotactile sensitivity with age has been documented by increased thresholds.[112] This decreased sensitivity is related to structural changes in the *Pacinian* corpuscle pathways. Meissner's corpuscles and Merkel cells decrease progressively with aging.[113] Meissner corpuscles change relative to whether we have performed physical labor. With manual labor, the corpuscles become winding and large; without manual labor, they develop neurofibrillary networks. Structural changes include reduced elasticity of the skin in older people, as well as reduced numbers and altered morphology of skin tactile receptors. Effects of aging on the peripheral system and CNS also include demyelination, which affects the timing of neural signals, as well as reduced numbers of peripheral nerve fibers.[111] Regardless of structural changes, older adults can lose up to 90% of these receptors. *Merkel cells*, another type of pressure receptor, also display changes in size and structure during aging.[113] With the loss of pressure and light touch receptors, valuable feedback about the environment is decreased, and balance responses may be impaired.

Tactile acuity declines with age.[111] Touch thresholds in the fingers of older adults were found to be elevated 2½ times over younger adults.[114] Spatial acuity as tested by two-point discrimination has been found to be impaired with age. Stevens and colleagues[115] documented a lower ability to detect gap discrimination on five body areas (plantar and dorsal surfaces of the forefoot, volar forearm, and upper and lower surfaces of the forefinger) in older adults compared with young adults. The rate of deterioration of spatial acuity is slower in the proximal parts of the body compared with the distal parts.[116] However, the upper and lower surfaces of the fingertips and feet show identical declines in tactile acuity so that it is incorrect to attribute this effect of aging to wear and tear.[117] Interestingly, studies have found that the pleasantness of being touched increases with age over 60 years in contrast to the decrease in perceived intensity.[111,118] Pleasant touch, such as experienced during a caress, appears to be even more pleasant in old age.[111]

Vibration. One of the most common sensory losses documented in older adults is the loss of vibratory sensation. The decline in the Pacinian and Meissner corpuscles correlates with impairments in detecting vibration seen in older adults. Awareness of vibration begins to decline after 60 years of age,[110,111] with the lower extremities more affected than the upper extremities.[9] Perry[119] studied vibration perception on the plantar surface of older and younger adults using monofilaments. Older adults were less sensitive at all sites tested compared with young adults. Vibration perception thresholds were found to double in the early 70s. Clinically it is important to include vibratory testing of the lower extremity in older adults when screening for sensory impairments because losses may be related to impaired balance.[120] See Table 9.2 for a summary of the age-related changes in cutaneous somatosensation.

Proprioception. Joint position sense (JPS) definitely declines with age,[121] especially in the lower extremities. Distal joints are more affected than proximal joints with the differences possibly being related to weight bearing. A decrease in JPS has been documented in the big toe and in the ankle in weight bearing and non–weight bearing.[122,123] Yang and colleagues[94] found that ankle proprioception decreased from middle age to older age with the sharpest decline occurring in the 75- to 90-year-old group. There were no gender differences. Knee proprioception was poorer in subjects with knee osteoarthritis than in subjects with unaffected knees in an age-matched control group.[124] Hip JPS and kinesthesia were significantly decreased in older adults compared with middle aged and younger adults.[125] Functionally, the decline in proprioception in the lower extremities has tremendous implications for compromising balance in older adults.[120,126]

Temperature. Aging is associated with a progressive decrease in thermal perception in the elderly. Typically, the reduction in thermosensitivity due to aging follows a distal-proximal pattern. Loss of warmth sensation outpaces loss of cold in the extremities. The primary cause of these losses is reduced thermoreceptor density and superficial skin blood flow. Changes in the peripheral nerve system, particularly fiber loss and decreased conduction velocity, may also be involved in this loss.[127]

Compromised thermoregulation can predispose older adults to hypothermia or heat stroke. Control of body temperature regulation by the hypothalamus is altered significantly with age. The ability of the sympathetic nervous system to cause vasoconstriction and impede heat loss is impaired. As a result, mild hypothermia occurs in a large number of older adults in cooler rooms, which is why older people accommodate by more often wearing sweaters, coats, and hats. Thermoregulatory deficiency is also a result of a decline in temperature perception.[128]

Body Temperature

Stanford researchers have determined that average adult human body temperature in the United States has decreased since the 1800s. This study has called the "normal" human temperature of 37°C (or 98.6°F) as too high. They determined that mean body temperature

TABLE 9.2 **Age-Related Changes in Somatosensation**

Function	Receptor	Nature of Change
Touch/pressure	Fewer free nerve endings ↓ number of Pacinian corpuscles ↓ concentration of Meissner corpuscles	Significant increase in thresholds after age 60 years Lower thresholds in fingers than toes Light touch thresholds significantly increase in the hands and feet Men are generally less sensitive than women
Vibration	↓ number of Pacinian corpuscles ↓ concentration of Meissner corpuscles	Increased vibration threshold for perception Lower extremities more affected than upper extremities Greatest decline after 60 years
Proprioception (passive joint position)	↓ number of intrafusal fibers in the spindle ↓ in all joint receptor types	Decreased joint position sense in the big toe and ankle Thresholds for lower extremity joints twice as great after 50 years of age than before 40 years
Kinesthesia (active joint motion)	Demyelination and decreased peripheral nerve fibers	Decreased timing of neural signals Age-related changes increase with greater memory demands

Data from Cavazzana A, Röhrborn A, Garthus-Niegel S, et al. Sensory-specific impairment among older people. An investigation using both sensory thresholds and subjective measures across the five senses. *PloS One.* 2018;13(8):e0202969; McIntyre S, Nagi SS, McGlone F, Olausson H. The effects of ageing on tactile function in humans. *Neuroscience.* 2021;464:53-58; Shaffer SW, Harrison AL. Aging of the somatosensory system: a translational perspective. *Phys Ther.* 2007;87:193-207; Williams HG. Aging and eye-hand coordination. In: Bard C, Fleury J, Hay L, eds: *Development of Eye-Hand Coordination.* Columbia: University of South Carolina Press; 1990:352.

in men and women, after adjusting for age, height, weight, and, in some models, date and time of day, has decreased monotonically by 0.03°C per birth decade.[129] Resting metabolic rate is the largest component of a typical modern human's energy expenditure, comprising around 65% of daily energy expenditure for a sedentary individual which has decreased. This analysis found that body temperatures have been dropping consistently over the past 170 years, with the new normal being closer to 97.5 degrees, when taken orally.[129] Other studies have found the human body temperature averaging out differently, including at 97.7°F, 97.9°F, and 98.2°F.[130] This may affect what we now consider a fever during illness.

Pain. How aging leads to changes in pain perception and brain functional connectivity that can lead to chronic pain is not completely understood. Aging seems to be associated with increased pain thresholds and poor functioning of endogenous pain inhibition mechanisms.[131] Additionally, age-related changes in the spontaneous organization of the brain have been linked to the cognitive, perceptual, and motor alterations that frequently accompany aging. Older participants display enlarged cortical representations of the body and enhanced cortical excitability of the primary somatosensory cortex that can lead to reduced tactile perception.

Older adults may have a reduced functional connectivity between key nodes of the descending pain inhibitory pathway. This suggests that, in aging, the pain system is activated slightly later, but over time, the dysfunction of the pain modulatory and evaluation processes could lead to increased pain perception.[131] The loss of descending inhibitory control is thought to be critical to the development of chronic pain, but what causes this loss (of inhibitory control) in function is not well understood. The loss of cortical drive to the descending pain modulatory system underpins the expression of neuropathic sensitization after peripheral nerve injury.[132] In other words, pain perception is altered over years due to the appearance of certain changes in the brain structure. The inhibitory mechanisms that gradually reduce pain in younger individuals do not work as efficiently in an older person. Taken together, these results could explain why older adults are more vulnerable to developing chronic pain disorders.

Vestibular Sense

Dizziness and vertigo are common disturbances in persons older than 50 years. Structures of the vestibular system such as the hair cells undergo degeneration.[133] A 20%–40% reduction in hair cells has been reported in the saccule and utricle and in the semicircular canals. Current evidence suggests that certain aspects of this multifaceted system may deteriorate with age and sometimes with severe consequences, such as injurious falls. The number of nerve cells in the vestibular system decreases from about age 55.[134] Blood flow to the inner ear also decreases with age. Idiopathic bilateral vestibular loss can become more severe as age progresses due to these changes. Another factor in balance dysfunction may be changes in the strength of peripheral vestibular signaling in older adults. How this decreased sensory information is unable to be accurately processed by central circuits is also a contributing factor. Older adults tend to use the proprioceptive sense rather than visual and vestibular cues for postural motor control.[134] Neuronal and hair cell losses in the inner ear are the two other factors affecting the peripheral vestibular system. These losses affect both the function of the otolith organs and the semicircular canals, which affect balance reactions. Overall, there is an age-related decline of peripheral vestibular sensing[135] and the central combination of different sensory signals for balance.[134]

Neuronal loss has been documented in parts of the vestibular nuclear complex that receive input from the semicircular canals.[136] Anson et al.[137] linked slower gait speed in older adults who had lost horizontal semicircular canal function. Loss of synapses is postulated to occur in response to constant stimulation of this sensory system.[138] Neural changes in the vestibular nerve are evident in older adults and may begin as early as 40 years of age. By 75 years, the number of myelinated vestibular nerve fibers declines almost 40%.[139] Older individual may exhibit disequilibrium from age-related changes in the peripheral or central vestibular system. There is an increased gain in the VOR in older adults, which can result in the person perceiving movement of the environment when the head is moved. The nervous system compensates for age-related deterioration of the vestibular system as evidenced by not all older adults exhibiting vestibular disorders. However, dizziness and vestibular dysfunction may manifest themselves when the nervous system is no longer able to compensate.[140] "Data from the National Health and Nutrition Examination Survey (NHANES) indicate a high prevalence of difficulties with vestibular function among the elderly, with 69% among those aged 70–79 years and 85% among those aged 80+ years having vestibular dysfunction."[141]

Presbystasis is the age-related decline in equilibrium or dynamic balance seen when no other pathology is noted.[142] Reliance on vestibular input alone may result in loss of balance and even falls in the older adult.[134,143] Healthy older adults without general sensory deficits do not exhibit as much of an increase in postural sway as do older adults who show sensory deficits. The latter group is more likely to experience falls.[144,145] Postural sway is described in Chapter 11.

Special Senses

Vision. Visual acuity increases in the 20s and 30s, remains stable in the 40s and 50s, and then declines.[146] The most rapid decrease in acuity occurs between 60 and 80 years of age. By 85, there is an 80% loss from the acuity level present at 40 years of age.[147] Structural changes in the optical part of the eye contribute to these age-related changes in function. The cornea and lens thicken, the lens curvature decreases, and a yellowish pigment accumulates. Aging changes in the lens protein may be a result of oxidative damage.[128] Table 9.3 lists some age-related changes in vision.

Central vision can be impaired by cataracts, a decrease in the transparency of the lens. The increase in lens density is due to accumulation of pigments. Cataracts begin to form in everyone older than 30 years,[148] and a little over 17% of those older than 40 years have at least one cataract.[149] The rate of progression, however, is different for every individual. Most cataracts develop bilaterally in those older than 50 years and are present to some degree in all 70-year-olds.[150] Fully developed cataracts are documented in one-third of persons 80 years old.[148] Visual acuity of 20/50 or worse is an indication for surgical removal. Those with diabetes have a higher incidence of cataracts than do the rest of the population.

Color discrimination in the green-blue end of the spectrum becomes more difficult as the lens of the eye yellows with aging. Pupil size declines with age, allowing less light into the eye. By 60 years of age, retinal illumination is reduced by one-third, and the older adult is less able to detect low levels of light. Because of the lens changes, light may be scattered over more of the retinal surface, resulting in glare. Glare introduces extraneous

TABLE 9.3	Age-Related Changes in Vision
Function	**Nature of Change**
General	Density of the lens increases and may lose transparency (cataract)
	Stiffening of the lens causes an inability to change shape (presbyopia)
	Decreased number and orientation of photoreceptors in the macula
Binocular vision	Decreases
Color vision	Becomes difficult to differentiate between similar colors
Contrast sensitivity	Declines
Dark adaptation	Takes an older adult longer to adjust to changes in light levels
Depth perception	Decreases
Glare adaptation	Becomes more difficult to adapt
Visual acuity	Usually remains stable until the age of 65, then declines
	Dynamic visual acuity or detention of moving objects becomes more difficult
Visual fields	Size of visual field decreases and peripheral vision decreases after age 45
Visual processing	Slows down

Data from Erdinest N, London N, Lavy I, Morad Y, Levinger N. Vision through healthy aging eyes. Vision (Basel). 2021;5(4):46. Petrash JM. Aging and age-related diseases of the ocular lens and vitreous body. *Invest Ophthalmol Vis Sci.* 2013;54(14):ORSF54-9. Lord SR, Delbaere K, Sturnieks DL. Aging. *Handb Clin Neurol.* 2018;159:157–171. Saftari LN, Kwon O-S. Ageing vision and falls: a review. J Physiol Anthropol. 2018;37:11.

light into the eye and may be particularly troublesome for older adults. Because of retinal sensitivity loss, the elder's eyes are overstimulated by oncoming headlights or sudden flashes of light.

Contrast sensitivity and dark adaptation decline with age. Contrast sensitivity loss causes a loss of depth perception, which can be especially dangerous when going up or

down the stairs. Adaptation to dim light decreases with age, which can be hazardous when entering a darkened house or a less well-illuminated room. A teenager needs only 6–7 minutes to adapt to darkness, but an 80-year-old may need more than 40 minutes.[151] These changes are related to a decline in the number of receptors and a decreased regeneration capacity of photoreceptor pigment.[152]

Presbyopia is the diminished ability to focus clearly at normal reading distances. One contributing cause is the thickening of the lens due to continued growth of lens fibers.[148] The ciliary muscle normally acts to change the curvature of the lens to focus the image. With aging, the ciliary muscles become less able to adequately accommodate to distance changes; those over 40 years often complain, "My arms are not long enough to read the print of the newspaper." Accommodation difficulties may also impair the older person's ability to read the speedometer in the car because of a decreased ability to change the lens size when switching from far to near vision. Corrective lenses such as bifocals or trifocals become necessary. By the age of 60 years, when the lens can no longer accommodate, presbyopia exists.

Hearing. *Presbycusis*, an age-related decline in hearing acuity, is due to a loss of sensory cells in the inner ear or, more specifically, the organ of Corti. Structural changes that contribute to age-related hearing loss include degeneration of the hair cells at the base of the cochlea, degeneration of nerve cells in the spiral ganglia, atrophy of associated vascular and connective tissue, and loss of neurons in the cortical auditory centers.[152] Because the loss typically occurs at the base of the structure, hearing is initially impaired for high-frequency tones such as the whistle of a tea kettle or a doorbell. Speech perception is preserved because speech is heard at lower sound frequencies. This type of hearing loss is associated with aging and can begin as early as 30 years of age and progress until 80 years.

Presbycusis is more than a simple hearing loss of pure tones. It also involves speech processing and discrimination. Although speech perception is preserved, the ability to discriminate or recognize what is being said decreases. The loss of discrimination is greater than would be expected from the hearing loss alone. Seventy-five percent of adults older than 70 years will exhibit hearing loss of this type. The environment and heredity can contribute to the onset of presbycusis, so it is important to know the risk factors. Noise exposure, smoking, ototoxic medications, hypertension, and family history have been identified by Gates and Mills[153] in their review of presbycusis as risk factors.

Taste and smell. Certain diseases and conditions as well as normal aging and dietary intake can be associated with taste disorders.[154] Each taste bud contains a number of specialized epithelial cells, including taste receptor cells for recognizing sweet, bitter, umami, sour, and salty compounds. The number of taste buds decreases as one ages. Each remaining taste bud also begins to lose volume.[155] In addition, salivary glands produce less saliva during the aging process. This can cause dry mouth, which can directly affect the sense of taste. The increase in the use of medication in elderly people may also affect the oral conditions influencing the sense of taste. Taste sensitivity that decreases with age may also be influenced by insufficient dietary intake, especially iron and thiamin. Although the exact mechanism of the effect of aging on taste sensation is not well understood, aging appears to clearly influence taste sensation.

The loss of smell is greater than that of taste.[156] In an earlier review, Schiffman[157] noted that there is a modest loss of taste in normal healthy aging. Smell identification declines progressively with age.[158] Identification of tastes declines with age. Memory distortion, changes, or both in the social and emotional context in which eating occurs may also contribute to a decreased perception of the flavor and appeal of food for older adults. Poor appetite can cause a decline in energy and activity and ultimately lead to a decline in overall function. The sense of smell, which also diminishes, may be related to a loss of nerve endings and less mucus production in the nose. Mucus helps odors stay in the nose long enough to be detected by the nerve endings. Mucus also helps clear odors from the nerve endings. Certain things can speed up the loss of taste and smell. These include diseases, smoking, and exposure to harmful particles in the air. An impaired sense of smell, or olfactory dysfunction, is now recognized as a possible symptom of Alzheimer disease. Olfactory sensation decline has emerged as an early predictor of the condition. Olfactory dysfunction has also been determined to be a risk factor for other forms of dementia and cognitive decline in apparent cognitively healthy older adults.[159]

Functional Implications

Impairment of any one sensory system during early development can lead to difficulty in function. Hearing loss affects the development of motor skills and balance.[160] Because the eighth cranial nerve subserves both hearing and motion sense, it stands to reason that if one part is damaged, the other portion may also be damaged. Many children with hearing impairments have poor vestibular function, resulting in balance deficits.[161] Some children with primarily vestibular deficits are unsafe without protective headgear.

The effects of deficits in tactile, vestibular, and proprioceptive systems on sensory integration are also well documented. Deficits are linked to poor body scheme, self-image, difficulty in motor planning, or sequencing movement and balance. Sensory information is used to learn movement. The ability to process sensory information and thus integrate it with movement in a planned and organized manner is important for motor coordination.

The effects of visual deficits on the developmental course were documented by Jan and colleagues.[162] Visually impaired children must substitute auditory cues to direct movement; because so many movements are visually guided, their acquisition of motor milestones is delayed. Children with crossed eyes, or strabismus, may have difficulty in developing head control or midline reaching. The earlier that the visual alignment deficits are detected and corrected, the better off children are in terms of upper extremity control. The ability to prevent or detect visual deficits earlier may decrease the concomitant activity and participation limitations.

A decline in function of any one sensory system because of aging can have serious functional implications. For example, presbyopia makes it more difficult for the older adults to read dials on the stove or to do needle work. A decline in depth perception can contribute to an increased potential for falling while going up or down the stairs. Presbycusis may isolate an elder from a lively conversation or decrease awareness of a warning siren while driving the automobile with the radio turned on. Food preparation and mealtime may be less enjoyable because of age-related changes in smell and taste abilities. Changes in somatosensation in the lower extremities and motion sense may contribute to an increased likelihood of falling or an increased fear of falling, which can lead to hypoactivity. Any or all of the potential sensory changes with aging can curtail an individual's range of movement by increasing dependence on compensatory devices or strategies.

Because vision is so important to development across the life span, two conditions that affect vision, amblyopia and macular degeneration, are discussed in detail. One occurs early in development and is potentially reversible, whereas the other occurs at the end of the life span. Both are examples of sensory changes that can have significant functional implications. An important life skill that can be impeded by either of these conditions is driving. It is our most relied-on means of mobility and is prized as a reward by the adolescent, deemed almost as a right of passage. Adults depend on driving to get to and from jobs, appointments, shopping, and leisure activities. Driving becomes a significant quality-of-life issue as individuals reach older age and strive to maintain independence.

Amblyopia

Amblyopia is derived from the Greek word for "blunt or dull sight." The loss of sight can occur in childhood. The brain depends on receiving simultaneous clear focused images from both eyes (binocular) for the visual pathways to develop properly. Visual fields overlap in binocular vision because a part of the visual world is perceived by each eye. Binocularity allows us to see a three-dimensional image of our surroundings. When one eye is deprived of input, it is difficult to produce a single image. The person with amblyopia elects to see with only one eye in order to see only one image. The lazy eye, if deprived of visual input for sufficient time, will lose sight, and the child will become functionally blind because of a lack of visual cortex development.

Risk factors for amblyopia include strabismus and various refractive errors. Monocular deprivation can result when one eye is deviated in any direction—in, out, up, or down—a condition known as strabismus. Four types of refractive errors seen in children can put them at risk for amblyopia: myopia (nearsightedness) makes far-away objects blurry; hyperopia (farsightedness) makes nearby objects blurry; astigmatism makes both far-away and nearby objects blurry; and anisometropia (unequal refractive error). The severity of amblyopia is related to the age at which it started and the type of asymmetry. The critical period for amblyopia is the first 8 years. It is "relatively easy to correct until that age by improving the quality of the visual input in the affected eye."[163]

Amblyopia is the most common cause of blindness in infants and children.[164] The global prevalence of amblyopia is reported to be 4.3%,[165] while the prevalence in the United States remains stable at 2%–3%.[166] Despite global efforts to increase awareness, a large number of children with visual problems are not being identified. It is estimated that 5%–10% of preschoolers and 25% of school-aged children have visual problems that impact learning and quality of life.[166] Amblyopia not only affects visual acuity in the affected eye but produces deficits in positional acuity and contrast sensitivity along with perceptual deficits in the strong eye.[164] A range of visual-motor deficits can also occur as a result of the "lazy eye." Therefore, amblyopia is considered a binocular problem because the entire developing visual system is affected.[164]

A child's use of only one eye may not be apparent unless screening is conducted. "In January 2016, a new joint policy statement from the AAP, American Academy of Ophthalmology (AAO), American Association for Pediatric Ophthalmology and Strabismus (AAPOS), and the American Association of Certified Orthoptists (AACO) regarding the pediatric eye examination was published. The updated policy statement, published in the journal *Pediatrics*, incorporates earlier and routine visual assessments using instrument-based screening to help identify children who may benefit from early intervention to improve vision (or correct vision problems). Instrument-based screening technology is revolutionizing early detection and prevention of amblyopia by allowing screening of more children and at a younger age."[166]

Malalignment of the eye caused by strabismus may be corrected by surgery while refractive errors may be corrected with glasses or patching. Amblyopia is usually unilateral but it can be bilateral.[167] Traditionally, treatment of amblyopia consisted of occlusion or patching of the eye with corrective lenses being used as an adjunctive treatment. The treatment rationale was based on forcing the lazy eye to work harder. Correction of refractive errors can benefit children with amblyopia if the correction is used earlier in treatment, not just as an adjunct to occlusion.[168] In those children with refractive errors and amblyopia, one-fourth to one-third of the children treated first with corrective lenses did not require occlusion therapy.[169] A better understanding of the neural basis and sequela of amblyopia has led to exploring additional treatment options. These options include perceptual learning, playing video games, and binocular training. The premise of these treatments is to use sensory tasks to improve sight. Perceptual learning has been defined as "any relatively permanent or consistent change in perception of a stimulus array following practice or experience with this array...."[170]

Childhood amblyopia is also the leading cause of loss of vision in one eye in adults.[171] The potential for loss of vision occurs during critical periods in the postnatal development of the visual system. Maturation of the visual system is experience-dependent; that is, the eye must be exposed to sensory stimulation to complete the development of the entire visual system, which has significant impact on visual perception (Clinical Implications Box 9.1).

Macular Degeneration

The macula is the part of the eye where the most acute vision occurs because it contains the fovea, the central focusing point of the optic system. Age-related macular degeneration (AMD) is a degenerative disease that affects the macula and supporting retinal pigment epithelium (RPE). Approximately 11 million people in the United States are affected by AMD, a prevalence that is over double that of Alzheimer disease.[176] It is more likely to be seen after age 50.[177] The pathogenesis of AMD is not completely understood. It is thought to be the result of complex interactions between the environment and genetics. With aging, vascular and nutritional changes affect the function of the macula. Cellular senescence of

RPE endangers the health of the eye's photoreceptors.[178] RPE is a nondividing cell, which is essential for maintaining the eye's photoreceptors.[179] Senescent changes also occur in choroidal tissue cells, retinal neurons, and microglia. The aging body's immune response results in impaired inflammatory regulation, which also contributes to retinal degeneration. AMD results in painless, central vision loss. Loss of central vision can make it more difficult to see faces, drive, read, or do close-up work like puzzles or cooking.

Macular degeneration is the most common cause of irreversible loss of eyesight in adults over 50 years of age.[177-179] There are two types of AMD: a "wet" type and a "dry" type. The most common form is the "dry" type. Dry AMD occurs in three stages—early, intermediate, and late—and progresses slowly. Clinically, the early stage of AMD is marked by the presence of *drusen*, which is a yellow material found between the RPE and Bruch's membrane. Pigment abnormalities in the RPE can also be seen in AMD. The dry type of AMD accounts for 90% of all diagnosed cases.[179] The early stage is also called atrophic AMD and the advanced stage is referred to as *geographic atrophy*. There is no treatment as yet for late-stage dry AMD. It is responsible for a large number of cases of moderate visual loss in older adults. Treatment for early and intermediate dry type includes use of nutritional supplements, such as zinc and other antioxidants, and close observation. Because the loss

---

CLINICAL IMPLICATIONS BOX 9.1
Amblyopia: A Preventable Loss of Vision

Deprivation of visual input during a critical period can lead to a permanent visual deficit. There are three critical periods for visual acuity: during development from early gestation through 3–5 years of age; during a period of deprivation, possible from the first few months to 7–8 years of age;[172] and during the recovery period from the time of deprivation into adulthood.[173] Many motor and sensory conditions can lead to amblyopia, including strabismus, myopia, astigmatism, cataract, and refractive differences between the two eyes. Early recognition and referral can prevent vision loss. Photoscreening is a technique that uses a camera and a flash to identify refractive errors and risk factors for amblyopia.

Prevention Focuses
- Screening is recommended for children 1 through 5 years.[54,166]

- Instrument-based screening can detect risk factors for amblyopia such as high refractive errors and strabismus.[166]
- Photoscreening has been useful in detecting amblyogenic risk factors in children as young as 2 years.[174]
- Use of instrument-based screening improved the percentage of 3-, 4-, and 5-year-olds successfully screened compared to chart-based vision screening in pediatric primary care practices.[175]
- Treatment is effective if amblyopia is detected before age 8.[163]
- Treatment is still indicated if detected later than the limit of the critical period. Research is focusing on extending/manipulating the critical period.

of vision in the "dry" type is gradual, the person may not be aware of how much sight has been lost. It is recommended by the AAO that individuals with the "dry" type use an Amsler grid on a daily basis to check the status of their eyesight.

The wet type of AMD is a less common type of late AMD. It is also called advanced neovascular AMD because it is caused by the leakage of newly formed blood vessels that have grown into the eye. Severe vision loss can occur faster because of these new blood vessels, pigment epithelial detachment, and disciform scarring. The wet type can be treated by injecting anti-VEGF (vascular endothelial growth factor) medications in the affected eye or using photodynamic therapy, which is a combination of injections and laser treatment. The drugs are used to inhibit growth of the blood vessels causing damage. There are 200,000 new cases of this exudative type of AMD diagnosed annually in the United States.[180] AMD pathogenesis has been linked to oxidative damage of the RPE and immune-related intraocular inflammation. Dietary supplements, nutrients, and antioxidants have been used to reduce the risk of severe visual loss.

Macular degeneration begins differently in every person. Some common symptoms include a gradual loss of the ability to see objects clearly, distorted vision, a gradual loss of clear color vision, and a dark or empty area in the center of vision. These symptoms are not unique to AMD but do indicate the need to seek professional assessment. The Amsler grid is an early detection chart that may be used independently, alerting the clinician to changes in vision that should be assessed by an optometrist (Fig. 9.7). The Amsler grid continues to be the recommended method for monitoring vision in those at risk.[181] There is no way to restore central vision once it is lost, but peripheral vision is not damaged and low vision aids can be helpful. It is important to be aware of risk factors and potential prevention strategies (Clinical Implications Box 9.2).

Driving

Retention of the ability to drive in older adulthood is a significant quality-of-life issue. Driving is an example of an IADL. In a National Health and Aging Trends Study of over 6000 medicare beneficiaries 65 or older, those who chose to stop driving reported experiencing loneliness and isolation as consequences.[185] Depression is a common finding in older adults who cease driving.[186] Women are more likely to cease driving than men.[187] Men who are married or have more education are less

---

CLINICAL IMPLICATIONS BOX 9.2
Age-Related Macular Degeneration: Who Is at Risk?

Age-related macular degeneration (AMD) is the leading cause of legal blindness in adults over 50 years of age in the United States and the developed world.[177-179] Unfortunately, few of the many potential risk factors are modifiable. AMD is a major public health issue, as the number of individuals with this condition is expected to reach 288 million by 2040.[176,182] Research into prevention of the progression of AMD is focusing on inhibiting retinal cell senescence and decreasing drusen deposition.[178] Global cost of visual impairment relative to AMD is in the billions. Increased public awareness of AMD as a common cause of irreversible loss of eyesight in older adults may promote further research into the prevention of blindness.

Risk Factors
- *Age:* Risk increases with age after 50 years.[179,183] Individuals over 75 years have a threefold increase in risk. AMD cases were almost twice as prevalent in woman than men in 2010.[184]

- *Ethnicity:* Hispanic and Black populations have a lower prevalence rate than White population.[183] However, the rate in Hispanics is expected to rise nearly sixfold by 2050 because of expected changes in population demographics.[184]
- *Genetics:* A positive family history (parent or sibling with AMD) is a strong predictor.
- *Environment:* Cigarette smoking is the major modifiable risk factor for AMD.[183]
- *Previous cataract surgery.*[179]

Potential Prevention Strategies
- Stop smoking, or do not start.
- Get regular physical activity.
- Have regular vision assessments.
- Use an Amsler grid as a means to detect early AMD in those at risk and to recognize progression if already diagnosed with the dry type (see Fig. 9.7).
- Take prescribed dietary supplements if you have intermediate AMD in one or both eyes.[183]

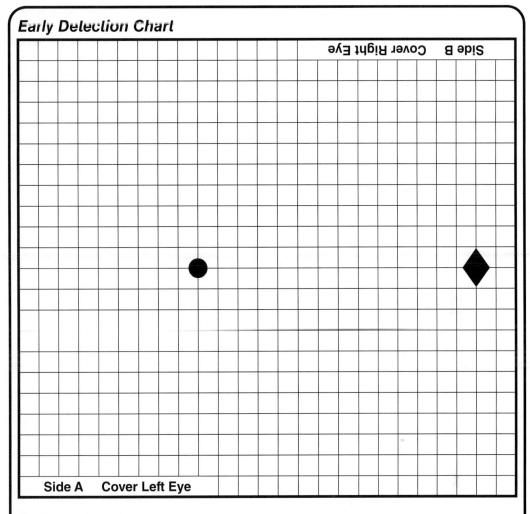

Early Detection Chart

Side B   Cover Right Eye

Side A   Cover Left Eye

Directions for using the chart:
1. Wear your reading glasses or bifocals and have good lighting on card. Hold card facing you so you can read side A. Cover your left eye.
2. Hold card at arm's length and stare only at small dot while bringing chart toward your eye.
3. Pull the card toward you until the large "♦" disappears from view. The lines should look straight and black.
4. If lines appear wavy, grey or fuzzy, draw on top of them and show chart to your optometrist.

5. Turn card upside down to read side B. Close your right eye and follow steps 2, 3 and 4.

Be sure to call your optometrist immediately if you notice a change, or if you don't understand how to use the chart. This screening test does not replace a thorough eye examination by your optometrist.

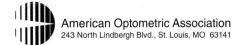

American Optometric Association
243 North Lindbergh Blvd., St. Louis, MO 63141

Fig. 9.7 Amsler grid: early detection chart. (From the American Optometric Association.)

likely to stop driving.[187] Healthy older adult drivers drive more slowly, which could reflect their insight into their own limitations.[188] Although some report driving skills are preserved in healthy older persons,[189] others have documented that healthy older drivers make fewer steering corrections and eye movement excursions than do younger drivers.[190] Four categories of age-related changes can affect driving in older adults: sensory, motor, cognitive, and physical functions. These changes are found in Table 9.4.

Driving is a very visual task. Decline in visual acuity, contrast sensitivity, visual attention, and useful field of view (UVOF) are frequently mentioned as reasons for impaired performance of motor vehicle operational skills.[191–193] A decline in function of any part of the visual system, whether peripheral (as in the eye with changes in lens accommodation) or central (as with processing of sensory information), results in the modification of motor behavior. A decline of visual acuity to 20/50 or less means restriction from driving. Ragland, Satariano, and MacLeod[194] found that poor vision was the most common reason given by older adults for limiting or stopping driving. The implications of visual difficulties for the ability of the individual to drive (especially at night), to be mobile on uneven terrain, or to be in unfamiliar environments are vast.

UVOF is defined as "the area of the visual field that is functional for an observer at a given time and for a given task."[73] The UVOF test assesses visual attention and processing speed. When distractions are present, the UVOF of older adults becomes smaller, making visual search less efficient. Using a new methodology called naturalistic driving, Huisingh and colleagues[193] found that severe impairment of UVOF in older adults resulted in an increased rate of near-crash involvement. Furthermore, their data suggest the contrast sensitivity and impaired visual processing speed increase the likelihood that an older adult will be involved in a near crash. Naturalistic driving study is dependent on observation of driving behavior in the real world. "Continuous high-resolution behavioral data, via video, GPS, accelerometers, are collected from a group of drivers with no experimental manipulation for an extended amount of time."[195,196] Use of this methodology as a way to assess driving in older adults appears promising despite needing significant resource allocations.

Cognitive impairments, especially those related to Alzheimer disease, are associated with an increased risk in driving.[197] Up to 30% of older adults with dementia continue to drive.[195] Individuals with Alzheimer disease can be easily distracted, cannot remember where they are going, and may even have a greater decrease in visual-spatial processing and orientation. In a study of more than 14,000 adults aged 70 or

TABLE 9.4   Age-Related Physiological Changes That May Affect Driving

Type of Change	Examples
Sensory	Reduced peripheral vision Reduced visual acuity Reduced UFOV Eye disease (cataracts, macular degeneration, glaucoma, diabetic retinopathy) Reduced contrast sensitivity Increased glare sensitivity Decreased lower extremity sensation Decreased ankle proprioception Hearing loss (horns, sirens, and noise from their own vehicle)
Motor	Decline in strength Decreased neck mobility (upward vertical vision, head turning) Decreased trunk mobility (trunk turning) Decreased reaction time Decreased endurance
Cognitive	Distracted by irrelevant stimuli Decreased visual searching Decreased hazard perception Decreased selective attention Decreased spatial navigation
Physical	Deeper set eyes (loss of fat in orbits) Loss of height Joint pain Loss of cervical range of motion Loss of upper extremity range of motion

Horswill MS. Hazard perception in driving. *Curr Dir Psychol Sci.* 2016;25:425-430; Huisingh C, Levitan EB, Irvin MR, et al. Visual sensory and visual-cognitive function and rate of crash and near-crash involvement among older drivers using naturalistic driving data. *Invest Opthalmol Vis Sci.* 2017;58:2959-2967; Karthaus M, Falkenstein M. Functional changes and driving performance in older drivers: assessment and interventions. *Geriatrics (Basel).* 2016;1:12; Kunishige M, Miyaguchi H, Fukuda H, et al. Spatial navigation ability is associated with the assessment of smoothness of driving during changing lanes in older drivers. *J Physiologic Anthropol.* 2020;39(1):25; Smither JA, Mouloua M, Hancock PA, et al. Aging and driving part I: implications of perceptual and physical changes. In: Vincenzi DA, Mouloua M, Hancock PA, eds. *Human Performance Situation Awareness and Automation: Current Research and Trends.* Mahwah, NJ: Erlbaum; 2004:315-319; Yang N, Waddington G, Adams R, Han J. Age-related changes in proprioception of the ankle complex across the lifespan. *J Sport Health Sci.* 2019;8:548-554.

older, Anstey and colleagues[191] reported that cognitive function and perceived self-health were stronger predictors of whether an older adult would cease driving than sensory function and medical conditions. Older adults with poor memory, slow processing speed, or poor self-rated health had a higher probability of driving cessation within a subsequent 5-year period. In a naturalistic driving study, older drivers with greater cognitive impairment drove more slowly than those with less cognitive impairment.[188] In a survey of older adults with dementia, 54% of participants ceased driving because of increasing cognitive deficits.[198] Driving is not advised for individuals who are in the moderate stage of Alzheimer disease.[197]

The evidence on whether individuals with mild cognitive impairment (MCI) are safe to drive is not as clear-cut as with individuals with Alzheimer disease or related dementia. In an observational study,[199] older drivers were assessed as safe or unsafe based on an on-road safety scale. Presence of MCI was based on diagnostic criteria. Safe MCI drivers exhibited a similar pattern of errors as the safe cognitively normal drivers, suggesting that driving restrictions based solely on the presence of MCI may be unwarranted. Feng and colleagues[199] found that drivers with suspected MCI changed their driving behavior when "making turns across oncoming traffic." Vardaki et al.[201] identified areas of driving difficulty of older drivers—an MCI group and an age-matched healthy control group. Both groups had difficulty switching tasks in new and unexpected situations. The driving performance in the healthy control group was only affected with unfamiliar tasks that required a higher cognitive demand. In the MCI group, cognitive overload occurred with easier tasks. Perceptual-motor performance declines in older adults as evidenced by a decrease in reaction time. This may be related to difficulty sustaining attention or managing divided attention for the many visually related driving tasks. The impact of the loss of mobility, both real and perceived, can substantially affect an individual's self-image. The ability to perceive road hazards and respond accordingly within a reasonable amount of time is related to crash and near-crash involvement in older adults.[193,202,203]

Safety is always a concern for older adults. As individuals live longer, there will be greater numbers of geriatric drivers. Remaining independent requires the ability to get to and from the physician's office, grocery store, and friends' and relatives' homes. Maintaining independence by being able to come and go whenever the need arises is important to the average elder. Older drivers are less likely to drive under compromising visual conditions, such as at night or in inclement weather. Are older drivers safe? According to the Insurance Institute for Highway Safety,[204] fewer older drivers died in crashes and were involved in collisions between 1998 and 2019 compared to earlier decades. Fatal crash rates for drivers ages 70–79 years are now less than those for drivers ages 35–45 years.[205] Some of this decline may be related to gender differences in the self-regulation and cessation of driving. Gender differences are seen in the crash risk, rate and types of crashes, driving patterns, self-regulation, and cessation of driving.

Health improvements and adoption of vehicles with improved safety features have contributed to increased survivability and reduced crashes.[206] Despite that fact, older drivers are more likely to be fatally injured when involved in a vehicular crash.[205] Difficulty with seeing instrument panels, dealing with glare and haze, and judging vehicle speed have also been reported by older drivers.[193,207] Because so many problems are related to visually related driving tasks, some states have initiated the use of state-mandated tests of visual acuity in 70-year-old drivers. The only two regulations associated with lower fatality rates among older drivers are in-person renewal or vison testing and only among drivers aged 85 and older.[208] According to the Insurance Institute for Highway Safety, an upswing in crashes due to the aging US populations has been prevented by better policies, safer vehicles, and better health of elders. All therapists can play a vital role in enhancing the mobility of older drivers. Driving is an extremely important and complex IADL, which can have a huge impact on the level of independence, health, and well-being of an older adult. Benefits of driving have to be weighed against the risk of injury to self and others. Physical and occupational therapists are uniquely qualified to assess an older individual's ability to drive or continue to drive. Intervention strategies are being identified to address age-related changes in sensory, motor, and function that can challenge older drivers.

SUMMARY

Sensory input plays an important role in the learning and refinement of movement. Early sensory combinations allow for development of body recognition and the ability to know where the body ends and the world begins. This integration of multiple sensory inputs and the association-coordination of sensory and motor information form the basis for cognition and perception. Sensory input from the external environment initiates the activity that shapes synaptic connections and sculpts learning pathways. The autonomic nervous system and the reticular system act as gatekeepers, determining which sensory information reaches consciousness and which is dampened. The thalamus is a central relay station that directs the flow of sensory information to association cortices. All sensory systems have similar characteristics: transduction and coding, representation, perception, and integration at all levels of the nervous system. Sensory systems develop early in utero and are therefore ready to function at birth. Some, such as vision and hearing, must have additional input to complete the development of their neural pathways. Sensory abilities change with age; deficits in any sensory system, whether from congenital absence, trauma, or declining with age, can result in functional impairment of movement. Many older adults exhibit multiple sensory system impairments.[209] Presbystasis, presbyopia, and presbycusis are all seen in older adults but not to the same degree in all individuals. A loss in one sensory modality does generalize to losses in all sensory modalities.[110] Age-related changes in the sensory systems, therefore, are neither uniform nor universal.

REFERENCES

1. Gibson JJ. *The Senses as Perceptual Systems*. Boston: Houghton-Mifflin; 1966.
2. Piaget J. *Origins of Intelligence*. New York: International University Press; 1952.
3. Dusing S.C. Postural variability and sensorimotor development in infancy. Dev Med Child Neurol. 2016;58(Suppl 4):17–21.
4. Hirabayashi S, Iwasaki Y. Developmental perspective of sensory organization on postural control. *Brain Dev*. 1995;17(2):111–113.
5. Nougier V, Bard C, Fleury M, et al. Contribution of central and peripheral vision to the regulation of stance: developmental aspects. *J Exp Child Psychol*. 1998;68:202–215.
6. Shumway-Cook A, Woollacott M. *Motor Control: Translation Research into Clinical Practice*. 5th ed. Philadelphia: Wolters Kluver; 2017.
7. Ferber-Viart C, Ionescu E, Morlet T, et al. Balance in healthy individuals assessed with Equitest: maturation and normative data for children and young adults. *Int J Pediatr Otorhinolaryngol*. 2007;71:1041–1046.
8. Mtui E, Gruener G, Dockery P. *Fitzgerald's Clinical Neuroanatomy and Neuroscience*. 8th ed. Elsevier Limited; 2021.
9. Shaffer SW, Harrrison AL. Aging of the somatosensory system: a translational perspective. *Phys Ther*. 2007;87:193–207.
10. Lephart SM, Fu FH. The role of proprioception in the treatment of sports injuries. *Sports Exer Inj*. 1995;1:96–102.
11. Proske U, Chen B. Two senses of human limb position: methods of measurement and roles in proprioception. *Exp Brain Res*. 2021;239:3157–3174. https://doi.org/10.1007/s00221-021-06207-4.
12. Bragonzoni L, Rovini E, Barone G, et al. How proprioception changes before and after total knee arthroplasty: A systematic review. *Gait Posture*. 2019;72:1–11. https://doi.org/10.1016/j.gaitpost.2019.05.005.
13. Fisher AG, Murray EA, Bundy AC, eds. *Sensory Integration: Theory and Practice*. FA Davis: Philadelphia; 1991.
14. Ayres AJ. *Sensory Integration and Learning Disorders*. Los Angeles: Western Psychological Services; 1972.
15. Breslin PA. An evolutionary perspective on food and human taste. *Curr Biol*. 2013;23:R409–R418. https://doi.org/10.1016/j.cub.2013.04.010.
16. Hooker D. *The Prenatal Origin of Behavior*. Lawrence: University of Kansas Press; 1952.
17. Lowrey GH. *Growth and Development of Children*, 8th ed. Chicago: Year Book; 1986.
18. Windle WF. *Physiology of the Fetus*. Philadelphia: WB Saunders; 1940.
19. Wyke B. The neurological basis of movement: a developmental review. In: Holt KS, ed. *Movement and Child Development*. Philadelphia: JB Lippincott; 1975: 19–33.
20. Anand KJ, Hickey PR. Pain and its effect in the human neonate and fetus. *N Engl J Med*. 1987;31:1321–1329.
21. Kostovic I, Rakic P. Developmental history of the transient subplate zone in the visual and somatosensory cortex of the macaque monkey and human brain. *J Comp Neurol*. 1990;297(3):44:1063-1073.

22. Gilles FH, Leviton A, Dooling EC. *The developing Human. Growth and Epidemiologic Neuropathy.* Boston: John Wright; 1983.

23. Goksan S, Hartley C, Emery F, et al. fMRI reveals neural activity overlap between adult and infant pain. *Elife.* 2015;4:e06356. https://doi.org/10.7554/eLife.06356.

24. Perry M, Tan Z, Chen J, et al. Neonatal pain: perceptions and current practice. *Crit Care Nurs Clin North Am.* 2018;30:549–561. https://doi.org/10.1016/j.cnc.2018.07.013.

25. Humphrey T. The embryologic differentiation of the vestibular nuclei in man correlated with functional development. In *International Symposium on Vestibular andOculomotor Problems*, Tokyo, 1965, p 51.

26. Hadders-Algra M. Neural substrate and clinical significance of general movements: an update. *Dev Med Child Neurol.* 2018;60:39–46.

27. Ornitz EM, Atwell CW, Walter DO, et al. The maturation of vestibular nystagmus in infancy and childhood. *Acta Otolaryngol.* 1979;88:244–256.

28. Meisami E, Timiras PS. *Handbook of Human Growth and Development Biology, Vol. 1, Part B.* Boca Raton, FL: CRC Press; 1988.

29. Dunn K, Reissland N, Reid VM. The functional foetal brain: a systematic preview of methodological factors in reporting foetal visual and auditory capacity. *Dev Cogn Neurosci.* 2015;13:43–52. https://doi.org/10.1016/j.dcn.2015.04.002.

30. Litovsky R. Development of the auditory system. *Handb Clin Neurol.* 2015;129:55–72. https://doi.org/10.1016/B978-0-444-62630-1.00003-2. PMID: 25726262; PMCID: PMC4612629.

31. Birnholz JC, Benacerraf BR. The development of human fetal hearing. *Science.* 1983;222:516–518.

32. Forestell CA. Flavor perception and preference development in human infants. *Ann Nutr Metab.* 2017;70(Suppl 3):17–25. https://doi.org/10.1159/000478759.

33. Paglia L. Taste development and prenatal prevention. *Eur J Paediatr Dent.* 2019;20:257. https://doi.org/10.23804/ejpd.2019.20.04.01.

34. Prechtl HFR. Behavioral states of the newborn infant (a review). *Brain Res.* 1974;76:185–212.

35. Smith SL, Gossman M, Canan BC. Selected primitive reflexes in children with cerebral palsy: consistency of response. *Phys Ther.* 1982;62:1115–1120.

36. Johnson SP. Development of visual-spatial attention. *Curr Top Behav Neurosci.* 2019;41:37–58. https://doi.org/10.1007/7854_2019_96.

37. White H, Jurbran R, Heck A, Chroust A, Bhatt RS. The role of shape recognition in figure/ground perception in infancy. *Psychon Bull Rev.* 2018;25:1381–1387. https://doi.org/10.3758/s13423-018-1476-z.

38. Rochat P, Hespos SJ. Differential rooting response by neonates: evidence for an early sense of self. *Early Dev Parent.* 1997;6:105–112.

39. Rochat P. Self-perception and action in infancy. *Exp Brain Res.* 1998;123:102–109.

40. Rochat P. Clinical pointers from developing self-awareness. *Dev Med Child Neurol.* 2021;63:382–386.

41. Kaye H, Lipsitt L. Relationship of electro to actual threshold to basal skin conductance. *Child Dev.* 1964;35:1307–1312.

42. Meltzoff AN, Borton R. Intermodal matching by human neonates. *Nature.* 1979;282:403–404.

43. Leed JE, Chinn LK, Lockman JJ. Reaching to the self: the development of infants' ability to localize targets on the body. *Psychol Sci.* 2019;30:1063–1073. https://doi.org/10.1177/0956797619850168.

44. Begum Ali J, Spence C, Bremner AJ. Human infants' ability to perceive touch in external space develops postnatally. *Current Biology.* 2015;25:R978–R979. https://doi.org/10.1016/J.CUB.2015.08.055.

45. Bremner AJ. Developing body representations in early life: combining somatosensation and vision to perceive the interface between the body and the world. *Dev Med Child Neurol.* 2016;58(Suppl 4):12–16. https://doi.org/10.1111/dmcn.13041.

46. Gottfried AW, Rose SA. Tactile recognition in infants. *Child Dev.* 1980;51:69–74.

47. Rose SA, Gottfried AW, Bridger WH. Cross-modal transfer in 6-month-old infants. *Dev Psychol.* 1981;17:661–669.

48. Freier L, Mason L, Bremner AJ. Perception of visual-tactile colocation in the first year of life. *Dev Psychol.* 2016;52:2184–2190. https://doi.org/10.1037/dev0000160.

49. Bremner AJ, Spence C. The development of tactile perception. *Adv Child Dev Behav.* 2017;52:227–268. https://doi.org/10.1016/bs.acdb.2016.12.002.

50. Salapatek P, Cohen L. *Handbook of Infant Perception: From Sensation to Perception.* New York: Academic Press; 1987.

51. Puchalski M, Hummel P. The reality of neonatal pain. *Adv Neonatal Care.* 2002;2(5):233–247.

52. Fitzgerald M, Walker SM. Infant pain management: a developmental neurobiological approach. *Nat Clin Pract Neurol.* 2009;5(1):35–50.

53. Simons SHP, Tibboel D. Pain perception development and maturation. *Semin Fetal Neonatal Med.* 2006;11:227–231.

54. AAP Committee on Fetus and Newborn and Section on Anesthesiology and Pain Medicine Prevention and Management of Procedural Pain in the Neonate: an update. *Pediatrics.* 2016;137(2):e20154271. https://doi.org/10.1542/peds.2015-4271.

55. Olsson E, Ahl H, Bengtsson K, et al. The use and reporting of neonatal pain scales: a systematic review of randomized trials. *Pain*. 2021;162:353–360. https://doi.org/10.1097/j.pain.0000000000002046.

56. Grunauer M, Mikesell C, Bustamante G, et al. PICU-MIC Research Group. Pain assessment and management in pediatric intensive care units around the world, an international, multicenter study. *Front Pediatr*. 2021;9:746489. https://doi.org/10.3389/fped.2021.746489.

57. Brummelte S, Grunau RE, Chau V, et al. Procedural pain and brain development in premature newborns. *Ann Neurol*. 2012;71:385–396.

58. Meltzoff AN, Murray L, Simpson E, et al. Re-examination of Oostenbroek et al.: evidence for neonatal tongue protrusion. *Dev Sci*. 2018;21(4):e12609. https://doi.org/10.1111/desc.12609.

59. Morgan R, Rochat P. Intermodal calibration of the body in early infancy. *Ecol Psychol*. 1997;9:1–24.

60. Atkinson J, Braddick O. Visual development. *Handb Clin Neurol*. 2020;173:121–142. https://doi.org/10.1016/B978-0-444-64150-2.00013-7.

61. Clifton RK, Rochat P, Robin DJ, Berthier NE. Multimodal perception in the control of infant reaching. *J Exp Pscyhol*. 1994;20:876–886.

62. von Hof P, van der Kamp J, Savelsbegh GJP. The relation between infants' perception of catchableness and the control of catching. *Dev Psychol*. 2008;44:182–194.

63. Butterworth GE, Ciccheti D. Visual calibration of posture in normal and motor retarded Down's syndrome infants. *Perception*. 1978;7:513–525.

64. Butterworth GE, Hicks L. Visual proprioception and postural stability in infants: a developmental study. *Perception*. 1977;6:255–262.

65. Lee DN, Aaronson E. Visual proprioceptive control of standing in infants. *Percept Psychophys*. 1974;15:529–532.

66. Sundermier L, Woollacott MH. The influence of vision on the automatic postural muscle responses of newly standing and newly walking infants. *Exp Brain Res*. 1998;120:537–540.

67. Eviatar L, Eviatar A, Naaray I. Maturation of neurovestibular responses in infants. *Dev Med Child Neurol*. 1974;16:435–446.

68. Ornitz EM. Normal and pathological maturation of vestibular function in the human child. In: Romand R, ed. *Development of Auditory and Vestibular Systems*. New York: Academic Press; 1983:479–536.

69. Eliot L. *What's Going on in There?. How the Brain and Mind Work the First Five Years of Life*. New York: Bantam; 1999.

70. Marmur R, Sabo E, Carmeli E, et al. Optokinetic nystagmus as related to neonatal position. *J Child Neurol*. 2007;22(9):1108–1110.

71. Weissman BM, DiScenna AO, Leigh RJ. Maturation of the vestibulo-ocular reflex in normal infants during the first 2 months of life. *Neurology*. 1989;39:534–538.

72. Fife TD, Tusa RJ, Furman JM, et al. Assessment. vestibular testing techniques in adults and children: Report of the Therapeutics and Technology Assessment Subcommittee of the American Academy of Neurology. *Neurology*. 2000;55(10):1431–1441.

73. Coren S, Ward LM, Enns JT. *Sensation and Perception*. 5th ed. Fort Worth, TX: Harcourt; 1999.

74. Nandi R, Luxon LM. Development and assessment of the vestibular system. *Int J Audiol*. 2008;47:566–577.

75. Bertenthal BI, Rose JL, Bai DL. Perception-action coupling in the development of visual control of posture. *J Exp Psych*. 1997;23:1631–1643.

76. Kandel ER, Koester JD, Mach SH, Siegelbaum S. *Principles of Neural Science*. 6th ed. London, UK: McGraw Hill; 2021.

77. Shimojo SJ, Bauer J, O'Connell KM, et al. Pre-stereoptic binocular vision in infants. *Vision Res*. 1986;26: 501–510.

78. Hyde ML, Riko K, Malizia K. Audiometric accuracy of the click ABR in infants at risk for hearing loss. *J Am Acad Audiol*. 1990;1:59–66. PMID: 2132587.

79. American Speech-Language-Hearing Association. Short latency auditory evoked potentials [Relevant Paper] 1989. https://www.asha.org/policy/rp1987-00024/#sec1.5.1 Accessed February 14, 2022.

80. Iverson JM. Developmental variability and developmental cascades: lessons from motor and language development in infancy. *Curr Dir Psychol Sci*. 2021;30:228–235. https://doi.org/10.1177/0963721421993822.

81. Lifter K, Bloom L. Object knowledge and the emergence of language. *Infant Behav Dev*. 1989;12:395–423.

82. Romero RR, Segaran J, Leonard JA, et al. Language exposure related to structural neural connectivity in childhood. *J Neurosci*. 2018;38:7870–7877. https://doi.org/10.1532/JNEUROSCI.0484-18.2018.

83. Rosenfeld RM, Tunkel DE, Schwartz SR, et al. Clinical practice guideline: tympanostomy tubes in children (update). *Otolaryngol Head Neck Surg*. 2022;166(1suppl):S1–S55. https://doi.org/10.1177/01945998211065662.

84. Rosenfeld RM, Tunkel DE, Schwartz SR, et al. Executive summary of clinical practice guideline on tympanostomy tubes in children (update. *Otolaryngol Head Neck Surg*. 2022;166(2):189–206. https://doi.org/10.1177/01945998211065661.

85. Casselbrant ML, Villardo RJ, Mandel EM. Balance and otitis media with effusion. *Int J Audiol*. 2008;47:584–589. https://doi.org/10.1080/14992020802331230.

86. Rosenstein D, Oster H. Differential facial responses to four basic tastes in newborns. *Child Dev*. 1988;59:1555–1568. PMID: 3208567.

87. Beauchamp GK, Mennella JA. Flavor perception in human infants: development and functional significance. *Digestion*. 2011;83(suppl 1):1–6. https://doi.org/10.1159/000323397.

88. MacFarlane A. Olfaction in the development of social preferences in the human neonate. *Ciba Found Symp*. 1975;33:103–113.

89. Coffield CN, Mayhew EM, Haviland-Jones JM, Walker-Andrews AS. Adding odor: less distress and enhanced attention for 6-month-olds. *Infant Behav Dev*. 2014;37:155–161. https://doi.org/10.1016/j.infbeh.2013.12.010.

90. Taylor S, McLean B, Falkmer T, et al. Does somatosensation change with age in children and adolescents? A systematic review. *Child Care Health Dev*. 2016;42:809–824. https://doi.org/10.1111/cch.12375.

91. Goble DJ, Lewis CA, Hurvitz EA, Brown SH. Development of upper limb proprioceptive accuracy in children and adolescents. *Hum Mov Sci*. 2005;24:155–170. https://doi.org/10.1016/j.humov.2005.05.004.

92. Hermann RP, Novak CB, Mackinnon SE. Establishing normal values of moving two-point discrimination in children and adolescents. *Dev Med Child Neurol*. 1996;38:255–261.

93. Visner J, Geuze RH. Kinaesthetic acuity in adolescent boys: a longitudinal study. *Dev Med Child Neurol*. 2000;42:93–96.

94. Yang N, Waddington G, Adams R, Han J. Age-related changes in proprioception of the ankle complex across the lifespan. *J Sport Health Sci*. 2019;8:548–554. https://doi.org/10.1016/j.jshs.2019.06.003.

95. Bigelow A. The correspondence between self and image movement as a cue to self-recognition for young children. *J Genet Psychol*. 1981;139:11–26.

96. Thelen E. Motor development: a new synthesis. *Am Psychol*. 1995;50:79–95.

97. Elliot JM, Connolly KJ, Doyle AJR. Development of kinaesthetic sensitivity and motor performance in children. *Dev Med Child Neurol*. 1988;30:80–92.

98. Livesey DJ, Parks NA. Testing kinaesthetic acuity in preschool children. *Aust J Psychol*. 1995;47(3):160–163.

99. Livesey DJ, Intili D. A gender difference in visual-spatial ability in 4-year-old children: effects on performance of a kinesthetic acuity task. *J Exp Child Psychol*. 1996;63:436–446.

100. Gabbard CP. *Lifelong Motor Development*. 5th ed. San Francisco: Pearson Benjamin Cummings; 2008.

101. Charpiot A, Tringali S, Ionescu E, Vital-Durand F, Ferber-Viert C. Vestibulo-ocular reflex and balance maturation in healthy children aged from six to twelve years. *Audiol Neurootol*. 2010;15:203–210. https://doi.org/10.1159/000255338.

102. Goulème N, Debue M, Spruyt K, et al. Changes of spatial and temporal characteristics of dynamic postural control in children with typical neurodevelopment with age: results of a multicenter pediatric study. *Int J Pediatr Otorhinolaryngol*. 2018;113:272–280. https://doi.org/10.1016/j.ijporl.2018.08.005.

103. Sinno S, Dumas G, Mallinson A, Najem F, Abouchacra KS, Nashner L, Perrin P. Changes in the sensory weighting strategies in balance control throughout maturation in children. *J Am Acad Audiol*. 2021;32:122–136. https://doi.org/10.1055/s-0040-1718706.

104. Williams HG. *Perceptual and Motor Development*. Englewood Cliffs, NJ: Prentice Hall; 1983.

105. Haywood KM. Eye movements during coincidence-anticipation performance. *J Mot Behav*. 1977;9:313–318.

106. Collins JK. Distance perception as a function of age. *Aust J Psychol*. 1976;28:109–113.

107. Simic N, Rovet J. [Formula: see text] Dorsal and ventral visual streams: typical and atypical development. *Child Neuropsychol*. 2017;23:678–691. https://doi.org/10.1080/09297049.2016.1186616.

108. Forster B, Cavina-Pratesi C, Aglioti SM, Berlucchi G. Redundant target effect and intersensory facilitation from visual-tactile interactions in simple reaction time. *Exp Brain Res*. 2002;43:480–487. https://doi.org/10.1007/s00221-002-1017-9.

109. Nickerson RS. Intersensory facilitation of reaction time. *Psychol Rev*. 1973;80:489–509.

110. Cavazzana A, Röhrborn A, Garthus-Niegel S, et al. Sensory-specific impairment among older people. An investigation using both sensory thresholds and subjective measures across the five senses. *PLoS One*. 2018;13(8):e0202969.

111. McIntyre S, Nagi SS, McGlone F, Olausson H. The effects of ageing on tactile function in humans. *Neurosci*. 2021;464:53–58.

112. Decorps J, Saumet JL, Sommer P, Siqaudo-Rossel D, Fromy B. Effect of ageing on tactile transduction processes. *Ageing Res Rev*. 2014;13:90–99. https://doi.org/10.1016/j.arr.2013.12.003.

113. García-Piqueras J, García-Mesa Y, Cárcaba L, et al. Ageing of the somatosensory system at the periphery: age-related changes in cutaneous mechanoreceptors. *J Anat*. 2019;234:839–852. https://doi.org/10.1111/joa.12983.

114. Bruce MF. The relation of tactile threshold to histology in the fingers of elderly people. *J Neurol Neurosurg Psychiatry*. 1980;43:730–734.

115. Stevens JC, Alvarez-Reeves M, Dipietro L, et al. Decline of tactile acuity in ageing: a study of body site, blood

flow, and lifetime habits of smoking and physical activity. *Somatosens Mot Res*. 2003;20:271–279.

116. Stevens JC, Choo KK. Spatial acuity of the body surface over the life span. *Somatosens Mot Res*. 1996;13: 153–166.

117. Wickremaratchi MM, Llewelyn JG. Effects of ageing on touch. *Postgrad Med J*. 2006;82:301–304.

118. Sehlstedt I, Ignell H, Backlund H, Wasling R, et al. Gentle touch perception across the lifespan. *Psychol Aging*. 2016;31:176–184.

119. Perry SD. Evaluation of age-related plantar-surface insensitivity and onset age of advanced insensitivity in older adults using vibratory and touch sensation test. *Neurosci Lett*. 2006;392:62–127.

120. Day BL, Lord SR. Aging. In: Lord SR, Delbaere K, Sturnieks DL, eds. *Handbook of Clinical Neurology*. 159. New York: Elsevier; 2018:157–171.

121. Chen X, Qu X. Age-related differences in the relationships between lower-limb joint proprioception and postural balance. *Hum Factors*. 2019;61:702–711. https://doi.org/10.1177/0018720818795064.

122. Kokmen E, Bossemeyer Jr RW, Williams WJ. Quantitative evaluation of joint motion sensation in an aging population. *J Gerontol*. 1978;33:62–67.

123. Verschueren SM, Brumagne S, Swinnen SP, et al. The effect of aging on dynamic position sense at the ankle. *Behav Brain Res*. 2002;136:593–603.

124. Lee SS, Kim HJ, Ye D, Lee DH. Comparison of proprioception between osteoarthritic and age-matched unaffected knees: a systematic review and meta-analysis. *Arch Orthop Trauma Surg*. 2021;141:355–365. https://doi.org/10.1007/s00402-020-03418-2.

125. Wingert JR, Welder C, Foo P. Age-related hip proprioception declines: effects on postural sway and dynamic balance. *Arch Phys Med Rehabil*. 2014;95:253–261. https://doi.org/10.1016/j.apmr.2013.08.012.

126. Henry M, Baudry S. Age-related changes in leg proprioception: implications for postural control. *J Neurophysiol*. 2019;122:525–538. https://doi.org/10.1152/jn.00067.2019.

127. Guergova S, Dufour A. Thermal sensitivity in the elderly: a review. *Ageing Res Rev*. 2011;10(1):80–92. https://doi.org/10.1016/j.arr.2010.04.009.

128. Timiras PS. *Physiological Basis of Aging and Geriatrics*. Boca Raton, FL: CRC Press; 1994.

129. Protsiv M, Ley C, Lankester J, Hastie T, Parsonnet J. Decreasing human body temperature in the United States since the industrial revolution. *Elife*. 2020;9:e49555. https://doi.org/10.7554/eLife.49555. Published 2020 Jan 7.

130. Gurven M, Kraft TS, Alami S, et al. Rapidly declining body temperature in a tropical human population.

Sci Advances. 2020;6(44):eabc6599. https://doi.org/10.1126/sciadv.abc6599.

131. González-Roldán AM, Terrasa JL, Sitges C, et al. Age-related changes in pain perception are associated with altered functional connectivity during resting state. *Front Aging Neurosci*. 2020;12:11. https://doi.org/10.3389/fnagi.2020.00116.

132. Drake RAR, Steel KA, Apps R, Lumb BM, Pickering AE. Loss of cortical control over the descending pain modulatory system determines the development of the neuropathic pain state in rats. *Neurosci*. 2021;10:e65156.

133. Rauch SD, Velazquez-Villasenor L, Dimitri PS, Mechant SN. Decreasing hair cell counts in aging humans. *Ann NY Acad Sci*. 2001;942:220–227.

134. Arshad Q, Seemungal BM. Age-related vestibular loss: current understanding and future research directions. *Front Neurol*. 2016;7:231.

135. Coto J, Alvarez CL, Dejas I, et al. Peripheral vestibular system: age-related vestibular loss and associated deficits. *J Otol*. 2021;16:258–265. https://doi.org/10.1016/j.joto.2021.06.001.

136. Smith PF. Age-Related neurochemical changes in the vestibular nuclei. *Front Neurol*. 2016;7:20. https://doi.org/10.3389/fneur.2016.00020.

137. Anson E, Pineault K, Bair W, Studenski S, Agrawal Y. Reduced vestibular function is associated with longer, slower steps in healthy adults during normal speed walking. *Gait Posture*. 2019;68:340–345. https://doi.org/10.1016/j.gaitpost.2018.12.016.

138. Wan G, Corfas G. No longer falling on deaf ears: mechanisms of degeneration and regeneration of cochlear ribbon synapses. *Hear Res*. 2015;329:1–10.

139. Bergstrom B. Morphology of the vestibular nerve: III. Analysis of the myelinated vestibular nerve fibers in man at various ages. *Acta Otolaryngol*. 1973;76: 331–338.

140. Matheson AJ, Darlington CL, Smith PF. Dizziness in the elderly and age-related degeneration of the vestibular system. *N Z J Psychol*. 1999;28(1):10–16.

141. Agrawal Y, Carey JP, Della Santina CC, Schubert MC, Minor LB. Disorders of balance and vestibular function in US adults: data from the national health and nutrition survey. *2001-2004/ Arch Int Med*. 2009;169: 938–944.

142. Kennedy R, Clemis JD. The geriatric auditory and vestibular system. *Otolaryngol Clin North Am*. 1990;23:1075–1082.

143. Sturnieks DL, George St R, Lord SR. Balance disorders in the elderly. *Neurophysiol Clin*. 2008;38(6):467–478.

144. Duncan G, Wilson JA, MacLennen WJ, et al. Clinical correlates of sway in elderly people living at home. *Gerontology*. 1992;38:160–166.

145. Ring C, Nayak USL, Isaacs B. The effect of visual deprivation and proprioceptive change on postural sway in healthy adults. *J Am Geriatr Soc.* 1989;37:745–749.

146. Pitts DG. Visual function as a function of age. *J Am Optom Assoc.* 1982;53:117–124.

147. Weale RA. Senile changes in visual acuity. *Trans Ophthalmol Soc UK.* 1975;95:36–38.

148. Duthie EH, Katz PR, eds. *Practice of Geriatrics.* Philadelphia: WB Saunders; 1998.

149. Duthie EH, Katz PR, Malone ML, eds. *Practice of Geriatrics.* Philadelphia: WB Saunders; 2007.

150. Cleary BL. Age-related changes in the special senses. In: Matteson MA, McConnell ES, Linton AD, eds. *Gerontological Nursing.* Philadelphia: WB Saunders; 1997:385–405.

151. Williams HG. Aging and eye-hand coordination. In: Bard C, Fleury M, Hay L, eds. *Development of Eye-Hand Coordination.* Columbia: University of South Carolina Press; 1990:327–357.

152. Meisami E. Aging of the sensory systems. In: Timiras PS, ed. *Physiological Basis of Aging and Geriatrics.* Boca Raton, FL: CRC Press; 1994:115–132.

153. Gates GA, Mills JH. Presbycusis. *Lancet.* 2005;366:1111–1120.

154. Jeon S, Kim Y, Min S, et al. Taste sensitivity of elderly people is associated with quality of life and inadequate dietary intake. *Nutrients.* 2021;13(5):1693.

155. Feng P, Huang L, Wang H. Taste bud homeostasis in health, disease, and aging. *Chem Senses.* 2014;39(1):3–16.

156. Schiffman SS, Graham BG. Taste and smell perception affect appetite and immunity in the elderly. *Eur J Clin Nutr.* 2000;54(Suppl 3):S54S63.

157. Schiffman SS. Effects of aging on the human taste system. *Ann N Y Acad Sci.* 2009;1170:725–729.

158. Ship J. The influence of aging on oral health and consequences for taste and smell. *Physiol Behav.* 1999;66:209–215.

159. Yaffe K, Freimer D, Chen H, et al. Olfaction and risk of dementia in a biracial cohort of older adults. *Neurol.* 2017;31(88):456–462.

160. Horak FB, Shumway-Cook A, Crowe TK, et al. Vestibular function and motor proficiency of children with impaired hearing or with learning disability and motor impairments. *Dev Med Child Neurol.* 1988;30:64–79.

161. Rine RM, Cornwall G, Gan K, et al. Evidence of progressive delay of motor development in children with sensorineural hearing loss and concurrent vestibular dysfunction. *Percept Mot Skills.* 2000;90:1101–1112.

162. Jan JE, Sykanda A, Groenveld M. Habilitation and rehabilitation of visually impaired and blind children. *Pediatrician.* 1990;17:202–207.

163. Hensch TK, Quinlan EM. Critical periods in amblyopia. *Vis Neurosci.* 2018;35:E014. https://doi.org/10.1017/S0952523817000219.

164. Levi DM. Rethinking amblyopia. *Vision Res.* 2020;176:118–129. https://doi.org/10.1016/j.visres.2020.07.014.

165. Mostafaie A, Ghojazadeh M, Hosseinifard H, et al. A systematic review of amblyopia prevalence among the children of the world. *Rom J Ophthalmol.* 2020;64:342–355. https://doi.org/10.22336/rjo.2020.56.

166. Children's Eye Foundation. *A Practical Guide for Primary Care Physicians: Instrument-Based Vision Screening in Children.* Grapevine, TX: Children's Eye Foundation; 2016.

167. Braverman R.S. Introduction to amblyopia. www.aao.org/disease-review/amblyopia-introduction. Accessed January 12, 2022.

168. Asper L, Watt K, Khuu S. Optical treatment of amblyopia: a systematic review and meta-analysis. *Clin Exp Optom.* 2018;101:431–442. https://doi.org/10.1111/cxo.12657.

169. Stewart CE, Moseley MJ, Fielder AR, et al. Refractive adaptation in amblyopia: quantification of effect and implications for practice. *Br J Ophthalmol.* 2004;88:1552–1556.

170. Gibson EJ. Perceptual learning. *Annu Rev Psychol.* 1963;14:29–56. https://doi.org/10.1146/annurev.ps.14.020163.000333.

171. Simmons K. Preschool vision screening: rationale, methodology and outcome. *Surg Ophthalmol.* 1996;41:3–30.

172. Lewis TL, Mauer D. Effects of early pattern deprivation on visual development. *Optom Vis Sci.* 2009;86:1–7.

173. Daw NW. Critical periods and amblyopia. *Arch Ophthalmol.* 1998;116:502–505.

174. Vilà-de Muga M, Van Esso D, Alarcon S, et al. Instrument-based screening for amblyopia risk factors in a primary care setting in children aged 18 to 30 months. *Eur J Pediatr.* 2021;180:1521–1527. https://doi.org/10.1007/s00431-020-03904-0.

175. Modest Jr Majzoub KM, Moore B, et al. Implementation of instrument-based vision screening for preschool-age children in primary care. *Pediatrics..* 2017;140:e20163745.

176. Handa JT, Rickman CB, Dick AD, et al. A systems biology approach towards understanding and treating non-neovascular age-related macular degeneration. *Nature Com.* 2019;10:3347. https://doi.org/10.1038/s41467-019-11262-1.

177. Lin JB, Tsubota K, Apte RS. A glimpse at the aging eye. *NPJ Aging Mech Dis.* 2016;10:16003. https://doi.org/10.1038/npjamd.2016.3.

178. Lee KS, Lin S, Copland DA, Dick AD, Liu J. Cellular senescence in the aging retina and developments of senotherapies for age-related macular degeneration. *J Neuroinflammation.* 2021;18:32. https://doi.org/10.1186/s12974-021-02088-0.

179. Al-Zamil W, Yassin SA. Recent developments in age-related macular degeneration: a review. *Clin Interv Aging.* 2017;12:1313–1330. https://doi.org/10.2147/CIA.S143508.

180. National Eye Institute. Age-related macular degeneration (AMD) tables. Last updated February 7, 2020. https://www.nei.nih.gov/learn-about-eye-health/outreach-campaigns-and-resources/eye-health-data-and-statistics/age-related-macular-degeneration-amd-data-and-statistics/age-related-macular-degeneration-amd-tables. Accessed January 26, 2022.

181. Boyd D. Have A.M.D.? Save your sight with an Amsler Grid. https://www.aao.org/eye-health/tips-prevention/facts-about-amsler-grid-daily-vision-test. Accessed January 18, 2022.

182. Congdon N, O'Colmain B, Klaver CC, et al. Causes and prevalence of visual impairment among adults in the United States. *Arch Ophthalmol.* 2004;122:477–485. https://doi.org/10.1001/archopht.122.4.477.

183. National Eye Institute. Age-related macular degeneration, last updated June, 22, 2021. https://www.nei.nih.gov/learn-about-eye-health/eye-conditions-and-diseases/age-related-macular-degeneration. Accessed January 26, 2022.

184. National Eye Institute. Age-related macular degeneration (AMD) data and statistics, last updated July 17, 2019. https://www.nei.nih.gov/learn-about-eye-health/outreach-campaigns-and-resources/eye-health-data-and-statistics/age-related-macular-degeneration-amd-data-and-statistics accessed January 24, 2022.

185. Quin W, Xian X, Taylor H. Driving cessation and social isolation in older adults. *J Aging Health.* 2020;32:962–971. https://doi.org/10.1177/0898264319870400.

186. Chihuri S, Mielenz TJ, DiMaggio CJ, et al. Driving cessation and health outcomes in older adults. *J Am Geriatr Soc.* 2016;64:332–341. https://doi.org/10.1111/jgs.13931.

187. Choi M, Mezuk B, Lohman MC, Edwards JD, Rebok GW. Gender and racial disparities in driving cessation among older adults. *J Aging Health.* 2013;25(8 Suppl):147S–162S. https://doi.org/10.1177/0898264313519886.

188. Wang S, Sharma A, Dawson J, Rizzo M, Merickel J. Visual and cognitive impairments differentially affect speed limit compliance in older drivers. *J Am Geriatr Soc.* 2021;69:1300–1308.

189. Carr D, Jackson WJ, Madden DJ, et al. The effect of age on driving skills. *J Am Geriatr Soc.* 1992;40:567–573.

190. Perryman KM, Fitten LJ. Effects of normal aging on the performance of motor-vehicle operational skills. *J Geriatr Psychiatry Neurol.* 1996;9:136–141.

191. Anstey KJ, Eramudugolla R, Ross LA, Lautenschlager NT, Wood J. Road safety in an aging population: risk factors, assessment, interventions, and future directions. *Int Psychogeriatr.* 2016;28:349–356. https://doi.org/10.1017/S1041610216000053.

192. Karthaus M, Falkenstein M. Functional changes and driving performance in older drivers: assessment and interventions. *Geriatrics (Basel).* 2016;1(12). https://doi.org/10.3390/geriatrics1020012.

193. Huisingh C, Levitan EB, Irvin MR, et al. Visual sensory and visual-cognitive function and rate of crash and near-crash involvement among older drivers using naturalistic driving data. *Invest Opthalmol Vis Sci.* 2017;58:2959–2967. https://doi.org/10.1167/iovs.17-21482.

194. Ragland DR, Satariano WA, MacLeod KE. Reasons given by older people for limitation or avoidance of driving. *Gerontologist.* 2004;44:237–244.

195. Toups R, Chirles TJ, Ehsani JP, et al. Driving performance in older adults: current measures, findings, and implications for roadway safety. *Innov Aging.* 2022;6:igab051. https://doi.org/10.1093/geroni/igab051.

196. Ehsani JP. Naturalistic driving studies: an overview and international perspective. In: Vickerman R, ed. *International Encyclopedia of Transportation.* Vol 7. Philadelphia: Elsevier; 2021:20–38.

197. Carr DB, Stowe JD, Morris JC. Driving in the elderly in health and disease. *Handb Clin Neurol.* 2019;167:563–573. https://doi.org/10.1016/B978-0-12-804766-8.00031-5.

198. Croston J, Meuser TM, Berg-Weger M, et al. Driving retirement in older adults with dementia. *Top Geriatr Rehabil.* 2009;25(2):154–162.

199. Eramudugolla R, Huque MH, Wood J, Anstey KJ. On-road behavior in older drivers with mild cognitive impairment. *J Am Med Dir Assoc.* 2021;22:399–405. https://doi.org/10.1016/j.jamda.2020.05.046. e1.

200. Feng YR, Meuleners L, Stevenson M, et al. A longitudinal study examining self-regulation practices in older drivers with and without suspected mild cognitive impairment. *Clin Interv Aging.* 2021;16:2069–2078. https://doi.org/10.2147/CIA.S336802.

201. Vardaki S, Dickerson AE, Beratis I, Yannis G, Papageorgiou SG. Driving difficulties as reported by older drivers with mild cognitive impairment and without neurological impairment. *Traffic Inj Prev.* 2019;20(6):630–635. https://doi.org/10.1080/15389588.2019.1626986.

202. Horswill MS. Hazard perception in driving. *Curr Dir Psychol Sci.* 2016;25:425–430.

203. Willstrand TD, Broberg T, Selander H. Driving characteristics of older drivers and their relationship to the useful field of view test. *Gerontology.* 2016;63:180–188.

204. Insurance Institute for Highway Safety – Older Drivers. https://www.iihs.org/topics/older-drivers Accessed January 27, 2022.

205. Cox AE, Cicchino JB. Continued trends in older driver crash involvement rates in the United States: Data through 2017-2018. *J Safety Res*. 2021;77:288–295. https://doi.org/10.1016/j.jsr.2021.03.013.

206. Cicchino JB. Effects of lane departure warning on police-reported crash rates. *J Safety Res*. 2018;66:61–70. https://doi.org/10.1016/j.jsr.2018.05.006.

207. Feng YR, Meuleners L, Stevenson M, et al. The impact of cognition and gender on speeding behavior in older drivers with and without suspected mild cognitive im-pairment. *Clin Interv Aging*. 2021;16:1473–1483. https://doi.org/10.2147/CIA.S319129.

208. Tefft BC. Driver license renewal policies and fatal crash involvement rates of older drivers, United States, 1986-2011. *Inj Epidemiol*. 2014;1:25. https://doi.org/10.1186/s40621-014-0025-0.

209. Correia C, Lopez KJ, Wroblewski KE, et al. Global sensory impairment in older adults in the United States. *J Am Geriatr Soc*. 2016;64:306–313. https://doi.org/10.1111/jgs.13955.

Endocrine and Integumentary System Changes

INTRODUCTION

The endocrine system and the integumentary system are the final two systems highlighted in the movement systems' foundation for optimizing movement across the life span. While these two systems seem disparate in nature, they are linked by the interaction of the inner and outer body. The endocrine system is responsible for homeostasis, which affects all body systems discussed up to this point in the text. Not all functions of the endocrine system will be discussed, but a sufficient representation of its actions and changes across the life span will be presented. The skin reflects changes in internal homeostasis and external exposure to the environment. The skin visibly denotes ethnicity and age. Touch conveys care in our profession and is an important part of the healing process. The integumentary system guides our first introduction into the world and provides sensory perception of that world and the individuals within society. Optimal functional movement across the life span depends on the efficient function of both the endocrine and integumentary systems.

Homeostasis is the process that keeps the internal environment constant or in balance. Homeostasis of functions such as breathing, sleeping, eating, and eliminating allows individuals to participate fully in all life roles such as play, work, and leisure. Circadian rhythms (from *circa*, which means "about," and *dies*, which means "day") are innately directed rhythms that occur every 24 hours. These rhythms affect all aspects of human physiology. Easily recognizable rhythms include the sleep-wake cycle and the cyclical release of hormones. Biologically, the cycles of change seen in these functions make it easier to adapt to different environments. The cyclical nature of these functions provides a clue to their control and a way to explain behavior. Hormonal control of cyclical functions is mediated by the autonomic nervous system (ANS) and the endocrine system, which together maintain the body's internal homeostasis. The site of the central circadian biological clock in humans is found in the suprachiasmatic nucleus (SCN) of the anterior hypothalamus. It responds to light cues. Peripheral clocks are found in other tissues throughout the body.[1]

Circadian rhythms provide an anticipatory facet to homeostasis. These rhythms are internally driven by hormones and entrained by external factors. One of the strongest of these cues is the duration of light and dark. Circadian rhythms and endocrine rhythms are tightly interconnected.[2] Hormones such as melatonin, cortisol, gonadal steroids, thyroid hormones, and growth hormone (GH) all show daily oscillations based on central and peripheral clocks. Peripheral clocks are present in peripheral organs and tissues such as the heart, liver, intestines, and retina that contribute to the metabolic process.[3] Secretion of nutrient-sensitive hormones such as insulin and leptin oscillates based, in part, on the timing of food intake and light-dark cycles. The bidirectional interaction of the circadian rhythms with hormones and other changing environmental variables involved in energy metabolism is very complicated and will not be discussed further.[1]

The skin is also important in maintaining homeostasis as it constitutes the outer protective covering of the body. It provides temperature regulation in response to both the internal and external environments. The skin protects against infection and contains immune cells.[4] Skin and brain are connected since the sensory receptors that provide perceptual information about the body are located in and surrounded by the skin. Touch is a means by which individuals communicate care and concern as exemplified by a mother rocking a baby.

ENDOCRINE SYSTEM

The endocrine system consists of a collection of glands that manufacture and secrete hormones into the bloodstream. These chemical messengers affect various cells of the body and regulate many aspects of physiological function. The endocrine system plays a role in the rate of growth, basal metabolic rate, immune response, stress responses, and reproduction. The endocrine system is second only to the nervous system in terms of its ability to act as a major communication system. It is composed of the hypothalamus, pituitary gland, thyroid, parathyroid, adrenal gland islet cells of the pancreas, and the gonads, ovaries, or testicles. The neuroendocrine system is the interaction between the nervous system and the endocrine system. Neuroendocrine cells are those that release hormones into the bloodstream in response to stimulation of the nervous system. The endocrine system meets the neuroendocrine system at the interface of the hypothalamus and pituitary gland. The hypothalamus releases hormones that control the activity of the pituitary gland and integrates endocrine and ANS functions to maintain homeostasis.

The hypothalamus and its related structures oversee the functions of the brain such as body temperature, thirst and satiation centers, and osmolality of body fluids. These functions are vital to the maintenance of homeostasis and represent basic physiological needs. The human species has a need to drink and to take in salt, to maintain body temperature, to eat, to reproduce, and to respond to stress. These basic physiological drives ensure the survival of the species.

The control of endocrine functions is therefore closely related to behavior. In addition to its major role in controlling endocrine functions of the body, the hypothalamus controls many aspects of emotional behavior. Because the hypothalamus is a major part of the limbic system, it is not surprising that our emotional state can and does affect basic bodily functions. Homeostasis is disrupted by our thoughts, emotions, and stress, which are manifested in physiological changes in bodily functions, as anyone nervously waiting for an important interview can attest. A brief description of the endocrine glands and their role in maintaining the body's homeostasis is presented below and in Table 10.1.

Pituitary

The main function of the pituitary gland is to produce and release several specific hormones that support critical bodily functions such as growth and metabolism. The pituitary gland is divided into an anterior and a posterior structure with the anterior constituting 80% of the entire pituitary gland. The anterior pituitary makes and releases several hormones, including but not limited to GH, thyroid stimulating hormone (TSH), follicle stimulating hormone (FSH), luteinizing hormone (LH), prolactin, and adrenocorticotropic hormone (ACTH). Insulin-like growth factors are produced in the liver in response to secretion of GH by the anterior pituitary. These hormones mediate responses to stress.[5,6] The posterior part of the pituitary gland is connected by neurons to the hypothalamus and stores oxytocin (OT) and arginine vasopressin (AVP), which can be released directly into the circulation. OT is required for lactation and AVP is involved in regulation of osmotic balance.[6,7] The pituitary gland is often referred to as the master gland because it controls other endocrine glands. In response to releasing factors from the hypothalamus, the pituitary gland controls the ANS.[8]

Thyroid

The thyroid gland is a two-lobed structure connected by an isthmus that looks like a butterfly. It is located at the base of the neck and releases hormones that control metabolism and regulate other vital functions such as

TABLE 10.1	**Main Human Hormones**	
Gland	**Hormones**	**Functions**
Pituitary	Trophic hormones	Stimulate thyroid, adrenal, gonadal, and pancreatic activities
Thyroid	Thyroid hormones Calcitonin	Regulate metabolism, growth and development, behavior, and puberty Promote deposition of calcium (Ca) in the bones
Parathyroid	Parathyroid hormone	Controls serum Ca ion concentration by increasing Ca absorption by the gut and kidneys and releasing Ca from bones
Adrenal	Aldosterone Epinephrine Corticosteroid hormones	Regulate metabolism and behavior
Pancreas	Insulin and glucagon	Regulate blood sugar levels
Hypothalamus	Releasing hormones	Stimulate pituitary activity Stimulate thyroid, adrenal, pancreatic, and gonadal activities
Thymus	Thymosin	Stimulates development of T cells
Gonads	**Sex steroid hormones (androgens and estrogens)**	**Regulate growth and development, reproduction, immunity, onset of puberty, and behavior**

breathing, heart rate, body temperature, central nervous system (CNS), and peripheral nervous system (PNS). The thyroid gland uses iodine from the food you eat to make its two main hormones: T3 and T4.[9] The hypothalamus and the pituitary monitor the balance between the two thyroid hormones. The hypothalamus produces thyroid-releasing hormone (TRH), which signals the pituitary to release more or less TSH, which in turn tells the thyroid gland to produce more or less thyroid hormones. For example, if levels of both T3 and T4 are high, the hypothalamus directs the pituitary to release less TSH to the thyroid gland to slow production. If both are low, the pituitary releases more TSH, which tells the thyroid to produce more thyroid hormones.

Parathyroid

These small pea-shaped pair of glands are located in the neck behind the thyroid gland. There are one pair on either side. Together, they regulate calcium and phosphate metabolism to maintain appropriate levels of both minerals by releasing parathyroid hormone (PTH). PTH helps the synthesis of active vitamin D and calcitriol in the kidneys.[10] PTH can produce resorption of calcium and phosphate from bone, resorption of calcium from the kidneys, excretion of phosphorus from the kidneys,

and absorption of calcium and phosphate from the GI tract with the help of vitamin D (see Chapter 5).[11]

Adrenal

The adrenal glands are located on top of both kidneys. They are small and triangular-shaped, each surrounded by a fibrous capsule. They help regulate metabolism, blood pressure, the immune system, and response to stress. Each gland is composed of an adrenal medulla and adrenal cortex derived from different embryonic origins. The adrenal medulla secretes epinephrine, which is important in the ANS response to stress, which is "fight or flight," a rapid response that results in increased heart rate and blood pressure, and sweating. The adrenal cortex produces and secretes mineralocorticoids, glucocorticoids, and adrenal androgens.[12] The adrenal cortex maintains fluid-electrolyte balance in the kidneys by secreting aldosterone, a mineralocorticoid, which coordinates the excretion of potassium and reabsorption of sodium by the kidneys. It is also important in regulating blood pressure. The adrenal cortex also secretes cortisol, a glucocorticoid, in response to stress. The adrenal glands supplement other glands by producing androgen precursors that can be converted to sex hormones (androgens and estrogen). Dehydroepiandrosterone

(DHEA) and DHEA-sulfate (DHEA-S) are androgen precursors.[13]

Pancreas

The pancreas is located behind the stomach and in front of the spine. It is an accessory digestive gland because it secretes gastrin, which stimulates the stomach to produce acid. The pancreas secretes hormones into the blood stream as part of its endocrine function and secretes digestive enzymes through ducts as an exocrine gland.[14] The endocrine part of the pancreas consists of four types of endocrine cells: alpha (α) cells produce glucagon, beta (β) cells produce insulin, delta (δ) cells produce somatostatin, and cells produce pancreatic polypeptide.[15] The endocrine cells of the pancreas are found in an area called the islets of Langerhans. The major function of the endocrine pancreas is to maintain the body's blood glucose balance. If blood glucose is too high, insulin is secreted; if blood glucose is too low, glucagon is secreted. Somatostatin can inhibit the release of insulin, glucagon, and pancreatic polypeptide.[15] Somatostatin can also inhibit release of GH from the pituitary gland. Pancreatic polypeptide can inhibit the release of glucagon.[16] Ghrelin cells make up a very small percentage of pancreatic islet cells and are mainly found in the gut.[17] These ghrelin cells play a role in glucose homeostasis because it is the hunger hormone and responds mainly to food intake. Glucose, the brain's metabolic food, is vital for brain metabolism and maintenance of body homeostasis.

Thymus

The thymus gland consists of two lobes and resides in the chest behind the sternum and just above and in front of the heart. It makes T lymphocytes (T cells) and white blood cells. The thymus gland is an integral part of the immune system as well as the endocrine system. Thymosin stimulates T cell development. Once mature, they migrate to the lymph nodes as vital parts of the immune system. The immune system is very complex and is divided into innate immunity, which is independent of the thymus, and adaptive immunity, which depends on the thymus.[18] Thymic output is highly controlled by age and stage of development.

Gonads

The testes and ovaries are endocrine glands involved in reproduction. They both synthesize and secrete hormones; the testes secrete testosterone and the ovaries secrete estrogen and progesterone. The hypothalamus triggers the release of gonadotrophic hormones that regulate the menstrual cycle once puberty is reached. Testosterone is secreted as early as the seventh week of gestation. Following menopause, the ovaries can produce testosterone and androstenedione, which can be converted to estrogens peripherally.

Hypothalamus

The hypothalamus monitors physiological set points for almost every internal body function. For example, there are set point values for body temperature, blood glucose levels, blood pressure, and salt concentration in the blood. If these values are under or over the normal range, sensing mechanisms relay information to the hypothalamus or subsystems under its control, and steps are taken to correct the error. Negative feedback is the most common way in which values are corrected. Set points for regulated variables can be changed or reset. Set points can be changed by external or internal stimuli. Some set points, such as body temperature, display a circadian rhythm; body temperature is higher during the day than during the night. Reflexes control some endocrine functions via the hypothalamus. A stimulus is received that is interpreted as an error by an integrating center. The integrating center stimulates an effector, which is typically a muscle or a gland, which in turn produces a response that corrects the error, reestablishing homeostasis. The muscle may act to change blood flow to an area to prevent heat loss. The hypothalamus relays commands to the ANS to activate heat gain or heat loss mechanisms. When an increase in blood sugar is detected, insulin is secreted by the pancreas. The level of glucose in the blood declines, and insulin secretion ceases. Negative feedback systems are corrective by nature. An error must be detected for the system to be engaged.

Hypothalamic Axes

Glands that signal each other in a specific order are referred to as an axis. There are several axes that are controlled by the hypothalamus. One very important one is the hypothalamic-pituitary-adrenal (HPA) axis. The HPA axis maintains physiological homeostasis by releasing several key regulatory molecules. For example, the hypothalamus releases corticotropin-releasing hormone (CRH), which in turn acts on the pituitary gland to synthesize and release ACTH into the circulation. ACTH acts on the adrenal gland to make and release corticosteroids, such as cortisol and corticosterone. These glucocorticoids modulate physiological processes such as metabolism, immune responses, stress response, and the ANS. The HPA axis can trigger a negative feedback loop by activating a glucocorticoid receptor (GR) in the brain to shut down corticosteroid production.[19]

The paraventricular nucleus of the hypothalamus acts as a regulator of the stress response.[6] Cortisol is necessary for survival under stress.[11] It attenuates the body's inflammatory response and helps preserve body cell integrity, which is the rationale for the use of steroids therapeutically. Chronic stress can decrease the sensitivity of the feedback system that oversees the HPA axis.

Other hypothalamic axes include the hypothalamic-pituitary-thyroid (HPT) axis and the hypothalamic-pituitary-somatotropic (HPS), which are critical for growth and development, and the hypothalamic-pituitary-gonadal (HPG) axis, which is critical for puberty and development of reproduction. HPT axis monitors the body's energy status and regulates energy expenditure.[20] The roles of these axes and hormones are discussed in the following age-related sections.

ENDOCRINE CHANGES ACROSS THE LIFE SPAN

Hormones and growth factors play varying roles in human growth and development beginning in utero and progressing through three stages of postnatal growth (infancy, childhood, and adolescence), which reflect different hormonal phases of the growth process.[21] The HPS axis directs the production of GH, a somatotropin, from somatotropes of the pituitary gland and secretes it into the circulation. The HPS via an effect of GH also stimulates production of insulin-like growth factor-1 (IGF-1).[22] Table 10.2 summarizes the hormones involved in growth.

Prenatal

The endocrine system develops in stages in utero after the second month of gestation.[23] The first endocrine gland to develop is the thyroid gland, at 24 days of gestation.[24] The pituitary forms at 4 weeks and is composed of ectoderm from two different sources, which explains why there are two different tissue types (glandular and

TABLE 10.2	Hormone Actions During Growth		
Type of Hormone/ Growth Factor	**Abbreviation**	**Secreted by**	**Influence on Growth**
Insulin	—	Pancreas	Stimulates fetal growth Increases growth velocity
Insulin-like growth factors	IGF-1, IGF-2	Liver	Affects both prenatal and postnatal growth Stimulates chondrogenesis in the growth plate
Thyroid hormones Thyroxine Triiodothyronine	T4 T3	Thyroid	Prenatally needed for CNS development Postnatally needed for GH secretion in childhood and adolescence
Growth hormone	GH	Anterior pituitary gland	Affects mainly postnatal growth Stimulates hepatic IGF-1 production and chondrogenesis in the growth plate Highest secretion in adolescence
Leptin		Adipocytes, placenta	Regulates GH secretion and stimulates chondrogenesis in the growth plate
Sex steroids	Estrogen Testosterone	Placenta, ovaries Placenta, testes	Both increase GH at puberty Estrogen causes closure of growth plates in males and females at the end of puberty Testosterone causes descent of the testes into the scrotum in the last 2–3 months of gestation

From Benyi E, Sävendahl L. The physiology of childhood growth: hormonal regulation. *Horm Res Paediatr.* 2017; 88:6-14; Murray PG, Clayton PE. Endocrine control of growth. *Am J Med Genet C Semin Med Genet.* 2013; 163 C(2):76-85; Hall JE, Hall ME. *Guyton and Hall's Textbook of Medical Physiology.* 14th ed. Philadelphia: Elsevier; 2020.

neural) composing the gland. The function of these tissues contributes to the maximum rate of growth in height of the fetus seen around the fourth month of gestation.[25] The fetal adrenal gland produces steroids that influence the maturation of the liver, epithelium of the digestive tract, and the lungs.[23]

Fetal growth is nutrition-dependent and therefore reliant on the mother's nutritional intake and the integrity of the placenta. Neither the sex hormones or GH play a role in fetal growth. Levels of insulin-like growth factors (IGF-1 and IGF-2) in umbilical cord blood correlate to the infant's size at birth.[26] The placenta is an endocrine gland that supplies the developing fetus with peptide hormones, neurohormones, and steroids. The placenta secretes leptin, a hormone, which is associated with fetal growth.[27] The placenta converts steroids produced by the fetus' adrenal gland to biologically active steroids such as estrogens. The placenta secretes substances autonomously without being regulated by fetal or maternal signals.[28] Placental insufficiency and poor maternal nutrition are causes of intrauterine growth retardation.[29]

Development of thymic epithelial cells (TECs) occurs during fetal development. TECs are necessary for formation of the thymus gland.[18] T cells, produced by the fetal thymus, ensure that a normal complement of T cells is in circulation and available at birth.[18,30]

Thyroid hormones play a major role in the development of the brain and nervous system. However, the fetal thyroid gland does not become functionally mature until 20 weeks gestation.[31] Prior to that time, the fetus must depend on the mother to supply thyroid hormones and iodine for growth and development. Maternal thyroid hormones assist the development of the HPT axis, which begins to mature in the second trimester.[32] Thyroid hormones regulate fetal growth by making certain hormones and growth factors are available. Thyroid hormones regulate the layering of the cerebral cortex and cell migration.[33] Thyroid hormones affect consumption of oxygen and glucose by fetal tissue and send developmental and maturational signals to the skin, heart, lungs, liver, bone, brown adipose tissue, and the ANS. As the fetus approaches term, thyroid hormones prepare fetal tissues to function in an extrauterine environment. Thyroid hormones are responsible for the activation of physiologic processes needed for survival at birth. For example, thyroid hormones direct deposition of brown fat and the synthesis of surfactant in the lungs.[34] Lack of thyroid hormones during early gestation is not reversible after birth, whereas the effects of congenital hypothyroidism can be prevented by thyroid hormone replacement therapy.[35] The role of thyroid hormones in fetal and infant development is depicted.

Infancy Through Adolescence

At birth, the transition from the warm uterine environment to the cool extrauterine one promotes the infant's hypothalamus to secrete TRH, which in turn stimulates the pituitary to secrete TSH and cause a rise in production of T3 and T4 by the thyroid gland.[31] In addition to activating thermogenesis, thyroid hormones are critical for glucogenesis, cardiac adaptations, and pulmonary gas exchange.[34] The HPT axis becomes fully functional a month or two after birth[36] and supports development of synapses, astrocytes, and glial support cells.[32] Screening for hypothyroidism is mandated at birth. Early detection and treatment of an affected newborn improves brain function and limits cognitive impairment.[31]

GH, produced by the anterior pituitary, mainly affects postnatal growth.[21] It exerts a profound effect on cell proliferation in target tissues. For example, GH sustains the normal rate of protein synthesis in the body needed for cartilage cell proliferation at the epiphyseal plates of bone. Too much GH can produce gigantism; too little, dwarfism. Postnatal growth rate averages 25 cm per year during the first year of life.[21] The hypothalamus regulates GH secretion by the anterior pituitary via GH-releasing hormone and the inhibitory hormone somatostatin.[21,37] Insulin and IGF-1 also continue to assist in postnatal growth in infancy.[21] GH works indirectly on cell division by influencing the liver to secrete IGF-1. This growth factor in turn stimulates protein synthesis and impedes protein degradation. IGF-1 is the main regulator of postnatal growth. Insulin binds to the IGF-1 receptor and increases growth velocity.[38] IGF-2 is also a growth hormone which plays a role in postnatal growth, but its exact function is unclear. A peak level of insulin-like growth factor is seen in adolescence. GH and IGF-1 levels are low during the day, but 1–2 hours after falling asleep, large amounts are secreted. GH is released in a pulsatile manner by the pituitary during the night. The amount of GH produced at night can represent 20%–40% of the day's total output. Nutritional status has a major impact on regulating growth during the first two years of life.[21,37] The importance of the first 1000 days (conception to age 2 years) has been well documented.[39–41] Growth during this time is dependent on nutritional status rather than hormone regulators. This may explain the growth curve variability seen in the first 2 years of life.[21]

Childhood growth is directed by GH, IGF-1, insulin, thyroid hormones, and leptin.[41] Leptin continues to influence postnatal growth as it is secreted by adipose tissue as well as the placenta. Leptin is produced by adipose tissue which is now recognized as an active endocrine gland.[42] It has been called the *"satiety hormone"* and is involved in weight regulation. Researchers are interested in discovering its potential role in development of childhood obesity.[43] Leptin levels in cord blood predicted adiposity in 3-year-old children in a prospective cohort study.[44] More recently, researchers found epigenetic changes in cord blood DNA to be associated with leptin levels, a measure of neonatal adiposity.[45]

Thymus-dependent immunity is critical in early life. Infants born with DiGeorge syndrome exhibit thymic hypoplasia or aplasia.[46] Abnormal development of the thymus gland and thymocytes results in life-threatening infections and early mortality due to an inability to develop adaptive immune responses. The thymus is largest at birth and is most active up until puberty.[18] Involution of the thymus begins in childhood.[18,47] Involution (or atrophy) is the process of replacing thymic epithelial tissue with fat. The thymus continues to produce T cells after puberty even though production wanes due to involution.[30]

Thyroid hormone and PTH are important for postnatal growth of bones. Thyroxine (T3), the physiologically active thyroid hormone, regulates bone turnover and bone mineral density. The amount of thyroid hormone secreted declines slightly from birth to puberty and then increases to support the adolescent growth spurt. Gender differences in thyroid function tests are reported in adolescence.[48] Hypothyroidism can cause delayed skeletal maturation in childhood or adolescence.

PTH is involved in maintaining calcium homeostasis by acting at three sites: the bones, the gastrointestinal tract, and the kidneys. This involvement continues throughout the life span. Levels of PTH in healthy children have been studied,[49] with a significant increase seen in girls between 8 and 10 years compared to between 10 and 12 years in boys consistent with bone and pubertal growth spurts. Thyroid hormones have an effect on dental development,[50,51] so it is not surprising to find that skeletal maturity and dental maturity are usually correlated.[52]

The earliest signs of puberty in both sexes—the acquisition of axillary and pubic hair—are a result of increased secretion of androgens by the adrenal gland.[53] The adrenal gland is directed to secrete androgens by corticotropin released from the anterior pituitary gland. The adrenal androgens also play a major part in directing the course of the adolescent growth spurt in both sexes. The remaining changes that occur during puberty are the result of increased activity within the HPG axis. The hypothalamus produces increased amounts of gonadotropin-releasing hormone (GRH) just before puberty. During childhood, only low levels of GRH, pituitary gonadotropins, and estrogen or testosterone are secreted. GRH is released in rhythmic bursts during the night at 2-hour intervals, causing nocturnal release of gonadotropins, which in turn stimulates the cells of the ovary or testicle to secrete estrogen or testosterone. Testosterone and the adrenal androgens produce greater growth of muscle in the male. Female growth for the most part is dependent on the androgens of the adrenal cortex alone.[25]

The rise in estrogen triggers menarche, the first menstrual period. On average, the onset of menarche in the United States decreased to 11.9 years.[54] A greater percentage of Hispanic women reached menarche at age 10 than non-Hispanic white women. Racial differences in timing of menarche may reflect differences in nutrition, socioeconomic status, poverty level, and family structure. Poor fetal nutrition and poor endocrine function have been associated with earlier onset of menarche.[55] Earlier onset of menarche has also been linked to childhood trauma and stress.[56] The advent of the first period is a late-stage phenomenon of puberty occurring after the development of the breast and pubic hair and growth spurt. Female athletes have a later onset of menarche than nonathletes.[57] Rising estrogen levels also cause the epiphyses to close, thus terminating skeletal growth. Because girls go through puberty earlier than do boys, they attain peak height earlier and develop secondary sex characteristics sooner than do boys.

Testosterone is critical to the attainment of sexual maturity in males. The first sign of puberty in boys is testicular enlargement. In males, the final puberty markers are spermarche, facial hair growth, and voice changes.[53] Spermatogenesis begins at puberty under the direction of testosterone which has negative feedback effects on the hypothalamus and anterior pituitary gland. Testosterone also induces changes in the male reproductive organs and development of the secondary sex characteristics and sex drive. Testosterone stimulates growth during puberty through its effect on GH secretion. It also causes the eventual closure of the epiphyses. Testosterone, unlike estrogen, has a strong anabolic effect on protein synthesis that can also account for the increased muscle mass in men compared with women. Anabolic steroids are synthetic agents that are converted into testosterone by the body. Some male and female athletes use anabolic steroids to build body mass and strength, but these drugs are potentially very dangerous and can have serious side effects such as liver damage.

Adulthood

The main role of GH in adults is to regulate metabolism.[58] GH is released in pulses and in a circadian rhythm during the night. Sleep is necessary to ensure release of GH. GH acts on the liver to produce IGF-1. GH release is correlated inversely with amount of intraabdominal fat present in a person's body composition. Physical fitness and adiposity were found to be the major determinants of decline in GH in healthy adults.[59] Body composition changes that include increased fat deposition can lead to more free fatty acids (FFAs) being available, which can cause increased insulin resistance. Higher levels of insulin, FFA, and free IGF-1 suppress pituitary release of GH and increase fat deposition.[58] GH and IGF-1 are the major hormones in the HPS axis. IGF-1 consistently declines, beginning at age 20 in men and women. GH, after peaking during puberty, declines by 1%–2% a year after puberty.[60] The decrease in IGF-1 and GH in healthy adults is related to the amount of GH secreted. Levels of IGF-1 may be maintained via GH effect on production and secretion by the liver throughout adulthood. See Fig. 10.1C for a graph depicting the age-related decline of IGF-1. The age-related decrease in GH and IGF-1 is termed somatopause and represents the decline in function of the HPS axis.

The pancreas increases in weight until between 30 and 40 years of age due to accumulation of fat.[61] The function of the islet cells of the pancreas is to release insulin. This ability gradually declines after age 40, which can affect blood sugar control. Secretion of insulin is triggered by rising levels of glucose such as after a meal. Once the levels of glucose decrease, insulin secretion decreases. Insufficient insulin secretion results in type 2 diabetes. Increased resistance to insulin at the target organ can also increase the risk of developing type 2 diabetes.

During adulthood, hormones are integrally associated with our normal physiological response to stress.

The hypothalamus and anterior pituitary coordinate the release of corticotropin, which stimulates the adrenal cortex to secrete cortisol, a glucocorticoid. The HPA axis synchronizes the human stress response with circadian rhythms. The activity of the sympathetic nervous system is also increased during stress. The familiar fight-or-flight reaction is accompanied by an increased secretion of epinephrine, additionally readying the body for physical activity and for coping with new situations. The paraventricular nucleus of the hypothalamus acts as a regulator of the stress response.[6] Cortisol is necessary for survival under stress.[11] It attenuates the body's inflammatory response and helps preserve body cell integrity, which is the rationale for the use of steroids therapeutically. "Good stress" is present during that new job interview, whereas "tolerable stress" might be more serious such as loss of a job but in a situation where the person has a support system to overcome the loss. Chronic stress can decrease the sensitivity of the feedback system that oversees the HPA axis (see Fig. 10.2). Chronic elevation of cortisol due to chronic stress may result in the HPA axis response becoming maladaptive, which can lead to metabolic syndrome, mental health disorders, cardiovascular disease, and immune dysfunction.[42,62]

The thymus gland in adulthood continues to actively produce T cells into the fourth decade. However, after 40 years of age, thymic output is reduced.[63] There are many peripheral mechanisms available for maintaining T cell numbers that have been studied in mice but not yet understood in humans. Once T cells are produced by the thymus gland, they move to peripheral lymphoid tissues and wait to be activated by the immune system. Epigenetic modifications are thought to be involved in thymic atrophy by causing senescence of the thyroid epithelial cells.[64]

Adults begin to show a progressive increase in TSH concentration with increasing age beginning in the third decade.[65] This finding came from the NHANES III study and was confirmed by a longitudinal study of a community-based group, mean age of 45.5 years at baseline, and followed for 13 years.[66] The mechanism and explanation for the need to produce more TSH is uncertain. Inadequate negative feedback or decreased receptor sensitivity has been suggested.[48]

The age-related decline of DHEA/DHEA-S is termed adrenopause[67,135] and is related to changes in the HPA and HPG axes with age. Age-related changes in gonadal

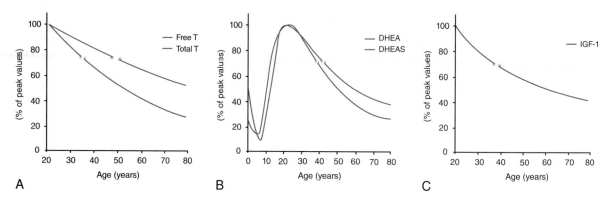

Fig. 10.1 Decline in hormone production with age. (**A**) Testosterone, total T *(red)* and free *(blue)*; (**B**) DHEA *(blue)* and DHEA-S *(red)*; and (C) IGF-1. *DHEA,* Dehydroepiandrosterone; *DHEA-S,* dehydroepiandrosterone sulfate; *IGF-1,* insulin-like growth factor-1. (From Pataky MW, Young WF, Nair S. Hormonal and metabolic changes of aging and the influence of lifestyle modifications. May Clin Proc. 2021: 96:788–814.)

hormones are termed menopause and andropause. Production of testosterone (T) gradually and consistently declines beginning around the third decade (see Fig. 10.1A).[68] Free T, which is the biologically active form, declines twice as fast. DHEA and its sulfated form DHEA-S are precursors of androgenic and estrogenic hormones.[69] They reach peak levels by the age of 30 years and then decline at a rate of 2%–3% a year in men and women (see Fig. 10.1B).[70,71] By the third decade, men and premenopausal women experience a decline in DHEA and DHEA-S.

Menopause is part of normal aging for a woman. On average, the menstrual cycles become less regular around late middle age with the onset of the menopausal transition reported as age 46 years (range 34–54).[22] The failure of the ovaries to produce estrogen affects the genitourinary tract, the skeletal system, and body composition and alters vasomotor regulation. A woman may experience an increased need to urinate and some urethral irritability. Loss of minerals from the bone puts a woman at risk for osteoporosis (see Chapter 5). Loss of estrogen also increases a woman's risk for cardiovascular disease. Physiological changes associated with menopause include thinning of the walls of the vagina and decreased lubrication, vasomotor changes leading to hot flashes or flushes, less immediate responses to sexual arousal, and fewer contractions during orgasm. There is a discernible decrease in function of the endocrine system in females at three levels. The decline at the organ level, the ovary, and effects of decline in circulating hormone levels have

been briefly described. Finally, target organs, the estrogen receptors in the body, are also affected. Estrogen receptors are plentiful in the skin. They are located in fibroblasts, keratinocytes, sebaceous and sweat glands, hair follicles, and blood vessels.[72] The breasts lose connective tissue; the skin becomes thin; and sweat glands and hair follicles become dry and less resilient due to the loss of estrogen.[73]

Estrogen replacement can ameliorate the genitourinary symptoms of menopause, such as vaginal dryness, and vasomotor symptoms, such as hot flashes, and prevent fracture caused by accelerated bone loss.[22,74] Benefits were found to exceed the risk for most women under 60 years of age and less than 10 years post-onset of menopause.[75,76] These practice guidelines and position statements additionally recommend that transdermal delivery of estrogen is less likely to produce risk of venous thromboembolism (VTE), stroke and coronary artery disease than other means of delivery.[75,76] The dosage and means of delivery of estrogen in hormone therapy can affect the ability of estrogen to produce a thrombotic environment. Estrogen causes conditions that are favorable to producing a clot by affecting platelets.[77] The exact mechanism is unclear.

Men undergo less dramatic changes relative to a reduction in circulating testosterone levels. Andropause has been replaced with the term late-onset hypogonadism (LOH).[78] Despite the fact that morning testosterone (T) levels decline steadily over time, only 20% of men over the age of 65 years have T levels below the normal range for young men.[22] Contrary to the very

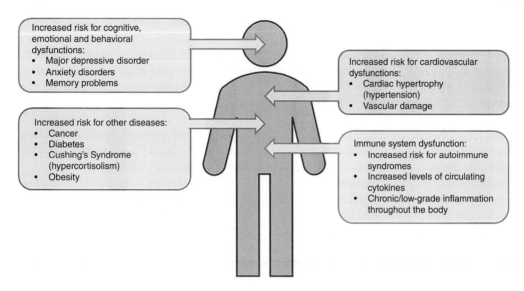

Fig. 10.2 Effects of chronic stress. (From Sheng JA, Bales NJ, Myers SA, et al. The hypothalamic-pituitary-adrenal axis: development, programming actions of hormones, and maternal-fetal interactions. *Front Behav Neurosci.* 2021;14:601939.)

recognizable symptoms of menopause, men with LOH exhibit few distinct signs and symptoms that can be differentiated from the effects of aging. The decline in the amount of testosterone in the circulation does not indicate a decrease in potency. Sperm continue to be produced but in smaller quantities. The decline in sperm production appears to be linked to connective tissue changes around the inside of the seminiferous tubules. This decline begins in the 40s and 50s, with a decrease in sperm motility noted after the age of 50 years. "Sexual dysfunction is consistently associated with low serum testosterone, and even more closely associated with low serum-free testosterone."[22] Androgen deficiency and erectile dysfunction are two separate clinical entities. The decline in testosterone with age does cause the libido to diminish but does not cause impotence (erectile dysfunction). An increase in gonadotropins in the serum with age indicates that the testes are less responsive to their effects.

T replacement therapy for age-related decline in testosterone is available in several forms: oral tablets, injections, and transdermal creams or patches. Regardless of how the testosterone is given, many health benefits have been documented. The benefits include improved physical and sexual function, cardiovascular and bone health, and cognitive function.[79] Other studies have found a lack of significant benefits in these same areas.[68] Furthermore, the majority of studies have been done in healthy older men, when the frail elderly may be able to benefit most from such replacement therapy.

A systematic review of the effects of work on symptoms of andropause and menopause identified work-related factors of psychologic stress, physical effort, and sleep disorders as being significantly correlated with andropause manifestations.[78] Age at menopause and severity of symptoms were associated with repetitive work, high job strain, and pesticide exposure in female workers. Sleep disorders were related to shift work, and both males and females indicated job-related stress as contributing to their symptoms. Modification of the workplace or the organization of the work may assist in developing health promotion programs.

Older Adulthood

As the body ages, it is less resilient to environmental stress. It becomes more difficult to maintain the status quo or homeostasis. There are four patterns of change in endocrine function during typical aging. The first pattern is related to endocrine gland failure, which is exemplified by the ovary during menopause. Risk for VTE is greater for women over 60 years of age or 10 years or more postmenopause than for women under

60 years.[80] The Women's Health Initiative, a large randomized control trial, was conducted by the National Heart, Lung and Blood Institute of NIH and studied postmenopausal women up to 79 years.[81] Their findings are part of the North American Menopause Society (NAMS) latest position statement (2022)[76] in which they concluded that hormone therapy reduced bone loss, fracture risk, and joint pain. Hormone therapy continues to be the gold standard for vasomotor symptoms. Additional findings in the NAMS's 2022 position statement include beneficial effects of estrogen on skin thickness, collagen, and elasticity; reduction in eye pressure related to glaucoma in Black women; and decreased risk of age-related macular degeneration. Relative to cognition, hormone therapy is not recommended to prevent cognitive decline. Beginning hormone replacement in women aged 65 years or older increases the risk for dementia. Risks for VTE, coronary heart disease, stroke, and dementia are greater for women who begin hormone therapy more than 10 or 20 years from menopause or are 60 years or older.[76]

The second pattern of change is associated with a decrease in sensitivity of target organs to the hormones secreted. An example is the age-related decline in peripheral tissue response to insulin. Changes in the endocrine part of the pancreas include an overall decrease in number of endocrine cells, specifically β cells, which produce insulin, deposition of amyloid, and a decrease in ductal structures.[61] As the pancreas decreases in weight in the elderly, the likelihood of developing pancreatic dysfunction or disease increases. Insulin receptor sensitivity decreases with age.[82] This decrease in sensitivity is associated with decline of T and reduction in GH with age.[83] Insulin is less effective in decreasing glucose production in the liver in older adults, and it takes longer for the insulin to be metabolized.[84] Rates of insulin action and pulsatility are higher in an elderly population compared to young adults.[85] Insulin-triggered glucose disposal is greater in aerobically trained old and young subjects than in their sedentary counterparts.[86] The researchers also found no age-related differences in insulin sensitivity and suggested that the commonly observed age-related reduction in insulin sensitivity may be due to reductions in physical activity rather than aging per se. Furthermore, insulin receptor sensitivity can be improved, irrespective of age, by either aerobic or resistance exercise.[87]

The third pattern is seen in the failure of an expected adaptive response, such as an insufficiency in the expected normal increase in blood pressure on standing from a supine or seated position caused by a lack of renin. Lack of renin is usually related to low blood volume. The renin-angiotensin-aldosterone system is responsible for the hormonal regulation of plasma volume (Hall and Hall, 2020).[88] This system tries to compensate for an inability of the sympathetic nervous to increase blood pressure. Jacob and colleagues[89] concluded that reduced plasma renin activity was a component of orthostatic intolerance.

The final pattern is marked by an increase in sensitivity within the endocrine system as seen when there is a more aggressive response to vasopressin (AVP), the antidiuretic hormone in older adults for a given level of osmolality. Older individuals tend to retain fluid more easily. AVP is secreted by the posterior pituitary and regulates the body's water balance. Plasma osmolality is maintained within a narrow range despite large swings in fluid intake. When plasma osmolality is low, AVP secretion is inhibited and water is excreted from the kidneys. Conversely, when plasma osmolality is high, AVP is secreted and water is retained or conserved. Three processes regulate this water metabolism: secretion of AVP, the renal response to AVP secretion, and control of thirst.[90] All three processes are affected by aging and therefore so is the physiologic mechanism of water metabolism.[90,91] In older adults, decreases in plasma osmoreceptors and arterial baroreceptors are accompanied by an increase in sensitivity to AVP. A greater augmentation of AVP secretion per unit change in plasma osmolality is demonstrated in elderly subjects compared to younger subjects.[90,92] Renal response to ADH is decreased. Older adults appear to have a higher set point to detect thirst and a blunted response to thirst signals.

In healthy older adults, the concentration of TSH increases with age without a decline in concentration of free T4 (free thyroxine).[22] This age-related change is indicative of a resetting of the TSH set point.[48] The change in thyroid function in older adults is highly variable between individuals. "Each individual has set points (individual means) for TSH and T4, and what is normal for one individual may not be normal for another...."[48] Other researchers have reported that thyroid function in older adults remained over a 5-year period.[93] The clinical significance of subclinical hyperthyroidism or hypothyroidism continues to be debated. From middle age up to 65 or 70 years of age, subclinical hypothyroidism is a risk factor for cardiovascular disease. It is not a risk for older individuals, and in those over 85 years of age, subclinical hypothyroidism may be linked to longer life.[94,136] Biondi et al. 2019 Age-related TSH reference ranges for older adults over the age of 80 need to be changed to reflect present knowledge.[95]

Women are at greatest risk for developing abnormal TSH levels after menopause.[96] Clinical hypothyroidism is six times more common in women than men.[97,138] Primary hypothyroidism prevalence increases in both men and women over 65 years of age.[98,99] Age-specific hormone reference values should be used to avoid over-treating older individuals. The goal of thyroid replacement therapy is to keep values of serum thyrotropin between 0.4 and 4 mIU/L.[100]

With aging, there are tissue changes but no change in levels of PTH.[11] Murthy and associates[101] reported higher numbers of falls, lower gait speed and grip strength, and higher BMI in a community dwelling group of older adults with high PTH. Vitamin D and PTH levels are associated with fall risk in middle age and older woman.[102] To summarize, high levels of PTH are associated with balance problems (see Chapter 11), sarcopenia (see Chapter 6), osteoporosis (see Chapter 5), and frailty in older adults (see Chapter 13).[103]

The thymus is the sole source of new T cells throughout life. T cell production declines with age due to progressive involution. Despite progressive atrophy of the thymus gland, thymic output has been detected until about 80 years of age.[104] Decline in T cell immunity is characterized by *immunosenescence* and *inflammaging*.[105] *Immunosenescence* is the term used to describe the changes in structure and function of the immune system due to aging.[106] *Immunosenescence* is linked to the thymic involution, which results in disruption of T cell homeostasis.[106] *Inflammaging* is an elevated reactivity seen in older adults, which results in systemic inflammation when there is no acute infection. These two processes predispose older individuals to autoimmune diseases and decreased vaccination response. Researchers are exploring the possibility of rejuvenating the immune system in older adults by epigenetic modification of TECs.[64]

The HPA axis tightly controls cortisol synthesis. ACTH, produced by the pituitary gland, controls the production of cortisol, a glucocorticoid, by the adrenal gland.[13] With aging, regulation of the HPA axis is altered, resulting in an elevated nocturnal peak of ACTH and cortisol, which affects sleep and memory function in the elderly.[107] In older adults, the HPA axis becomes more sensitive to secretion of CRH and more resistant to the effects of antiinflammatory steroids.[108] It is hard to separate aging changes in the adrenal gland from the age-related changes in hypothalamus-pituitary regulation.[13] The production of aldosterone, a mineralocorticoid produced by the adrenal gland, decreases with aging. The decline appears to be related to a decrease in plasma renin activity, not because of aging of the adrenal gland.[91] DHEA/DHEA-S, also products of the adrenal gland, decline beginning in early to middle adulthood and continue to decline until death (Fig. 10.1B).

The sensitivity of the HPA axis decreases with aging and changes the patterns of secretion and response to negative feedback from targeted tissues. One example of this disruption is glucose homeostasis. Glucose metabolism is disrupted with increasing age. The brain, specifically the hypothalamus and brain stem, receives peripheral metabolic signals from hormones such as insulin and leptin and nutrients such as glucose and fatty acids to regulate glucose metabolism.[109] Brain glucose metabolism declines significantly in old age.[110] Decline in glucose metabolism along with increased oxidative damage to the brain can impair cognition in older adults.[68] The ANS modulates pancreatic insulin/glucagon secretion, hepatic glucose production, and skeletal muscle glucose uptake. Insulin also modulates glucose metabolism in the liver and provides signals to the brain that assist with homeostasis. "Experimental evidence suggests that defective metabolic sensing in hypothalamic neurons may lead to dysregulation of glucose homeostasis and diabetes."[109] Leptin improves insulin receptivity and regulates glucose metabolism separately from its other roles in growth and reproduction.[111]

Age-related changes in other hormones produced by the HPG and HPS axes continue to decline from peaks in adulthood. Men maintain fertility and sex hormone production until old age. However, testicular volume decreases by 30% after age 75. A slow progressive decline in morning serum T concentrations of 25% occurs in healthy men from 25 to 75 years of age.[22] GH and IGF-1 begin to decline in early to middle adulthood and continue to decline until death (see Fig. 10.1C). GH, after peaking during puberty, declines by 1%–2% a year until death in men and women.[60] Potential age-related metabolic consequences of reduced testosterone, DHEA, and

GH are outlined in Table 10.3. The reduction of these hormones increases a person's risk for developing metabolic syndrome. Metabolic syndrome is a group of conditions that increase a person's risk for coronary heart disease, diabetes, and stroke.[112] Metabolic syndrome is also called insulin resistance syndrome.

On the positive side, lifestyle modifications can impact hormone production in aging.[68] While the level of physical activity often declines with retirement, that does not have to be the norm. Participation in a robust leisure activity or taking up a new sport such as pickle ball may provide sufficient exercise to counteract age-related changes in not only the endocrine system but also all the body systems impacted by hormones. Exercise and calorie restriction (CR) appear to be the most effective and modifiable lifestyle factors that result in health benefits during aging.[68] Both interventions can assist in maintaining muscle mass and preventing fat accumulation. Regular physical exercise involving aerobic and resistive training can positively influence hormone production in older adults.

INTEGUMENTARY SYSTEM

The integumentary system consists of skin, which makes up 15% of the body's weight and by area is the largest organ of the body, as well as hair, nails, and glands. The skin is made up of three layers: the epidermis, the dermis, and the hypodermis (also called subcutaneous tissue) (Fig. 10.3).

The outermost layer, the epidermis, is further divided into four sublayers—the stratum corneum, stratum granulosum, stratum spinosum, and stratum basalis—and four major cell types—keratinocytes, melanocytes, Langerhans cells, and Merkel cells.[4,72,113] The stratum corneum provides protection from injury and a barrier from loss of fluid and electrolytes. Keratinocytes produce keratin, a skin protein, which makes skin stronger and waterproof.[113] Melanocytes provide pigmentation to the skin by producing melanin, which helps protect the skin from ultraviolet (UV) light exposure.[113] Langerhans cells are involved in immune responses and antigen presentation. Merkel cells or disks respond to pressure (see Fig. 9.1). The epidermis has no blood supply of its own and depends on the dermis for nutrition. The epidermal-dermal junction, the border between the epidermis and dermis, is known as the basement membrane. Below this

membrane. The ducts of the eccrine sweat glands project to the skin surface through the epidermis.[112]

The dermis, provides nutrition, structural support, and circulation to the skin.[114] It also houses eccrine sweat glands which secrete water and electrolytes important to thermoregulation. In addition to sweat production, these glands also produce antimicrobials and are rich in stem cells. Eccrine sweat glands contribute to the immune response in the skin and function in repair of the epidermis after injury. They also provide a moisturizing layer at the skin surface to maintain skin hydration.[114,115]

The dermis provides tensile strength to the skin and provides support for the epidermis. It is composed of two layers, the papillary and reticular layers.[116,117] The papillary layer contains capillaries and nerves that nourish the epidermis. The reticular layer is made up of strong connective tissues containing collagen and elastic fibers primarily from fibroblasts, giving the dermis strength.[116] Structures within the dermis provide phagocytosis of foreign substances (macrophages) and histamine reaction for inflammatory response (mast cells). The dermis also contains a rich network of blood and lymph vessels, hair follicles, and sweat glands. In addition to eccrine sweat glands the dermis houses apocrine sweat glands. Apocrine sweat glands, which do not participate in thermoregulation, originate from hair follicles and secrete a milky, protein-rich sweat in response to stimuli such as stress and fear. They are found in the axilla and groin.[114,116] Sensory receptors present in the dermis include Ruffini end organs (stretch receptors), Meissner corpuscles (movement receptors), and Pacinian corpuscles (vibration sense).[72,116] Nerve endings that perceive pain and temperature (types A and C) can also be found in the dermis, and free nerve endings (type C) can cross the dermal epidermal junction to reach the epidermis. Autonomic (sympathetic) nervous system innervation of the dermis also assists in regulation of body temperature by its effect on the blood/lymph vessels, hair cells, and sweat glands.[72]

The hypodermis is made up of adipose (fat) which stores energy, provides thermal insulation, and serves to absorb trauma. It helps adhere the skin to underlying fascia, muscle, and bone.[72,116] Immune cells can be found in the hypodermis, which is also a site where growth factors are produced.[4]

The major functions of the skin are sensory perception, thermoregulation, protection, cell fluid maintenance, and vitamin D synthesis.

TABLE 10.3 Potential Age-Related Metabolic Consequences of Reduced Testosterone, DHEA, and Growth Hormone		
Potential Age-Related Metabolic Consequences of		
Reduced Testosterone (Andropause)	**Reduced DHEA (Adrenopause)**	**Reduced Growth Hormone (Somatopause)**
• ↑ subcutaneous and visceral fat • ↑ risk for obesity • ↓ insulin sensitivity • ↑ risk for type 2 diabetes • ↑ high blood pressure • ↑ triglycerides • ↑ risk of metabolic syndrome • ↓ muscle mass • ↓ strength • ↓ bone density	• ↑ body fat mass • ↑ waist to hip ratio • ↓ lean body mass • ↓ VO$_2$ max • ↑ risk of cardiovascular disease • ↑ risk of ischemic heart disease • ↓ bone density	• ↑ risk for obesity • ↑ visceral adipose tissue • ↓ lean body mass • ↓ strength • ↑ risk of metabolic syndrome • ↑ risk of cardiovascular disease • ↓ bone density

Based on both human observational studies and rodent studies.
↑, Increased; ↓, decreased; *DHEA*, dehydroepiandrosterone.
From Pataky MW, Young WF, Nair S. Hormonal and metabolic changes of aging and the influence of lifestyle modifications [Table 1]. *Clin Proc.* 2021: 96:788–814.

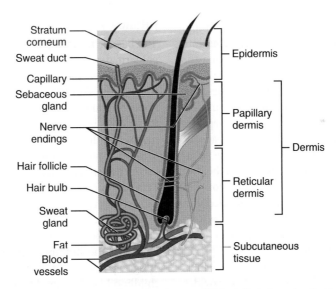

Fig. 10.3 Three layer structure of the skin. (From Goodman and Fuller's Pathology: Implications for the Physical Therapist, Fourth edition; Saunders, Elsevier).

Sensory Perception

The skin houses several sensory receptors, including mechanoreceptors, hair follicles, and free nerve endings. The mechanoreceptors include Meissner corpuscles (movement sensation and touch), Pacinian corpuscles (vibration), Ruffini endings (stretch), and Merkel cells (spatial imagery and touch).[4,116] Hair follicles perceive tactile stimulation, and free nerve endings sense noxious stimuli such as pain, itch, temperature, and touch.[4]

Thermoregulation

"Thermoregulatory mechanisms occurring in the skin include insulation, sweating, and control of blood flow."[117] Body heat is generated by organs deep in the body, such as the liver, heart, and brain, and in skeletal muscles during exercise. The skin and subcutaneous tissues, especially fat, act as insulation. Receptors in the skin detect temperature and send impulses to the hypothalamus to coordinate the ANS to control body temperature and maintain homeostasis. Sweat is produced by the eccrine sweat glands when the core temperature rises above 37°C. Fluid loss in sweat cools the body through evaporation via the sympathetic nervous system. Increased blood flow to the skin allows heat to be transferred from the core of the body to the skin surface where it can be dissipated by one of the four mechanisms: radiation (heat waves), conduction (to the air or to objects), convection (air currents), and evaporation (sweating).[88] Hair also assists with temperature regulation in that it traps air near the surface of the skin.[116]

Protection

The skin acts as a protective barrier across the life span beginning in utero. It provides a barrier between the external and internal environments. The barrier function both prevents foreign material from entering into the body through the skin and fluids from leaving the body and causing water loss.[4] The skin's immune functions include production of antimicrobial peptides, low pH (5.4–5.9), sweat production, and presence of several immune cells in the skin.[4] Antimicrobial peptides are produced by keratinocytes, sweat glands, sebaceous glands, and several other cells of the skin.[4] The sebaceous glands in the skin produce an oily film on the skin which contributes to both antimicrobial protection and prevention of fluid loss. Myeloid and lymphoid cells in the skin can also activate the body's immune system when necessary. Finally, hair prevents particles from entering the nose, ears, and eyes.[116]

Melanocytes, present in the epidermis, produce melanin, which is a photoprotective pigment that provides protection from ultraviolet light.[113] Keratin, produced in the epidermis, makes the skin stronger and waterproof, assisting in maintenance of hydration.[113] "Fitzpatrick skin phototype is a commonly used system to describe a person's skin type in terms of response to ultraviolet radiation (UVR) exposure."[118] There are six skin types: (1) pale white skin, (2) white skin, (3) light brown skin, (4) moderate brown skin, (5) dark brown skin, and (6) deeply pigmented dark brown to black skin. Photoaging, or the impact of exposure to UV radiation in sunlight,

varies in individuals based upon their skin type. UV light is less able to penetrate into the dermal layer of individuals with darker skin because of the protective effect of higher levels of melanin than that seen in light skin individuals. The dark epidermis of Black individuals approximates the protection of SPF 13.4 sunscreen.[119]

Vitamin D Synthesis

Vitamin D is synthesized when skin is exposed to UV light. It is essential for controlling the amount of phosphorus and calcium that is mobilized from the bone and absorbed through the small intestine. It regulates the proliferation and differentiation of keratinocytes and plays a role in fighting opportunistic infections.[120] The major natural source of vitamin D comes from the skin. When exposed to sunlight, cholesterol in the skin is converted to a vitamin D precursor, supporting vitamin D synthesis.[113] Many factors have been linked to low vitamin D ranging from skin type, gender, body mass index, physical activity, and alcohol intake.[121]

Infancy Through Adolescence

The barrier functions of the skin, as reflected by transepidermal water loss and stratum corneum thickness, develop over the first 4–5 years of life.[122,123] During infancy, the skin has more water content than in childhood or adulthood, but infants lose excess water faster than adults.[122] The infant skin's ability to moisturize and to produce lipid is also decreased compared to adults. This, in conjunction with the thinner stratus corneum, leaves infants and toddlers more susceptible to diaper rash and atopic dermatitis.[123] Bathing can damage the skin, so careful handling is required. Skin thickens during infancy and childhood as more subcutaneous fat is deposited. The amount of water in the skin decreases in childhood and the stratum corneum thickens to adult levels by age 4 years.[122] Skin surface moisture decreases through childhood, as measured by skin conductance, with skin hydration reaching adult values by age 5 years.[123]

Sweat gland development and function also develops in infancy and adolescence. Eccrine sweat glands, which play a major role in thermoregulation through evaporation, develop from 3–8 months gestation. By 2–3 years of age, children have developed the total number of sweat glands that will be formed.[124] These glands then grow in size as the body size increases, which also increases the amount of sweat that the gland can produce.[124] The small size of the sweat glands is thought to limit the amount of sweat production possible in children. Children sweat less during exercise than adolescents and adults, which may limit their ability to maintain thermoregulation through sweating and evaporation.[124,125] Children depend more on temperature regulation methods such as vasodilation and radiant heat loss between the skin and the air.[124,125] Because of these differences in thermoregulation ability between children and adults, children may become overheated when exercising in high-temperature climates.

The most noticeable skin changes in adolescence have to do with puberty. Androgenous hormone production of puberty activates sebaceous glands to produce more sebum, an oily moisturizer of the skin. Sebum production peaks in puberty and then slowly begins to decrease.[126] Eccrine sweat glands are stimulated to produce more sweat. Apocrine sweat glands also become active. With sweat production and oil gland production increased, skin problems of puberty such as excessive sweating and acne develop. The primary cause of acne is increased sebum production of the sebaceous glands. Acne affects 80% of individuals between 11 and 30 years of age and almost all teens and young adults, at least mildly.[126] Axillary and pubic hair growth is also seen as the adolescent develops secondary sexual characteristics.

Adulthood and Older Adulthood

The integumentary system continues to function as a protective barrier and maintains sensory, thermoregulatory, and other functions through adulthood. Alterations in skin structure and function begin to be seen by 60 years of age.[127] Because of decreases in estrogen levels, skin changes with aging become noticeable in women earlier than in men (Fig. 10.4).[128]

Structural and Functional Characteristics of Aging Skin

Both intrinsic and extrinsic factors influence skin aging. Both intrinsic and extrinsic factors can induce permanent senescence in skin cells, resulting from the shortening of telomeres, mitochondrial impairment, and upregulation of DNA damage response signaling, finally leading to the cell cycle arrest.[72,129–131] Intrinsic aging is determined by genetics and gender. Hormonal levels, race, and a decrease in antioxidant capacity are additional intrinsic factors that contribute to aging of all layers of the skin.[130,132] Cells are damaged due to a

buildup of by-products of cellular metabolism, reactive oxygen species (ROS), and inadequate cellular repair mechanisms because of a decrease in dermal mast cells, fibroblasts, and collagen.[113] Estrogen levels strongly influence skin aging in women. Extrinsic factors influencing skin aging include exposure to UV light (photoaging), cigarette smoke, environmental pollution, and trauma.[113,128,132,133] Stress and lack of sleep have also been identified as factors that influence skin aging.[130,133]

The number of layers of the skin remains the same with aging; however, changes in the structure and function of the epidermis, dermis, and hypodermis are seen. All layers of skin are affected by aging.[130] Common changes of the skin, such as wrinkle formation, dryness, increased pigmentation, and decreased firmness, are easily observable in older adults. The skin progressively thins at a rate of 6%–7% per decade over an adult's life time.[128]

Thinning of the epidermal layer occurs with aging.[130,133] The number of melanocytes and Langerhans cells in the epidermis also decreases,[113] with a loss of 6%–8% of melanocytes per decade after the age of 30 years.[72] The ability of the epidermis to proliferate new cells also diminishes by 50% between 20 and 70 years of age.[113,130] Thinning of the epidermis decreases the surface area of the epidermis. This thinning, with decreased dermal papillae and circulation and flattening of epidermal/dermal junction, diminishes effective nutrient and oxygen exchange to the epidermis.[72,113,128,130,133] The changes between the epidermal and dermal levels also make older skin less resistant to shearing forces.[128] Decreased function of keratinocytes and diminished ability of the epidermis to maintain its lipid content decrease the barrier function of the epidermis.[130] Decreased production of sebum by the sebaceous glands, sweat production, and decreased water content in the stratum corneum contribute to diminished ability of the epidermis to maintain water and lipid content, as well as decreasing protection from infection.[72,113,128] Other functional integumentary changes resulting from changes in the epidermis of older adults include dryness, increased healing time, and decreased ability to activate vitamin D production.[113,128] Wrinkles also develop as epidermal changes occur with age.[72,130] Because of racial differences in dermal thickness and lipid content, Asian and Black individuals experience less wrinkling than their White counterparts.[119,132] Loss of melanocytes contributes to pigment changes seen with aging.[72,128,130] Individuals with skin types III–VI (skin of color) are less susceptible to hypo- or hyperpigmentation with aging and often show signs of skin aging up to 10 years later than light skin individuals.[119]

Changes seen in the dermal layer include decreased number of cells, diminished vascularity, decreased collagen synthesis, and altered extracellular matrix.[128,130,132] Collagen, which contributes to the skin strength, decreases and becomes more disorganized with age.[113,128,133] Loss of fibroblasts with aging decreases the ability of the skin to maintain dermal extracellular matrix and collagen, which increases wrinkling and loss of elasticity.[113,128,134] Fibroblast loss also impacts the immune function of the integument with aging.[133] The number of mast cells in the dermis decreases by 50%, impacting immune function and blood flow decreases up to 60% diminishing the ability of the dermis to respond to injury or infection.[113] The diminished blood flow also lowers the effectiveness of integumentary

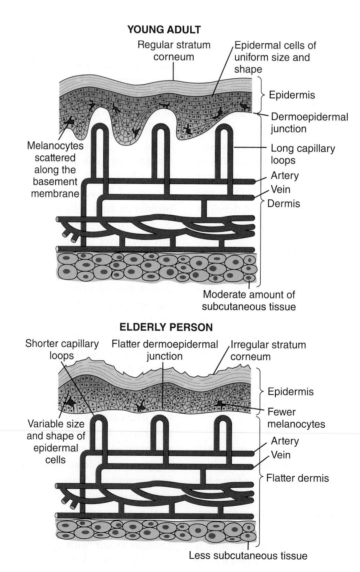

Fig. 10.4 Differences in skin structure between younger and older skin. (From Banasik, Jacquelyn L. Edition: Pathophysiology Seventh edition.)

thermoregulatory functions. As the dermis changes, torsional/tear injuries of the skin are more likely, skin becomes less elastic, and wrinkling is seen.[128,130,133] Dermal changes in collagen and extracellular matrix contribute to deep wrinkle formation of the skin.[72]

Changes in the hypodermis of older adults are primarily seen in fat atrophy and changes in subcutaneous fat distribution.[72,132] Functional implications of these changes are loss of shock absorption, resistance to trauma, and thermal insulation.[113]

Changes in Sensory Function of the Integument With Aging

Sensory function of the integument also decreases with aging, due to decreased function of sensory receptors in both the epidermis and dermis. Decreased sensitivity to touch has been identified in individuals over the age of 60 years.[127] Older adults are less able to detect light touch, vibration, texture, distance between two points and direction of movement, pain, and temperature.[113,127] Factors that contribute to these sensory changes include decreased number of nerve fibers in the epidermis and dermis; decreased nerve conduction velocity of sensory neurons; decrease in the number of Merkel cells and Meisner corpuscles; and an increase in size, with decreased axonal innervation of Pacinian corpuscles.[127]

SUMMARY

Hormones and their receptors are found in every tissue in the body. They maintain and regulate everyday functions: waking and sleep, metabolism, immunity, adaptation to stress through complicated networks called axes. The endocrine system coordinates its actions with the circadian rhythms of our bodies. Changes due to aging begin in middle adulthood and continue into older adulthood and are related to changes in hormone production, hormone effectiveness, and hormone receptor sensitivity. "Aging results in a decline in anabolic hormone production."[68] This decline when coupled with a habitual decline in physical activity can produce a cascade of aging changes from loss of muscle mass (sarcopenia), less energy expenditure, obesity, and insulin resistance to increased risk for type 2 diabetes, cardiovascular disease, hypertension and dementia.[68]

The integumentary system provides a protective covering for the body and carries out temperature regulation, immune functions, sensory perception and repair when damaged. Skin covers the entire body and is subject to intrinsic and extrinsic risk factors with aging.[139] Contrast and compare the soft smooth skin of an infant, the potential facial acne of an adolescent and the presence of wrinkles of the older adult. With aging the skin loses elasticity and its immune function may break down. All functions of the skin are affected by aging. Older adults are more suspectable to overheating and have some deficits in sensory discrimination. The older adult can also be at greater risk for skin tearing and skin breakdown from prolonged immobility.

REFERENCES

1. Serin Y, Acar Tek N. Effect of circadian rhythm on metabolic processes and the regulation of energy balance. *Ann Nutr Metab.* 2019;74(4):322–330. https://doi.org/10.1159/000500071.
2. Gnocchi D, Bruscalupi G. Circadian rhythms and hormonal homeostasis: pathophysiologic implications. *Biology (Basel).* 2017;6:10. https://doi.org/10.3390/biology6010010.
3. Richards J, Gumz ML. Advances in understanding the peripheral circadian clocks. *FASEB J.* 2012;26(9):3602–3613. https://doi.org/10.1096/fj.12-203554.
4. Nguyen AV, Soulika AM. The dynamics of the skin's immune system. *Int J Mol Sci.* 2019;20(8):1811. https://doi.org/10.3390/ijms20081811.
5. Scanes CG. *Pituitary Gland. Sturkie's Avian Physiology.* 6th ed. Milwaukee, WI: Academic Press; 2015.
6. Sheng JA, Bales NJ, Myers SA, et al. The hypothalamic-pituitary-adrenal axis: development, programming actions of hormones, and maternal-fetal interactions. *Front Behav Neurosci.* 2021;14:601939. https://doi.org/10.3389/fnbeh.2020.601939.
7. Borrow AP, Stover SA, Bales NJ, Handa RJ. Posterior pituitary hormones. In: Litwack G, ed. *Hormonal*

Signaling in Biology and Medicine: Comprehensive Modern Endocrinology. Cambridge: Academic Press; 2019: 203–226.

8. Shahid Z, Asuka E, Singh G. *Physiology, Hypothalamus. StatPearls [Internet].* Treasure Island (FL): StatPearls Publishing; 2022. PMID: 30571001.

9. Brady B. Thyroid gland: overview. 2019. www.endocrineweb.com/conditions/thyroid-nodules/thyroid-gland-controls-bodys-metabolism-how-it-works-symptoms-hyperthyroi. Accessed April 29, 2022.

10. Khan M, Jose A, Sharma S. *Physiology, Parathyroid Hormone. [Updated 2022 Jun 28]. StatPearls [Internet].* Treasure Island (FL): StatPearls Publishing; 2022 Jan.

11. Goodman CC, Pariser G. The endocrine and metabolic systems. In: Kellogg CCC, Fuller KS, eds. *Goodman and Fuller's Pathology: Implications for the Physical Therapist.* 5th ed. Elsevier; 2021.

12. Gao X, Yamazaki Y, Tezuka Y, et al. Gender differences in human adrenal cortex and its disorders. *Mol Cell Endocrinol.* 2021;526:111177. https://doi.org/10.1016/j.mce.2021.111177.

13. Tezuka Y, Atsumi N, Blinder AR, et al. The age-dependent changes of the human adrenal cortical zones are not congruent. *J Clin Endocrinol Metab.* 2021;106:1389–1397. https://doi.org/10.1210/clinem/dgab007.

14. Sargis R.M. Overview of the pancreas. https://www.endocrineweb.com/endocrinology/overview-pancreas 2015 Accessed April 29, 2022.

15. Xavier GdS. The cells of the islets of Langerhans. *J Clin Med.* 2018;7:54. https://doi.org/10.3390/jcm7030054.

16. Tan TM, Bloom SR. *Pancreatic Polypeptide.* 2nd ed. Cambridge, MA: Academic Press; 2013.

17. Rindi G, Savio A, Torsello A, et al. Ghrelin expression in gut endocrine growths. *Histochem Cell Biol.* 2002;117:521–525. https://doi.org/10.1007/s00418-002-0416-0.

18. Thapa P, Farber DL. The role of the thymus in the immune response. *Thorac Surg Clin.* 2019;29:123–131. https://doi.org/10.1016/j.thorsurg.2018.12.001.

19. DeMorrow S. Role of the hypothalamic-pituitary-adrenal axis in health and disease. *Int J Mol Sci.* 2018;19(4):986. https://doi.org/10.3390/ijms19040986.

20. Parra-Montes de Oca MA, Sotelo-Rivera I, Gutiérrez-Mata A, et al. Sex dimorphic responses of the hypothalamus-pituitary-thyroid axis to energy demands and stress. *Front Endocrinol (Lausanne).* 2021;12:746924. https://doi.org/10.3389/fendo.2021.746924.

21. Benyi E, Sävendahl L. The physiology of childhood growth: hormonal regulation. *Horm Res Paediatr.* 2017;88:6–14. https://doi.org/10.1159/000471876.

22. van den Beld AW, Kaufman JM, Zillikens MC, Lamberts SWJ, Egan JM, van der Lely AJ. The physiology of endocrine systems with ageing. *Lancet Diabetes Endocrinol.* 2018;6:647–658. https://doi.org/10.1016/S2213-8587(18)30026-3.

23. Carlson DM. *Human Embryology & Developmental Biology.* 6th ed. Philadelphia: Elsevier; 2019.

24. Moore LK, Persaud TVN, Torchia MG. Pharyngeal apparatus, face, and neck. In: Moore KL, Persaud TVN, Torchia MG, eds. *Before We Are Born: Essential of Embryology and Birth Defects.* 10th ed. Philadelphia: Elsevier; 2020:91–116.e1.

25. Sinclair D, Dangerfield P. *Human Growth After Birth.* 6th ed. New York: Oxford University Press; 1998.

26. Verhaeghe J, Van Bree R, Van Herck E, Laureys J, Bouillon R, Van Assche FA. C-peptide, insulin-like growth factors I and II, and insulin-like growth factor binding protein-1 in umbilical cord serum: correlations with birth weight. *Am J Obstet Gynecol.* 1993;169:89–97. https://doi.org/10.1016/0002-9378(93)90137-8.

27. Koistinen HA, Koivisto VA, Andersson S, et al. Leptin concentration in cord blood correlates with intrauterine growth. *J Clin Endocrinol Metab.* 1997;82(10):3328–3330. https://doi.org/10.1210/jcem.82.10.4291.

28. Costa MA. The endocrine function of human placenta: an overview. *Reprod Biomed Online.* 2016;32(1):14–43. https://doi.org/10.1016/j.rbmo.2015.10.005.

29. Cetin I, Alvino G. Intrauterine growth restriction: implications for placental metabolism and transport. *A review. Placenta.* 2009;30(Suppl A):S77–S82. https://doi.org/10.1016/j.placenta.2008.12.006.

30. Haynes BF, Sempowski GD, Wells AF, Hale LP. The human thymus during aging. *Immunol Res.* 2000;22(2-3):253–261. https://doi.org/10.1385/IR:22:2-3:253.

31. Eng L, Lam L. Thyroid function during the fetal and neonatal periods. *Neoreviews.* 2020;21:e30–e36. https://doi.org/10.1542/neo.21-1-e30.

32. Klosinska M, Kaczynska A, Ben-Skowronek I. Congenital hypothyroidism in preterm newborns—the changes of diagnostics and treatment: a review. *Front Endocrinol.* 2022;13:860862. https://doi.org/10.3389/fendo.2022.860862.

33. Bernal J. Thyroid hormone regulated genes in cerebral cortex development. *J Endocrinol.* 2017;232(2):R83–R97. https://doi.org/10.1530/JOE-16-0424.

34. Forhead AJ, Fowden AL. Thyroid hormones in fetal growth and prepartum maturation. *J Endocrinol.* 2014;221:R87–R103. https://doi.org/10.1530/JOE-14-0025.

35. Moog NK, Entringer S, Heim C, et al. Influence of maternal thyroid hormones during gestation on fetal brain development. *Neuroscience.* 2017;342:68–100. https://doi.org/10.1016/j.neuroscience.2015.09.070.

36. Kratzsch J, Pulzer F. Thyroid gland development and defects. *Best Pract Res Clin Endocrinol Metab.* 2008;22(1):57–75.

37. Murray PG, Clayton PE. Endocrine control of growth. *Am J Med Genet C Semin Med Genet.* 2013;163C(2): 76–85. https://doi.org/10.1002/ajmg.c.31357.

38. Zhang F, He Q, Tsang WP, Garvey WT, Chan WY, Wan C. Insulin exerts direct, IGF-1 independent actions in growth plate chondrocytes. *Bone Res.* 2014;2:14012. https://doi.org/10.1038/boneres.2014.12.

39. Schwarzenberg SJ, Georgieff MK. Committee on Nutrition. Advocacy for improving nutrition in the first 1000 days to support childhood development and adult health. *Pediatrics.* 2018;141(2):e20173716. https://doi.org/10.1542/peds.2017-3716.

40. Mameli C, Mazzantini S, Zuccotti GV. Nutrition in the first 1000 days: the origin of childhood obesity. *Int J Environ Res Public Health.* 2016;23;13(9):838. https://doi.org/10.3390/ijerph13090838.

41. Matonti L, Blasetti A, Chiarelli F. Nutrition and growth in children. *Minerva Pediatr.* 2020;72(6):462–471. https://doi.org/10.23736/S0026-4946.20.05981-2.

42. Russel G, Lightman S. The human stress response. *Nat Rev Endocrinol.* 2019;15:525–534. https://doi.org/10.1038/s41574-019-0228-0.

43. Karr JL, Brinton JT, Crume T, Hamman RF, Glueck DH, Dabelea D. Leptin levels at birth and infant growth: the EPOCH study. *J Dev Orig Health Dis.* 2014;5:214–218. https://doi.org/10.1017/S204017441400021X.

44. Mantzoros CS, Rifas-Shiman SL, Williams CJ, Fargnoli JL, Kelesidis T, Gillman MW. Cord blood leptin and adiponectin as predictors of adiposity in children at 3 years of age: a prospective cohort study. *Pediatrics.* 2009;123:682–689. https://doi.org/10.1542/peds.2008-0343.

45. Kadakia R, Zheng Y, Zhang Z, Zhang W, Josefson JL, Hou L. Association of cord blood methylation with neonatal leptin: an epigenome wide association study. *PLoS One.* 2019;14(12):e0226555. https://doi.org/10.1371/journal.pone.0226555.

46. Bernstock JD, Totten AH, Elkahloun AG, Johnson KR, Hurst AC, Goldman F, Groves AK, Mikhail FM, Atkinson TP. Recurrent microdeletions at chromosome 2p11.2 are associated with thymic hypoplasia and features resembling DiGeorge syndrome. *J Allergy Clin Immunol.* 2020;145(1):358–367.e2. https://doi.org/10.1016/j.jaci.2019.09.020.

47. Chinn IK, Blackburn CC, Manley NR, Sempowski GD. Changes in primary lymphoid organs with aging. *Semin Immunol.* 2012;24:309–320. https://doi.org/10.1016/j.smim.2012.04.005.

48. Walsh JP. Thyroid function across the lifespan: do age-related changes matter? *Endocrinol Metab (Seoul).* 2022;37(2):208–219. https://doi.org/10.3803/EnM.2022.1463.

49. Stagi S, Cavalli L, Ricci S, Mola M, Marchi C, Seminara S, Brandi ML, de Martino M. Parathyroid

50. hormone levels in healthy children and adolescents. *Horm Res Paediatr.* 2015;84(2):124–129. https://doi.org/10.1159/000432399.

50. Vucic S, Korevaar TIM, Dham B, et al. Thyroid function during early life and dental development. *J Dent Res.* 2017;96(9):1020–1026. https://doi.org/10.1177/0022034517708551.

51. Leitch VD, Bassett JHD, Williams GR. Role of thyroid hormones in craniofacial development. *Nat Rev Endocrinol.* 2020;16(3):147–164. https://doi.org/10.1038/s41574-019-0304-5.

52. Jourieh A, Khan H, Mheissen S, Assali M, Alam MK. The correlation between dental stages and skeletal maturity stages. *Biomed Res Int.* 2021;9:9986498. https://doi.org/10.1155/2021/9986498.

53. Abreu AP, Kaiser UB. Pubertal development and regulation. *Lancet Diabetes Endocrinol.* 2016;4:254–264. https://doi.org/10.1016/S2213-8587(15)00418-0.

54. Martinez GM. Trends and patterns in menarche in the United States: 1995 through 2013-2017. Nat Health Stat Rep. 146: September 10, 2020. ww.cdc.gov/nchs/data/nhsr/nhsr146-508.pdf. Accessed July 15, 2022.

55. Calcaterra V, Ccna H, Rcgalbuto C, Vinci F, Porri D, Verduci E, Chiara M, Zuccotti GV. The role of fetal, infant, and childhood nutrition in the timing of sexual maturation. *Nutrients.* 2021;13:419. https://doi.org/10.3390/nu13020419.

56. Colich NL, Platt JM, Keyes KM, Sumner JA, Allen NB, McLaughlin KA. Earlier age at menarche as a transdiagnostic mechanism linking childhood trauma with multiple forms of psychopathology in adolescent girls. *Psychol Med.* 2020;50(7):1090–1098. https://doi.org/10.1017/S0033291719000953.

57. Calthorpe L, Brage S, Ong KK. Systematic review and meta-analysis of the association between childhood physical activity and age at menarche. *Acta Paediatr.* 2019;108(6):1008–1015. https://doi.org/10.1111/apa.14711.

58. Olarescu NC, Gunawardane K, Hansen TK, Møller N, Jørgensen JOL. Normal physiology of growth hormone in adults. 2019 Oct 16. In: Feingold KR, Anawalt B, Boyce A, et al., eds. *Endotext [Internet].* South Dartmouth (MA): MDText.com, Inc.; 2000.

59. Vahl N, Jorgensen JO, Jurik AG, Christiansen JS. Abdominal adiposity and physical fitness are major determinants of the age associated decline in stimulated GH secretion in healthy adults. *J Clin Endocrinol Metab.* 1996;81(6):2209–2215. https://doi.org/10.1210/jcem.81.6.8964853.

60. Corpas E, Harman SM, Blackman MR. Human growth hormone and human aging. *Endocr Rev.* 1993;14:20–39. https://doi.org/10.1210/edrv-14-1-20.

61. Matsuda Y. Age-related pathological changes in the pancreas. *Front Biosci (Elite Ed).* 2018;10:137–142.

https://doi.org/10.2741/e813. PMID: 28930609.McEwen BS. Redefining neuroendocrinology: epigenetics of brain-body communication over the life course. *Front Neuroendocrinol*. 2010, 19.0 30. doi: 10.1016/j.yfrne.2017.11.001.

62. McEwen BS. Redefining neuroendocrinology: epigenetics of brain-body communication over the life course. *Front Neuroendocrinol*. 2018;49:8–30. https://doi.org/10.1016/j.yfrne.2017.11.001.2018.

63. Thome JJ, Grinshpun B, Kumar BV, et al. Longterm maintenance of human naive T cells through in situ homeostasis in lymphoid tissue sites. *Sci Immunol*. 2016;1:eaah6506. https://doi.org/10.1126/sciimmunol.aah6506.

64. Hu C, Zhang K, Jiang F, Wang H, Shao Q. Epigenetic modifications in thymic epithelial cells: an evolutionary perspective for thymus atrophy. *Clin Epigenetics*. 2021;13(1):210. https://doi.org/10.1186/s13148-021-01197-0.

65. Surks MI, Hollowell JG. Age-specific distribution of serum thyrotropin and antithyroid antibodies in the US population: implications for the prevalence of subclinical hypothyroidism. *J Clin Endocrinol Metab*. 2007;92:575–4582.

66. Bremner AP, Feddema P, Leedman PJ, et al. Age-related changes in thyroid function: a longitudinal study of a community-based cohort. *J Clin Endocrinol Metab*. 2012;97(5):1554–1562. https://doi.org/10.1210/jc.2011-3020.

67. Lamberts SW, Van den Beld AW, Van Der Lely A-J. The endocrinology of aging. *Science*. 1997;278:419–424.

68. Pataky MW, Young WF, Nair S. Hormonal and metabolic changes of aging and the influence of lifestyle modifications. *May Clin Proc*. 2021;96:788–814. https://doi.org/10.1016/j.mayocp.2020.07.033.

69. Turcu AF, Rege J, Auchus RJ, Rainey WE. 11-Oxygenated androgens in health and disease. *Nat Rev Endocrinol*. 2020;16:284–296. https://doi.org/10.1038/s41574-020-0336-x.

70. Feldman HA, Longcope C, Derby CA, et al. Age trends in the level of serum testosterone and other hormones in middle-aged men: longitudinal results from the Massachusetts male aging study. *J Clin Endocrinol Metab*. 2002;87:589–598. https://doi.org/10.1210/jcem.87.2.8201.

71. Rainey WE, Carr BR, Sasano H, Suzuki T, Mason JI. Dissecting human adrenal androgen production. *Trends Endocrinol Metab*. 2002;13:234–239. https://doi.org/10.1016/s1043-2760(02)00609-4.

72. Bonte F., Girard D., Archambault J.C., Desmouliere A., 2019. Ch 10: Skin changes during aging. In Harris JR and Korolchuk VI (eds). Biochemistry and cell biology of aging. Part II: clinical science, Subcellular biochemistry 91, doi.10.10007/978-981-13-3681-2_10. Pp 249-280.

73. Wilkinson HN, Hardman MJ. The role of estrogen in cutaneous ageing and repair. *Maturitas*. 2017;103:60–64. https://doi.org/10.1016/j.maturitas.2017.06.026.

74. Stuenkel CA, Davis SR, Gompel A, et al. Treatment of symptoms of the menopause: an Endocrine Society clinical practice guideline. *J Clin Endocrinol Metab*. 2015;100(11):3975–4011. https://doi.org/10.1210/jc.2015-2236.

75. Cobin RH, Goodman NF. AACE Reproductive Endocrinology Scientific Committee. American Association of Clinical Endocrinologists and American College of Endocrinology position statement on menopause-2017 update. *Endocr Pract*. 2017;23(7):869–880. https://doi.org/10.4158/EP171828.PS. Erratum in: *Endocr Pract*. 2017; 23(12):1488.

76. "The 2022 Hormone Therapy Position Statement of The North American Menopause Society" Advisory Panel. The 2022 hormone therapy position statement of The North American Menopause Society. Menopause. *Menopause*. 2022;29:767–794.

77. Abou-Ismail MY, Citla Sridhar D, Nayak L. Estrogen and thrombosis: a bench to bedside review. *Thromb Res*. 2020;192:40–51. https://doi.org/10.1016/j.thromres.2020.05.008.

78. Martelli M, Zingaretti L, Salvio G, Bracci M, Santarelli L. Influence of work on andropause and menopause: a systematic review. *Int. J Environ Res Public Health*. 2021;18:10074. https://doi.org/10.3390/ijerph181910074.

79. Snyder PJ, Bhasin S, Cunningham GR, et al. Effects of testosterone treatment in older men. *New Engl J Med*. 2016;374:611–624. https://doi.org/10.1056/NEJMoa1506119.

80. Boardman HM, Hartley L, Eisinga A, et al. Hormone therapy for preventing cardiovascular disease in post-menopausal women. *Cochrane Database Syst Rev*. 2015;10(3):CD002229. https://doi.org/10.1002/14651858.CD002229.pub4.

81. Women's Health Initiative. National Heart, Lung and Blood Institute of National Institute of Health. www.whi.org. Accessed August 14, 2022.

82. Davidson MB. The effect of aging on carbohydrate metabolism: a review of the English literature and a practical approach to the diagnosis of diabetes mellitus in the elderly. *Metabolism*. 1979;28:688–705. https://doi.org/10.1016/0026-0495(79)90024-6.

83. Johansson J-O, Fowelin J, Landin K, Lager I, Bengtsson B-Å. Growth hormone-deficient adults are insulin-resistant. *Metabolism*. 1995;44:1126–1129. https://doi.org/10.1016/0026-0495(95)90004-7.

84. Basu R, Dalla Man C, Campioni M, et al. Effects of age and sex on postprandial glucose metabolism: differences in glucose turnover, insulin secretion, insulin action,

and hepatic insulin extraction. *Diabetes*. 2006;55:2001–2014. https://doi.org/10.2337/db05-1692.

85. Meneilly GS, Veldhuis JD, Elahi D. Disruption of the pulsatile and entropic modes of insulin release during an unvarying glucose stimulus in elderly individuals. *J Clin Endocrinol Metab*. 1999;84:1938–1943. https://doi.org/10.1210/jcem.84.6.5753.

86. Lanza IR, Short DK, Short KR, et al. Endurance exercise as a countermeasure for aging. *Diabetes*. 2008;57:2933–2942. https://doi.org/10.2337/db08-0349.

87. Robinson MM, Dasari S, Konopka AR, et al. Enhanced protein translation underlies improved metabolic and physical adaptations to different exercise training modes in young and old humans. *Cell Metab*. 2017;25:581–592. https://doi.org/10.1016/j.cmet.2017.02.009.

88. Hall JE, Hall ME. *Guyton and Hall Textbook of Medical Physiology*. 14th ed. Philadelphia: Elsevier; 2020.

89. Jacob G, Robertson D, Mosqueda-Garcia R, Ertl AC, Robertson RM, Biaggioni I. Hypovolemia in syncope and orthostatic intolerance role of the renin-angiotensin system. *Am J Med*. 1997 Aug;103(2):128–133. https://doi.org/10.1016/s0002-9343(97)00133-2.

90. Cowen LE, Hodak SP, Verbalis JG. Age-associated abnormalities of water homeostasis. *Endocrinol Metab Clin North Am*. 2013;42(2):349–370. https://doi.org/10.1016/j.ecl.2013.02.005.

91. Koch CA, Fulop T. Clinical aspects of changes in water and sodium homeostasis in the elderly. *Rev Endocr Metab Disord*. 2017;18(1):49–66. https://doi.org/10.1007/s11154-017-9420-5.

92. Tamma G, Goswami N, Reichmuth J, De Santo NG. Valenti G. Aquaporins, vasopressin, and aging: current perspectives. *Endocrinology*. 2015;156(3):777–788. https://doi.org/10.1210/en.2014-1812.

93. Roberts L, McCahon D, Johnson O, Haque MS, Parle J, Hobbs FR. Stability of thyroid function in older adults: the Birmingham Elderly Thyroid Study. *Br J Gen Pract*. 2018;68(675):e718–e726. https://doi.org/10.3399/bjgp18X698861.

94. Razvi S, Shakoor A, Vanderpump M, Weaver JU, Pearce SH. The influence of age on the relationship between subclinical hypothyroidism and ischemic heart disease: a metaanalysis. *J Clin Endocrinol Metab*. 2008;93(8):2998–3007. https://doi.org/10.1210/jc.2008-0167.

95. Biondi B, Cappola AR, Cooper DS. Subclinical hypothyroidism: a review. *JAMA*. 2019;322:153–160.

96. Gietka-Czernel M. The thyroid gland in postmenopausal women: physiology and diseases. *Prz Menopauzalny*. 2017;16(2):33–37. https://doi.org/10.5114/pm.2017.68588.

97. Nygaard B. Hypothyroidism (primary). *BMJ Clin Evid*. 2014;21(2014):0605.

98. Stott DJ, Rodondi N, Kearney PM, et al. Thyroid hormone therapy for older adults with subclinical hypothyroidism TRUST Study Group. *N Engl J Med*. 2017;29; 376(26):2534–2544. https://doi.org/10.1056/NEJMoa1603825.

99. Garber JR, Cobin RH, Gharib H, et al. American Association of Clinical Endocrinologists and American Thyroid Association Taskforce on Hypothyroidism in Adults. Clinical practice guidelines for hypothyroidism in adults: cosponsored by the American Association of Clinical Endocrinologists and the American Thyroid Association. *Endocr Pract*. 2012;18(6):988–1028. https://doi.org/10.4158/EP12280.GL.

100. Thayakaran R, Adderley NJ, Sainsbury C, et al. Thyroid replacement therapy, thyroid stimulating hormone concentrations, and long term health outcomes in patients with hypothyroidism: longitudinal study. *BMJ*. 2019;366:l4892. https://doi.org/10.1136/bmj.l4892.

101. Murthy L, Dreyer P, Suriyaarachchi P, et al. Association between high levels of parathyroid hormone and frailty: The Nepean Osteoporosis and Frailty (NOF) Study. J Frailty. *Aging*. 2018;7(4):253–257. https://doi.org/10.14283/10.14283/jfa.2018.22.

102. Bird ML, El Haber N, Batchelor F, Hill K, Wark JD. Vitamin D and parathyroid hormone are associated with gait instability and poor balance performance in mid-age to older aged women. *Gait Posture*. 2018;59:71–75. https://doi.org/10.1016/j.gaitpost.2017.09.036.

103. Murthy L, Duque G. Parathyroid hormone levels and aging: effect on balance. *Vitam Horm*. 2021;115:173–184. https://doi.org/10.1016/bs.vh.2020.12.009.

104. Mitchell WA, Lang PO, Aspinall R. Tracing thymic output in older individuals. *Clin Exp Immunol*. 2010;161(3):497–503. https://doi.org/10.1111/j.1365-2249.2010.04209.x.

105. Thomas R, Wang W, Su DM. Contributions of age-related thymic involution to immunosenescence and inflammaging. *Immun Ageing*. 2020;17:2. https://doi.org/10.1186/s12979-020-0173-8.

106. Pawelec G. Age and immunity: What is "immunosenescence"? *Exp Gerontol*. 2018;105:4–9. https://doi.org/10.1016/j.exger.2017.10.024.

107. Buckley TM, Schatzberg AF. Aging and the role of the HPA axis and rhythm in sleep and memory-consolidation. *Am J Geriatr Psychiatry*. 2005;13(5):344–352. https://doi.org/10.1176/appi.ajgp.13.5.344.

108. O'Brien JT, Schweitzer I, Ames D, Tuckwell V, Mastwyk M. Cortisol suppression by dexamethasone in the healthy elderly: effects of age, dexamethasone levels, and cognitive function. *Biol Psychiatry*. 1994;36(6):389–394. https://doi.org/10.1016/0006-3223(94)91214-9.

109. Roh E, Song DK, Kim MS. Emerging role of the brain in the homeostatic regulation of energy and glucose metabolism. *Exp Mol Med*. 2016;11;48(3):e216. https://doi.org/10.1038/emm.2016.4.

110. Bentourkia M, Bol A, Ivanoiu A, et al. Comparison of regional cerebral blood flow and glucose metabolism in the normal brain: effect of aging. *J Neurol Sci*. 2000;1;181(1-2):19–28. https://doi.org/10.1016/s0022-510x(00)00396-8.

111. Obradovic M, Sudar-Milovanovic E, Soskic S, et al. Leptin and obesity: role and clinical implication. *Front Endocrinol (Lausanne)*. 2021;12:585887. https://doi.org/10.3389/fendo.2021.585887.

112. National Heart, Lund and Blood Institute, National Institute of Health. Metabolic syndrome. What is metabolic syndrome? www.nhlbi.nih.gov/health/metabolic-syndrome Accessed August 9, 2022

113. Nigam Y, Knight J. Anatomy and physiology of aging 11: the skin. *Nursing Times*. 2017;113(12):51–55.

114. Lin Y, Chen L, Zhang M, et al. Eccrine sweat gland and its regeneration: current status and future directions2021. *Front Cell Dev Biology*. 2021;9:667765. https://doi.org/10.3389/fcell.2021.667765.

115. Cui CY, Schlessinger D. Eccrine sweat gland development and sweat secretion. *Exp Dermatol*. 2015;24(9):644–650. https://doi.org/10.1111/exd.12773.

116. Kim JY, Dao H. *Physiology, Integument*. In *Stats Pearls (Internet)*. Treasure Island (FL): Stats Pearls publishing; 2022. Available from www.ncbi.nlm.nih.gov/books/NBK554386? Accessed June 18, 2022.

117. McLafferty E, Hendry C, Alistair F. The integumentary system: anatomy, physiology and function of skin. *Nurs Stand*. 2012;27(3):35–42. https://doi.org/10.7748/ns2012.10.27.7.35.c9358.

118. Australian Radiation Protection and Nuclear Safety Agency www.arpansa.gov.au/sites/default/files/legacy/pubs/RadiationProtection/FitzpatrickSkintype.pdf Accessed May 24, 2022.

119. Vashi NA, de Castro Maymone MB, Kundu RV. Aging differences in ethnic skin. *J Clin Aesthet Dermatol*. 2016;9:31–38.

120. Bergqvist C, Ezzedine K. Vitamin D and the skin: what should a dermatologist know? *G Ital Dermatol Venereol*. 2019;154(6):669–680. https://doi.org/10.23736/S0392-0488.19.06433-2.

121. Kechichian E, Ezzedine K. Vitamin D and the skin: An update for dermatologists. *Am J Clin Dermatol*. 2018;19(2):L223–L235. https://doi.org/10.1007/s40257-017-0323-8.

122. Walters RM, Khanna P, Chu M, Merck MC. Developmental changes in skin barrier and structure during the first 5 years of life. *Skin Pharmaco/Physiol*. 2016;29:111–118. https://doi.org/10.1159/000444805.

123. Kong F, Galzote C, Duan Y. Changes in skin properties over the first 10 years of life: a cross-sectional study. *Arch Dermatol Res*. 2017;309:653–658. https://doi.org/10.1007/s00403-017-1764-x

124. Gomes LH, Carneiro-Júnior MA, Marins JCB. Thermoregulatory responses of children exercising in a hot environment. *Rev Paul Pediatr*. 2013;31(1):104–110. https://doi.org/10.1590/s0103-05822013000100017.

125. Arlegui L, Smallcombe JW, Fournet D, Tolfrey K, Havenith G. Body mapping of sweating patterns in pre-pubertal children during intermittent exercise in a warm environment. *Eur J Appl Physiol*. 2021;121(12):3561–3576. https://doi.org/10.1007/s00421-021-04811-4.

126. Bergler-Czop B, Brzezinska-Wcislo L. Dermatological problems of the puberty. *Postep Derm Alergol*. 2013;3:178–187. https://doi.org/10.5114/pdia.2013.35621.

127. McIntyre S, Nagi SS, McGlone FM, Olausson H. The effects of aging on tactile function in humans. *Neuroscience*. 2021;464:53–58. https://doi.org/10.1016/j.neuroscience.2021.02.015.35-42.

128. Farage MA, Miller KW, Elsner P, Maibach HI. Characteristics of the aging skin. *Adv Wound Care (New Rochelle)*. 2013;2(1):5–10. https://doi.org/10.1089/wound.2011.0356.

129. Birch-Machin MA, Tindall M, Turner R, Haldane F, Rees JL. Mitochondrial DNA deletions in human skin reflect photo rather than chronologic aging. *J Invest Dermatol*. 1998;110:149–152. https://doi.org/10.1046/j.1523-1747.1998.00099.x.

130. Csekes E, Račková L. Skin aging, cellular senescence and natural polyphenols2021. *Int J Med Sci*. 2021;22:12641. https://doi.org/10.3390/ijms222313641.

131. Harley CB, Futcher AB, Greider CW. Telomeres shorten during ageing of human fibroblasts. *Nature*. 1990;345:458–460.

132. Venkatesh S, Maymone MBC, Vashi NA. Aging in skin of color. *Clin Dermatol*. 2019;37:351–357. https://doi.org/10.1016/j.clindermatol.2019.04.010.

133. Russell-Goldman E, Murphy GF. The pathobiology of skin aging. *Am Journal of Pathology*. 2020;190(7):1356–1369. https://doi.org/10.1016/j.ajpath.2020.03,007.

134. Wang AS, Dreesen O. Biomarkers of cellular senescence and skin aging. *Front Genet*. 2018;9:247. https://doi.org/10.3389/fgene.2018.00247. 9, 247.

135. Anawalt BD, Merriam GR. Neuroendocrine aging in men: andropause and somatopause. *Endocrin Metab Clin North Am*. 2001;30:647–669. https://doi.org/10.1016/s0889-8529(05)70206-1.

136. Biondi B, Cooper DS. The clinical significance of subclinical thyroid dysfunction. *Endocr Rev*. 2008;29(1):76–131. https://doi.org/10.1210/er.2006-0043.

137. Szoke E, Shrayyef MZ, Messing S, et al. Effect of aging on glucose homeostasis: accelerated deterioration of beta-cell function in individuals with impaired glucose tolerance. *Diabetes Care*. 2008;31(3):539–543. https://doi.org/10.2337/dc07-1443.

138. Wilson SA, Stem LA, Bruehlman RD. Hypothyroidism: diagnosis and treatment. *Am Fam Physician*. 2021;15;103(10):605–613. PMID: 33983002.

139. Wong QYA, Chew FT. Defining skin aging and its risk factors: a systematic review and meta analysis. *Sci Rep*. 2021;11:22075. https://doi.org/10.1038/s41598-021-01573-z.

11

Posture, Balance, and Locomotion

Timothy Hanke,* PhD, PT

OBJECTIVES

After studying this chapter, the reader will be able to:
1. Define posture and balance.
2. Differentiate between static and dynamic balance.
3. Differentiate types of postural control: steady-state, reactive, anticipatory, and adaptive.
4. Describe locomotor patterns, especially gait.
5. Understand theoretical approaches to the study of posture, balance, and locomotion.
6. Describe posture, balance, and locomotion changes across the life span.

Posture is defined as the attitude or position of the body.[1] As such, being in a prone position and in a sitting position are both postures. When talking about someone's posture, most of us think of the alignment of body segments with respect to each other as well as with respect to the outside world. Posture has three functions. First, posture functions to maintain alignment of the body's segments in any position: supine, prone, sitting, quadruped, and standing. Second, posture as a position can function to anticipate change to allow the body to engage in voluntary, goal-directed movements. When reaching or stepping, the body may make postural adjustments before, during, and after a movement. Third, posture changes in reaction to unexpected perturbations. This last function requires quick adaptation. Thus posture is more than just maintaining a position of the body such as standing. Posture is active, whether it is sustaining an existing posture or moving from one posture to another.

Balance is the ability to maintain a posture while at rest and during activity. "Normal balance requires control of both gravitational forces to maintain posture and acceleration forces to maintain equilibrium."[2,3] Balance requires the integration of multiple systems: musculoskeletal,

neuromuscular, and sensory. Each system can be evaluated as contributing to balance or balance can be assessed by evaluating the performance of a functional activity. Using the International Classification of Functioning, Disability and Health framework balance can be described as both a structure/function and an activity.[4] Balance is postural control and control of posture is balance. The two terms are used interchangeable throughout this chapter.

Postural control and balance are linked processes. They provide the foundation for development of gross motor skills that enable children to participate in complex movements and play. Furthermore, postural control and balance are integral to performance of all voluntary movements that enable individuals to participate in daily life. Postural control is defined as achieving a certain body position such as upright standing and maintaining that position in any static (maintaining a posture) or dynamic (performing a motor skill) situation.[5,6] Balance cannot be separated from the task and the environment in which it is performed.

MODELS OF POSTURAL ORGANIZATION

Posture is organized at two different levels.[7] The first level is that of the body scheme. The body scheme includes posture as a reference to gravity, its anatomical relationships,

---

*Contributing author

and the concept of support. The postural body scheme represents the body's structures such as the head, trunk, and feet and the sensory receptors that provide information about gravity and the external environment.

The second level organizes postural control on the basis of the information from the representational level to form postural networks. The internal representation of the body segments involved in a posture makes up the representational level. The ways in which the various segments of the body relate to one another and how the relationships change based on sensory information are also represented within the *postural networks* in the central nervous system (CNS). Posture is represented as a whole entity rather than as just its component parts.

Postural networks are formed during development. For example, when a child experiences sitting, postural muscles are activated. The large number of muscle combinations that are initially available are eventually narrowed to those combinations that are most functional. The process of selection forms networks and is illustrated in Fig. 3.3. The neural basis for the development of these postural networks is discussed in Chapter 3.

Assaiante and Amblard[8] proposed an ontogenetic model for the sensorimotor organization of postural control for balance. Their model is based on two functional principles. One principle assumes that the organization of balance depends on which frame of reference is used by the body. The two possible frames of reference are the support surface and gravity. If the support surface is the frame of reference, postural control is organized in an ascending direction from the feet to the head (as seen in a quiet standing posture) or from the hip to the head (as seen in locomotion). If the vertical line of gravity is the frame of reference, postural control is organized in a descending direction from head to feet. A second functional principle is that children learn to control increasing degrees of freedom during a movement. The linkage between the head and trunk can be "en bloc" or articulated. When the head and trunk are en bloc, they move as a unit so that the head is stable on the trunk. When the linkage between the head and neck is articulated, the head is stable in space.

The model of Assaiante and Amblard[8] is based on typical, natural movement activities of children when balance is not disturbed. Four periods of development of postural control have been identified across the life span (Fig. 11.1). In the figure, the direction of the organization is listed across the top along with the organization of the

head and trunk linkage. From birth to the achievement of an upright stance, a cephalocaudal or descending type of organization is predominant. Control appears first in the muscles of the neck, then in the trunk, and finally in the legs. The second period lasts from the achievement of upright bipedal posture up to 6 years of age. During this second period, control is ascending from the support surface, that is, from the feet during standing or ascending from the hips up during locomotion.

At age 7, there is a return to a descending organization with an articulated linkage between the head and the trunk. This is not a return to the original condition found in the first period but rather a progression to the establishment of head stabilization in space strategy (HSSS). HSSS is a basic means of organizing descending temporal control of balance. By being able to master the degrees of freedom allowed by the neck joint, the child improves the accuracy of the visual and vestibular messages received relative to balance or postural control. The final period of postural development adds a measure of selectivity to the articulated operation of the head and trunk unit. This selective control of the degrees of freedom is presumed to be task dependent. The fourth period is present in adulthood.

TYPES OF BALANCE/POSTURAL CONTROL

Balance is the key to functional movement. From a biomechanical perspective, there are two major types of balance: static and dynamic. Static balance is the ability to maintain an upright posture and to keep the line of gravity within the limits of the base of support (BOS). When static posture is controlled, we are said to have good static balance in a particular position such as sitting or standing. No external support is needed. Dynamic balance is the ability to maintain postural control when mobile.

Balance performance can be classified into the following categories of postural control: static steady-state (i.e., maintaining a "quasi-static" position while standing/sitting), dynamic steady-state (i.e., maintaining a steady position while walking), proactive/anticipatory (i.e., anticipation of a predicted postural disturbance), and reactive balance (i.e., compensation of a postural disturbance).[9] *Steady-state postural control* ensures stability by maintaining the body's center of mass (COM) within its BOS. All of the forces acting on the body are balanced when the COM is within its limits of stability; that is, within the boundaries of the BOS, such as in

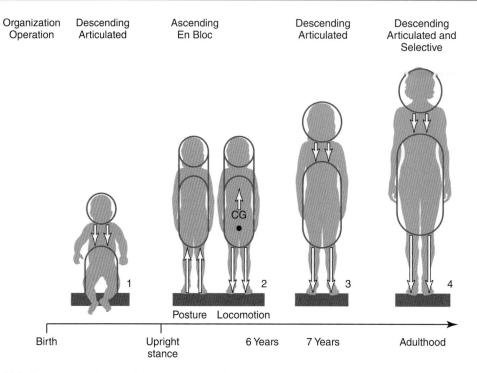

Fig. 11.1 Ontogenetic scheme of the organization of posturokinetic activities. (Adapted and reprinted from Assaiante C, Amblard B. An ontogenetic model of the sensorimotor organization of balance control in humans. *Hum Mov Sci.* 1995;14:13-43, p. 13, with permission from Elsevier Science.)

sitting or standing. *Steady-state* postural control is used when the ground is stationary and the BOS does not change. Postural control in quiet standing is also considered static *steady-state* balance because the movement of the COM that occurs when we gently sway over our ankles remains within the BOS. The area circumscribed by the sway represents a cone of stability (Fig. 11.2). The cone represents the functional limits of stability for that posture.

Reactive postural control governs the unexpected movement of the COM within or outside the BOS. Various balance responses are possible given the speed of the displacement or perturbation and whether the displacement results in the COM exceeding the BOS. Righting or equilibrium reactions are produced in response to weight shifts within the BOS. When the COM moves out of the BOS, as in a slip or fall, additional automatic postural responses occur. An unexpected perturbation on a force platform is an example of reactive postural control or balance. In this case, the movement of the platform shifts the person's COM, resulting in the need for a postural correction.

Postural adjustments made before a movement are classified as *anticipatory*. These adjustments are also called *proactive* as they anticipate a disturbance of posture before it happens. We typically make such postural adjustments before reaching, lifting, and stepping. Anticipatory postural adjustments (APAs) require that the nervous system feed information forward to postural muscles to prepare for the movement to follow. Think of being a water skier in the water, waiting for the first pull of the rope. You may hear the acceleration of the boat before you feel the pull, but you had better be ready to successfully achieve your goal of being lifted to an upright position. When you prepare to lift a box of heavy books, you expect the load and you prepare your posture accordingly. Experience is important in acquiring *anticipatory postural control.*

Another type of postural control is *adaptive postural control.* Adaptive postural control is demonstrated when we modify a motor response because of a change in environmental conditions or task demands. Most individuals change their speed and step width when walking on slippery ground. Aspects of cognition, such as attention,

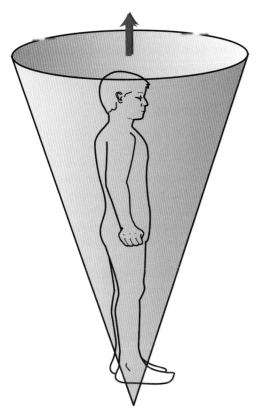

Fig. 11.2 Cone of stability. (From Martin ST, Kessler M. *Neurologic Intervention for Physical Therapist Assistants.* Philadelphia: WB Saunders; 2000:37.)

motivation, and intention, influence anticipatory and adaptive postural control. When attention is directed away from the balance task, it may be more difficult to adapt. Adaptive postural control seems to be a special condition of the three main types of postural control. Think of adaptive postural control as that learned by experience. The more experience with variable tasks or environmental conditions, the better the adaptation.

COMPONENTS OF A POSTURAL CONTROL SYSTEM

"The multicomponent nature of balance is reflected in the postural control theory."[10] Postural control theory describes balance as the product of integrated sensory inputs, the mechanical constraints of the body, and the nervous system's ability to process the task requirements within an environmental context. There are six major components of postural control using a systems framework:[11] (1) Biomechanical constraints, (2) orientation in space, (3) sensory strategies, (4) movement strategies, (5) dynamic control, and (6) cognitive processing.[11,12]

Biomechanical Constraints

The body is a mechanically linked structure that supports posture and provides a postural response. The viscoelastic properties of the muscles, joints, tendons, and ligaments can act as inherent constraints to posture and movement. The flexibility of body segments such as the neck, thorax, pelvis, hip, knee, and ankle contributes to attaining and maintaining a posture or making a postural response. Each body segment has mass and grows at a different rate. Each way in which a joint can move represents a degree of freedom. Because the body has so many individual joints and muscles with many possible ways in which to move, certain muscles work together in synergies to control the degrees of freedom.

Normal muscle tone is needed to sustain a posture and to support normal movement. *Muscle tone* has been classically defined as the resting tension in the muscle and the stiffness in the muscle as it resists being lengthened.[13] Muscle tone is determined by assessing the resistance felt during passive movement of a limb. Resistance is due mainly to the viscoelastic properties of the muscle. On activating the stretch reflex, the muscle proprioceptors, the muscle spindles, and Golgi tendon organs contribute to muscle tone or stiffness. The background level of activity in antigravity muscles during stance is described as postural tone by Shumway-Cook and Woollacott.[9] Together, the viscoelastic properties of muscle, the spindles, Golgi tendon organs, and descending motor commands regulate muscle tone.

All postures have a BOS. The BOS is that area of the body in contact with the support surface. The perimeter of the BOS is the typical limit of stability. When the mass of the body is maintained within the limits of the BOS, the posture is maintained. Developmental postures such as sitting, quadruped, and standing all have a different BOS. For example, standing has a smaller BOS than being in quadruped (hands and knees). Static postural control/balance in standing is measured by postural sway.[14] Keeping the COM of the body within the BOS constitutes balance. During quiet stance, as the body sways, the limits of stability depend on the interaction of the position and velocity of movement of the COM. We are more likely to lose balance if the velocity of the

COM is high and at the limits of the BOS. The body perceives changes in the COM in a posture by detecting amplitude of center of pressure (COP) motion. The COP is the point of application of the ground reaction force. In standing, there would be a COP under each foot. Feel how the COP changes as you shift weight forward and back while standing.

Orientation in Space

The head carries two of the most influential sensory receptors for posture and balance: the eyes and labyrinths. These two sensory systems provide ongoing sensory input about the movement of the surroundings and head, respectively. The eyes and labyrinths provide orientation of the head in space. The eyes must be able to maintain a stable visual image even when the head is moving, and the eyes have to be able to move with the head as the body moves. The labyrinths relay information about head movement to ocular nuclei and about position, allowing the mover to differentiate between *egocentric* (head relative to the body) and *exocentric* (head relative to objects in the environment) motion. Lateral flexion of the head is an egocentric motion. The movement of the head in space while walking or riding in an elevator is an example of exocentric motion.

Verticality is the ability to correctly orient to gravity.[12] The perception of visual verticality is separate from the perception of postural (proprioceptive) verticality.[15] Individuals with unilateral vestibular loss have disturbed visual but not postural verticality, while people exhibiting hemineglect due to a stroke have impaired postural verticality.[16] Either situation can lead to postural instability and increased fall risk.[17]

Children's ability to orient in space based on sensory input and gravity develops over time. See the previous discussion on Assaiante and Amblard. Early on children utilize gravity to define orientation in space but later as the vestibular system develops, the older child begins to use a more mature HSSS. HSSS is present only after 11 months of independent walking and is not complete until 6 years of age.[18]

HSSS involves an anticipatory stabilization of the head in space before body movement. When walking the head leads the motion. In adults, head orientation anticipates walking direction. Head anticipation, like head stabilization, aligns vestibular and visual receptors allowing for feed-forward control over postural-movement synergies.[19] By maintaining the angular position of the head with regard to the spatial environment, vestibular inputs can be better interpreted. Older adults have been shown to adopt this strategy when faced with distorted or incongruent somatosensory and visual information.[20]

Sensory Strategies

The maturation of the sensory systems and their relative contribution to balance have been extensively studied.[14,21-24] The visual, vestibular, and somatosensory systems provide the body with information about movement and cue postural responses. The incoming sensory information must be organized and integrated by the CNS to maintain or restore balance in static and dynamic conditions. The visual system provides information about the body's position in the environment. The peripheral vestibular system detects angular and linear velocity and analyzes spatial orientation. The somatosensory system and cutaneous input provide information about the body parts' relationship to the support surface and each other. The process of adjusting the sensory contributions to postural control is termed sensory reweighting.[21] The three sensory systems mature at different rates so the CNS reweights sensory inputs based on their availability.[24] Sensory integration has been described as the ability to reweight sensory information when input is altered.

Strategies for weighting sensory information change during development.[22] Using computerized dynamic posturography (CDP), healthy children from 3 to 6 years of age changed from using primarily visual-vestibular input to using somatosensory-vestibular input for balance control.[25,26] Adolescents use different sensory strategies than adults.[27] Adolescents do not handle visual conflicts as well as adults. Slow maturation of sensorimotor representations of proprioception and vision account for differences in strategies.[28] Proprioceptive processing continues to improve into late adolescence.[29]

Vision is very important for the development of head control. Newborns are sensitive to the flow of visual information and can even make postural adjustments in response to this information.[30] Input from the visual system is mapped to neck movement initially and then to trunk movement as head and trunk control is established. The production of spatial maps of the position of various body parts seems to be linked to muscular action. The linking of posture at the neck to vision forms before somatosensation is mapped to neck muscles.[9]

Most researchers agree that vision is the dominant sensory system for the first 3 years of life and that infants rely on vision for postural control in the acquisition of walking.

Vestibular information is also mapped to neck muscles at the same time as somatosensation is mapped. Eventually, mapping is done of combinations of sensory input such as visual-vestibular information.[31] This bimodal mapping allows for comparisons to be made between previous and present postures. The mapping of sensory information from each individual sense proceeds from the neck to the trunk and on to the lower extremities.[9] Information from vision acts as feedback when the body moves and as an anticipatory cue in a feedforward manner before movement. As a child learns to make use of somatosensory information from the lower extremities, somatosensory input emerges as the primary sensory input on which postural response decisions are made. Adults use somatosensation as their primary source for postural response. When there is a sensory conflict, the vestibular system acts as a tiebreaker in making the postural response decision. If somatosensation says you are moving and vision says you are not, the vestibular input should be able to resolve the conflict to maintain balance. Vestibular function relative to standing postural control continues to mature through the age of 15–17 years.[22,32]

Movement Strategies

Postural control/balance is the process by which the CNS, sensory system, and musculoskeletal system produce muscular strategies to regulate the relationship between the COM and BOS.[33] Stability involves the use of two mechanisms. The first involves development of torques at the joints of the supporting leg or legs and trunk to control COM motion without changing the BOS. More recently this strategy has been identified as a feet-in-place strategy. The second mechanism involves stepping or grasping movements of the limbs to alter the BOS when a person's balance is disturbed. This is a change in support strategy. If the source of the destabilization is recognized, it can be anticipated. Sensory information about the body's orientation and motion is also needed and may not be available ahead of an unexpected disturbance in balance. In that case, the sensory information of the instability can be either fed forward or fed back for postural correction. The way in which the postural system may operate is shown in Fig. 11.3.

There are three types of perturbations possible: physiological, mechanical, and informational. Physiological events can disrupt the operation of the nervous system control such as loss of posture due to orthostatic hypotension. Examples of mechanical disturbances of balance are changes in the forces acting on the body, such as a push or shove, slip, or trip. Another example could come from a change in range of motion at the ankle that could change the available BOS in standing. A change in the ambient light, as when walking into a dark room, is an example of an informational perturbation. Changes in sensory information coming in from the environment can affect reactive balance. Sensory information can be used proactively to adapt one's walking path to avoid an obstacle.

Motor coordination is the ability to coordinate muscle activation in a sequence that preserves posture. The use of muscle synergies in postural reactions and sway strategies in standing are examples of this coordination and are described in the upcoming section on neural control. Determination of the muscles to be used in a synergy is based on the task to be done and the environment in which the task takes place. Strength and muscle tone are prerequisites for movement against gravity and motor coordination. Head and trunk control require sufficient strength to extend the head, neck, and trunk against gravity in prone; to flex the head, neck, and trunk against gravity in supine; and to laterally flex the head, neck, and trunk against gravity in side-lying.

Postural responses are made in reaction to internally and externally perceived needs. Movement performance is changed when we encounter ice on a sidewalk. A young child may change the manner in which stairs are descended based on perception of safety. Developmentally, the sensorimotor system of an infant must adapt to gravity. The nervous system generates movement solutions to the problems the infant encounters during the attainment of an upright erect posture. The sensory systems also signal the need for automatic postural reactions to preserve posture. With the development of postural networks in the CNS, anticipatory postural control develops and is used to preserve posture (see Chapter 4). Adaptive postural control allows changes to be made to movement performance in response to internally or externally perceived needs.

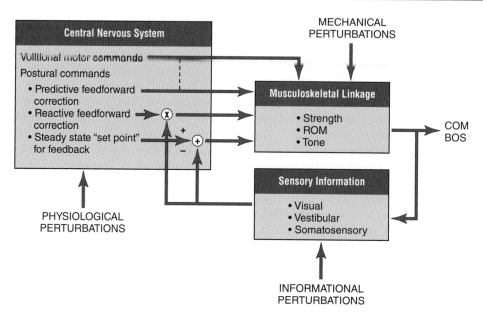

Fig. 11.3 A conceptual model of the postural control system. In feedback control, sensory information is used to continuously update the corrective changes to the center of mass or base of support. In feedforward control, preprogrammed stabilizing reactions are released, either predictively (anticipatory postural adjustments) or in reaction to sensory information pertaining to the state of instability (triggered postural reactions). Mechanical perturbations involve changes in the forces acting on the body (due to movement of the body or interaction with the environment). Informational perturbations pertain to transient changes in the nature of the orientational information available from the environment. Physiological perturbations refer to transient internal events that disrupt the operation of the neural control system. *ROM*, Range of motion. (Adapted from Maki BE, McIlroy WE. Postural control in the older adult. *Clin Geriatr Med.* 1996;12(4):635-658.)

Dynamic Control

Dynamic postural control is also seen when transitioning from one posture such as four-point to tall kneeling. Where does the center of the body's mass have to move to attain a kneeling position from being on hands and knees? If no posterior weight shift happens, it is impossible for a person to attain an upright position in tall kneeling. Gait is even more complex to control than a single movement transition. During gait, the COM has to be controlled while the BOS changes with each step. The reader is referred to a later discussion in the Locomotion section.

Dynamic postural control improves with age but is not completely achieved until 16 years of age. In a multicenter posturography study, Goulème and collegues[24] saw changes in temporal and spatial characteristics of dynamic postural control in children from ages 3 to 16 years. Spatial parameters measured included the surface area of the COP and its mean velocity. Time and frequency of postural sway were also measured.

All postural parameters declined with age, indicating improved dynamic postural control. The postural control system continues to reweight sensory input through adolescence. Gender differences are present, with girls exhibiting better postural control.[22,24] The gender difference may be linked to pubertal maturation.[24]

Depending on the literature, there are two trains of thought as to when mature postural control is achieved in children. Traditionally, postural control was thought to be mature at 7[34,35] or 8 years.[36] Others report adult-like sensory integration during stance at 12 years.[37,38] The discrepancies in age may be related to the elements of postural sway that were used to assess postural control. In Verbecque and associates' study,[5] adult-like postural control was seen in children as young as 6 years of age based on postural sway area results, whereas adult-like responses based on sway velocity were not achieved until 12 years of age.[5]

Voss and associates[39] studied individuals from 5 to 30 years of age using inertial sensors. They found "a nonlinear decrease with age in total sway area, RMS [root mean square] sway, Jerk, and mean velocity across six conditions." Jerk is the measurement of the rate at which the COP moves through a given BOS (TA Hanke, personal communication-email to editor Suzanne "Tink" Martin, October 2022). "The most significant transition for total sway area and jerk appears between ages 8 and 9, with children demonstrating adult-like postural responses by ages 9–10."[39] "In contrast, RMS sway and velocity achieved adult-like patterns by ages 11−13 across all EO and tandem stance conditions."[39] Based on these results, postural control continues to develop gradually throughout adolescence.

Cognitive Processing

Postural control is influenced by the attentional demands of the task as well as the environment in which the task occurs. Even quiet standing requires cognitive processing. Information that is salient to the task will be attended to while other incoming information may be ignored. Maintaining static or dynamic stability while responding to commands is dual-tasking. Individuals with cognitive processing problems may have difficulty controlling their posture when occupied with a secondary cognitive task. As noted later in this chapter, balance requires anticipatory planning to negotiate in the environment. When a person feels particularly stressed, anxious, angry, or fearful, they may be more likely to experience lack of concentration necessary for stability. When a person is tired or doing other things that they need to think about, it can affect their balance both in forethought and reactions such as an uneven surface or a perturbation. If someone is concentrating on a mental task, the brain has less capacity to spare for other tasks, such as maintaining balance. It takes mental effort and capacity for the brain to cope with conflicting information about balance, and so if a person becomes tired and unable to concentrate, it can cause a decreased balance response.

NEURAL BASIS FOR POSTURAL CONTROL AND BALANCE

There are two ways to view the neural basis of postural control, the reflex/hierarchical model and the systems model. One is the traditional reflex and hierarchical model of postural control already discussed in Chapter 4. The development of postural control does appear to follow a hierarchy and to proceed in a cephalocaudal sequence. Head control is developed before trunk control. Once an erect posture is achieved, however, it is more beneficial to use a systems approach to analyzing postural control. The six elements of the systems model of postural control have already been described. The reflex/hierarchical model of postural control is CNS-dependent and focused on reactive postural control. The systems model encompasses the maturation of the musculoskeletal system as well as the CNS and focuses on all aspects of postural control/balance: reactive, anticipatory, and adaptive.

Postural Reflexes

Cervicospinal and vestibulospinal reflexes assist in maintaining postural stability. The reticular formation within the brain stem contributes to postural tone by balancing the activation of flexor and extensor muscles to allow us to express these reflexes. Vestibular responses are used primarily to stabilize the head in space. Therefore the brain stem is involved in postural control. It coordinates information from the spinal cord, cerebellum, cortex, and special senses (vision, vestibular, and somatosensation). Central postural commands are relayed to motor neurons via the reticulospinal, vestibulospinal, and medial corticospinal tracts.[40] Output is modified by sensory input that conveys environmental context.

Reactive Postural Control

Righting reactions begin at birth and exhibit peak occurrence at 10–12 months. These reactions can be elicited by any one of a number of sensory stimuli: vestibular, proprioceptive, visual, or tactile. Righting reactions become incorporated into equilibrium reactions and therefore persist as part of our automatic reactive balance mechanism (Table 11.1). *Righting* is defined as maintenance or restoration of the proper alignment of the head or trunk in space. One category of righting reactions produces movement in one plane; these movements are described as anterior, posterior, or lateral head-righting or trunk-righting. When held upright in vertical and tilted in any direction, the head and trunk right or tilt in the opposite direction. Likewise, when we are in side-lying position, the somatosensory cue of the trunk on the supporting surface cues lateral head-lifting (righting). Head-righting develops during the first several months in response to gravity's effect on the vestibular system and through the body's contact (somatosensation) with the supporting surface.

TABLE 11.1   Postural Reactions

Reaction	Age at Onset	Age at Integration
Head-Righting		
Neck (immature)	34 weeks of gestation	4–6 months
Labyrinthine	Birth to 2 months	Persists
Optical	Birth to 2 months	Persists
Neck (mature)	4–6 months	5 years
Trunk-Righting		
Body (immature)	34 weeks of gestation	4–6 months
Body (mature)	4–6 months	5 years
Landau	3–4 months	1–2 years
Protective		
Downward lower extremity	4 months	Persists
Forward upper extremity	6–7 months	Persists
Sideways upper extremity	7–8 months	Persists
Backward upper extremity	9 months	Persists
Stepping lower extremity	15–17 months	Persists
Equilibrium		
Prone	6 months	Persists
Supine	7–8 months	Persists
Sitting	7–8 months	Persists
Quadruped	9–12 months	Persists
Standing	12–24 months	Persists

Data from Barnes MR, Crutchfield CA, Heriza CB. *The Neurophysiological Basis of Patient Treatment.* Vol. 2. Atlanta: Stokesville; 1982.

A second category of righting reactions produces rotation around the body axis, as in rolling to maintain alignment of body segments. These righting reactions of the head and trunk function to produce rotation around the long axis of the body and are an integral part of producing a smooth movement transition from one posture to another. Mature neck- and body-righting allow for the developmental change from log rolling to segmental rolling seen in the 4- to 6-month-old infant.

Equilibrium reactions are more sophisticated than righting reactions and involve a total body response to a slow shift of the center of gravity outside the BOS. In a lateral sitting equilibrium reaction, the head and trunk right, and the arm and leg abduct opposite the weight shift, followed by head and trunk rotation toward the abducted extremities (Fig. 11.4). Equilibrium reactions begin to appear at 6 months of age in the prone position,

even as the infant is experiencing supported sitting. The remaining equilibrium reactions appear in an orderly sequence: prone, supine, sitting, quadruped, and standing. The maturation of reactions in developmental postures lags behind the attainment of movement in the next higher developmental posture. For example, equilibrium reactions mature in the sitting position when the child is creeping and mature in the quadruped position when the child is walking.

Righting and equilibrium reactions are triggered by sensory cues such as visual recognition of a changing horizon. Vestibular or somatosensory cues are also used to perceive that a postural response is needed. Head-righting occurs before trunk-righting. Reactive postural control is mastered in developmental positions sequentially but with some overlap. For example, equilibrium reactions may mature in a lower developmental position

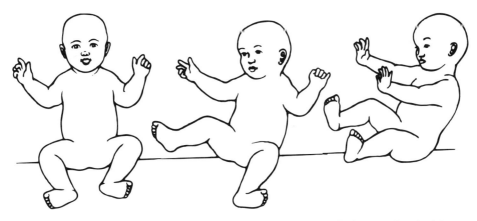

Fig. 11.4 Sitting equilibrium reaction in response to lateral weight shift. Equilibrium reactions in sitting mature when the infant begins creeping.

such as sitting as the child crawls around in quadruped and mature in the quadruped position when the child is walking. Reactive balance occurs when moving from one posture to another and is used to attain/maintain an erect standing posture or move safely across a room.

A protective reaction is an extremity response to a quick displacement of the center of gravity out of the BOS. A downward response of the legs is seen at 4 months. Protective extension of the upper extremities becomes evident when the infant begins to sit with support. Displacement in sitting results in brisk extension of an arm to catch and protect against falling. The infant can prop forward on extended arms if placed around the same time. Upper extremity protective reactions begin at 6 months in sitting and develop sequentially forward, sideways, and backward. Haley[41] found that this order of acquisition is not always followed. Protective reactions are generally completely developed by 10 months of age. These reactions become our backup system if we fail to regain our balance by the use of an equilibrium reaction. Unfortunately, the use of these automatic responses can result in unintentional injury, as when an older adult sustains a Colles fracture from falling on an outstretched arm.

Postural control can be changed through learning and experience. One of the most basic premises of a systems perspective is that with practice and repetition, motor behavior can change. The more a pattern of movement, in this case, a postural adjustment, is repeated, the more adaptable it becomes. Practice and experience allow the organization of postural responses to accomplish a functional end such as support of movement. Learning requires that all perceptual systems contribute useful information to the control of posture. Infants are capable of using perceptual information from many different senses after 6 months of age. Therefore the development of postural control as viewed within a systems model is also suggestive of mapping or associating sensory input from sensory systems to a particular action, such as head lifting. Experience strengthens connections between sensory and motor pathways controlling balance. When learning is compromised, as in persons with mental disabilities, it may be possible to make postural adjustments but not in a timely manner. The implementation of the muscular response is slower due to nervous system immaturity. Also, anticipatory postural control, which requires experiential learning, is inadequate or delayed in children with Down syndrome.[42]

Two systems models of the control of standing balance have been proposed.

Nashner Model of Postural Control of Stance

Nashner[43] formulated a model for the control of standing balance. His model describes three common sway strategies seen in steady-state standing: the ankle strategy, the hip strategy, and the stepping strategy. Depending on the characteristics of the support surface, the speed of perturbation, and the degree of displacement, different strategies emerge.

Adults sway about the ankle when the foot is fully supported during quiet stance (Fig. 11.5A). This strategy depends on solid contact under the foot to provide

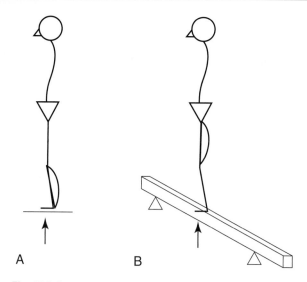

Fig. 11.5 Sway strategies. (A) Postural sway about the ankle in quiet standing, with the foot fully supported. (B) Postural sway about the hip in standing on a balance beam, with the foot partially supported. (From Martin ST, Kessler M. *Neurologic Intervention for Physical Therapist Assistants*. Philadelphia: WB Saunders; 2000:38.)

a resistive force, enabling the ankle muscles to exert their effect through "reverse action." With the foot fixed on the ground, either the plantar flexors or the dorsiflexors contract to pull the leg backward and forward with respect to the foot, keeping the COM within the BOS. If we sway backward, the anterior tibialis fires to bring us forward; if we sway forward, the gastrocnemius fires to bring us back to the midline. This strategy depends on having a solid surface under the feet and intact vision, vestibular system, and somatosensation. The ankle strategy is used when the perturbations or disturbances to balance are small.

Adults sway about the hip when standing crosswise on a narrow balance beam, as shown in Fig. 11.5B. An ankle strategy cannot be used in this situation because there is no support under the toes and heels to provide a reactive force to the ankle motion. Therefore the only successful strategy is the hip strategy, in which hip flexion and extension combine with knee extension and flexion to ensure balance. Larger perturbations elicit a hip strategy if the feet are supported, as when performing a postural stress test.

The last sway strategy, that of stepping, occurs when the speed and strength of the balance disturbance are sufficient to produce a protective step. By taking a step,

the BOS is widened and balance is regained because the COM is once again within the BOS. It had been thought that the COM had to exceed the BOS for stepping to occur, but such is not the case. Some researchers have found that the directions given to subjects during a balance task may constrain them from stepping.[14]

Children 18 months old are able to demonstrate an ankle strategy in quiet standing when balance is disturbed.[35] Their response time is longer than that of adults. According to Shumway-Cook and Woollacott,[34] children 4–6 years old displayed varying strategies to the same type of perturbations in standing; sometimes a hip strategy was used, and sometimes an ankle strategy was used. A consistent ankle strategy performed in a timely manner was not evident until 7–10 years of age. This coincides with the maturation of nervous system myelination of major tracts by age 10.

Winter Stiffness Model of Postural Control of Stance

Research has looked at how the body's COM is controlled during quiet stance. Winter and colleagues[44] proposed a straightforward model that gives an almost immediate corrective response. "The model assumes that muscles act as springs to cause the COP to move in phase with the COM as the body sways about some desired position."[44] The stiffness control in the sagittal plane comes from the torque produced by the ankle plantar flexors/dorsiflexors. In the frontal plane, the stiffness comes from the hip abductor/adductor torque. The model of Winter and colleagues[44] is also an inverted pendulum. Movement of the COP under the feet regulates the body COM. The difference between the body COM and the COP is proportional to the acceleration of the body COM. The researchers showed that the torque needed to restore posture was set by the joint stiffness.

In a review of proprioceptive control of posture, Allum and colleagues[45] questioned whether the proprioceptive cues from the ankles do trigger balance responses in standing and during locomotion. The research reviewed supports the idea that postural strategies other than sway strategies are possible. Input to the trunk and hip may be more important than input to the ankle in triggering balance correction in standing. This may reflect the fact that the hip is the joint in the lower extremity that is used to recover stability when posture/ balance is disturbed in a mediolateral direction. Hip abductor and adductor muscles are preferentially active when balance is disturbed in the mediolateral direction and their rate of activation is impaired in older versus younger individuals.[46] Responses to mediolateral postural disturbances activate muscles in a proximal-to-distal order.

POSTURE AND BALANCE ACROSS THE LIFE SPAN

Balance performance is very task specific rather than a general ability.[47] Balance is a component of health and activity-related fitness and is therefore important across the life span. Kiss and associates[47] reviewed 26 studies of balance in healthy individuals aged 6 and over. They included studies that measured static/dynamic steady-state, reactive, and/or proactive balance. The systematic review and meta-analysis found small-sized correlations between types of balance and age. Dynamic steady-state balance was correlated with reactive balance in children and older adults.[48,49] This correlation was not found in any other age group. "Significant age differences were found for the associations between dynamic and static steady-state balance in children compared to old adults."[47] Proactive and reactive balance were correlated in young and old adults.[50,51] Further research is indicated to explore whether significant age differences do exist or if there are methodological inconsistencies.

For physical therapists, the study of posture and balance development is an integral part of the study of motor development. Posture, like movement, varies characteristically with age. *Balance* is a developmental characteristic related to posture. In this chapter, the specific changes in human postural function are examined from a life span perspective. A real constraint to a broad and systematic study of posture is the lack of information about posture during large periods of the human life span. Typically, research and collections of literature regarding posture, even when claiming a life span perspective, skip important life periods. We know most about very young infants, children, and older adults. Less is known about postural development in later childhood, adolescence, and young and middle adulthood.

Infancy and Childhood

Postural control develops in a cephalocaudal and proximal-distal sequence in infants. Head control is achieved before trunk control, shoulder control before finger control, and pelvic control before foot control. Once an erect stance is achieved, the relationship with the support surface initiates a caudocephalic sequence of responses or distal to proximal as described by Nashner.[43] Postural control is essential to developing skilled actions such as locomotion and manipulation. Bertenthal and Von Hofsten[52] stated that eye, head, and trunk control are the foundation for reaching and manipulation.

Development of Spinal Curves

Static postural alignment is dependent to some extent on the spinal curves seen when viewing upright posture from the side. Everyone is familiar with the anatomical landmarks used to determine alignment. Spinal curves develop over the life span. Although the adult spine has sagittal curves in the cervical, thoracic, lumbar, and pelvic regions, the infant has only two curves. The flexed posture of the newborn is the result of physiological flexor tone and the need to conform to the mother's uterus. The infant's two curves are concave forward: one in the thoracic region and the other in the pelvic region. The latter is formed by the curve of the sacrum, which is composed of separate vertebral components at this stage of development.

As the infant grows and develops sufficient strength to lift the head, the cervical curve develops and is convex forward. This curve becomes more noticeable as the infant holds the head up at 3–4 months. The lumbar curve is also convex forward and develops when the baby begins to sit up. The curves could fail to develop if the child is unable to develop head control and sitting.

Development of Postural Control

Postural development proceeds from head control to trunk control. The infant assumes a prone on elbows posture at approximately 3 months when the head and upper back are extended sufficiently to allow the freeing of the arms from under the infant. Weight bearing in the posture is important for developing proximal shoulder girdle stabilization. The prone progression of developmental postures consists of achieving a prone-on elbows position and then moving to prone on extended arms and finally moving up to quadruped or all fours. From a hands and knees posture, the infant pulls to stand and achieves an upright posture. Initially, support of hands or tummy may be required.

With the achievement of upright stance, erect posture is precarious. Because the newly erect infant's center of gravity is relatively high (T12 compared with

L5-S1 in an adult), the BOS is widened. The center of gravity is also forward due to a large liver. For the upper trunk to achieve a vertical position, the lumbar lordosis is increased, and the arms are brought into a high guard position (see Fig. 3.25).

Sensory contributions to balance in infants. Jouen and colleagues[30] showed that 3-day-old infants made postural adjustments of the head in response to optical flow patterns. These are patterns of light associated with movement. The brain uses this information to know where the head and the body are relative to the surrounding environment. Spontaneous head control is noted in infants at 10 weeks of age when electromyographic responses can be recorded in reaction to being tilted.[53] Bertenthal and associates[54] investigated the developmental changes in postural control of 5-, 7-, 9-, and 13-month-old infants in response to optical flow. The infants were able to scale their postural responses to the visual information. The scaling was even possible in presitters but improved with practice and the development of sitting. The ability to use visual information for postural responses increased from 5 to 9 months of age. Vestibular and somatosensory systems can also trigger balance responses in infants and toddlers in sitting.[55]

Sitting. Sitting is a new posture in which the COM is suspended above the BOS. Fairly rapid postural adjustments are needed to resist or to compensate for sudden losses of balance. Even infants who were unable to sit alone were able to integrate visual information and make a motor response (postural adjustment) without having the strength and coordination to maintain a sitting posture independently. Improvement in muscle activation patterns is a function of experience with perceptual modulation of posture.[56,57]

Balance strategies in sitting. Infants develop directionally specific postural responses before being able to sit.[58] These responses appear to be innate and are guided by an internal representation of the limits of stability, such as orientation of the vertical axis and relationship of COM to BOS. This is consistent with the hypothesis of a central pattern generator being the source of initial postural responses.[55] This circuitry determines the spatial characteristics of muscle activation that is triggered by afferent information. During this period of time, the infant demonstrates a large number of postural responses. With further development, "a gradual selection process emerges from 3 months onwards."[58] With experience, the initial variability is reduced and the temporal and spatial features of responses are fine-tuned to match task-specific demands. This process is consistent with the neuronal group selection theory, where experience continues to shape postural networks by changing the synaptic strength of nervous system connections.

Development of sitting postural control has been studied using COP data. Researchers[59] longitudinally assessed the postural sway of infants at three stages of sitting. The first stage begins when the infant holds the head and upper trunk up but does not sit alone. The second stage involves the infant sitting alone briefly and is followed by the third stage of the infant being able to sit alone. Nonlinear measurement showed significant changes in COP distribution over time. This method is a moderately reliable way to assess the development of sitting postural control in typically developing infants and those at risk for cerebral palsy.[60] Nonlinear dynamics provide an alternate explanation for the development of postural control. Rather than being the result of a central pattern being generated and subsequently modulated, the infant's ability to control the body's degrees of freedom to master postural control in sitting is a result of a dynamic process.[61]

Multisensory afferent input is used to shape adaptive postural responses. Chen and associates[57] studied postural sway in sitting infants in response to anterior-posterior oscillations in a virtual moving room. Newly sitting infants displayed variable postural behavior, and within a few months post-sitting, infants demonstrated postural control in response to various amplitudes and frequencies of visual motion. They concluded that sensory reweighting occurs to support visual-postural adjustments a few months after learning to sit. Arnold and colleagues[62] studied changes in postural sway while infants either visually attended to a toy held by another person or when holding a toy. Different support surfaces were used but the surfaces did not affect sway. Visually attending to a toy was associated with lower sway velocity and less sway.

Most studies of the development of anticipatory postural control have been conducted in sitting, using reaching as the task. Postural activity in the trunk is measured while an infant reaches from a seated posture. Trunk muscles are activated before muscles used for reaching. Researchers concluded that anticipatory postural control occurs before voluntary movements and is present in infants by 6–8 months of age.[63] Children appear to tolerate more imbalance as they grow up. Anticipatory control of posture increases from 2 to 11 years of age, with older children demonstrating more refined scaling of responses.[64] In other words, children become better at matching the amount of postural preparation needed for a specific task. Less postural activation is needed when picking up a light object versus picking up a heavy object.

Sit to stand transition. Moving from sitting to standing is an everyday occurrence and a necessary prerequisite for walking. Cahill and colleagues[65] studied three age groups of children on a sit-to-stand task. The children were grouped as follows: 12–18 months, 4–5 years, and 9–10 years. The movement became more coordinated as measured by the smoothness of phase-plane plots. The youngest group could perform the movement but could not cease moving once a standing posture was attained and either took steps or raised onto their toes. The oldest group generated a pattern of vertical ground reaction force like that of adults when coming to stand but could not do so consistently. Differences in performance were attributed to developmental differences in the children's ability to control the horizontal momentum of the body mass, use sensory input for balance, and understand the task.

Standing posture in childhood. Children 2–3 years of age exhibit a characteristic lumbar lordosis that ranges between 30 and 40 degrees.[66,67] When infants begin to stand and walk, their feet are flat and they begin to exhibit a longitudinal arch only as the fat pad in the foot diminishes. Changes in lower extremity alignment in the stance posture occur over a 6-year period. The 18-month-old child stands with bow legs (genu varum), but by 3 years of age, the legs may exhibit genu valgus or knock knees. The legs straighten out by 6 years.[68]

Balance on two feet increases as independent locomotion is achieved. Once double limb support is mastered in standing, the next challenge is to develop balance while standing on one foot. Single-leg standing (SLS) begins at approximately age 3 years with momentary to 3 seconds and progresses sequentially to 10-plus seconds at 6 years (Table 11.2). SLS reaches adult levels by approximately 10 years.[69,70] Momentary to 3-second one-foot standing balance is needed to ascend a step or to step over an object. Longer unilateral standing balance is a prerequisite for fundamental motor skills, such as hopping, galloping, and skipping (see Chapter 3).

TABLE 11.2 Age-Related Expectations for One-Foot Standing Balance

Age (years)	Time
3	Momentary to 3 s
4	4–6 s
5	8–10 s
6	10+ s eyes open and eyes closed

Sensory contributions to standing balance. The maturation of the sensory systems and their relative contribution to balance have been extensively studied with some conflicting findings. As children master independent walking, the primacy of vision for postural control lessens gradually. Balance control changes from being primarily visual-vestibular to being somatosensory-vestibular by age 3.[26] Proprioception function matures by 3–4 years of age.[32] Therefore within the 4- to 6-year-old range, vision is still important for balance, but proprioception and touch are being used more. Sinno and associates found that children between 5 and 8 years old had adult-like somatosensory function when tested using the Sensory Organization Test (SOT). The SOT uses six different sensory conditions to assess balance (see Fig. 11.6). Spontaneous sway is measured under specific sensory conditions that force the individual to reweight another sensory input in order to maintain postural control (conditions 2 through 6). The SOT assesses how vision, somatosensation, and vestibular inputs are used by an individual for balance. In normal support conditions, children 6–10 years old are more stable with vision.[71] Use of specific sensory inputs develops at different ages.[22] Somatosensation develops early, vision matures around 11–12 years old, and vestibular continues to mature through 15–17 years.

For 8-year-olds, central vision produced greater postural stability than peripheral vision. Peripheral visual cues were more important for postural stabilization in children 11 to 13 years old.[72] This finding is consistent with Sinno and colleagues'[22] findings that visual function in children demonstrated a peak around 12 years. When studying one-foot standing balance, static balance was also found to be dependent on visual information. However, dynamic destabilization in a medial-lateral (ML) direction was linked to motor response speed. Static single-leg postural control was studied in children aged 6–12 years using accelerometric technology.[73] The

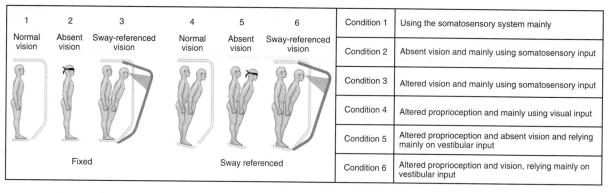

						Condition 1	Using the somatosensory system mainly
1	2	3	4	5	6	Condition 2	Absent vision and mainly using somatosensory input
Normal vision	Absent vision	Sway-referenced vision	Normal vision	Absent vision	Sway-referenced vision	Condition 3	Altered vision and mainly using somatosensory input
						Condition 4	Altered proprioception and mainly using visual input
						Condition 5	Altered proprioception and absent vision and relying mainly on vestibular input
Fixed			Sway referenced			Condition 6	Altered proprioception and vision, relying mainly on vestibular input

Fig. 11.6 Sensory Organization Test. (From Sinno S, Dumas G, Mallinson A, Najem F, Abouchacra KS, Nashner L, Perrin P. Changes in the sensory weighting strategies in balance control throughout maturation in children. *J Am Acad Audiol.* 2021; 32:122-136, Fig. 1, p. 125.)

children were tested with eyes open and eyes closed. Balance improved more with increasing age when visual information was present. Sex differences in balance were seen when the children performed single-leg stance without vision. Lack of vision had a greater impact on the boys than girls aged 6–11 years. The discrepancy was not present in the 12-year-olds. The researchers concluded that boys preferred visual strategies while the girls preferred using somatosensory information.

Conner and colleagues[14] studied static standing balance and dynamic standing balance reactions in typically developing children from 5.8 to 12.7 years of age. They were interested in the relationship of static (postural sway) and dynamic (stepping thresholds) standing balance performance. Children stood on a force platform for 30 seconds with eyes open and eyes closed. No age-related decline in sway was observed. Single-stepping threshold in the children was assessed by perturbing their balance while wearing a harness on a treadmill. Age was significantly related to improved stepping thresholds but not to reduced postural sway. The researchers concluded that postural control in quiet standing and after external perturbation are two unique tasks.

Postural sway in standing on a moveable platform under normal vestibular and somatosensory conditions is greater for children 4–6 years of age than for children 7–10 years of age.[34] By 7–10 years of age, an adult sway strategy is demonstrated wherein the child has been thought to depend primarily on somatosensory information. Vestibular information is also being used, but the system is not yet mature. Interestingly, children with

visual impairments are not able to minimize postural sway to the same extent as nonvisually impaired children. Rogge and colleagues[74] found larger postural sway and lower single-leg stance time in children and adolescents who were blind or visually impaired compared to matched sighted individuals who were blindfolded. According to Rogge and associates' results, the absence of visual cues affects postural stability irrespective of the age of the person.

Research supports that there is a transition period of around 7–8 years that can be explained by the use of the HSSS.[73] By 7 years of age, children are able to make effective use of HSSS that depends on dynamic vestibular cues. However, the transition to adult postural responses in standing is not complete by 12 years of age. Children at 12–14 years of age are still not able to handle misleading visual information to make appropriate adult balance responses.[75] These researchers found that although the somatosensory inputs and scores in the 6- to 14-year-old subjects were as good as the young adults studied, their sensory organization was different. They concluded that children prefer visual input to vestibular input for determining balance responses and that vestibular information is the least effective for postural control.

It is generally accepted that visual, vestibular, and somatosensory information must be integrated to control standing balance; however, there are conflicting findings about their relative contributions to balance. In a large study using the SOT, Steindl and colleagues[76] tried to shed light on some of the conflicting data on the effect of age and maturation of sensory systems on balance.

They reconfirmed that the proprioceptive system is fully developed in 3 to 4-year-olds and that visual input appears to be more crucial to balance under conditions of support surface instability. Visual afference of postural control is mature at approximately 15 or 16 years of age. Vestibular maturation occurs in adolescence and is the last sensory system involved with postural control to mature. The ability to solve intersensory conflicts requires that all three sensory systems be mature, and one can assume this happens in adolescence.

In summary, visual input dominates posture and balance during the first 3 years of life. The 4- to 6-year-old child is able to make more use of proprioceptive information, but the balance responses in standing are highly variable. By 7–10 years of age, the child is able to demonstrate adult-like reactive postural control strategies in response to perturbations in standing, such as swaying over the ankles like an inverted pendulum. Balance responses are not completely mature, however, until 15–16 years.

Anticipatory Control

Anticipatory postural control occurs before a movement takes place. Postural muscles prepare for the movement. Infants (10–17 months old) demonstrate anticipatory action in the calf muscles when trying to pull open a drawer in standing.[77] Consistency of anticipatory postural responses in standing and reaching tasks increases during childhood and into early adolescence. A study in 3- to 5-year-olds[78] found that the functional reach test could be used reliably in 4- and 5-year-olds. Donahoe and associates[79] tested children between 5 and 15 years of age using the functional reach test. Balance was seen to improve with age up to the 11- to 12-year-old age category and then appeared to stabilize. The ability to anticipate the postural adjustments needed to allow for reaching forward is used on a daily basis in childhood activities. The task is an example of feedforward control of balance and is a test of anticipatory control. Lower extremity strength especially in the hip and knee flexors was found to be important in controlling balance in all directions in children 7–12 years of age when tested using the multidirectional reach test.[80]

Adaptive Control

Motor adaptation was studied in 6- to 8-year-old children using a split-belt treadmill.[81] The children's ability to adapt to the new motor task and to recalibrate perceptual information was compared to adults performing the same task. The children adapted to the new movement more slowly than the adults. Perceptual recalibration was also reduced in the children compared to the adults. The study concluded that the capacity to learn new perceptual and motor calibrations develops together in childhood. Children from 6–8 years of age demonstrate reliable adaptation but show an immature time-course of learning compared to adults. Children over the age of 9 years demonstrate adult-like adaptation patterns.

Adolescence and Transitional Movements

The spatial and temporal characteristics of dynamic postural control change with age. Using posturography, Goulème and associates[24] found that mature postural control "is not completely achieved but is still ongoing beyond 16.08 years old." The postural control system continues to reweight all sensory inputs based on the situation and their functional activation. Gender differences are present. Girls allocate less energy to maintain postural control in a more challenging balance condition than boys by using their vestibular input. The ability to reweight sensory inputs is based on their availability with adult-like sensory integration during stance being present at 12 years of age. The postural control system continues to reweight sensory input through adolescence. Vestibular input is the last to mature.

Lebiedowska and Syczewska[82] looked at the relationship between body size and its effect on postural sway in children 7–18 years of age. They wanted to know if the structural changes in body height and mass affected spontaneous sway parameters. They found no significant correlations between the postural sway and developmental factors of age, body height, and body mass. However, there was a decrease in sway parameter when values were normalized to body height that indicated a small improvement in static equilibrium with taller children. Conner and associates[14] found no reductions in postural sway in children between 5 and 12 years even though they adjusted for height. Stepping thresholds in the study improved with age. The researchers concluded that balance reaction capabilities in children are related to age and should be further studied. A study of rising from the floor movements in teenagers revealed what appears to be a peak in the incidence of symmetrical movement patterns around the age of 15 years.[83] Younger and older teens were found to exhibit more asymmetry while rising than did middle teens. This is particularly true for lower limb movements. It may be that peak performance in a task occurs when most individuals demonstrate the greatest ability to control force within this task. Although children seem to have difficulty controlling force production in this task, and as a result demonstrate asymmetry in their rising actions, teens exhibit a refined competence in simultaneously controlling the upper limb, trunk, and lower limb movements. They move from recumbency by flexing the trunk and moving the feet directly in front of their buttocks while balancing in a sitting position, and then they transfer weight from the buttocks to the feet with ease. Control of the force and direction of movement in the righting task is impressive at this age.

Adulthood and Transitional Movements

The midteen peak in symmetrical performance is diminished slightly during the late-teen period and into the early 20 s. Although symmetrical performance is the most common form of rising, it is the mode of action of approximately one-fourth of young adults. The remainder demonstrate asymmetry in at least one component of body action, be it the upper limbs, the trunk, or the lower limbs. This is when individuals are making the transition from high school to college or the workforce. Compared with the high school years, young adulthood presents fewer formalized opportunities to participate in physical activity. Green and Williams[84] found that the activity level is related to performance in the rising from the floor task during the middle adult years. More active adults are more likely to use symmetrical patterns.

Patterns of movement change with age, and movement patterns used by older adults are variable.[85,86] Posture and balance may decline as an individual ages because of changes in a static posture, loss of flexibility and muscle strength, vestibular impairments affecting postural awareness and head stabilization, tone changes resulting from medications or pathologies, changes in sensorimotor input and integration, decreased neural transmission, and visual changes. Many of the changes in movement patterns seen in older adults are the result of inactivity and the lack of motor practice.[87,88]

Balance in Older Adults

Effect of Sensory Changes With Age

Sensory input for balance changes with advancing age. The three sensory systems (visual, vestibular, and somatosensory) responsible for posture undergo age-related changes. The visual system is less able to pick up contours and depth cues because of a decline in contrast sensitivity. Both of these losses can impair postural control. The problems can be intensified if there are cataracts, retinopathy, glaucoma, or macular degeneration. The vestibular system loses hair cells that detect changes in the direction of flow of the endolymph within the semicircular canals and saccule and utricle. The eighth cranial nerve (vestibulocochlear) may show a reduced number of nerve fibers. Both of these changes can affect otolith function and result in positional vertigo. Vibratory sense and proprioception in the lower extremities decline and could contribute to a decrease in somatosensory input from the support surface and awareness of the degree of postural sway. Older adults exhibit an increased postural sway when standing on a foam surface. The researchers associated the increased sway with a decline in visual contrast sensitivity and visual acuity in older adults because they could not compensate for decreased somatosensation with vision.[89] Scovil and associates[90] found that stored visuospatial information from the environment is needed for planning and executing a stepping reaction. These and other findings demonstrate the importance of vision for maintaining balance under challenging conditions.[91]

Older adults appear to have more difficulty using the built-in redundancy of the sensory systems linked to postural responsiveness.[92] Under typical circumstances, an adult will use vestibular input to resolve a conflict situation in which somatosensory cues indicate the body is moving and the visual cues do not indicate movement or vice versa. The vestibular system acts as the deciding vote as to whether we need to respond. Hay and colleagues[92] found that older adults were less stable in standing than younger adults when visual cues were removed. Both groups had difficulty when a vibratory stimulus was applied at the ankle, thus altering proprioceptive input. However, the older adults responded less well to having normal proprioceptive input restored than the younger adults. It appears that in addition to age-related changes in sensory receptors producing peripheral deficits, there also may be a slowing of central control mechanisms responsible for postural regulation. Conflicting sensory inputs were presented to the older adults to test the hypothesis that central processing is also involved in age-related changes of postural responsiveness. The older adults were much more affected by a combined conflicting situation that involved proprioceptive and visual information than were young adults.

Steady-State Balance

Humans exhibit a degree of spontaneous postural activity or sway when "standing still." Typically, this sway is considered an ongoing adjustment to or compensation for the effects of gravity and other subtle movements such as breathing, looking, and those associated with maintaining comfort through modulating weight bearing beneath the feet. Alternatively, this spontaneous sway may not be so spontaneous at all. If postural activity is an emergent feature imposed by the constraints of the individual and the environment, it may be that the variable sway serves an informational role as a search strategy providing postural control mechanisms in the CNS with continuous information about the individual's location in space via the stimulation of sensory systems.[93] In this case, spontaneous sway provides information in an a priori fashion rather than being something that is completely compensatory in nature.

Older adults have more spontaneous sway than younger persons.[33,94] This is a common finding in the research literature. However, it is important to understand that sway can be measured in a variety of ways. Most appropriately, sway implies body movement. This is often represented by the motion of the body's COM. However, most sway measurements capture dynamic aspects of the COP. COP is the point of application of the ground reaction force. As a location, the COP can be characterized by its amplitude (average position, path, and speed) or frequency (mean frequency of sway). With respect to the former, numerous studies have identified greater speed and range of COP motion in older adults as compared with younger adults.[33,95] On the other hand, frequency measures have shown mixed results.[95] Larger sway by older adults has been shown to be correlated with changes in sensory function as well as lower extremity muscle strength. However, it is unclear which is the cause and which is the effect: for example, are the changes in lower extremity muscle activity producing increased sway or is this activity in response to increased spontaneous sway?

Altering the sensory conditions during static standing affects older and younger adults differently. For example, older persons shift to a more asymmetrical standing posture when their eyes are closed than younger persons.[96] There are numerous studies that have identified increases in postural instability as a result of decreasing vision during standing.

ML sway is increasingly being used as a predictor of fall status in older adults. Maki and colleagues[97] found that lateral spontaneous sway under an eyes-closed condition was the single best predictor of falls in older persons when compared with a variety of postural control measures. Interestingly, lateral sway in older adults with a history of falling is more pronounced than in age-matched adults without a history of falling.[33] Standing in a near-tandem stance is particularly challenging to lateral balance, and older adults with a history of falling have difficulty with this task. ML sway increases with eyes closed, particularly for older people who have prospectively been determined to exhibit multiple falls. ML sway appears to be especially sensitive in this subgroup of elders. Impaired lower extremity proprioception, decreased quadriceps strength, and slow reaction time are the best predictors of increased sway in this posture.[98,99]

Anterior posterior sway as measured by COP velocity and Rhomberg quotient (RQ) increases when visual input is removed. This occurs more in people who fall rather than nonfallers. Therefore older adults' increased reliance on vision is an important feature of age-associated changes and puts older adults at increased risk of falls when RQ is higher.[100] RQ is the ratio between eyes closed and eyes open values for a sway variable. It measures a person's reliance on vision and quantifies the degree to which balance worsens when vision is removed.

Dynamic Balance

The interaction between posture and voluntary movement is what delineates dynamic standing balance from static standing balance. Internally generated, voluntary movements are perturbations to posture. That is, a self-generated, voluntary movement such as raising one's arm may be destabilizing. So-called APAs before or concomitant with an arm raise are necessary to prevent postural instability. In contrast, a voluntary movement of the lower extremity, such as during the process of standing on one foot, requires a lateral shift of the body's COM to unweight the stepping limb to achieve a new unipedal posture without a loss of balance. Evidence exists that for both arm and leg movements, older adults exhibit differences in postural control compared with younger adults.

Compared with movements of the arm, voluntary movements of the lower extremity pose additional and greater balance challenges to older persons. Gait initiation, stepping on or over an object, or sport-related actions such as kicking all require the transition from a bipedal to a unipedal stance configuration. The requisite postural adjustment in these examples is a lateral weight transfer before limb liftoff. Additionally, forward-oriented actions such as gait initiation also include an anterior-posterior postural adjustment.

Older adults are known to exhibit both delays in the reaction time of the prime mover and longer onset latencies of responses in the postural muscles necessary for stabilizing balance.[101] Rogers and associates[102] examined self-initiated and reaction time arm movements in older and younger adults. They found that when older adults were asked to raise an arm at their own pace, they were less likely to demonstrate the necessary lower extremity postural muscle activity before activating the shoulder prime mover. Moreover, older adults exhibited a significantly shorter interval between the contraction of the postural muscles and those responsible for the focal shoulder movement. Collectively, this suggests that aging may alter necessary APAs and affect the timing between postural and focal movement elements during voluntary arm movements.

Besides prolonged reaction time to initiating the focal movement, older adults exhibit a prolonged weight transfer time. Weight transfer is the postural adjustment, and weight transfer time represents the time to complete the postural adjustment. It has been determined that the prolonged time taken to transfer body weight off the stepping foot is actually of greater importance than the delays seen in reaction time for initiating the task itself.[103]

It is unclear why older adults generally take longer to perform the postural adjustment for lateral weight transfer during tasks such as step initiation. It may be partially attributable to changes in the torque-generating capacity of muscles important in accelerating the body's COM laterally, namely the hip abductors.[104] However, Jonsson and associates[105] suggest alterations in weight transfer are a function of the sequencing of forces during this phase as compared with the ability to generate absolute force. This suggests that problems of coordination between posture and movement may lie at the heart of the age-related changes in postural adjustments associated with leg movements. Data from a rhythmic

stepping in place task appear to support the contention that older persons adapt coordination to maintain balance and step performance during time-critical stepping.[106] "Specifically, both the excursion of COM motion and step length were reduced in older persons compared to younger and middle-aged adults in order to keep pace at higher metronome-paced stepping frequencies. Such change with age may reflect strategic adaptations to prolonged weight transfer times and to preserve balance during time-critical stepping."[106]

There is evidence that changes in step performance with age may be dependent on the type of step executed and the specific step-related conditions. Older adults take smaller steps than younger adults under voluntary step initiation conditions, but apparently do not take smaller steps during self-paced rhythmical stepping in place.[107-109] Additionally, protective steps induced by a large external perturbation also appear not to exhibit an age-related difference in step length.[103]

Step direction affects the amount of lateral weight transfer necessary to step or initiate gait. The COM does not need to be shifted as far for a lateral step versus a forward step. Therefore a side step requires less postural adjustment, that is step limb vertical ground reaction force, than a forward step.[110] Older adults, however, produce a greater peak vertical ground reaction force for lateral stepping than younger adults. This greater force results in a greater shift of the COM toward the stance limb. Older adults shift their weight toward the support limb more than younger adults. Collectively, a greater force combined with a longer time to produce the weight shift may be reflective of a safer, more conservative strategy being opted for by older persons. It is safer because the weight shift is greater and more conservative because the time taken to accomplish the postural adjustment is longer.

Previous and present level of activity or function also affects the postural adjustment necessary for step initiation in older persons. Physically active older adults exhibit postural and balance changes when initiating a step. Henriksson and Hirschfeld[111] found that older persons stand more asymmetrically than younger adults before initiating gait. The asymmetry may be an active compensation for the prolonged weight transfer times in older persons. Being more asymmetrical so that the stepping limb is relatively unloaded before a step requires less weight transfer during step initiation. Not surprisingly, weight transfer time is also prolonged during step initiation for lower-functioning older persons.[112]

As a response to an external perturbation, stepping was once thought to be a balance strategy of last resort.[113] This is no longer the case. Rogers and associates[114] found that stepping is a common balance strategy, and this response is conditioned by the context of the perturbation parameters applied to the subject. That is, the combination of perturbation direction, displacement, direction, and speed influences whether or not a stepping response occurs. However, instruction is also very important. Too often, research studies have instructed subjects to try not to step. Instructing a person to either "react naturally" or "try not to step" will elicit very different responses. A person is far more likely to step when given the instruction "react naturally."[115]

Pai, colleagues,[116] and associates[117] evaluated a dynamic mechanical model of the COM-BOS relationship and found that externally induced, protective stepping frequently occurred before the COM reached the limits of the BOS. Evidently, protective stepping does not depend solely on the mechanical constraint of the position of the COM exceeding the BOS. Stepping can no longer be considered a balance strategy of last resort, and it may actually be a preferred response under real-world conditions. Therefore clinical physical therapists should strongly consider focusing efforts toward the evaluation and treatment of stepping strategies over so-called ankle and hip strategies typically observed during very small perturbations or when the BOS is altered in an artificial manner such as standing perpendicular on a balance beam.

Older adults respond differently to external perturbations than do younger adults. Older persons tend to step more frequently, step to lower perturbation magnitudes, take multiple steps in response to larger perturbations, and often take a more laterally directed forward step than do younger adults given the same perturbation amplitude.[118,119] Importantly, the later second step, often laterally, is made because of a primary problem in arresting the COM velocity or terminating the step to regain a stable stance position.[103,120] The more laterally directed step is particularly evident for those older persons with a history of falling.

The timing of a protective step is also affected by age and fall status. Older persons tend to step as fast as younger persons when given an external perturbation.[121,122] However, older adult fallers have been shown to step *earlier* than older adults without a history of falling. This may be due to older adult fallers preplanning a step or, on the other hand, willingness by younger persons and older persons without a history of falling to be displaced further before initiating a step under similar conditions.

Lateral stability in the face of a lateral perturbation has continued to be studied in older adults.[118,119] As with anterior-posterior perturbations, older adults are more likely to step and take multiple steps to a lateral perturbation. When younger adults step, they typically respond with a side step of the limb in the direction of the perturbation (ipsilateral limb). The stepping limb is being passively loaded due to the direction of the perturbation. Stepping with the ipsilateral loaded limb requires significant power in order to unweight the limb and abduct it laterally to control the COM motion. Older adults, in contrast, tend to step with the opposite unloaded limb first and then take either a crossover step to the front or back or take a medial step followed by a second lateral step with the ipsilateral limb. While this affords a rapid response to the perturbation, the consequences include possible limb collision during a crossover step or smaller margins of stability at step termination.[118,119]

SUMMARY OF POSTURE AND BALANCE

Posture and balance rely on the sensory and motor subsystems of the CNS and the musculoskeletal system to influence age-related changes in the various types of postural control. In addition, the somatosensory, visual, and vestibular systems play a pivotal role in organizing responses to external disturbances of posture. It is important to recognize that many types of balance (static, dynamic, and reactive), as well as anticipatory and adaptive postural control, can be exhibited within a task-specific context. The ability to maintain a posture, whether standing still or while moving, is an ongoing challenge. Balance requires reacting to challenges appropriately and generating an anticipatory posture before the onset of overt movement. Lastly, adaptive postural control allows us to adapt to changing tasks and environmental conditions, including gravity, which protects us from losing balance.

Postural networks evolve during the course of early development. Changes in synaptic strength within the nervous system occur at a relatively rapid rate early and later in the human life span. These changes, which seem influenced by use, contribute to both the acquisition of postural abilities and their decline. The neural control of posture varies with age, and the acquisition and modulation of posture are dynamic processes that involve more than just the nervous system.

The effects of the musculoskeletal system on posture are related to physical growth. We grow when we are young. We get bigger and taller, and our body proportions change. These physical changes challenge the postural systems across the growing years. The anatomical structures of bone and muscle also change with age. These changes contribute to our ability to generate force, to be flexible, and to attain a certain stature. The acquisition and loss of spinal curves provide a perfect example of age-related change. The ability of the body to control the degrees of freedom of its segments changes over time as has been demonstrated in the development of postural control in sitting and standing.

During adulthood, activity level and experiences with different movements influence our weight and body dimensions, which then affect postural control. Physical dimensions vary with age, not only because of internally mediated growth processes but also psychological and sociocultural factors related to work, lifestyle, mental status, and activity level. The factors that contribute to age-related change in posture and balance are widely and richly varied. They range from decreased physical activity, sedentary behavior, lower extremity weakness, and poor balance to negative perception of health-related quality of life.[87,88] Understanding these various factors and their relationships leads to increased understanding not only of postural development but also of all motor development throughout the human life span.

LOCOMOTION

Locomotion is the act of moving from place to place by means of one's own mechanisms or power.[123] It is a task critical to independent function, reflecting our ability to move safely and efficiently from one place to another. Locomotion contributes to the ability to participate in meaningful work, leisure, and community activities. The essential elements of locomotion include progression, stability, and adaptation. We must have the strength and control necessary to progress toward a location, sufficient dynamic balance to maintain our posture and to overcome the force of gravity or other external forces,

and the ability to adapt the locomotor pattern to meet our needs and the demands of the environment.[9]

Exactly how we accomplish the task of getting from point A to point B depends on many factors: the exact task to be done, the interaction of our body systems that will perform the task, and the environment in which the task is to take place. For example, walking uphill, walking downhill, and walking in water are very different tasks than walking on a level, firm surface. Children, young adults, and older adults will all perform these tasks differently, depending on their size, strength, and balance. We will present the development of locomotion across the life span, focusing on walking (gait). Further, we will examine the interrelationships among the body systems of the individual, the environment, and the task. All three are equally important to an individual's ability to accomplish the desired movement.

The traditional method used to describe the development of locomotion patterns has been to divide the particular pattern into specific phases or component parts. Although the descriptive method of analysis has been beneficial, biomechanical analysis has provided a more in-depth and objective method for analyzing movements. Another consideration in recognizing the variety of movement patterns used by infants and children, as well as the rapid acquisition of new locomotor skills, takes into account the role of experience and practice on acquisition of efficient locomotor patterns. Description of locomotor patterns such as rolling, crawling and creeping, and walking are found in Chapter 3. The locomotor patterns that evolve after upright walking such as running, hopping, galloping, and skipping, otherwise known as fundamental motor skills, are also presented in Chapter 3. Present research into locomotor patterns has focused less on phases of skill acquisition and focused more on how the body and the environment develop together.[124] Motor behaviors are seen as providing the raw material for social interaction, perception, and cognition.[125–128]

Erect Walking

Walking is the act of moving on foot. *Ambulation* is another term that is used synonymously with walking. A third term, *gait*, refers to the manner in which a person walks. Gait can be described by several parameters of time and distance, including stride length, step length, cadence, and velocity. A complete *gait cycle* is defined as one complete stride of one limb. *Stride length* is the distance from the heel strike of one foot to the heel strike of that same foot. *Step length* is the distance from the heel strike of one foot to the heel strike of the other foot. *Cadence* or step frequency refers to the number of steps taken per unit of time and is usually reported as the number of steps per minute. *Walking velocity* is the measurement of distance per unit of time. It can be measured in several ways, for example, velocity in m/s = stride length (m/step) × cadence (steps/s) × 0.5. In the clinic, the term walking (gait) speed is used synonymously with walking velocity, but it is important to note that velocity is a vector quantity while speed is a scalar quantity. This means that all measurements made within the clinic expressed in distance per unit of time represent gait speed. It is simply the time taken to walk a known distance. Dividing the known distance by the time taken to traverse that distance gives a value in meters per second or sometimes feet per minute. Gait speed is the sixth vital sign and is considered a major measure of function.[129]

Walking is a complex task, where we must use all parts of the body in a coordinated manner. The muscular and skeletal systems provide the support and mechanical mechanisms to move, whereas the nervous system assists in controlling the walking pattern. Sensory information from the visual, proprioceptive, and vestibular systems allows us to navigate through an environment.

The erect walking pattern is defined as a two-phase pattern of movement in the upright position: the *stance phase*, which is approximately 60% of a complete gait cycle, and the *swing phase*, which is approximately 40% of a complete gait cycle. The stance phase provides stability, maintaining the body in an upright position against the force of gravity, whereas the swing phase is responsible for progressing the body forward through space. At the beginning and end of the stance phase, both lower extremities are in contact with the floor, referred to as *double limb support*. In a mature gait pattern, double limb support occurs in the first and last 10% of the stance phase.[9] The percent of time spent in double limb support varies as we walk slowly or quickly and at various times across the life span.

The upper and lower extremities move in a reciprocal pattern during walking and help to propel the body forward or backward in space. A 50% temporal and distance-phasing relationship exists between the lower limbs. As stated earlier, 50% phasing between the limbs indicates that when one limb is 50% completed with its cycle, the contralateral limb starts its cycle. According to Clark and Whitall,[130] newly walking infants coordinate their limbs in a 50% temporal phasing relationship, just like adults. These researchers revealed, however, that the young walkers exhibited significantly increased variability compared with infants who had been walking for 3–6 months. Once toddlers have a few months of walking experience, variability in their walking pattern decreases, and gait pattern characteristics, such as step length (normalized for limb length), step width, and walking skill, begin to resemble the gait of an older child or adult.[131] Most spatiotemporal gait parameters are significantly different across adults from 18–89 years old.[132] "Elderly populations show a reduction of preferred walking speed, cadence, step and stride length, all related to a more cautious gait, while gait variability measures remain stable over time."[132]

Body System Impact on Walking Control

How do we control the act of walking? Arm, leg, trunk, and head movements all work together to maintain balance as our center of gravity moves outside of the BOS, but how do we organize and control this finely coordinated movement?

The nervous system plays a key role in the control of walking. Early stepping movements and locomotor patterns are controlled by pattern generators in the spinal cord or the brain stem.[133,134] Initially, stepping, controlled only by these pattern generators, is stereotypic. The early stepping pattern that is produced is related to the pattern seen in reflex stepping and kicking in the infant.[135] Descending nervous system influences from the cerebellum contribute to the modulation of the gait pattern and error correction. This level of control helps fine-tune the gait pattern and assists us in walking over uneven terrain. The cortex also assists in the development of spatially directed movement. The visual cortex processes information from the environment so that perception and action can be linked.[136]

Sensory information is also critical to control locomotion, assisting in the adaptation of the gait pattern to the environment in which it is occurring. Visual information is an important stimulus for locomotion. The infant is first enticed to move and explore by seeing something or someone to move toward. Visual orientation also is important in aligning the body with the support surface. Visual flow information helps align the body in reference to the environment and helps in the assessment of walking speed. Self-produced loco-motion increases target-directed behavior in infants.[137] Walking infants travel farther to access a toy compared to crawlers.[138]

The somatosensory system contributes to the control of walking. Information from the muscle spindles and joint receptors contributes to the rhythm of walking, whereas the Golgi tendon organ influences timing of the transition from stance to swing phase of the gait cycle. Information from cutaneous receptors may also contribute to the ability to negotiate over obstacles. The vestibular system assists in alignment of the head in relationship to gravity, and the vestibulo-ocular reflex (VOR) is important for head stabilization in space. The vestibular system does not appear to contribute to head stabilization during walking until age 7 years. Children up to age 6 depend primarily on visual and somatosensory information to organize and control walking. This sensory information allows them to use an ascending temporal organization of balance control (feet/pelvis to head). As the visual and vestibular systems become more functional in modulating ambulation, descending temporal organization of balance control (from head to toe) is seen in the walking child.[139]

In adults, the lack of coordination between eye movements and locomotion may contribute substantially to the occurrence of falls. During normal ambulation and head movement, the VOR stabilizes gaze and therefore helps to keep the image of the environment stable on the retina. Looking down on the ground while walking to step over an obstacle is made possible by a highly coordinated fast eye-head movement. To perform such a movement, larger eye-head gaze shifts beyond the normal oculomotor range, which necessitates that the saccadic and vestibular signals be well coordinated. A saccade is a rapid eye movement that shifts the line of sight between points of fixation. Evidence indicates that age influences the function of VOR performance and suppression. According to Srulijes, older adults have a decreased ability to enhance and suppress the VOR, compared to young adults, which can make them more susceptible to falls.[140] In summary, the collective interactive effects of the neuromusculoskeletal system reveal a set of essential factors or requirements for safe and successful walking. These requirements include progression, stability, adaptability, long-term viability, and long-distance navigation.[141] Progression, the ability to walk from point A to point B, includes the generation of

a locomotor rhythm and the ability to produce sufficient joint torque and ground reaction forces to propel the body forward. Therefore stride characteristics and force or torque production are all relevant outcome variables associated with progression.

The COM is outside of the BOS during 80% of the walking cycle. Therefore stability is a major requirement for walking. Stability in walking implies an ability to proactively coordinate the body COM motion with stepping, adjust posture to environmental demands, and reactively adjust step length, height, and/or width to perturbations from the environment. The sensory system is integral to successful gait stability as are ongoing and rapid motor responses.

Adaptability is needed to take walking into real-world, functional contexts. Adjustments to the locomotor pattern are needed to accommodate and interact with the spaces, places, structures, and surfaces in the environment. Obstacles, stairs, ramps, curbs, grass, gravel, or other terrains all require an adaptable locomotor pattern. Vision is the primary sensory modality for the adjustment of the walking path and pattern when obstacles are present or terrain changes.[141,142]

Progression, stability, and adaptability are important for the short-term success of walking. To walk successfully for longer periods requires long-term viability. Long-term viability implies the minimization of stress on tissue and the minimization of energy expenditure. Stress on tissue is a factor when the musculoskeletal changes affect the gait pattern, as is sometimes the case when pain accompanies osteoarthritic changes to load-bearing lower extremity joints. Cardiovascular and strength changes also impact one's ability to maintain energy cost within a reasonable range. The use of assistive devices, more common with increased age, may also impact energy expenditure. Energy expenditure, more formally the metabolic cost of walking, has been reported to be greater in older adults than younger adults, with the difference appearing in the seventh decade.[143] The increase in metabolic cost in older adults appears to be due to age-related changes in muscles and the cardiovascular system.[144]

Metabolic cost is related to walking speed. Das Gupta and associates[145] found no difference in metabolic cost in healthy, fit older adults (mean age 75 years) and young adults (mean age 26 years) when using preferred overground walking speed. Older adults did have a higher metabolic cost when walking on a treadmill than young adults using the same preferred walking speed. Fitness levels and age related changes in muscles and the cardiovascular system can limit an older adult's mobility. Finally, to possess a truly successful gait pattern, one must be able to walk to locations where the destination is not seen at the outset. This ability to navigate long distances to unseen locations is not possible without adequate perception, memory, judgment, and cognitive spatial mapping.[18,146]

Developmental Stages

Infants and Toddlers

Independent ambulation is attained by 12.1 months of age in 50% of infants.[147] Until this point, the infant does not have sufficient strength or balance control of the head and trunk for independent walking. Extensor muscle strength is thought to be the critical variable in the development of independent locomotion.[135] Until sufficient strength is present, the stability component necessary for upright locomotion is absent. Infants also need to be able to coordinate their limb segments and adaptively deal with the challenges of environmental changes before they have sufficient control for the progression and adaptability components needed to walk.

The gait pattern of toddlers and children changes rapidly over the first months of walking and then continues to mature into childhood. The initial gait pattern is characterized by a wide BOS, arms held in a high guard position, short swing phase, lack of heel strike or push-off, and a need for the infant to propel themselves forward by leaning forward at the trunk. In addition, the new walker demonstrates less knee flexion in stance than an experienced walker and keeps the legs externally rotated during the swing phase. As the new walker gains balance and control of the upright position during movement, the gait pattern changes slowly into the mature gait pattern of the adult. At 2–3 years of age, the child walks with a reciprocal arm swing and demonstrates a heel strike. By approximately 3–4 years of age, the child's BOS has decreased to levels seen in mature walking, and time spent in single-limb stance during walking increases.[9,148,149] According to Sutherland and coworkers,[150] 98% of toddlers have a mature gait pattern by age 4. The gait pattern continues to be refined through 7 years of age. As previously described, the child initially uses somatosensory information and an ascending temporal organization of balance control during walking; then after age 7, a descending organization of balance is seen.[139]

The gait parameters of time and distance—step length and width, stride length, cadence, and walking velocity—all change as the physical characteristics of the child change. Step length increases as there is growth in stature and leg length. The taller and longer-legged a person, the bigger is the step length. Cadence of the infant is much greater than that of the adult. The number of steps taken per minute decreases gradually throughout childhood, with the biggest reduction seen during the first year of walking. Walking velocity increases with age in a linear manner from 1–3 years of age. From ages 4–7, the rate of change of walking velocity diminishes, but the relationship to age remains linear.[150] Changes in walking speed, cadence, and stride length from ages 1–12 are found in Table 11.3.

McGraw's[151] early observations and definitions of the development of erect locomotion reflect the gait changes discussed previously. She defined seven phases for the development of erect locomotion, which are illustrated in Fig. 11.7, using a hierarchical theoretical framework of motor control. In phase A, the *newborn or reflex stepping*, the infant is in a flexed posture when held upright, and attempts to step are the result of elicitation of the stepping reflex, a primitive reflex movement pattern. In phase B, *inhibition*, or the *static phase*, elicitation of the stepping reflex is not readily observed. The infant moves the body up and down, holding the feet in position. In phase C, *transition*, the infant may stand in position and stamp the feet, but there is no progression forward. In phase D, *deliberate stepping*, the infant attempts to step when held upright. In phase E, *independent stepping*, the infant takes steps independently. The early walker maintains hips and knees in slight flexion to bring the COM closer to the ground. At about 12–13 months of age, infants are learning to walk alone. In phase F, heel-toe progression, the more mature walker ambulates with a narrower BOS. Feet are closer together and show a heel-toe progression. The upper extremities are in low guard (shoulders in more of a neutral position with the elbows in extension), and the hips and knees are extended more. Phase G, *integration*, or *maturity of erect locomotion*, finds the arms down and moving reciprocally, synchronous with the movements of the lower extremities; out-toeing has been reduced, and pelvic rotation is present, along with the double knee lock pattern. In the double knee lock pattern, there is knee extension just before heel contact, but at the moment of heel contact, there is knee flexion to help absorb impact shock; then, as the

TABLE 11.3 Gait Parameters of Children From 1–12 Years of Age

Age (years)	Cadence (steps/min)	Cycle Time (s)	Stride Length (m)	Speed (m/s)
1	127–223	0.54–0.94	0.29–0.58	0.32–0.96
1.5	126–212	0.57–0.95	0.33–0.66	0.39–1.03
2	125–201	0.60–0.96	0.37–0.73	0.45–1.09
2.5	124–190	0.63–0.97	0.42–0.81	0.52–1.16
3	123–188	0.64–0.98	0.46–0.89	0.58–1.22
3.5	122–186	0.65–0.98	0.50–0.96	0.65–1.29
4	121–184	0.65–0.99	0.54–1.04	0.67–1.32
5	119–180	0.67–1.01	0.59–1.10	0.71–1.37
6	117–176	0.68–1.03	0.64–1.16	0.75–1.43
7	115–172	0.70–1.04	0.69–1.22	0.80–1.48
8	113—169	0.71–1.06	0.75–1.30	0.82–1.50
9	111–166	0.72–1.08	0.82–1.37	0.83–1.53
10	109–162	0.74–1.10	0.88–1.45	0.85–1.55
11	107–159	0.75–1.12	0.92–1.49	0.86–1.57
12	105–156	0.77–1.14	0.96–1.54	0.88–1.60

From Richards J, Levine D, Whittle MW. *Whittle's Gait Analysis*. 5th ed. Elsevier: 2012.
Approximate range (95% limits) for general gait parameters in free-speed walking by normal children of different ages (ages 1–7 years based on Sutherland et al., 1988).

body moves forward over the foot, the knee returns to extension for weight bearing during the stance cycle. These characteristics indicate a mature gait pattern and usually have developed by age 3 or 4.

From a motor control perspective, the development of the nervous system, and other factors such as strength and balance, contribute to the development of walking in infants and toddlers. Biomechanical factors influence the infant's acquisition of upright locomotion. Infants must have sufficient strength of the lower limbs and trunk to support themselves upright against gravity and sufficient balance control and coordination to maintain an upright body position. By 2–3 months, the infants' legs increase in weight to the degree that there is insufficient strength for moving them in a stepping pattern against gravity.

The COM of the beginning walker is located at the lower thoracic level, making balance control more difficult. The new walker attempts to improve balance control by using a wide BOS, with the hips abducted and externally rotated. This provides ML stability, but if the new walker's head moves out of the BOS in an anteroposterior direction, loss of balance occurs. There is more mediolateral movement than anteroposterior

movement in the gait pattern of new walkers. New walkers not only demonstrate more mediolateral motion but also more of a "stepping in place" pattern of movement, with more hip flexion than is seen in mature walking.[152,153] This pattern helps the new walker safely clear the foot during gait. With experience, the walker's BOS narrows, and forward progression over a planted foot is possible. The new walker uses muscle coactivation to stabilize an upright position and to decrease the degrees of freedom that have to be controlled. The gait pattern becomes more fluid and reciprocal as this muscle coactivation is released. Within a few months of walking, toddlers use the more mature model of walking, in which they efficiently and synchronously control posture over the stance leg as they swing the other leg forward. The pendulum action of the lower extremities in this more mature walking pattern is related to limb length but also depends on strength and intersegmental coordination of the limbs.[152] By 18–24 months the COM descends closer to the BOS, allowing the body to become more stable and begin reciprocal muscle action.

From a cognitive, motor learning perspective, experience and learning also make a significant contribution to the development of locomotor patterns. The infant

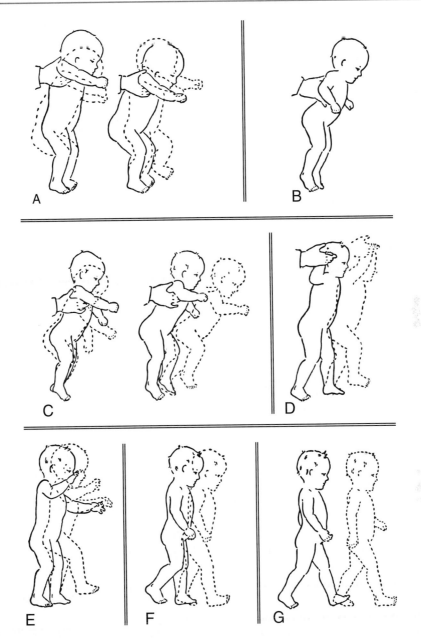

Fig. 11.7 The seven phases (A–G) of the assumption of the upright position. (From McGraw MB. *The Neuromuscular Maturation of the Human Infant.* New York: Hafner Press; 1945.)

demonstrates the ability to modify locomotor patterns as body size and body weight increase. With practice, the infant gains better control of intersegmental coordination of the limbs and body, making walking against the force of gravity more efficient.[152] The infant also must learn to adapt locomotor patterns when changing from quadruped patterns (creeping and plantigrade) to bipedal walking. In addition, they must adapt walking and locomotor skills to meet the challenges of a variety of support surfaces (tile, wood, carpet, grass, etc.), to adjust to obstacles in their path, and to meet challenges such as ascending/descending a sloped surface, uneven terrain, and so on. This learning is supported by the infant's development of information-processing strategies and by spending vast amounts of time practicing skills. Infants have demonstrated that they practice walking an accumulated 6 hours per day, taking approximately 9000 steps over the length of approximately 29 football fields.[131] These infants use a distributed practice model interspersing short bursts of walking with rest periods.[131] The infant also practices over approximately a dozen different types of surfaces in a day, which introduces the model of variable and random practice schedules into the learning of walking.[131] Infants learn from their experiences while creeping and walking to adapt to challenging situations. Experience helps infants adapt to situations and safely move through their environment.[124,154]

Children and Adolescents

A child demonstrates a mature gait pattern between 3 and 4 years of age and continues to use an ascending organization of postural control with somatosensory information. On level surfaces, some influence of vestibular control is noted as the child begins to use an HSSS.[155] Consistent heel strike and knee flexion in early stance are present. A mature muscle activation pattern is also exhibited in electromyography. Further refinements in the temporal and spatial aspects of the gait pattern occur between 5 and 6 years of age and continue to change with child growth until adult values are reached at approximately 15 years of age.[148] Step speed and step length are greater in the 6-year-old than in the 5-year-old. The 5-year-old also spends more time in double limb support than the older child. By the age of 7 years, the time spent in a single-limb stance during gait is nearly that seen in the adult.[9] Ground reaction forces generated during gait may also continue to increase into the sixth year.[156]

Dynamic balance is associated with interlimb coordination. Mani and associates[157] studied interlimb coordination and torso coordination during gait in children aged 3–10 years of age. Contralateral coordination involves movement of the ipsilateral arm and contralateral leg together. Contralateral coordination gradually changed to an in-phase pattern with increasing age until age 9 years. Contralateral coordination and trunk/pelvis coordination were significantly correlated in the 5- to 6-year-olds and in the 7- to 8-olds. More than half the body mass is represented by the trunk and pelvis which

greatly affects balance and gait stability.[158] "Development of COM displacement during gait is a gradual process, evolving until 7 years of age."[159] At this age, the child's COM has descended to the level of the L_5 vertebra.[160] Mani and associates[157] "found no significant difference between young adults and 3–10 year [old] children in phase coupling movement between the trunk and pelvic twist movement." The range of motion in the trunk and pelvis becomes adult-like at 7–8 years of age.

The HSSS is used in a variety of walking environments by 7 years of age.[155] The gain of the vestibular ocular reflex does not reach adult levels until at least 7 years of age.[161] With this level of visual and vestibular maturation, the child is now able to stabilize using a descending temporal organization of postural control.

Anticipatory control of locomotion is not fully developed until early adolescence.[18] APAs are defined as muscle activation and COP displacements that occur before a movement.[162] APAs are often studied when the person is standing and performs a reaching task[163] or when the person is walking toward a target. Belmonti and associates[146] studied individuals from 4 to 35 years of age while performing a simple locomotor reaching task driven by target location. Locomotor trajectories were assessed during the task. They found that head anticipation of walking direction and head stabilization to gravity are fully developed around 11–13 years of age. Anticipatory, trajectory-based locomotor control becomes smoother in adolescence and is consistent with having an accurate representation of external space. This appears to be a crucial achievement of adolescence.[146]

Adults

The gait pattern of the adult was presented earlier when erect walking was introduced. The adult efficiently uses walking as a primary means of locomotion and to carry out daily tasks. Being able to walk is the most fundamental mobility task and is the key criteria for functional independence. Preferred walking speed of healthy adults between the ages of 30 and 59 is about 1.43 m/s.[164] An adult can vary gait velocity when dashing across a busy street, walking up or down a hill, or walking for long distances. While maintaining an erect posture and when normal muscle strength and endurance are present, the adult easily performs walking. In adulthood, the COM has descended to the sacral level, further improving gait stability. The walking adult easily changes pace, initiates and stops, and changes direction.

Mobility characteristics are being used to discriminate between young, middle age, and older adults. Researchers Swanson and Fling[165] found that only one mobility test, the 360-degree turn discriminated between young and middle-aged adults. Numerous walking and turning measures were able to discriminate between middle-aged and older adults. The significant differences in mobility between middle-aged and older adults in this study[165] support Terrier and Reynard's conclusions[166] that gait instability starts to increase as early as ages 40–50.

Older Adults

Does the gait pattern change as we age? A decline in mobility is initiated in the fifth decade of life with further decline seen with increased age.[165] The gait pattern of older adults differs from that of younger individuals in several areas. Some of the common changes are listed in Table 11.4. Are similar gait pattern changes seen in all older adults? Although many of the body systems that support walking change with age (see Chapters 5–9), it should also be noted that psychosocial factors, perception of one's own abilities, or others' expectations of older adults' abilities may also contribute to changes in gait pattern. Much variation exists within the older adult population. Healthy, active older adults in their 60s–70s may walk using the same pattern as a younger population. Twenty percent of adults in their 80s walk normally, so gait abnormalities are not necessarily inevitable.[167] Older adults who have a chronic illness, such as arthritis, diabetes, or heart disease, may demonstrate pathological gait deviations or exaggerated gait changes. The pain of arthritis, the sensory loss accompanying diabetes, and the lack of endurance seen in patients with cardiac disease will all affect the gait pattern. Gait impairments often coexist with cognitive decline in people with neurodegenerative disease such as Parkinson disease. Gait is an activity that requires attention and executive function.[168]

Falling is more of a problem as adults continue to age and its effects translate to a major health issue for the older adult population. See Clinical Implications Box 11.1. Attempts to clarify the relationship between aging and walking date back to at least the early 1940s and continue today. This is quite difficult due to the multifactorial nature of the gait process. Research provides conflicting information about exactly how the gait of older adults changes with age. It is necessary to carefully study

TABLE 11.4 Gait Pattern Changes in the Older Adult

Gait Changes	Characteristics
Associated with normal aging	Decreased gait velocity Decreased stride length Decreased peak hip extension Decreased peak knee extension range of motion Decreased peak knee flexion in swing Decreased ankle plantar-flexion power
Associated with decreased strength	Increased pelvic tilt, due to abdominal weakness Decreased vertical displacement of body Decreased gait velocity Decreased cadence, due to ankle dorsiflexion weakness Concentric weakness of ankle plantar flexors
Associated with decreased stability and balance	Increased base of support Decreased gait velocity Decreased dynamic stability Increased time in double limb support Increased step width Increased use of visual scanning Inability to ignore erroneous visual information Decreased somatosensory signals

From Berard J, Fung J, Lamontagne A. Impact of aging on visual reweighting during locomotion. *Clin Neurophysiol.* 2012;123L1422-1428; Franz JR, Francis CA, Allen MS, O'Connor SM, Thelen DG. Advanced age brings a greater reliance on visual feedback to maintain balance during walking. *Hum Mov Sci.* 2015;40:381-392; Terrier P, Reynard F. Effect of age on the variability and stability of gait: a cross-sectional treadmill study in healthy individuals between 20 and 69 years of age. *Gait Posture.* 2015;41:170-174; Osaba MY, Rao AK, Agrawal SK, Lalwani AK. Balance and gait in the elderly: a contemporary review. *Laryngoscope Investig Otolaryngol.* 2019;4:143-153; and Yamaguchi T, Masani K. Effects of age on dynamic balance measures and their correlation during walking across the adult lifespan. *Nature.* 2022;12:14301.

healthy older adults and to try to separate out the gait pattern changes that are related solely to increasing age.

Progression. The most commonly reported findings when studying the gait of older persons is a slower

CLINICAL IMPLICATIONS BOX 11.1
Falling in Older Adults and Its Prevention

Falling is a common problem in older adults, often resulting in injury and hospitalization. Older adults with a history of falling exhibit some differences in their gait pattern when compared with older adults without a history of falling. These gait pattern differences can be exacerbated because after a fall, the older adult may become less active, fearing and trying to prevent another fall. Further changes in the gait pattern may be made in an attempt to increase safety during ambulation. Decreased activity levels may eventually lead to decreased levels of functional independence, and limited mobility may negatively affect quality of life.

Several factors have been identified that contribute to the increased incidence of falling in older adults, some of which are summarized here. There are also several strategies that can help in the prevention of falls in the older adult, improving functional independence and health status.

Characteristics of Gait Pattern in Older Adults Who Have Fallen
- Decreased stride length compared with nonfallers.[169]
- Decreased walking speed compared with nonfallers.[169]
- Decreased walking speed and cadence with increased double support time, especially when the person is concerned about a fall[170] and under dual task (e.g., walking when talking) conditions.[171]
- A conservative approach (i.e., taking numerous small steps) when approaching an obstacle.[169]
- Mediolateral instability in standing (more predictive of falls than anteroposterior instability).[172]
- Greater stride frequency across a range of imposed gait speeds and an inability to obtain the highest imposed gait speed.[173]
- Increased stride to stride variability.[115,173]

Kinematics
- Reduced hip extension[173]
- Reduced plantar flexion[173]
- Decreased trunk rotation and increased knee flexion[169]

Kinetics
- Increased hip flexion moment in stance; decreased hip extension moment in stance; decreased knee flexion moment in preswing; decreased knee power absorption in preswing.[174]

Possible Factors Contributing to Falls in Older Adults
- Difficulty corralling the body COM in response to a perturbation requiring multiple steps.[103]
- Disproportionately greater medial-lateral instability compared with nonfallers.[175]
- Difficulty modulating step length quickly enough to avoid an obstacle.[176]
- Speed and length of the step are less than they are in younger adults.[107]
- Slower rate of ankle torque development in response to a trip, making it more difficult to regain balance.[177]
- Increased difficulty performing another task while walking.[171,178]
- Impairments in hip abductor torque-generating capacity and decreased trunk axial rotation.[175]

Intervention Strategies for Fall Prevention
- Reduce risk factors for falls.[179,180]
- Multifactorial fall risk assessment and management programs.[181–183]
- Physical activity and specific exercise programs that include a balance training component.[183–185]
- For the individual at high risk for falls, it may be beneficial to include a home hazard assessment and modification.[183]
- Shoes with low heels and firm slip-resistant soles should be worn both inside and outside the home.[186]
- Therapeutic exercise and balance training for positive outcomes of increased balance, increased lower extremity strength and balance, increased safety, increased physical and functional capacity, and increased ability to perform instrumental and basic activities of daily living.[187,188]

---

walking speed compared with younger adults.[164,189–191] Gait velocity decreases about 1% annually after age 60.[167] Recalling that gait velocity is the product of stride length and cadence, it is important to evaluate all three gait parameters of progression together. Coinciding with a slower walking velocity is a shorter step length, longer stance phase, and shorter swing time than younger adults.[132,192] Gait speed decreases from approximately 1.43 m/s for adults aged 30–59 years to 0.95 m/s for individuals in their 80s.[167] At self-selected walking speeds, the stride of older adults is typically shorter than that of younger adults. Cadence, on the other hand, has not always demonstrated a significant change with age in healthy older persons.[167] Older adults may choose to walk slower for stability purposes, but more likely, there are multiple factors that play a role in the progressive slowing of gait with age.[191] These factors include a decline in the strength and integrity of the musculoskeletal system,[193] decline in aerobic capacity,[194] and psychological changes.[195] The most often used cutoff score for slow gait speed is 0.8 m/s.[196] This same cutoff value is an indicator of sarcopenia and an increased mortality risk.[197,198]

The decline in gait velocity at comfortable walking speeds is not the same across decades. Persons in their 60s and 70s generally maintain a stable gait speed but then show more marked decline in their 80s and 90s.[164,191] Maximum walking speed declines more steadily throughout adulthood.[167]

Kinematics. Changes in gait speed and stride length are associated with reductions in joint motion. Changes in ankle range of motion and pelvic obliquity have been noted in older adults.[199] Ankle plantar flexion at terminal stance can be decreased and the anterior pelvic tilt increased.[200,201] Peak knee extension range of motion is also significantly decreased in the older adult compared with the younger adult.[199,202]

A significant reduction in hip extension motion is seen even during faster walking in healthy older persons.[203] This is an important finding because it implies that the reduced range of motion is not simply a function of walking slower. An even greater reduction in hip extension is associated with older persons who have a history of falls. In both cases, this reduction in hip extension has been attributed to hip joint tightness.[204,205] However, simply stating it is a problem of static tightness at the hip is an insufficient explanation because this tightness is not manifested in the standing position. That is, the reduced hip extension is observed only during gait.[201]

Kinetics. Reductions in gait speed and stride length are associated with reductions in joint torque and ground reaction forces. However, it is unclear which finding is the cause and which is the effect. The difficulty with maintaining maximum walking speed appears to be related to an older adult's inability to generate as great a peak ankle plantar-flexor moment as a younger adult.[200] Winter and colleagues[206] found that even fit, healthy older persons exhibit a decreased plantar-flexor push-off power burst. Power is the rate of doing work over time, or put simply, it is force times velocity. They

also found a reduction in knee absorption power. No differences were noted for hip kinetics. Judge and colleagues[200] also found reduced ankle plantar-flexor power. After adjusting for step length differences between older and younger adult groups, they found that older adults tend to rely instead on increasing hip flexion power in late stance to increase speed.[200] Interestingly, the age-related differences in ankle kinetics disappeared when the step length was accounted for. It appears that older persons may increase hip kinetics as a compensation for reductions in distal joint kinetic function.[207,208]

Stability. Dynamic stability in gait depends on predictive, anticipatory, and reactive strategies. Age-related decline in anticipatory postural responses occurs during gait initiation. Gait initiation from a standing position involves a preparatory weight shift and forward lean.[209] Older adults demonstrate a decreased quality of the anticipatory weight shift prior to stepping that increases their fall risk.[210] Laundini and colleagues[209] found that older adults used a more cautious stepping strategy than young adults in response to an external waist perturbation applied during gait initiation. The younger adults were able to delay the timing of their APAs to preserve balance of the upcoming step.

Balance control differs between young and old while performing steady-state walking.[211] Older adults, as has been previously noted, walk with a wider step width. Wider foot placement during a single-limb stance combined with vertical ground reaction forces results in rotation of the body toward the contralateral leg. Older adults do not shift their COM as close to their stance foot as young adults, making ML balance more challenging. Exercise programs should target strengthening hip abductors and ankle plantar flexors and practice appropriate lateral weight transfer to improve frontal plane balance in older adults.[211] According to Nnodim and colleagues,[167] at least 33% of community-dwelling older adults have difficulty with gait, requiring medical equipment or assistance of another person to safely ambulate. The assistance or assistive device use increases with age from approximately 15% at age 60 to 82% by age 85.

The balance capabilities of older persons have been extensively studied, and there are numerous studies that suggest many of the gait adaptations observed during progression (e.g., reduced speed and stride length) are manifested to maintain balance or stability. For example, Shkuratova and associates[212] had a small group of healthy older adults change speed and walk in a figure eight pattern and assessed walking stability via temporal gait parameters. A major finding was that older persons did not adjust their maximal walking speed to the same extent as younger persons. Older persons were able to walk faster than their comfortable gait speed, but speed and stride length were reduced compared with younger adults. There were nonsignificant reductions in speed and stride length by older persons compared with younger persons during turns within the figure eight walking task. Collectively, these adaptations were seen as modifications to gait to maintain stability. Given that Maki and McIlroy[33] had shown a significant relationship between slower gait and smaller steps and fear of falling in older persons, it is reasonable to argue that these temporal and spatial gait changes are adaptive in order to maintain stability.

Menz and colleagues[213] also suggested that reductions in gait speed and step length (along with an increased step timing variability) by older persons are representative of a more conservative gait pattern. Stability was thought to be preserved because such a pattern reduces the magnitude of accelerations at the head and pelvis. Accelerations of major body segments near the body COM (pelvis) and segments containing important sensors for the successful maintenance of the gait pattern (vision and vestibular apparatus within the head segment) could be potentially destabilizing to an older person. Anterior-posterior trunk accelerations at push-off have also been observed to be lower in older persons.[214] As such, reductions in gait speed and step length may be a compensatory mechanism to preserve stability.

Mazza and colleagues[215] used upper body accelerations and the analysis of harmonic ratio as a means to understand how younger and older persons stabilize the head during walking. It is likely that younger persons synchronize accelerations in the upper body and attenuate these accelerations to maintain a stable head and thus a stable gaze during walking. A stable gaze is clearly an important feature of a stable gait because it enables the effective use of vision to adjust the gait pattern. Older adult women in the study did not attenuate head accelerations to the same extent as younger adult women.

Pavol and associates[216,217] used an innovative research paradigm to investigate the nature of balance during walking in older adults. They induced a trip during mid- to late swing using a concealed, mechanical obstacle that rose from the floor 5.1 cm. Those older adult subjects who walked faster and/or had less response time to recover were more likely to trip than those who walked slower. This was true irrespective of the effectiveness of the reactive stepping response elicited as a result of the trip. They concluded that not hurrying reduced the likelihood of falling as a result of a trip. In a follow-up study using modeling techniques, van den Bogert and associates[218] contended that there is a critical body lean angle (26 degrees) beyond which recovery from a trip is not possible. That is, the tripped foot must contact the ground before this forward body tilt is reached. Moreover, response time is an important determinant of the potential for a recovery from a trip. Response time is made up of several neuromuscular processes such as detection of the perturbation via sensory channels, reflexes in the lower extremities, and the actual execution of the protective stepping response.

The findings highlighted here imply that with respect to the requirements of walking, stability is a key requirement for successful walking in older persons. It is likely that the neuromusculoskeletal system is marshaled in such a way as to preserve stability during gait for older persons. Walking slower may be an adaptive strategy for the preservation of stability in older adults. However, much remains to be evaluated with respect to the assessment of balance control during walking in older adults. Specifically, much more needs to be done to assess both the anticipatory and reactive balance mechanisms necessary for a safe and efficient walking pattern.

Adaptability. Adaptability of gait is important when encountering varying terrains or surfaces in the environment and/or when encountering obstacles in the walking path. Several studies[219–222] have identified differences in the adaptability of gait in older persons. Swing foot clearance was the same for older and younger adults, but older adults used a more conservative strategy for obstacle clearance. This strategy included slower speed, shorter steps, and a shorter obstacle-heel strike distance. One study found decreased toe clearance of the lead foot,[220] but this was not a ubiquitous finding in the literature. Finally, older adults appear to increase hip flexion on the leading swing leg to maintain a safe distance between the foot and the obstacle.[219] Differences in findings between these studies may be related to the nature and form of the to-be-avoided obstacle.

The use of a conservative strategy was borne out in a systematic review of obstacle-crossing deficits in older adults.[223] Young and old adults were less likely to contact obstacles when adequate time was available to adapt foot placement. Older adults were slower and utilized greater hip flexion, hip adduction, and ankle dorsiflexion of the lead and trail limbs. There is emerging evidence that poor stepping accuracy and stepping errors are more common in older adults under unpredictable obstacle and stepping conditions.[176] Older adults' adaptations include slow, short steps and increased multiple steps while spending more time in double support. The ability to adjust gait is crucial for safe performance of activities of daily living. Reduced gait adaptability puts older adults at increased risk for falls when negotiating unexpected hazards.

Long-term viability. Walking is one of the most often recommended exercises for health promotion in older individuals. It is recommended that older adults walk at least 5000 steps daily to decrease their risk for falling.[224] Others encourage even more steps (7000–10,000) to gain health benefits.[225] Older adults who exhibit slower gait speed and increased walking variability may be at increased risk for falls.[226] Fear of falling and fatigue can be barriers for older adults walking long distances for health. Gait variability and gait asymmetry have been used as indirect ways to measure fatigue.[227] At 30 minutes of treadmill walking, older adults displayed significantly higher variability and asymmetry at the ankle, implying greater instability. Walking for an additional 30 minutes further increased the variability. Zhang and colleagues[228] documented changes in walking kinematics in older adults after a continuous 60-minute brisk walk using inertial measurement units. Sixteen of the 18 participants reported fatigue. Significant differences were found in kinematic variables that could indicate walking instability.

Long-distance navigation. Long-distance navigation refers to the ability to navigate to an unseen destination. This requirement for successful walking is not related to energy expenditure but to the development and maintenance of cognitive spatial maps for navigating through realistic environments. Visual perturbations and lighting changes within the environment being traversed can negatively impact gait parameters even in healthy older adults.[229,230]

BODY SYTEM INTERACTIONS RELATED TO LOCOMOTION

Structural and functional changes occur in all of the body systems with aging (see Chapters 5–10). The musculoskeletal, cardiovascular, pulmonary, neurological, and sensory systems contribute most to walking. Changes in these systems, seen from infancy through older adulthood, affect the development and refinement of the gait pattern.

Musculoskeletal System

Infants cannot support themselves in a standing position or walk because of insufficient strength to support the body against gravity and insufficient range of motion to fully extend their hips in the standing position. Through infancy, muscle mass increases and the infant achieves the ability to stand and walk. Changes from lower extremity varus in the beginning walker to a more valgus posture in the 3-year-old influence heel and foot position during gait. In children, the gait pattern changes with increasing length of the limbs and increasing muscle strength. With increasing lower extremity length, the stride length increases. Increasing strength allows the infant to exert greater forces when pushing off from the support surface. As toddlers gains more strength for push-off, they take longer steps and walk faster.[231] Running cannot occur until the child can generate sufficient force to push into a flight phase.

Changes in the musculoskeletal system with aging are described in detail in Chapter 5. Alterations in muscle spindle structure and function (increased capsular thickness, decreased number of intrafusal fiber, and reduced spindle diameter) result in reduced muscle spindle sensitivity in older adults.[98] There is also a decrease in type II muscle fibers, a decrease in the number of functional motor units, and changes in the muscle tissue with increased fat content and fibrin within the muscle fibers.[232] Muscle strength loss is one of the main causes of a decline in activities of daily living in the older adult population.[233] It has been suggested that the changes observed in the locomotion patterns and reduced gait velocity of older adults are most likely the result of decreases in muscular strength and flexibility.[189,200,234,235] Strengthening exercise programs have been shown to increase walking speed, cadence, and stride length of older adults.[234,236–239] Gait speed correlates with maximum voluntary plantar flexion strength and knee extension strength in older adults.[238] Increased cadence was found to be related to increased ankle dorsiflexion strength, whereas increased stride was found to be related to increased hip extension strength.[240] Decreased plantar flexion strength has also been thought to reduce step length and increase time in double limb support.[241] Decreased knee extension strength affects maximum walking speed, whereas hip abductor strength affects comfortable walking speed.[242]

The coordination of musculature within the locomotor pattern may undergo adaptive changes with aging. Therefore older adults should be evaluated both at the component level of walking (e.g., individual muscle activity) and at the locomotor pattern level. This level of control is clearly influenced by changes in sensory and motor systems but also possesses its own unique dynamic properties with respect to coordination among the segments within the lower extremity (intralimb coordination) and between limbs (interlimb coordination). Age-related deterioration has been observed in interlimb coordination.[243] Performing interlimb coordination at slow speeds increases attentional demand in older adults.[244]

Cardiovascular and Pulmonary Systems

The cardiovascular and pulmonary systems are important for providing fuel to the body tissues active in walking. Under normal conditions, cardiovascular and pulmonary function should be adequate to support walking. Typical cardiovascular changes in older adults reduce maximum aerobic capacity, peak exercise cardiac response, and maximum heart rate, but in healthy, nonfrail older adults do not impact nonmaximum activities such as gait.[245,246] In general, physically active and fit individuals of any age should be able to easily walk and complete their daily activities. In deconditioned individuals, walking uses a much higher proportion of the energy reserve than when we are conditioned, and everyday functional activities and walking may become too strenuous for someone with severe deconditioning.

Nervous System

The nervous system is crucially important for postural control, balance, and provision of sensory information needed for walking. Children begin to walk at approximately 1 year of age, but their gait pattern becomes more refined and coordinated over the next 6 years. Factors such as myelination of the nervous system, dendritic formation, and the number of functional motor units contribute to the development and quality of walking. Mobile infants are motivated to explore their environment and seek social and perceptual experiences. Through infancy and young childhood, biopsychosocial factors contribute to movement skill acquisition. In older adulthood, the number of dendrites and functional motor units decreases, as does nerve conduction velocity as a result of changes in myelin and the motor unit itself. These changes with age can contribute to increased reaction time and changes in the gait pattern.

The ability to perceive and use sensory input is critical to functional gait. In older adults, cutaneous sensory receptors are not as efficient as in younger adults. Overall, there is decreased foot position sense with age. Diminished proprioception is seen, especially at the ankles. Reduced proprioceptive acuity is associated with decreased lateral stability.[99] Touch sensitivity threshold can more than double in adults 62–83 years of age.[98] Vibration sense in lower extremity joints is also reduced. Balance is almost four times more impaired by reduced proprioception than by visual input.[98] Reduced reaction time will also affect gait.

Visual and vestibular function also decrease especially after age 65. The VOR and vestibulo-spinal reflexes deteriorate.[98] Loss of both visual and proprioceptive input can occur. Likely, loss of vision has a greater impact, as Jeka and colleagues[247] found older adults with high fall risk tended to weight visual stimuli higher than fall-prone older adults. More than one sensory input can be used to direct or modify balance. However, with aging, this built-in redundancy is reduced due to a decline in central processing ability. Poor sensory integration may increase the cognitive load needed to control balance in older adults. All these factors are thought to contribute to decreased gait velocity, increased gait variability, and increased risk of falls.

"Cautious" gait is characterized by slower walking speed, reduced step length (short stride), increased variability in timing of steps, wide base, and short swing phase.[213,226] Older subjects were more likely to exhibit this gait adaptation when walking on an irregular surface.[213] The researchers postulated that older adults in this study used adaptation to stabilize the head and pelvis to compensate for lower extremity weakness. Herman and colleagues[248] found that older individuals with a cautious gait had a significantly increased gait variability compared with age-matched older adults without a cautious gait pattern. Variability was associated with scores on the Geriatric Depression Scale and a measure of fear of falling.

Gait speed is associated with falls in community-dwelling older adults.[249] Lower gait speed is associated with indoor falls and higher gait speed with outdoor falls and higher activity levels.[250] Kyrdalen and colleagues'[249] study found that gait speed with a cutoff of 1.0 m/s could be useful in identifying older adults at risk for falls. A systematic review of measurement protocols for assessing gait speed in older adults found differences in equipment used, walking distance, timing points, use of walking aids, and number of trials as well as units of measurement.[251] The "gold standard" for recording speed is a stopwatch because it is simple and produces accurate results.[252] Based on their systematic review, Mehmet and associates[251] "recommend the following protocol for the measurement of gait speed in older adults: the person proceeds at a normal walking pace (walking aids permitted) in a straight line on a flat surface from a standing start over a distance of 9.0 m. The first 2.5-m distances are untimed (acceleration phase), the time taken to traverse the next 4.0 m is recorded with a handheld stopwatch, and

then the patient has a further 2.5 m to come to a standstill (deceleration phase). The fastest of two consecutive trials is recorded and is expressed as meters per second." The recommended protocol is suitable for clinical and community settings and would provide comparable outcome measurements. If clinic space allows, a majority of the research involves a similar test that utilizes a longer distance. The 10-Meter Walk Test is considered the gold standard for gait speed.[129,253] The 10-Meter Walk Test requires a 20-meter (m) straight path, with 5 m for acceleration, 10 m for steady-state walking, and 5 m for deceleration. Only the 10-m middle distance is timed.[129] Fig. 11.8 provides additional information regarding physical function as it relates to gait speed.

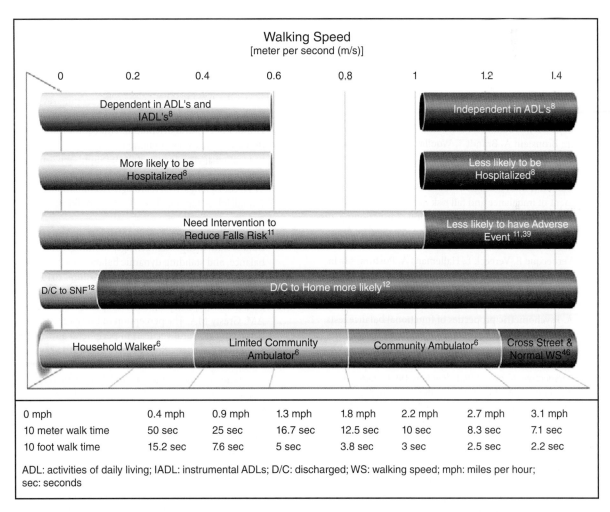

Fig. 11.8 Walking speed. (From Fritz S, Lusardi M. White paper: "walking speed: the sixth vital sign". *J Geriatr Phys Ther*. 2009;32:46-49.)

SUMMARY OF LOCOMOTION

Locomotion is a functional necessity of our lifestyle as humans. Parents celebrate and remember the first time their baby rolls, crawls, creeps, and takes a step, marking these functions as sociocultural milestones. The ability to move independently from one place to another is important to our independence and identity. In a rehabilitation setting, the first question a patient or their family often asks is, "When will the person walk again?" The person may need assistance in the form of a cane, walker, or a wheelchair.

Locomotion develops across the life span. The transition from using one form of locomotion to another depends on a number of factors: the interactions of the tasks to be accomplished, body systems' function, and the environment in which the behavior is to be produced. The change in locomotor patterns across the life span charts a bell curve, first becoming more efficient and then potentially becoming less efficient and possible unsafe. The challenges to locomotion for the older adult may include trips and falls, or failure to negotiate obstacles. Balance and gait instability are health risks that can negatively impact a person's quality of life. Therapists can better help individuals of all ages improve their functional independence and quality of life when they appreciate factors that contribute to efficient locomotion at all points across the life span.

REFERENCES

1. Venes D. Taber's Cyclopedic Medical Dictionary. 24th ed. Philadelphia: FA Davis; 2021.
2. Huxham FE, Goldie PA, Patla AE. Theoretical considerations in balance assessment. *Aus J Physiother.* 2001;47:89–100.
3. Massion J, Woollacott MH. Posture and equilibrium. In: Bronstein A, Brandt T, Woollacott M, eds. *Clinical Disorders of Balance Posture and Gait.* London: Arnold; 1996:1–18.
4. Cameron MH, Nilsagård YE. Measurement and treatment of imbalance and fall risk in multiple sclerosis using the international classification of functioning, disability and health model. *Phys Med Rehabil Clin N Am.* 2013;24:337–354.
5. Verbecque E, Vereeck L, Hallemans A. Postural say in children: a literature review. *Gait Posture.* 2016;49: 402–410.
6. Verbecque E, Lobo Da Costa PH, Vereeck L, Hallemans A. Psychometric properties of functional balance tests in children: a literature review. *Dev Med Child Neurol.* 2015;57:521–529.
7. Massion J. Postural control systems in developmental perspective. *Neurosci Biobehav Rev.* 1998;22:465–472.
8. Assaiante C, Amblard B. An ontogenetic model of the sensorimotor organization of balance control in humans. *Hum Mov Sci.* 1995;14:13–43.
9. Shumway-Cook A, Woollacot MH. *Motor Control: Translating Research into Clinical Practice.* 5th ed. Philadelphia: Wolters Kluwer; 2017.
10. Sibley KM, Beauchamp MK, Van Ooteghem K, Paterson M, Wittmeier KD. Components of standing postural control evaluated in pediatric balance measures: a scoping review. *Arch Phys Med Rehabil.* 2017;98:2066–2078. e4.
11. Sibley KM, Beauchamp MK, Van Ooteghem K, Straus SE, Jaglal SB. Using the systems framework for postural control to analyze the components of balance evaluated in standardized balance measures: a scoping review. *Arch Phys Med Rehabil.* 2015;96:122–132. e29.
12. Horak FB. Postural orientation and equilibrium: what do we need to know about neural control of balance to prevent falls? *Age Ageing.* 2006;35(Suppl 2):ii7–ii11.
13. Campbell WW, Barohn RJ. Muscle tone. In: Campbell WW, ed. *DeJong's The Neurologic Examination.* 7th ed. Philadelphia: Lippincott Williams & Wilkins; 2019:467–474.
14. Conner BC, Petersen DA, Pigman J, et al. The cross-sectional relationships between age, standing static balance, and standing dynamic balance reactions in typically developing children. *Gait Posture.* 2019;73: 20–25.
15. Bisdorff AR, Wolsley CJ, Anastasopoulos D, Bronstein AM, Gresty MA. The perception of body verticality (subjective postural vertical) in peripheral and central vestibular disorders. *Brain.* 1996;119(Pt 5):1523–1534.
16. Karnath HO, Fetter M, Niemeier M. Disentangling gravitational, environmental, and egocentric reference frames in spatial neglect. *J Cogn Neurosci.* 1998;10: 680–690.
17. Dieterich M, Brandt T. Perception of verticality and vestibular disorders of balance and falls. *Front Neurol.* 2019;10:172.
18. Belmonti V, Cioni G, Berthoz A. Anticipatory control and spatial cognition in locomotion and navigation through typical development and in cerebral palsy. *Dev Med Child Neurol.* 2016;58(Suppl 4):22–27.

19. Berthoz A. *The Brain's Sense of Movement.* Cambridge, MA: Harvard University Press; 2002.

20. DiFabio RP, Emasithi A. Aging and the mechanisms underlying head and postural control during voluntary action. *Phys Ther.* 1997;77:458–475.

21. Assländer L, Peterka RJ. Sensory reweighting dynamics in human postural control. *J Neurophysiol.* 2014;111:1852–1864.

22. Sinno S, Dumas G, Mallinson A, Najem F, Abouchacra KS, Nashner L, et al. Changes in the sensory weighting strategies in balance control throughout maturation in children. *J Am Acad Audiol.* 2021;32:122–136.

23. Cumberworth VL, Patel NN, Rogers W, Kenyon GS. The maturation of balance in children. *J Laryngol Otol.* 2007;121:449–454.

24. Goulème N, Debue M, Spruyt K, Vanderveken C, De Siati RD, Ortega-Solis J, et al. Changes of spatial and temporal characteristics of dynamic postural control in children with typical neurodevelopment with age: results of a multicenter pediatric study. *Int J Pediatr Otorhinolaryngol.* 2018;113:272–280.

25. Charpiot A, Tringali S, Ionescu E, Vital-Durand F, Ferber Viart C. Vestibulo-ocular reflex and balance maturation in healthy children aged from six to twelve years. *Audiol Neurotol.* 2010;15:203–210.

26. Foudriat BA, DiFabio RP, Anderson JH. Sensory organization of balance responses in children three to six years of age: a normative study with diagnostic implications. *Int J Paediatr Otorhinol.* 1993;27:255–271.

27. Barozzi S, Socci M, Soi D, Di Berardino F, Fabio G, Forti S, et al. Reliability of postural control measures in children and young adolescents. *Eur Arch. Otorhinolaryngol.* 2014;271:2069–2077.

28. Assaiante C, Barlaam F, Cignetti F, Vaugoyeau M. Body schema building during childhood and adolescence: a neurosensory approach. *Neurophyiol Clin.* 2014;44:3–12.

29. Cignetti F, Fontan A, Menant J, Nazarian B, Anton JL, Vaugoyeau M, et al. Protracted development of the proprioceptive brain network during and beyond adolescence. *Cereb Cortex.* 2017;27:1285–1296.

30. Jouen F, Lepecq JC, Gapenne O, et al. Optic flow sensitivity in neonates. *Infant Behav Dev.* 2000;23: 2761–2784.

31. Jouen F. Visual-vestibular interactions in infancy. *Infant Behav Dev.* 1984;7:135–145.

32. Hirabayashi S, Iwasaki Y. Developmental perspective of sensory organization on postural control. *Brain Dev.* 1995;17:111–113.

33. Maki BE, McIlroy WE. Postural control in the older adult. *Clin Geriatr Med.* 1996;12:635–658.

34. Shumway-Cook A, Woollacott MH. The growth of stability: postural control from a developmental perspective. *J Mot Behav.* 1985;17:131–147.

35. Forssberg H, Nashner LM. Ontogenic development of postural control in man: adaptation to altered support and visual conditions during stance. *J Neurosci.* 1982;2:545–552.

36. Rival C, Ceyte H, Olivier I. Developmental changes of static standing balance in children. *Neurosci. Lett.* 2005;376:133–136.

37. Libardoni TC, Silveira CBD, Sinhorim LMB, Oliveira AS, Santos MJD, Santos GM. Reference values and equations reference of balance for children of 8 to 12 years. *Gait Posture.* 2018;60:122–127.

38. Peterson ML, Christou E, Rosengren KS. Children achieve adult-like sensory integration during stance at 12-years-old. *Gait Posture.* 2006;23:455–463.

39. Voss S, Zampieri C, Biskis A, Armijo N, Purcell N, Ouyang B, et al. Normative database of postural sway measures using inertial sensors in typically developing children and young adults. *Gait Posture.* 2021;90:112–119.

40. Lundy-Ekman L. *Neruosocience: Fundamentals for Rehabilitation.* 5th ed. St Louis, MO: Elsevier; 2018.

41. Haley SM. Sequential analysis of postural reactions in non-handicapped infants. *Phys Ther.* 1986;66:531–536.

42. Liang H, Ke X, Wu J. Transitioning from the level surface to stairs in children with and without Down syndrome: motor strategy and anticipatory locomotor adjustments. *Gait Posture.* 2018;66:260–266.

43. Nashner L.M. Sensory, neuromuscular and biomechanical contributions to human balance. In Duncan P, ed. *Balance: Proceedings of the APTA Forum.* Alexandria, VA; 1990:5-12.

44. Winter DA, Patla AE, Prince F, Ishac M, Gielo-Perczak K. Stiffness control of balance in quiet standing. *J Neurophysiol.* 1998;80:1211–1221.

45. Allum JH, Bloem RF, Carpenter MG, et al. Proprioceptive control of posture: a review of new concepts. *Gait Posture.* 1998;8:214–242.

46. Inacio M, Creath R, Rogers MW. Effects of aging on hip abductor-adductor neuromuscular and mechanical performance during the weight transfer phase of lateral protective stepping. *J Biomech.* 2019;82:244–250.

47. Kiss R, Schedler S, Muehlbauer T. Associations between types of balance performance in healthy individuals across the lifespan: a systematic review and meta-analysis. *Front Physiol.* 2018;9:1366.

48. Muehlbauer T, Besemer C, Wehrle A, Gollhofer A, Granacher U. Relationship between strength, power and balance performance in seniors. *Gerontology.* 2012;58:504–512.

49. Muehlbauer T, Besemer C, Wehrle A, Gollhofer A, Granacher U. Relationship between strength, balance and mobility in children aged 7-10 years. *Gait Posture.* 2013;37:108–112.

50. Owings TM, Pavol MJ, Foley KT, Grabiner MD. Measures of postural stability are not predictors of recovery from large postural disturbances in healthy older adults. *J Am Geriatr Soc.* 2000;48:42–50.

51. Ringhof S, Stein T. Biomechanical assessment of dynamic balance: specificity of different balance tests. *Hum Mov Sci.* 2018;58:140–147.

52. Bertenthal B, Von Hofsten C. Eye, head and trunk control: the foundation for manual development. *Neurosci Biobehav Rev.* 1998;22:515–520.

53. Prechtl HFR, Hopkins B. Developmental transformations of spontaneous movements in early infancy. *Early Hum Dev.* 1986;14:233–238.

54. Bertenthal B, Rose JL, Bai DL. Perception-action coupling I the development of visual control of posture. *J Exp Psychol Hum Percept Perform.* 1997;23:1631–1643.

55. Hirschfeld H, Forssberg H. Epigenetic development of postural responses for sitting during infancy. *Exp Brain Res.* 1994;97:528–540.

56. Rachwani J, Soska KC, Adolph KE. Behavioral flexibility in learning to sit. *Dev Psychobiol.* 2017;59:937–948.

57. Chen LC, Jeka J, Clark JE. Development of adaptive sensorimotor control in infant sitting posture. *Gait Posture.* 2016;45:157–163.

58. Hadders-Algra M. Typical and atypical development of reaching and postural control in infancy. *Dev Med Child Neurol.* 2013;55(Suppl 4):5–8.

59. Kyvelidou A, Harbourne RT, Stuberg WA, Sun J, Stergiou N. Reliability of center of pressure measures for assessing the development of sitting postural control. *Arch Phys Med Rehabil.* 2009;90:1176–1184.

60. Wickstrom J, Stergiou N, Kyvelidou A. Reliability of center of pressure measures for assessing the development of sitting postural control through the stages of sitting. *Gait Posture.* 2017;56:8–13.

61. Kyvelidou A, Stuberg WA, Harbourne RT, Deffeyes JE, Blanke D, Stergiou N. Development of upper body coordination during sitting in typically developing infants. *Pediatr Res.* 2009;65:553–558.

62. Arnold AJ, Liddy JJ, Harris RC, Claxton LJ. Task-specific adaptations of postural sway in sitting infants. *Dev Psychobiol.* 2020;62:99–106.

63. Van Der Fits IB, Hadders-Algra M. The development of postural response patterns during reaching in healthy infants. *Neurosci Biobehav Rev.* 1998;22:521–526.

64. van der Heide JC, Otten B, van Eykern LA, Hadders-Algra M. Development of postural adjustments during reaching in sitting children. *Exp Brain Res.* 2003;151:32–45.

65. Cahill BM, Carr JH, Adams R. Inter-segmental co-ordination in sit-to-stand: an age cross-sectional study. *Physiother Res Int.* 1999;4:12–27.

66. Abitbol MM. Evolution of the lumbosacral angle. *Am J Phys Anthropol.* 1987;72:361–372.

67. Ascher C. *Postural Variations in Childhood.* Boston: Butterworth; 1975.

68. Staheli LT. *Fundamentals of Pediatric Orthopedics.* 5th ed. Philadelphia: Wolters Kluwer; 2016.

69. Kakebeeke TH, Locatelli I, Rousson V, Caflisch J, Jenni OG. Improvement in gross motor performance between 3 and 5 years of age. *Percept Mot Skills.* 2012;114:795–806.

70. Condon C, Cremin K. Static balance norms in children. *Physiother Res Int.* 2014;19:1–7.

71. Nougier V, Bard C, Fleury M, Teasdale N. Contribution of central and peripheral vision to the regulation of stance: developmental aspects. *J Exp Child Psychol.* 1998;68:202–215.

72. Hatziki V, Ziai V, Kollias I, Kioumourtzoglou E. Perceptual-motor contributions to static and dynamic balance control in children. *J Mot Behav.* 2002;34:161–170.

73. García-Liñeira J, Leirós-Rodríguez R, Chinchilla-Minguet JL, García-Soidán JL. Influence of visual information and sex on postural control in children aged 6-12 years assessed with accelerometric technology. *Diagnostics (Basel).* 2021;11:637.

74. Rogge AK, Hamacher D, Cappagli G, Kuhne L, Hötting K, Zech A, et al. Balance, gait, and navigation performance are related to physical exercise in blind and visually impaired children and adolescents. *Exp Brain Res.* 2021;239:1111–1123.

75. Ferber-Viart C, Ionescu E, Morlet T, Froehlich P, Dubreuil C. Balance in healthy individuals assessed with Equitest: maturation and normative data for children and young adults. *Int J Pediatr Otorhinolaryngol.* 2007;71:1041–1046.

76. Steindl R, Kunz K, Schrott-Fischer A, Scholtz AW. Effect of age and sex on maturation of sensory systems and balance control. *Dev Med Child Neurol.* 2006;48:477–482.

77. Witherington DC, von Hofsten C, Rosander K, Robinette A, Woollacott MH, Bertenthal BI. The development of anticipatory postural adjustments in infancy. *Infancy.* 2002;3495-317.

78. Norris RA, Wilder E, Norton J. The functional reach test in 3-5 year-old children without disabilities. *Pediatr Phys Ther.* 2008;19:20–27.

79. Donahoe B, Turner D, Worrell T. The use of functional reach as a measurement of balance in boys and girls without disabilities ages 5-15 years. *Pediatr Phys ther.* 1994;6:189–193.

80. Hirunyaphinun B, Taweetanalarp S, Tantisuwat A. Relationships between lower extremity strength and

the multi-directional reach test in children aged 7 to 12 years. *Hong Kong Physiother J.* 2019;39:143–150.

81. Rossi C, Chau CW, Leech KA, Statton MA, Gonzalez AJ, Bastian AJ. The capacity to learn new motor and perceptual calibrations develops concurrently in childhood. *Sci Rep.* 2019;9:9322.

82. Lebiedowska MK, Syczewska M. Invariant sway properties in children. *Gait Posture.* 2000;12:200–204.

83. Sabourin P. *Rising From Supine to Standing: A Study of Adolescents* [thesis]. Virginia Commonwealth University; 1989.

84. Green LN, Williams K. Differences in developmental movement patterns used by active versus sedentary middle-aged adults coming from a supine position to erect stance. *Phys Ther.* 1992;75:560B–568B.

85. Kowalski E, Catelli DS, Lamontagne M. Gait variability between younger and older adults: An equality of variance analysis. *Gait Posture.* 2022;95:176–182.

86. Thomas R, Williams AK, Lundy-Ekman L. Supine to stand in elderly persons: relationship o age, activity level, strength, and range of motion. *Issues Aging.* 1998;21:9–18.

87. de Malo Nascimento M, Gouveia BR, Gouveia ÉR, Campos P, Marques A, Ihle A. Muscle strength and balance as mediators in the association between physical activity and health-related quality of life in community-dwelling older adults. *J Clin Med.* 2022;11:4857.

88. Garcia Meneguci CA, Meneguci J, Sasaki JE, Tribess S, Júnior JSV. Physical activity, sedentary behavior and functionality in older adults: a cross-sectional path analysis. *PLoS One.* 2021;16e0246275.

89. Lord SR, Clark RD, Webster IW. Visual acuity and contrast sensitivity in relations to falls in an elderly population. *Age Ageing.* 1991;20:175–181.

90. Scovil CY, Zettel JL, Maki BE. Stepping to recover balance in complex environments: is online visual control of the foot motion necessary or sufficient? *Neurosci Lett.* 2008;445:108–112.

91. Lord SR, Menz HB. Visual contributions to postural stability in older adults. *Gerontology.* 2000;46:302–310.

92. Hay L, Bard C, Fleury M, Teasdale N. Availability of visual and proprioceptive afferent messages and postural control in elderly adults. *Exp Brain Res.* 1996;108:129–139.

93. Carpenter MG, Murnagham CD, Inglis JT. Shifting the balance: evidence of an exploratory role in postural sway. *Neurosci.* 2010;171:196–204.

94. Sturienks St DL, George R, Lord SR. Balance disorder in the elderly. *Clin Neurophysiol.* 2008;38:467–478.

95. Maki BE, Holliday PJ, Fernie GR. Aging and postural control. A comparison of spontaneous- and induced-sway balance tests. *J Am Geriatr Soc.* 1990;38:1–9.

96. Blaszcyk IW, Prince F, Raiche M, Hébert R. Effect of ageing and vision on limb load asymmetry during quiet stance. *J Biomech.* 2000;33:1243–1248.

97. Maki BE, Holliday PJ, Topper AK. A prospective study of postural balance and risk of falling in an ambulatory and independent elderly population. *J Gerontol.* 1994;49:M72–M84.

98. Lord SR, Delbaere K, Sturnieks DL. Aging. *Handb Clin Neurol.* 2018;159:157–171.

99. Lord SR, Rogers MW, Howland A, Fitzpatrick R. Lateral stability, sensorimotor function and falls in older people. *J Am Geriatr Soc.* 1999;47:1077–1081.

100. Howcroft J, Lemaire ED, Kofman J, McIlroy WE. Elderly fall risk prediction using static posturography. *PLoS ONE.* 2017;12e0172398.

101. Inglin B, Woollacott MH. Age-related changes in anticipatory postural adjustments associated with arm movements. *J Gerontol.* 1988;43:M105–M113.

102. Rogers MW, Kukulka CG, Soderberg GL. Age-related changes in postural responses preceding rapid self-paced and reaction time arm movements. *J Gerontol.* 1992;47:M159–M165.

103. Rogers MW, Hedman LD, Johnson ME, Cain TD, Hanke TA. Lateral stability during forward-induced stepping for dynamic balance recovery in young and older adults. *J Gerontol A Biol Sci Med Sci.* 2001;56A:M589–M594.

104. Addison O, Inacio M, Bair WN, Beamer BA, Ryan AS, Rogers MW. Role of hip abductor muscle composition and torque in protective stepping for lateral balance recovery in older adults. *Arch Phys Med Rehabil.* 2017;98:1223–1228.

105. Jonsson E, Henriksson M, Hirschfeld H. Age-related differences in postural adjustments in connection with different tasks involving weight transfer while standing. *Gait Posture.* 2007;26:508–515.

106. Hanke TA, Kay B, Turvey M, Tiberio D. Age-related differences in postural and goal-directed movements during medial-lateral rhythmic stepping. *Motor Control.* 2019;23:81–99.

107. Medell JL, Alexander NB. A clinical measure of maximal and rapid stepping of older women. *J Gerontol A Biol Sci Med Sci.* 2000;55:M429–M433.

108. Halliday SE, Winter DA, Frank JS, Patla AE, Prince F. The initiation of gait in young, elderly, and Parkinson's disease subjects. *Gait Posture.* 1998;8:8–14.

109. Hanke TA, Tiberio D. lateral rhythmic unipedal stepping in younger, middle-aged, and older adults. *J Geriatr Phys Ther.* 2006;29:20–25.

110. Patla AE, Frank JS, Winter DA, Rietdyk S, Prentice S, Prasad S. Age-related changes in balance control sys-

tem: initiation of stepping. *Clin Biomech (Bristol, Avon)*. 1993;8:179–184.

111. Hendriksson M, Hirschfeld H. Physically active older adults display alterations in gait initiation. *Gait Posture*. 2005;21:289–296.

112. Mbourou GA, Lajoie Y, Teasdale N. Step length variability at gait initiation in elderly fallers and non-fallers, and young adults. *Gerontology*. 2003;49:21–26.

113. Horak FB, Nashner LM. Central programming of postural movements: adaptation to altered support-surface configurations. *J Neurophysiol*. 1986;55:1369–1381.

114. Rogers MW, Hain TC, Hanke TA, Janssen I. Stimulus parameters and inertial load: effects on the incidence of protective stepping responses in healthy human subjects. *Arch Phys Med Rehabil*. 1996;77:363–368.

115. Maki BE. Gait changes in older adults: predictors of falls or indicators of fear. *J Am Geriatr Soc*. 1997;45:313–320.

116. Pai YC, Rogers MW, Patton J, Cain TD, Hanke TA. Static versus dynamic predictions of protective stepping following waist-pull perturbations in young and older adults. *J Biomech*. 1998;31:1111–1118.

117. Pai YC, Maki BE, Iqbal K, McIlroy WE, Perry SD. Thresholds for step initiation induced by support-surface translation: a dynamic center-of-mass model provides much better prediction than a static model. *J Biomech*. 2000;33:387–392.

118. Mille M-L, Johnson-Hilliard M, Martinez KM, Zhang Y, Edwards BJ, Rogers MW. One step, two steps, three steps more… directional vulnerability to falls in community-dwelling older persons. *J Gerontol A Biol Med Sci*. 2013;68:1540–1548.

119. Rogers MW, Mille M-L. Balance perturbations. *Handb Clin Neurol*. 2018;159:85–105.

120. McIlroy WE, Maki BE. Age-related changes in compensatory stepping in response to unpredictable perturbations. *J Gerontol A Biol Sci Med Sci*. 1996;51:M289–M296.

121. Luchies CW, Wallace D, Pazdur R, Young S, DeYoung AJ. Effects of age on balance assessment using voluntary and involuntary step tasks. *J Gerontol A Biol Sci Med Sci*. 1999;54:M140–M144.

122. Rogers MW, Kukulka CG, Brunt D, Cain TD, Hanke TA. The influence of stimulus cue on the initiation of stepping in young and older adults. *Arch Phys Med Rehabil*. 2001;82:619–624.

123. Hamilton N. Locomotion: solid surface. In: Hamilton N, Weimar W, Luttgens K, eds. *Kinesiology: Scientific Basis of Human Motion*. McGraw Hill; 2008. https://accessphysiotherapy.mhmedical.com/content.aspx?bookid=446&sectionid=41564598.

124. Adolph KE, Franchak JM. The development of motor behavior. *Wiley Interdiscip Rev Cogn Sci*. 2017;810.1002/wcs.1430.

125. Keen R. The development of problem solving in young children: a critical cognitive skill. *Ann Rev Psychol*. 2011;62:1–21.

126. Piaget J. *The Construction of Reality in the Child*. New York: Basic Books; 1954.

127. Adolph KE, Karasik LB, Tamis-LeMonda CS. Motor skills. In: Bornstein MH, ed. *Handbook of Cultural Development Science. Vol 1. Domains of development across cultures*. New York: Taylor and Francis; 2010: 61–88.

128. Gibson EJ. Exploratory behavior in the development of perceiving, acting, and the acquiring of knowledge. *Ann Rev Psychol*. 1988;39:1–41.

129. Fritz S, Lusardi M. White paper: "walking speed: the sixth vital sign." *J Geriatr Phys Ther*. 2009;32:46–49.

130. Clark JE, Whitall J. Changing patterns of locomotion: from walking to skipping. In: Woollacott M, Shumway-Cook A, eds. *Development of Posture and Gait Across the Life Span*. Columbia, SC: University of South Carolina Press; 1989:128–151.

131. Adolph KE, Vereijken B, Shjrout PE. What changes in infant walking and why. *Child Dev*. 2003;72:475–497.

132. Herssens N, Verbecque E, Hallemans A, Vereeck L, Van Rompaey V, Saeys W. Do spatiotemporal parameters and gait variability differ across the lifespan of healthy adults? A systematic review. *Gait Posture*. 2018;64: 181–190.

133. Connolly KJ, Forssberg H. *Neurophysiology and Neuropsychology of Motor Development*. London, UK: Mac Keith Press; 1997.

134. Grillner S. Control of locomotion in bipeds, tertrapods, and fish. In: Geiger SR, ed. *Handbook of Physiology*. vol 2. Bethesda, MD: American Psychological Society; 1981:1179–1236.

135. Thelen E, Ulrich BD, Jensen JL. The developmental origins of locomotion. In: Woollacott MH, Shumway-Cook A, eds. *Development of Posture and Gait Across the Life Span*. Columbia, SC: University of South Carolina; 1989:25–47.

136. Atkinson J, Braddick O. Visual development. *Handb Clin Neurol*. 2020;173:121–142.

137. Thurman SL, Corbetta D. Changes in posture and interactive behaviors as infants progress from sitting to walking: a longitudinal study. *Front Psychol*. 2019;10:822.

138. Karasik LB, Tamis-LeMonda CS, Adolph KE. Transition from crawling to walking and infants' actions with objects and people. *Child Dev*. 2011;82:1199–1209.

139. Assaiante C. Development of locomotor balance control in healthy children. *Neurosci Biobehav Rev.* 1998;22:527–532.

140. Srulijes K, Mack DJ, Klenk J, Schwickert L, Ihlen EA, Schwenk M, et al. Association between vestibulo-ocular reflex suppression, balance, gait, and fall risk in ageing and neurodegenerative disease: protocol of a one-year prospective follow-up study. *BMC Neurol.* 2015;15:192.

141. Patla AE. A framework for understanding mobility problems in the elderly. In: Craik RL, Oatis CA, eds. *Gait Analysis: Theory and Application.* St Louis, MO: Mosby; 1995:437–449.

142. Simoneau GG, Cavanagh PR, Ulbrecht JS, Leibowitz HW, Tyrrell RA. The influence of visual factors on fall-related kinematic variables during stair descent by older women. *J Gerontol.* 1991;46:M188–M195.

143. Waters RL, Lunsford BR, Perry J, et al. Energy-speed relationship of walking: standard tables. *J Orthop Res.* 1988;6:215–222.

144. Gaesser GA, Tucker WJ, Sawyer BJ, Bhammar DM, Angadi SS. Cycling efficiency and energy cost of walking in young and older adults. *J Appl Physiol.* 2018;124:414–420.

145. Das Gupta S, Bobbert M, Faber H, Kistemaker D. Metabolic cost in healthy fit older adults and young adults during overground and treadmill walking. *Eur J Appl Physiol.* 2021;121:2787–2797.

146. Belmonti V, Cioni G, Berthoz A. Development of anticipatory orienting strategies and trajectory formation in goal-oriented locomotion. *Exp Brain Res.* 2013;227:131–147.

147. WHO Multicentre Growth Reference Study Group. WHO Motor Development Study: windows of achievement for six gross motor development milestones. *Acta Paediatr Suppl.* 2006;450:86–95.

148. Levine D, Richards J, Whittle MW. *Whittle's Gait Analysis.* 5th ed. Philadelphia, PA: Elsevier; 2012.

149. Chambers HG. Pediatric gait analysis. In: Perry J, Burnfield JM, eds. *Gait Analysis: Normal and Pathological Function.* 2nd ed. Thorofare, NJ: Slack Inc.; 2010:341–364.

150. Sutherland DH, Olshen RA, Biden EN, Wyatt MP. *The Development of Mature Walking. Clinics in Developmental Medicine series, No 104/105.* London, UK: Mac Keith Press; 1988.

151. McGraw MB. *The Neuromuscular Maturation of the Human Infant.* New York: Hafner Press; 1945.

152. Ivanenko YP, Dominici N, Lacquaniti F. Development of independent walking in toddlers. *Exerc Sport Sci Rev.* 2007;35:67–73.

153. Dominici N, Ivenenko YP, Loacquaniti F. Control of foot trajectory in walking toddlers: adaptation to load changes. *J Neurophysiol.* 2007;97:2790–2801.

154. Adolph KE, Hoch JE. Motor development: embodied, enculturated, and enabling. *Annu Rev Psychol.* 2019;70:141–164.

155. Assaiante C, Amblard B. Ontogenesis of head stabilization in space during locomotion in children: influence of visual cues. *Exp Brain Res.* 1993;93:499–515.

156. Pellico LG, Torres RR, Mora CD. Changes in walking pattern between five and six years of age. *Dev Med Child Neurol.* 1995;37:800–806.

157. Mani H, Miyagishima S, Kozuka N, Takeda K, Taneda K, Inoue T, et al. Development of temporal and spatial characteristics of anticipatory postural adjustments during gait initiation in children aged 3-10 years. *Hum Mov Sci.* 2021;75:102736.

158. Shih HS, Gordon J, Kulig K. Trunk control during gait: walking with wide and narrow step widths present distinct challenges. *J. Biomech.* 2021;114.110135.

159. Dierick F, Lefebvre C, van den Hecke A, Detrembleur C. Development of displacement of centre of mass during independent walking in children. *Dev Med Child Neurol.* 2004;46:533–539.

160. Palmer DE. Studies of the center of gravity in the human body. *Child Dev.* 1944;15:99–180.

161. Assaiante C, Amblard B. Visual factors in the child's gait: effects on locomotor skills. *Percept Mot Skills.* 1996;83:1019–1041.

162. Bouisset S, Do MC. Posture, dynamic stability, and voluntary movement. *Neurophysiol Clin.* 2008;38:345–362.

163. Hay L, Redon C. Development of postural adaptation to arm raising. *Exp Brain Res.* 2001;139(2):224–232.

164. Bohannon RW, Williams Andrews A. Normal walking speed: a descriptive meta-analysis. *Physiotherapy.* 2011;97:182–189.

165. Swanson CW, Fling BW. Discriminative mobility characteristics between neurotypical young, middle-aged, and older adults using wireless inertial sensors. *Sensors (Basel).* 2021;21:6644.

166. Terrier P, Reynard F. Effect of age on the variability and stability of gait: a cross-sectional treadmill study in healthy individuals between 20 and 69 years of age. *Gait Posture.* 2015;41:170–174.

167. Nnodim JO, Nwagwu CV, Opara IN. Gait disorders in older adults – A structured review and approach to clinical assessment. *J Geriatr Med Gerontol.* 2020;6:101.

168. Amboni M, Barone P, Hausdorff JM. Cognitive contributions to gait and falls: evidence and implications. *Mov Disord*. 2013;28:1520–1533.

169. Newstead AH, Walden JG, Gitter AJ. Gait variables differentiating fallers from nonfallers. *J Geriatr Phys Ther*. 2007;30:93–101.

170. Delbaere K, Sturnieks DL, Crombez C, Lord SR. Concern about falls elicits changes in gait parameters in conditions of postural threat in older people. *J Gerontol A Biol Sci Med Sci*. 2009;64A:237–242.

171. Beauchet O, Annweiler C, Dubost V, Allali G, Kressig RW, Bridenbaugh S, et al. Stops walking when talking: a predictor of falls in older adults? *Eur J Neurol*. 2009;16:786–795.

172. Maki BE, Perry SD, Norrie RG. McIlroy. Effect of facilitation of sensation from plantar foot-surface boundaries on postural stabilization in young and older adults. *J Gerontol A Biol Sci*. 1999.

173. Barak Y, Wagenaar RC, Holt KG. Gait characteristics of elderly people with a history of falls: a dynamic approach. *Phys Ther*. 2006;86:1501–1510.

174. Kerrigan DC, Lee LW, Nieto TJ, Markman JD, Collins JJ, Riley PO. Kinetic alterations independent of walking speed in elderly fallers. *Arch Phys Med Rehabil*. 2000;81:730–735.

175. Hilliard MJ, Martinez KM, Janssen I, Edwards B, Mille ML, Zhang Y, Rogers MW. Lateral balance factors predict future falls in community-living older adults. *Arch Phys Med Rehabil*. 2008;89:1708–1713.

176. Caetano MJ, Lord SR, Schoene D, Pelicioni PH, Sturnieks DL, Menant JC. Age-related changes in gait adaptability in response to unpredictable obstacles and stepping targets. *Gait Posture*. 2016;46:35–41.

177. Thelen DG, Ashton-Miller JA, Schultz AB, Alexander NB. Do neural factors underlie age differences in rapid ankle torque development? *J Am Geriatr Soc*. 1996;44:804–808.

178. Toulotte C, Thevenon A, Watelain E, Fabre C. Identification of healthy elderly fallers and non-fallers by gait analysis under dual-task conditions. *Clin Rehabil*. 2006;20:269–276.

179. Peel NM. Epidemiology of falls in older age. *Can J Aging*. 2011;30:7–19.

180. Rubenstein LZ. Falls in older people: epidemiology, risk factors and strategies for prevention. *Age Ageing*. 2006;35(Suppl 2):ii37–ii41.

181. Morello RT, Soh SE, Behm K, Egan A, Ayton D, Hill K, et al. Multifactorial falls prevention programmes for older adults presenting to the emergency department with a fall: systematic review and meta-analysis. *Inj Prev*. 2019;25:557–564.

182. Tricco AC, Thomas SM, Veroniki AA, Hamid JS, Cogo E, Strifler L, et al. Comparisons of interventions for preventing falls in older adults: a systematic review and meta-analysis. *JAMA*. 2017;318:1687–1699.

183. Costello E, Edelstein JE. Update on falls prevention for community-dwelling older adults: review of single and multifactorial intervention programs. *J Rehabil Res Dev*. 2008;45:1135–1152.

184. Sherrington C, Michaleff ZA, Fairhall N, Paul SS, Tiedemann A, et al. Exercise to prevent falls in older adults: an updated systematic review and meta-analysis. *Br J Sports Med*. 2017;51:1750–1758.

185. Thomas E, Battaglia G, Patti A, Brusa J, Leonardi V, Palma A, Bellafiore M. Physical activity programs for balance and fall prevention in elderly: a systematic review. *Medicine (Baltimore)*. 2019;98:e16218.

186. Menant JC, Steele JR, Menz HB, Munro BJ, Lord SR. Optimizing footwear for older people at risk of falls. *J Rehabil Res Dev*. 2008;45:1167–1181.

187. Avin KG, Hanke TA, Kirk-Sanchez N, McDonough CM, Shubert TE, Hardage J, Hartley G. Academy of Geriatric Physical Therapy of the American Physical Therapy Association. Management of falls in community-dwelling older adults: clinical guidance statement from the Academy of Geriatric Physical Therapy of the American Physical Therapy Association. *Phys Ther*. 2015;95:815–834.

188. Nikitas C, Kikidis D, Bibas A, Pavlou M, Zachou Z, Bamiou DE. Recommendations for physical activity in the elderly population: a scoping review of guidelines. *J Frailty Sarcopenia Falls*. 2022;7:18–28.

189. Kang HG, Dingwell JB. Effects of walking speed, strength and range of motion on gait stability in healthy older adults. *J Biomech*. 2008;41:2899–2905.

190. Kang HG, Dingwell JB. Separating the effects of age and walking speed on gait variability. *Gait Posture*. 2008;27:572–577.

191. Dommershuijsen LJ, Ragunathan J, Ruiter R, Groothof D, Mattace-Raso FUS, Ikram MA, et al. Gait speed reference values in community-dwelling older adults—Cross-sectional analysis from the Rotterdam Study. *Exp Gerontol*. 2022;158:111646.

192. Lord SR, Lloyd DG, Li SK. Sensori-motor function, gait patterns and falls in community-swelling women. *Age Ageing*. 1996;25:292–299.

193. Evans W. Functional and metabolic consequences of sarcopenia. *J Nutr.* 1997;127(5 Suppl):998S–1003S.

194. Coen PM, Goodpaster BH. Role of intramyocellular lipids in human health. *Trends Endocrinol Metab.* 2012;23:391–398.

195. Brandler TC, Wang C, Oh-Park M, Holtzer R, Verghese J. Depressive symptoms and gait dysfunction in the elderly. *Am J Geriatr Psychiatry.* 2012;20:425–432.

196. Castell MV, Sánchez M, Julián R, Queipo R, Martín S, Otero Á. Frailty prevalence and slow walking speed in persons age 65 and older: implications for primary care. *BMC Fam Pract.* 2013;14:86.

197. Studenski S, Perera S, Patel K, Rosano C, Faulkner K, Inzitari M, et al. Gait speed and survival in older adults. *JAMA.* 2011;305:50–58.

198. Cruz-Jentoft AJ, Bahat G, Bauer J, Boirie Y, Bruyère O, Cederholm T, et al. Writing Group for the European Working Group on Sarcopenia in Older People 2 (EWGSOP2), and the Extended Group for EWGSOP2. Sarcopenia: revised European consensus on definition and diagnosis. *Age Ageing.* 2019;48:16–31.

199. Hageman PA, Blanke DJ. Comparison of gait of young women and elderly women. *Phys Ther.* 1986;66:1382–1387.

200. Judge JO, Ounpuu S, Davis RB. Effects of age on the biomechanics and physiology of gait. *Clin Geriatr Med.* 1996;12:659–678.

201. Lee LW, Zavarei K, Evans J, Lelas JJ, Riley PO, Kerrigan DC. Reduced hip extension in the elderly: dynamic or postural? *Arch Phys Med Rehabil.* 2005;86:1851–1854.

202. Ostrosky KM, VanSwearingen JM, Burdett RG, Gee Z. A comparison of gait characteristics in young and old subjects. *Phys Ther.* 1994;74:637–644. discussion 644-646.

203. Kerrigan DC, Lee LW, Collins JJ, Riley PO, Lipsitz LA. Reduced hip extension during walking: healthy elderly and fallers versus young adults. *Arch Phys Med Rehabil.* 2001;82:26–30.

204. Kerrigan DC, Xenopoulos-Oddsson A, Sullivan MJ, Lelas JJ, Riley PO. Effect of a hip flexor-stretching program on gait in the elderly. *Arch Phys Med Rehabil.* 2003;84:1–6.

205. Watt JR, Jackson K, Franz JR, Dicharry J, Evans J, Kerrigan DC. Effect of a supervised hip flexor stretching program on gait in elderly individuals. *PM R.* 2011;3:324–329.

206. Winter DA, Patla AE, Frank JS, Walt SE. Biomechanical walking pattern changes in the fit and healthy elderly. *Phys Ther.* 1990;70:340–347.

207. Riley PO, DellaCroce U, Kerrigan DC. Effect of age on lower extremity joint moment contributions to gait speed. *Gait Posture.* 2001;14:264–270.

208. DeVita P, Hortobagyi T. Age causes a redistribution of joint torques and powers during gait. *J Appl Physiol (1985).* 2000;88:1804–1811.

209. Laudani L, Rum L, Valle MS, Macaluso A, Vannozzi G, Casabona A. Age differences in anticipatory and executory mechanisms of gait initiation following unexpected balance perturbations. *Eur J Appl Physiol.* 2021;121:465–478.

210. Robinovitch SN, Feldman F, Yang Y, et al. Video capture of the circumstances of falls in elderly people residing in long-term care: an observational study. *Lancet.* 2013;381(9860):47–54.

211. Vistamehr A, Neptune RR. Differences in balance control between healthy younger and older adults during steady-state walking. *J Biomech.* 2021;128:110717.

212. Shyuratova N, Morris ME, Huxham F. Effects of age on balance control during walking. *Arch Phys Med Rehabil.* 2004;85:582–588.

213. Menz HB, Lord SR, Fitzpatrick RC. Age-related differences in walking stability. *Age Ageing.* 2003;32:137–142.

214. Kavanagh JJ, Barrett RS, Morrison S. Upper body accelerations during walking in healthy young and elderly men. *Gait Posture.* 2004;20:291–298.

215. Mazzà C, Iosa M, Pecoraro F, Cappozzo A. Control of the upper body accelerations in young and elderly women during level walking. *J Neuroeng Rehabil.* 2008;5:30.

216. Pavol MJ, Owings TM, Foley KT, Grabiner MD. Gait characteristics as risk factors for falling from trips induced in older adults. *J Gerontol A Biol Sci Med Sci.* 1999;54:M583–M590.

217. Pavol MJ, Owings TM, Foley KT, Grabiner MD. Mechanisms leading to a fall from an induced trip in healthy older adults. *J Gerontol A Biol Sci Med Sci.* 2001;56:M428–M437.

218. van den Bogert AJ, Pavol MJ, Grabiner MD. Response time is more important than walking speed for the ability of older adults to avoid a fall after a trip. *J Biomech.* 2002;35:199–205.

219. Lu TW, Chen HL, Chen SC. Comparisons of the lower limb kinematics between young and older adults when crossing obstacles of different heights. *Gait Posture.* 2006;23:471–479.

220. McFadyen BJ, Prince F. Avoidance and accommodation of surface height changes by healthy, community-dwelling, young, and elderly men. *J Gerontol A Biol Sci Med Sci.* 2002;57:B166–B174.

221. Chen HC, Ashton-Miller JA, Alexander NB, Schultz AB. Effects of age and available response time on ability

to step over an obstacle. *J Gerontol*. 1994;49:M227–M233.

222. Chen HC, Schultz AB, Ashton-Miller JA, Giordani B, Alexander NB, Guire KE. Stepping over obstacles: dividing attention impairs performance of old more than young adults. *J Gerontol A Biol Sci Med Sci*. 1996;51:M116–M122.

223. Galna B, Peters A, Murphy AT, Morris ME. Obstacle crossing deficits in older adults: a systematic review. *Gait Posture*. 2009;30:270–275.

224. Aranyavalai T, Jalayondeja C, Jalayondeja W, Pichaiyongwongdee S, Kaewkungwal J, Laskin JJ. Association between walking 5000 step/day and fall incidence over six months in urban community-dwelling older people. *BMC Geriatr*. 2020;20:194.

225. Tudor-Locke C, Craig CL, Aoyagi Y, Bell RC, Croteau KA, De Bourdeaudhuij I, et al. How many steps/day are enough? For older adults and special populations. *Int J Behav Nutr Phys Act*. 2011;8:80.

226. Osaba MY, Rao AK, Agrawal SK, Lalwani AK. Balance and gai in the elderly: a contemporary review. *Laryngoscope Investig Otolaryngol*. 2019;4:143–153.

227. Wong DW, Lam WK, Lee WC. Gait asymmetry and variability in older adults during long-distance walking: implications for gait instability. *Clin Biomech (Bristol, Avon)*. 2020;72:37–43.

228. Zhang G, Wong IK, Chen TL, Hong TT, Wong DW, Peng Y, et al. Identifying fatigue indicators using gait variability measures: a longitudinal study on elderly brisk walking. *Sensors (Basel)*. 2020;20:6983.

229. Figueiro MG, Plitnick B, Rea MS, Gras LZ, Rea MS. Lighting and perceptual cues: effects on gait measures of older adults at high and low risk for falls. *BMC Geriatr*. 2011;11:49.

230. Francis CA, Franz JR, O'Connor SM, Thelen DG. Gait variability in healthy old adults is more affected by a visual perturbation than by a cognitive or narrow step placement demand. *Gait Posture*. 2015;42:380–385.

231. Badaly D, Adolph KE. Beyond the average: walking infants take steps longer than their leg length. *Infant Behav Dev*. 2008;31:554–558.

232. Wiedmer P, Jung T, Castro JP, Pomatto LCD, et al. Sarcopenia: molecular mechanisms and open questions. *Aging Research Reviews*. 2021;65:101200.

233. Malmstrom TK, Miller DK, Simonsick EM, Ferrucci L, Morley JE. SARC-F: a symptom score to predict persons with sarcopenia at risk for poor functional outcomes. *J Cachexia Sarcopenia Muscle*. 2016;7:28–36.

234. Keating CJ, Cabrera-Linares JC, Parraga-Montilla JA, Latorre-Román PA, Del Castillo RM, García-Pinillos F. Influence of resistance training on gait and balance parameters in older adults: a systematic review. *Int. J. Environ Res Public Health*. 2021;18:1759.

235. Kerrigan DC, Todd MK, Della Croce U, Lipsitz LA, Collins JJ. Biomechanical gait alterations independent of speed in the healthy elderly: evidence for specific limiting impairments. *Arch Phys Med Rehabil*. 1998;79:317–322.

236. Hortobágyi T, Lesinski M, Gäbler M, VanSwearingen JM, Malatesta D, Granacher U. Effects of three types of exercise interventions on healthy old adults' gait speed: a systematic review and meta-analysis. *Sports Med*. 2015;45:1627–1643.

237. Papa EV, Dong X, Hassan M. Resistance training for activity limitations in older adults with skeletal muscle function deficits: a systematic review. *Clin Interv Aging*. 2017;12:955–961.

238. Uematsu A, Hoerobagyi T, Tsuchiya K, et al. Lower extremity power training improves healthy older adults' gain biomechanics. *Gait Posture*. 2018;62:303–310.

239. Van Abbema R, DeGreef M, Crajc C, et al. What type or combination of exercise can improve gait speed in older adults? A meta-analysis. *BMCC Geriatrics*. 2015;15:72.

240. Lord SR, Lloyd DG, Nirui M, et al. The effect of exercise on gait patterns inolder women: a randomized controlle dtrial. *J Gerontol A BIol Sci Med Sci*. 1996;51:M64–M70.

241. Winter DA. The Biomechanics and Motor Control of Human Gait: Normal, Elderly, and Pathological. Waterloo, Canada: Waterloo Press; 1991. 2nd ed.

242. Bohannon RW. Comfortable and maximum walking speed of adults aged 20-79 years: reference values and determinants. *Age Ageing*. 1997;26:15–19.

243. Van Hoornweder S, Mora DAB, Depestele S, Frieske J, van Dun K, Cuypers K, Verstraelen S, Meesen R. Age and interlimb coordination complexity modulate oscillatory spectral dynamics and large-scale functional connectivity. *Neuroscience*. 2022;496:1–15.

244. Fujiyama H, Hinder MR, Garry MI, Summers JJ. Slow and steady is not as easy as it sounds: interlimb coordination at slow speed is associated with elevated attentional demand especially in older adults. *Exp Brain Res*. 2013;227:289–300.

245. Jakovljevic DG. Physical activity and cardiovascular aging: physiologic and molecular insight. *Experimental Gerontology*. 2018;109:67–74.

246. Ruberto K, Ehsani H, ParVeneh S, et al. The association between heart rate behavior and gait perfor-

mance: the moderating effect of frailty. *PLosONE.* 2022;17(2):e0261013.

247. Jeka JJ, Allison LK, Kiemel T. The dynamics of visual reweighting in healthy and fall-prone older adults. *J Mot Beh.* 2010;42:197–208.

248. Herman T, Giladi N, Gurevich T, Hausdorff JM. Gait instability and fractal dynamics of older adults with a "cautious" gait: why do certain older adults walk fearfully? *Gait Posture.* 2005;21:178–185.

249. Kyrdalen IL, Thingstad P, Sandvik L, Ormstad H. Associations between gait speed and well-known fall risk factors among community-dwelling older adults. *Physiother Res Int.* 2019;24:e1743.

250. Quach L, Galica AM, Jones RN, Procter-Gray E, Manor B, Hannan MT, et al. The nonlinear relationship between gait speed and falls: the maintenance of balance, independent living, intellect, and zest in the elderly of Boston study. *J Am Geriatr Soc.* 2011;59:1069–1073.

251. Mehmet H, Robinson SR, Yang AWH. Assessment of gait speed in older adults. *J Geriatr Phys Ther.* 2020;43:42–52.

252. Maggio M, Ceda GP, Ticinesi A, De Vita F, Gelmini G, Costantino C, et al. Instrumental and non-instrumental evaluation of 4-meter walking speed in older individuals. *PLoS One.* 2016;11:1–10.

253. Middleton A, Fritz SL, Lusardi M. Walking speed: the functional vital sign. *J Aging Phys Act.* 2015;23:314–322.

Prehension

The human hand enhances our life through its dexterity and serves to express our intelligence, as well as our emotions, through gesture. *Prehension*, or the ability to use our hands and upper limbs effectively, can be a strong determinant of functional independence. Upper limb dysfunction limits the degree to which we use our prehensile skills even during simple tasks. To understand dysfunction, it is important to first review normal capabilities and explore prehension at different phases of the life span.

COMPONENTS OF PREHENSION

Imagine yourself supported in a chair, gazing at a cup of tea resting in front of you. Reach for the cup and secure the handle. As you drink the tea, adjust the handle within your hand. Now set the cup down on the table and let go of the handle. This simple task of drinking tea exemplifies the primary components of prehension: visual regard, reach, grasp, manipulation, and release. *Regard* is the visual attention held on an object; you perceive the location, size, and shape of the cup of tea and the handle. *Reach*, or transport, incorporates directing and grading arm position and preshaping the hand to match the location, size, and shape of an object, such as the handle of the cup. *Grasp* involves the act of closing and stabilizing the hand on an object; you secure the cup handle in your hand. *Manipulation* incorporates movement of an object while it is being held, as noted by the adjustment of the handle within

your hand. *Release* is the manner in which an object leaves the hand; you let go of the cup handle. If necessary, you may also lift and carry an objessct, such as the cup, with both hands. The cooperative effort of both hands is termed *bimanual coordination*. The act of drinking a cup of tea, like other prehensile tasks, reflects the interaction between goal-directed movement and environmental constraints.

Prehension uses anticipatory or feedforward control and feedback allowing us to prepare the hand, arm, and body in advance of intended movement or to respond to perturbations. Other inherent features of prehension are postural control and biomechanical components.[1,2]

Postural Control

Visual exploration and functional reaching are closely linked to postural control. Under *feedforward* or *proactive control*, stabilizing muscle contractions or anticipatory postural adjustments (APAs) are elicited in anticipation of upcoming disturbances in equilibrium. APAs prevent undesired movement and allow for adjustment in our center of gravity before the upper limb moves in space. Under *reactive control*, muscle responses are also elicited after perturbations induced by a prehensile act such as reaching to a distant target.

Core stability is the ability to control the trunk's position and motion over the pelvis to optimize force control and motion in distal segments as needed for athletics and other tasks.[3] It provides stability of the trunk while an individual uses their arms and legs in performing functional activity. Core stability has been found to correlate with fine-motor precision and integration tasks in children between 6 and 10 years of age.[4] Correlations have also been found between core strength and hand grip strength in young adults[5] and between core stability and upper extremity performance in athletes.[6,7] Participating in a core stability exercise program has also been found to improve upper extremity function in children with hemiplegic cerebral palsy.[8]

Although core stability is essential for efficient distal coordination, it is possible to have good fine-motor control despite insufficient proximal control or shoulder stability. For example, we find that children who have sustained injuries to the upper brachial plexus at birth (Erb palsy, C5–C6 spinal nerves) often have shoulder weakness and instability, yet despite some residual hand weakness have good distal coordination.

The extent of proximal and distal muscle activation is task-dependent.[9,10] Typically, the joint to be stabilized is determined by the goal of the activity. Proximal trunk muscles stabilize the body during reach-to-grasp movements, whereas sustained pinch and grip provide distal stabilization that frees the proximal joints to move. For

example, when we hold a toothbrush, the wrist, forearm, and elbow are free to move while the fingers and thumb stabilize the toothbrush for use. Thus the goal and constraints of the task dictate which muscles serve as stabilizers.

Biomechanics

Flexible postural control that adheres to select biomechanical principles allows us to use prehensile skills effectively. Certain biomechanical principles are inherent components of efficient muscle function, including length-tension relationships and related active and passive insufficiency of muscle-tendon units. The length-tension curve compares the tension produced in a muscle with its resting length at the time of contraction (Fig. 12.1). *Resting muscle length* is the length of the resting muscle when it is measured from attachment to attachment. Peak tension, which is necessary for a strong contraction, can be developed when the sarcomere filaments overlap between 80% and 120% of their resting length.[11] A contracting muscle or agonist demonstrates active insufficiency when its attachments are too close together, limiting tension development.

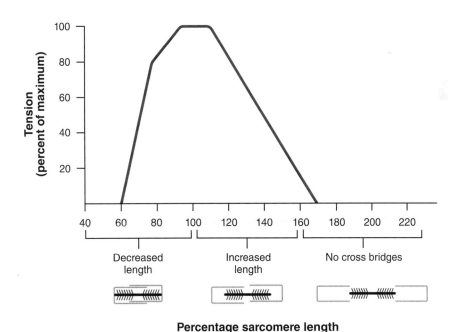

Percentage sarcomere length

Fig. 12.1 Length-tension diagram for a skeletal muscle. The ideal length of a sarcomere to produce maximum tension. (From Nervous system control of muscle tension. Lumenlearning.com. https://courses.lumenlearning.com/suny-ap1/chapter/nervous-system-control-of-muscle-tension/ Accessed December 31, 2022.)

Passive insufficiency results when the attachments of the agonist are too far apart for the muscle to generate adequate tension for effective contraction.

Based on these principles, many manipulative tasks are best performed with the wrist stabilized in approximately 20–30 degrees of extension and 10 degrees of ulnar deviation.[12,13] Wrist extension keeps the finger flexors within the useful range of the length-tension curve, allowing for adequate tension development during grip and pinch activities. When the wrist is extended, the thumb can move into a plane of opposition in relation to the other digits, and the fingers can achieve full flexion. These and other biomechanical principles play a significant role in manual acts.

Friction at the digit-object interface helps to maintain a secure grip on objects.[14] If the friction and fingertip forces are insufficient, objects will slip and may be dropped. To prevent object drops, feedback obtained from tactile receptors causes an increase in grip force at the fingertips. Any deficiency in tactile feedback will alter the response to slips.

Visual Regard

Visual regard and perception prompt us to reach for and grasp objects. These functions depend on the strength of our attention, visual acuity, and ocular control, including accommodation and convergence (see Chapter 9). *Visual perception* is the ability to use visual information to recognize, recall, discriminate, and understand what we see. As infants and children gain experience through play involving various systems, perceptual constructs are developed. Visual memory is established and complex processes develop with exposure to and interaction with different environments. Visual regard and perception also guide reach and refine manipulation skills in terms of accuracy and control. Selected visuoperceptual constructs, such as depth perception, figure-ground, and visuoconstruction, play key roles in reach, grasp, and manipulation. Depth perception allows us to localize objects in space and to estimate size and distance. For example, we can discriminate how far an object is out of reach before retrieving it. Figure-ground refers to the ability to visually focus on specific details in the foreground by selectively screening out competing background stimuli. Visuoconstruction is also related to the spatial planning process involved in building up and breaking down two- and three-dimensional objects.

This skill is used in putting together a puzzle or copying a three-dimensional design.

Visual-motor control, or *eye-hand coordination*, is the ability of an individual to use visual information for precise guidance of movement. Visual information is used to amend an internal representation or model of an object's physical properties and location before reaching for it and to enhance accuracy before object contact during an unfolding reach. Reach transports the hand to the object and grasp shapes the hand to the object. In *central vision*, the reach and grasp are integrated. *Central* vision supports grasp and manipulation because it provides information about object size and shape required for grip calibration and dexterous hand movement. Reaching for objects in a peripheral visual field is an everyday occurrence. However, when the object is not seen, the reach and grasp are changed. When using peripheral vision, proprioception is used to assist the reach. Grasp is delayed until the object is touched.[15] Sighted individuals use vision to guide reaching in many everyday tasks, such as retrieving a specific shirt hanging in the closet. Early object manipulation and development of concepts related to objects is delayed when there is a lack of vision.[16] When our vision is compromised, we rely on proprioceptive and tactile cues or visual memory to guide reach-to-grasp movements.

Reach and Grip Formation

The entire upper extremity is involved in the act of reaching and grasping an object. During reach-to-grasp movements, the shoulder moves the hand in space over a wide area, and the elbow places it closer to or further away from the body. The forearm and wrist position the hand before grasp of an object or receipt of a weight-bearing surface. The fingers and thumb adjust their position to accommodate the perceived spatial properties of an object during grip formation, such as its size and shape. This can be exemplified when reaching for a cup visualized at chest level. There are many ways to perform the task as exemplified below. To approach the cup, the shoulder may flex to about 80 degrees, while the scapula rotates up and protracts, and the elbow extends. As the cup handle is approached, the wrist may extend and the forearm may rotate into neutral. As the handle is approximated, the fingers may extend and the thumb may abduct in preparation. The fingers may close in on the handle by flexing, and the thumb may adduct. The trunk can also assist in reaching for an object. Reaching for an object requires coordination of the shoulder, elbow, and trunk motion.[17,18]

The *trajectory* of a reaching movement can be defined by the extent, orientation, and speed of the hand path as it moves the hand to a new position.[19] In adults, reaching behaviors include smooth bell-shaped velocity profiles and relatively continuous, straight hand paths with and without visual feedback (see Fig. 12.2).[20] Conversely, during early reaching, the hand paths are characterized by accelerations and decelerations resulting in indirect hand paths until about 2 years of age.[21]

Studies examining reaching differences between the dominant and nondominant arm reveal distinct neural control mechanisms for each arm.[22] For example, during planar reaching movements, the dominant arm typically displays a straighter hand path to the target than the nondominant arm. Furthermore, the dominant arm seems to employ anticipatory strategies during arm movements, while the nondominant arm seems to rely more on feedback.

Reach and grasp are associated with two visuomotor channels activated in parallel.[23] One channel relays information about an object's extrinsic properties, such as location, and activates proximal shoulder musculature used in the reach. The second channel is related to

preshaping the grip and provides intrinsic information about the object such as its location and contour. This information activates distal finger musculature. Reach and grasp follow different developmental paths but are thought to achieve near-adult precision and integration by 12 months of age.[24]

Preshaping of the hand, termed *grip formation*, can be divided into finger opening and finger closure or aperture. Maximum finger opening adjusts in anticipation of the size and shape of an object, based on an internal representation of the object's physical properties. As a reach-to-grasp movement unfolds, previous information is retrieved from memory, and the internal representation is updated via current sensory information. In typical adults, peak aperture occurs within 70%–75% of total movement time at the point of peak deceleration (see Fig. 12.2).[20,25] Inadequate timing between reach and grasp may extend the movement time and alter the path of the reach, compromising appropriate grip formation. In essence, the timing and size of peak aperture within a reach-to-grasp movement indicate whether it is planned for the expected target object's location and spatial properties. Furthermore, the speed of a reach and the shape of the hand as it grasps an object are dependent on the end goal or what will be done after the object is grasped.[23,26]

Impairments in central vision clearly impede grip formation. Studies of transport and grasp have reported maximal finger aperture and velocity of finger aperture to be greater when the vision of healthy subjects was restricted.[27] Without a clear idea of the size or shape of an object, individuals overestimated grip aperture to ensure successful grasp. Grasp duration and time to engage in a threading task are prolonged in children with amblyopia.[28] Binocular vision and visual feedback are crucial for controlling reach and grasp.[29]

Grasp

Classification of Adult Grasp Patterns

Once an object is approached, one of a variety of grip patterns will be used to secure it. The location, size, and shape of an object determine the type of pattern used. Traditionally, adult prehension patterns have been classified according to the work of Napier[30] and Landsmeer.[31] Napier[30] described two types of grip: power and precision. *Power grips* are defined as forcible activities of the fingers and thumb that act against the palm to transmit a force to an object. Examples include the cylindrical,

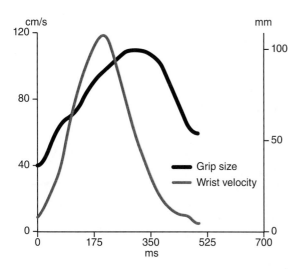

Fig. 12.2 Sample velocity profile with imbedded grip aperture. (Redrawn from Paulignan Y, Jeannerod M. Visuomotor channels in prehension. In: Wing AM, Haggard P, Flanagan JR, eds. *Hand and Brain: The Neurophysiology and Psychology of Hand Movements*. New York: Academic Press; 1996:268.)

spherical, and hook grip (Fig. 12.3). During *precision grip* and *pinch* activities, forces are directed between the thumb and fingers, not against the palm. Examples of precision grip or pinch include pad-to-pad prehension, tip-to-tip prehension, and pad-to-side, or lateral, prehension (Fig. 12.4). Sustained hold of power and precision grips require isometric muscular contractions. Typical grip and pinch patterns and the joints and muscles involved are listed in Table 12.1.

Despite their wide acceptance, the classic prehension patterns continue to be challenged and further examined. In his classification scheme, Landsmeer[31] kept the expression power grip but used the phrase "precision handling" to describe the manipulative quality of

prehensile function. *Precision handling* requires changes in position of the handled object, either in space or about its own axes, as well as exact control of finger and thumb position. Muscular contractions will vary between isometric and isotonic. Precision grip and handling exemplify the strong connection present between the motor cortex and the pyramidal tract. Wong and Whishaw[32] examined the precision grip in terms of the high degree of variability in contact strategies of the digits, purchase patterns, and the digits used between and

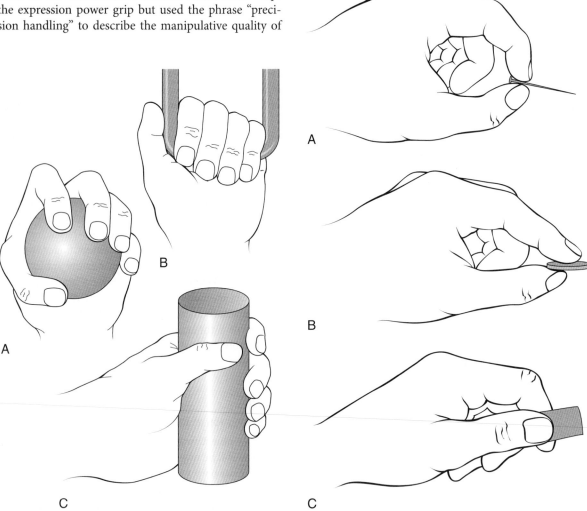

Fig. 12.3 Three varieties of power grip. (**A**) Spherical grip. (**B**) Hook grip. (**C**) Cylindrical grip. (Redrawn from Norkin CC, Levangie PK. *Joint Structure and Function: A Comprehensive Analysis.* Philadelphia: FA Davis; 1983.)

Fig. 12.4 Three varieties of precision pinch and handling. (**A**) Tip-to-tip. (**B**) Pad-to-pad. (**C**) Pad-to-side (lateral). (Redrawn from Norkin CC, Levangie PK. *Joint Structure and Function: A Comprehensive Analysis.* Philadelphia: FA Davis; 1983.)

TABLE 12.1	Classification of Prehension Patterns		
Patterns	**Joint Motion**	**Muscles Used**	**Function**
Cylindrical grasp	Thumb opposition, finger adduction, and flexion	FPL and thenar group, AdP, select interossei (task-dependent), fourth lumbrical and FDP (FDS for more power)	Holding on to a cylindrically shaped object such as a soda can
Spherical grasp	Thumb opposition, finger flexion, and abduction	FPL and thenar group, AdP, FDP (FDS for more power), fourth lumbrical interossei (except second)	Holding on to a round object such as a baseball
Hook grasp	MCPs neutral, finger flexion at PIPs and DIPs, thumb extension	Finger FDS and FDP, thumb, EPL and EPB, EDC, fourth lumbrical and fourth dorsal interossei	Holding on to a brief case handle
Pad-to-pad prehension	Thumb opposition and slight flexion of all thumb joints; finger flexion at MCP and PIP; flexion or extension of DIP of involved fingers	Thenar group, FPL, select interossei and FDS of involved fingers (FDP if DIP flexion is present)	Holding on to a coin
Tip-to-tip prehension	As in pad-to-pad prehension, with greater thumb and finger flexion, including DIP flexion	As in pad-to-pad prehension, with greater FDP force; FDP secondary to DIP flexion, interossei of involved fingers	Holding a needle
Pad-to-pad prehension (lateral)	Thumb adduction with IP flexion, index finger flexion, and abduction	Thumb, FPL, FPB, and AdP; involved fingers; FDS and FDP; reduced interossei and lumbricals except first dorsal interossei	Holding a key

AdP, Adductor pollicis; *DIP*, distal interphalangeal; *EDC*, extensor digitorum communis; *EPB*, extensor pollicis brevis; *EPL*, extensor pollicis longus; *FDP*, flexor digitorum profundus; *FDS*, flexor digitorum superficialis; *FPB*, flexor pollicis brevis; *FPL*, flexor pollicis longus; *IP*, interphalangeal; *MCP*, metacarpophalangeal; *PIP*, proximal interphalangeal.
Data from Landsmeer JMF. Power grip and precision handling. *Ann Rheum Dis*. 1962;21:164-169; Long C, Conrad PW, Hall EA, et al. Intrinsic-extrinsic muscle control of the hand in power grip and precision handling. *J Bone Joint Surg*. 1970;52(5):853-867; Napier JR. The prehensile movement of the human hand. *J Bone Joint Surg*. 1956;38:902-913; Napier JR. Function of the hand. In: Napier JR, ed. *Hands*. New York: Pantheon Books; 1980:68-83.

within individuals. They provided further support that innate or adaptive neural factors make important contributions to the grasping patterns used.

After an extensive survey of the literature, Casanova and Grunert[33] introduced their own classification system based on anatomical nomenclature and contact surfaces. They proposed the use of the terms "static prehension" and "dynamic prehension." *Static prehension* refers to any form of prehension in which the object does not move within the hand, although proximal joint movement may occur. An example of static prehension is isometrically holding a key using a lateral pinch. *Dynamic prehension* resembles Landsmeer's term of precision handling[31] because it is associated with positional changes of an object that occur within the hand rather than at the proximal joints. This is exemplified

when a needle is rolled between the fingers to visualize its eye before threading it. The force used during static or dynamic prehension may be strong or light in magnitude. For example, during precise static prehension, as in turning a key in a tough lock, a strong steady force is needed, whereas a light force is sufficient to secure a cotton ball.

We usually grade the fingertip forces we use during prehension. This ability to grade forces is based on previous learning and memory of the weight, texture, and other properties of the object.[34,35] Sensorimotor memories help form internal representations of the physical properties of objects and are used to scale the grip (squeeze) and load (vertical) forces in advance. This ability to scale fingertip forces in advance of object contact is a form of *anticipatory control*. Improvement in fingertip force control occurs throughout childhood and into adolescence.[36]

Significance of Thumb Opposition

Although prehension is evident in many forms of animal life, it attains maximum function in humans given the addition of thumb opposition. *Opposition* involves rotation at the carpometacarpal joint of the thumb to place the thumb pad diametrically opposite to the pad of one or all of the other digits (see Fig. 12.4). The thumb, because of its unique ability to oppose, is a common feature in most grip classifications, contributing 40%–50% of total hand function.[37] The comparative length of the index finger to the thumb is a major factor when attempting opposition or pad-to-pad contact. A reduction in thumb length, seen in an individual whose distal thumb phalanx has been amputated, limits the ability to fully rotate the thumb to the index pad. Thumb opposition in conjunction with movement at other digits is used to execute functional prehension, such as turning a doorknob or buttoning a shirt.

Significance of Other Digits

The index finger is considered the most important digit after the thumb because of its mobility and independent muscle attachments. It has been found to be the most dominant of the four fingers and accounts for 20% of lateral pinch, 20% of power grip from a supinated position of the forearm, and 50% of power grip from a pronated forearm position.[38,39] The long finger is the strongest and longest and has significant functional value. In some individuals, it replaces the index as the dominant finger and is used for pointing and manipulating small objects.[38] The index and long fingers are considered the prehensile digits and are the most anatomically stable. The small and ring fingers are recruited for power grip prehension. Although they are considered the most anatomically mobile, they also are the weakest digits.[39] Both the index and small fingers can produce isolated extension via the extensor indicis and the extensor digiti minimi, respectively. Because all of the digits are important in prehension, the loss of any one of them will limit prehensile ability to some degree.

Manipulation

Manipulation involves a series of tasks used to achieve a specific goal. Once we pick up an object through grasp, we may either sustain a hold on it or manipulate it with one or both hands to accomplish a task. All forms of manipulation demand the use of the small intrinsic and extrinsic muscles of the fingers or thumb.

Sustained Grip and Pinch

Once the index finger and thumb contact a target object with a stable grip, the goal is to generate sufficient fingertip forces to lift it. Sustaining a grip or pinch on an object or tool is done primarily with isometric contractions and intermittent isotonic contractions, as when writing with a pencil over a long period.

During object manipulation, a dynamic lift is generally combined with static hold and release of an object. The sequential tasks involved in grasping and lifting an object are triggered by discrete mechanical events that relay information from somatosensory receptors.[34] Experience aids in the development of internal representations of object properties. This information is used for anticipatory control or planning before lifting and manipulating an object. Without anticipatory control or scaling of fingertip forces, objects may slip from grasp or be squeezed too tightly because the feedback mechanisms are too slow to upgrade or to downgrade forces quickly.

In-Hand Manipulation

The ability to move objects within one hand, termed *in-hand manipulation*, is divided into three components, called shift, rotation, and translation.[40] *Shift* refers to the movement of an object on the finger pads or between the fingers. *Rotation* is the movement of an object around its axis using the fingers. *Translation* is the movement of an object from fingers to palm or from palm to fingers.

To translate objects such as a raisin from the palm to the fingertips, finger flexion and extension are used. Shift incorporates the pads of the fingers with thumb opposition as when turning thin pages in a book. Simple rotation involves turning an object on its axis 90 degrees, such as when turning a pencil to write. Complex rotation is defined as 180–360 degrees of object rotation, as when using the pencil eraser (Fig. 12.5A). In-hand manipulation skills can also incorporate stabilization of one object or part of an object within the hand while another object or object part is simultaneously being manipulated within the same hand.[40] Typically, if two objects are held in the same hand, the ring and small (ulnar) fingers stabilize one object while the index and long (radial) fingers manipulate the other object or part.

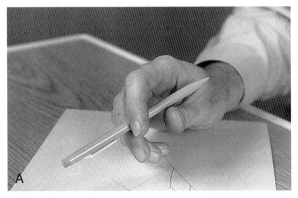

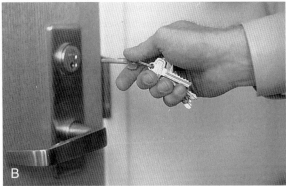

Fig. 12.5 Examples of in-hand manipulation. **(A)** Rotation component used to access the eraser of a pencil. **(B)** Shift component with ulnar stabilization used to manipulate a key when opening a lock.

Shift with stabilization is used to separate a group of keys from a single key when opening a lock (Fig. 12.5B). All three forms of in-hand manipulation can be exemplified with the use of a penny. For example, a penny can be translated from the palm up to the fingertips and then shifted across the finger pads to end with a hold between the index finger and the thumb. If you turned the penny over from heads to tails with your fingertips, that would be considered a rotation.

Stereognosis

Haptic perceptual exploration, or *stereognosis*, is the ability to recognize the names and properties of objects without vision through sensory cues and in-hand manipulation. Manipulation abilities, as well as sensibility, foster object identification, yet it is the memory of an object that makes it recognizable. Reach into your purse or pocket and retrieve a quarter. How did you know it was a quarter

and not a nickel? You probably used tactile cues and proprioceptive-kinesthetic input to judge the size and weight of the coin, based on the memory of a previous visual or other sensory experience. Although visual memory is a strong component of stereognosis, individuals without sight can develop this ability once they are taught, demonstrating that memory based on haptic exploration also plays a significant role in object recognition.

The vast number of receptors in our fingertips, muscles, joints, and skin provides the tactile and proprioceptive cues used to identify characteristics of an object. The slow and fast adapting mechanoreceptors in the fat pads and ridges of our fingers supply varied tactile information.[41] Proprioception conveys information regarding muscle force, limb movement, and changes in limb position. Afferent input contributing to proprioception includes information from muscle spindles, Golgi tendon organs, joint receptors, and cutaneous mechanoreceptors.[42] All of the receptors contribute to stereognosis. Without sensory input, the ability of humans to identify objects without vision is significantly impaired.

Release

Release is the process of letting go of a held object or taking pressure off an object. Release can be crude, as when we drop the hot handle of a frying pan, or it can be graded and controlled, as when we set a crystal glass onto a counter. Graded release is mastered and refined individually through the practice of specific tasks. Playing a musical instrument is a beautiful demonstration of how graded release is achieved. A master jazz pianist holds and releases pressure on the keys in such a controlled and graded fashion that the result is a varied sound combination of loud or soft, sustained or short-lasting tones. A novice player may not exhibit the same degree of finesse when holding or releasing the pressure on the piano keys, perhaps making all the tones loud and sustained. Tool use also demonstrates graded release. When using a screwdriver to drive in screws, a series of quick, graded grasps and releases are used to turn the handle effectively without engaging the whole shoulder girdle. Imagine a 5-year-old performing the same task. The child would probably display an alternating lateral trunk tilt or engage the shoulder girdle in the movement. This may be due to weakness, reduced ability to supinate the forearm, or insufficiently graded grasp and release. As control of release improves, our repertoire of fine-motor activities grows.

Bimanual Coordination

Bimanual coordination requires the spatial and temporal cooperation of both hands. Bimanual skills can be separated into *symmetrical* tasks in which there is a strong coupling between limbs, as when we throw a ball with two hands, and *asymmetrical* tasks or differentiation, as when one hand stabilizes an object while the other manipulates it. Examples of asymmetrical bimanual tasks include opening small containers (Fig. 12.6) or playing musical instruments, such as the guitar or violin. The neural organization associated with these two types of bimanual tasks varies depending on task goals and constraints.[43,44]

Bimanual coordination is a task-specific and active assembling procedure where two hands are restricted to act cooperatively by virtue of mutual coupling.[45] Coupling is the term used for the mutual attraction of the two limbs. Motion of the limbs can be coordinated in discrete or cyclical movements. Some patterns are spontaneously produced and others are learned after practice. Rhythmical movements or alternating movements of limbs have been identified as spontaneous coordination patterns.[46] The tendency to synchronize the two limbs can be overcome to perform tasks with different spatial or temporal requirements, such as rubbing your stomach and patting your head at the same time. Coupling of interlimb interactions is controlled at different level of the CNS.[47] Bimanual coordination is essential for performance of activities of daily living across the life span.[48,49]

PREHENSION DEVELOPMENT ACROSS THE LIFE SPAN

Prenatal Period
Growth of the Upper Limb

The limb buds, which represent the earliest form of the upper limb, begin to appear between the 26th and 27th days of gestation. By the end of the seventh week, the fingers are defined and the upper limb has rotated medially to its typical position at birth. Table 12.2 describes and illustrates upper limb growth until the seventh week of gestation. The dermatomes of the skin, which influence both the tactile and proprioceptive systems, begin to develop as early as 7 weeks of gestation. The classic proprioceptive system also begins to develop in utero with the differentiation of the articular skeleton and muscular systems around the seventh week of gestation.[50] The prenatal period ends with full development of the upper limbs.

Prenatal Action Development

Upper limb actions do not develop in isolation from the environment in which they occur. Therefore the uterine environment plays a significant role in early prehension development. The fetus responds to touch as early as 8 weeks and exhibits lateralized behavior from 10 weeks gestation. Hepper[51] and deVries and colleagues[52] noted hand-to-face contacts by fetuses at 10–12 weeks gestation which provide the possibility for thumb-to-mouth contact. Over 90% of fetuses were seen to suck their right thumb[53] and 83% of arm movements in utero were exhibited with the right versus the left arm.[54] There is clear evidence for a right-sided preference prenatally that continues after birth.[51]

Infancy and Toddlerhood

Upper limb and hand movements are present at birth, yet continued development is strongly influenced by maturation, task goals, and the ever-changing interaction between the environment and the characteristics of an individual infant.[55-57] While neuromaturation occurs,

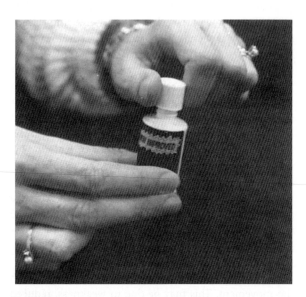

Fig. 12.6 Asymmetrical bimanual coordination demonstrating two prehension patterns: three-fingered palmar pinch (three-jaw chuck) to hold the base and dynamic lateral pinch to turn the top of the bottle.

TABLE 12.2 Development of the Upper Limb in the Embryonic Period

Age of Embryo	Upper Limb Development	Illustration
28–30 days	Upper limb buds "flipper-like" Lower limb buds appear	
31–32 days	Upper limb buds "paddle-like"	
33–36 days	Hard plates formed	
41–43 days	Digital or finger rays appear	
44–46 days	Elbow region visible, notches appear between finger rays	
47–48 days	All limb buds extend ventrally	
49–51 days	Upper limb longer and bent at elbow Fingers distinct but webbed	
52–53 days	Hands and feet approach each other Fingers are free and longer	
7th week	Upper limb rotates 90 degrees laterally in longitudinal axis (elbows face posterior) Lower limb rotates 90 degrees medially (knees face anterior) Tissue breaks down between digits from the circumference inward, producing fingers and toes	

Adapted from Moore KL, Persund TVN. *The Developing Human: Clinically Oriented Embryology*. 6th ed. Philadelphia: WB Saunders; 1998.

it is the development of perception-action loops that are thought to allow the infant to develop mature reach and grasp behavior.[24] There are four key perception-action loops which mirror the four adult phases of reach to grasp: (1) transport the hand to the general location of the target, (2) make precise contact with the target, (3) preshape the hand prior to target contact, and (4) close the hand to grasp the target using an appropriate grip configuration.[24] All components of prehension undergo a great deal of development during infancy.

Visual Regard

At birth, vision is limited. Newborns seem to have 20/800 vision, a fixed gaze of 7.8 inches (20 cm), and little accommodation.[58] Because vision needs the stimulation of light to develop, it is not until the second month of life that the structures associated with accommodation, oculomotor function, and convergence are established. Despite having low vision, newborns can fixate or sustain their gaze for brief periods and follow or track a moving target through a small range. As the newborn follows moving visual information (visual flow) from birth to 1 month of age, visual gaze typically lags behind a moving stimulus. Vestibular control over smooth gaze stabilization and adjustment, while the head and body are moving, functions earlier than visual control.[59] This is not surprising, because ocular movements induced by vestibular input in the fetus occur several months earlier than ocular movements stimulated by light postnatally. By 2–3 months of age, visual control improves as convergence and accommodation enable the infant to fixate for sustained periods and to follow a moving target through a wider range.[23,59] Visual lag while tracking a moving stimulus is diminished at 3 months. By about 5 months of age, the infant begins to demonstrate anticipatory tracking and can project the gaze ahead of a moving object.[60] Infants usually reach for objects in their visual field by 4–5 months. As visual memory develops over the next few months, infants realize that an object still exists even if it falls out of their visual field and will search for it. Binocular vision, accommodation, and acuity progress over an infant's second year of life, strengthening eye-hand coordination. It is not until 2 years of age that the infant can attend to stimuli presented in two visual fields, simultaneously demonstrating interhemispheric coordination.[61] The importance of visual tracking and reaching skills is demonstrated by studies in which these skills have predicted neurodevelopment in preterm infants.[62-64]

Reaching

Reaching proceeds grasping developmentally. Reaching involves the shoulder and grasping involves the hand. The nerves to the proximal joint musculature myelinate approximately 1 month ahead of the small hand muscles, which may be one reason why reaching behaviors precede the development of grasp patterns.[57,65] Although reaching behaviors in young infants are quite variable,

they become more refined and consistent with age and experience.

Early reaching is typically jerky, with several directional changes. Being able to successfully contact a toy during a reach occurs between 11 and 24 weeks of age.[66-68] Visually guided, anticipatory reaching behaviors begin to emerge about 4 months of age. Four-month-old infants can predict the future position of a moving ball and direct their reach toward the point of contact between the hand and the moving object. Although vision provides a stimulus to reach forward, initially, infants rely on proprioceptive feedback to adjust their hand trajectory.[67] Despite the ability of infants to reach by 3 or 4 months of age, it is not until 2 years of age that more stereotypic adultlike reaching patterns are displayed (see Fig. 4.6).[68] With experience and gains in motor control, children's reach becomes smooth, straight, and less variable.[66]

Factors that influence the type of reach an infant performs include the degree of postural control, the location of the target object, task goals, motivation, and cognition. Rochat[69] reported that when infants initially began to reach, even if they could not sit independently, they tended to do so with two hands. Older infants who sit independently prefer unimanual reaches.[69-71] Changing coordination in other behaviors, however, may also influence how reaching movements are executed. Corbetta and Thelen[72] found unimanual and bimanual reaching to fluctuate during the first year. During periods of strong bimanual reach, nonreaching interlimb activity tended to be synchronous. Yet, no specific form of interlimb coordination was observed during periods of unimanual reach. The authors postulated that changing coordination tendencies seem to influence the organization of goal-oriented reaching behaviors during the first year of life.

Toddlers can perform touch gestures and manually interact with touchscreen devices.[73] Over several days, 2- and 3-year-olds were able to operate tablets to purposively reach a goal. Two apps, shape matching and a storybook, were used in the study. Performance using the storybook app was compared to a paper book. An adult provided minimal scaffolding throughout. Three-year olds outperformed 2-year-olds on all measures. Mobile devices are common in young children's lives. Rideout[74] reported that 98% of the homes in the United States with children younger than 8 years had some type of mobile device, including a smartphone, e-reader, tablet, or gaming console. These devices may be a valuable addition to play/learning activities for children.[75,76]

Grip Formation

As reviewed earlier, we preshape our hand to the contour and size of target objects during reaching. Crude preshaping of the hand or anticipatory grip formation has been documented in infants as young as 18 weeks.[77] Von Hofsten and Ronnqvist[78] later examined grip formation during reaching in older infants of 5–6, 9, and 13 months of age. Opening aperture was adjusted to target size in the 9- to 13-month-old infants but not in the 5- to 6-month-old infants. In addition, finger opening was initiated earlier in the reach in 13-month-olds than in 9-month-olds, yet the timing did not vary for different-sized objects. Adults showed an earlier onset of opening for larger objects, or greater anticipatory grip formation. The progression in anticipatory grip formation or preshaping of the hand develops in infancy yet does not become adultlike until late childhood.[79]

Grasp and Manipulation

Many newborn reflexes are triggered by tactile stimuli. Within the first 6 months of life, early reflexes and random responses develop into voluntary prehension. These hand reflexes/reactions control finger closure via palmar stimulation and grasping, groping movements (Table 12.3). The grasp reflex is modified by the texture of the object grasped,[80] providing an example of early adaptation. Mass movement patterns are exemplified through elicitation of a traction response, in which stretching of one of the flexor muscle groups induces flexion of the entire upper limb.

When the newborn enters infancy, the hand reflexes are gradually integrated and progress into voluntary prehensile patterns. The 3-month-old infant can hold a toy if placed but release is limited. Hand play occurs when the infant brings both hands together for midline hand play at 4 months. Initial grasp patterns typically involve the fingers only, leaving the thumb passive. As the motor cortex develops postnatally, independent finger movements or fractionation emerges. Until that occurs and thumb opposition develops, infants use the hand like a rake to bring objects toward them. Thumb function, including opposition, progressively develops between 3 and 12 months and is responsible for the development of varied prehensile patterns. Anticipatory control of grasping is based on visually derived information about object size, orientation, and substance. It is evident after the infant begins reaching between 5 and 7 months.[81] During this same time period, the control of grasping shifts from tactile feedback to visual feedback.

Finger isolation, the ability to use fingers one at a time, may begin at 6 months[82] Isolation of the index finger typically begins between 9 and 12 months of age, which contributes to development of a pincer grasp at 9 months (see Table 12.4).[83,84] In an inferior pincer grasp, the thumb adducts and applies pressure on the lateral side of the index finger near the tip. The infant can pick up a cheerio using this immature pincer grasp. The thumb moves from adduction to opposition to produce a superior or neat pincer grasp around 11 months of age. The infant demonstrates pad-to-pad opposition of the

TABLE 12.3 Hand Reflexes/Reactions

Reflex	Onset	Integration	Stimulus	Response
Grasp	Birth (may be elicited in preterm infants at 25 weeks)	3–6 months	Touch to infant's palm	Flexion of fingers into the palm "catching phase"
Traction	28 weeks gestation	2–5 months	Stretch to shoulder flexors and adductors when pulled to sitting, the head lags at first	Infant flexes, lifting the head to midline of the rest of the body before falling forward
Instinctive grasp reaction	4–5 months	Replaced by voluntary grasp	Touch to any part of the palm of the hand	Movement toward stimulus, "forced groping" or "forced grasping"

From Anekar AA, Bordoni B. Palmar Grasp Reflex. [Updated 2022 Oct 24]. In: StatPearls [Internet]. Treasure Island (FL): StatPearls Publishing; Schott JM, Rossor MN. The grasp reflex and other primitive reflexes. *J Neurol Neurosurg Psychiatry.* 2003;74:558-560; Swaiman KF, Phillips J. *Swaiman's Pediatric Neurology.* 6th ed. Elsevier; 2017:14–19.

thumb to the index finger in a "tip" pinch, like an "ok" sign. This mature pincer grasp can be used to explore small objects and in self feeding. Prehension patterns become more adultlike as the infant approaches 1 year of age. By the end of the first year, the infant is able to isolate the index finger as a dominant pointer. Finger isolation and thumb to finger opposition are important developmentally as they support later functional activities such as counting one finger at a time, tying shoes, and typing on a keyboard. A 1-year-old infant can position the hand in space to achieve horizontal or vertical orientation before grasping and releasing an object.[84] Further development and experience with objects in play expand the infant's repertoire of grasp patterns.

Table 12.4 depicts a historical sequence of prehension development. Some researchers have begun to view this sequence as conservative and inflexible because it does not accurately reflect the functionally adaptive prehension seen in infants given various task constraints such as object size, shape, and texture.[85] In a longitudinal study of very young infants, Lee, Liu, and Newell[85] concluded that infant's prehension is a function of the object's properties. This is counter to Halverson's classic observations that grip forms emerge over time due to maturation.[86] Development of prehension is task-dependent.

The ability to use anticipatory control to coordinate fingertip forces during grasp and manipulation of objects is not innate.[87] It develops gradually over the first 2 years of life, as the young child interacts with various objects. Infants from 5 to 15 months utilize visual information about an object's structure to plan how they will grasp the object.[88] Infants in this study used a power handshape for rigid balls and a precision handshape for nonrigid balls, indicating that they anticipated the object's properties before grasping.

Observing the ability to grasp and lift before 2 years of age, Forssberg and colleagues[87] found that infants and toddlers increase grip and load forces sequentially, using a feedback strategy. After the second year, grip and load forces begin to be generated in parallel, demonstrating a transition to anticipatory control. Such coordination of fingertip forces is important to smooth prehension and development of in-hand manipulation and stereognosis.

In-hand manipulation skills develop gradually from infancy to childhood. The easiest skills are those of finger to palm translation and simple rotation, seen before 2 years of age. Complex rotation is still being refined in the 6- to 7-year-old child. Stereognosis also develops gradually after birth. In early infancy, the mouth and hands are used to gain information about objects. Intramodal and intermodal exploration and integration begin to develop in infancy and continue through adolescence. Intramodal integration is the ability to recognize objects by one modality (touch) after learning about the object using the same modality (touch). This ability appears first in infants as young as 2–3 months of age.[89] Intermodal integration develops next and is the ability to recognize an object by a different modality (vision) from which it was first explored (touch). Infants as young as 6 months can visually recognize a shape after only tactile contact with it.[90] Recognition of common objects through haptic exploration is relatively good by 2–3 years of age and seems to mature around 4–5 years of age.[91-93]

Stereognosis

Use of touch to recognize objects is an active "haptic" process.[94] Six exploratory procedures are pictured in Fig. 12.7.[95] Each exploratory process is associated with a different object property which is deduced from touching the object. For example, static contact assesses temperature, and pressure assesses hardness. Perception of shape is one of the last skills to develop haptically. The last exploratory procedure, contour following, is not expected in children under 5 years of age.[95] Proprioceptive information from the hand is combined with touch to learn about the substance and structural properties of objects.[96]

Release

The ability to release objects progresses in early infancy, as voluntary control over wrist, finger, and thumb extensors emerges. Release develops off a point of stability. For example, mutual fingering in midline by the 4-month-old and transferring of objects from hand to hand in the 5- to 6-month-old infant are possible because one hand can release off the stability provided by the other hand. Voluntary release typically emerges around 7–9 months of age. It is initially achieved through stabilization provided by an external surface, such as the tray of a highchair or from the stable hand of someone attempting to take an object from the infant. Once infants accurately release objects into a container without external support, they can develop graded release patterns. An infant can usually release a block into a small container by 12 months and release a pellet into a small container

TABLE 12.4 Historical Sequence of Prehension Development From Birth to 1 Year

Description	Age	Illustration	Stimulation
Recognizes hands	8 weeks (2 months)		Hand enters visual field assisted by the asymmetrical tonic neck reflex
Reflexive ulnar group	12 weeks (3 months)		Ulnar placement of objects encourages grasp; hanging toys may promote visual tracking
Retains objects placed in hand: Midline fingering; mouthing of fingers; swiping in visual field	16 weeks (4 months)		Placing objects anywhere in hand will encourage grasp; hanging toys will encourage swiping if they are within visual field and reach
Primitive squeeze grasp (wrist flexed); raking	20 weeks (5 months)		Introduction of toys of varied textures, sizes, and shapes will promote voluntary grasp and raking
Palmar grasp (no thumb participation, wrist moving into neutral)	24 weeks (6 months)		Placing toys in different positions will encourage eyes and hands to search before reach and grasp
Radial palmar grasp (thumb adduction begins); mouthing of objects	28 weeks (7 months)		Ideal toys are washable and those that can be picked up and transferred easily from one hand to the other
Scissors grasp (thumb adduction stronger)	32 weeks (8 months)		Introduction of toys with a thin circumference will strengthen thumb adductor
Radial-digital grasp (beginning opposition)	36 weeks (9 months)		Pliable materials such as clay or finger food will encourage opposition of thumb
Inferior pincer grasp (volar hold vs. pad to pad; hand supported before grasping); isolated index pointing	36–52 weeks (9–12 months)		Small objects varied in shape will promote exploration via poking, feeling, and manipulation
Pincer grasp—pad to pad (some support before grasping)	38–52 weeks (10–12 months)		Tiny objects, such as raisins, to pick up and drop will encourage development
Superior pincer grasp—tip to tip (hand unsupported before grasping)	52–56 weeks (1 year)		Thin yet safe objects the size of a pin will encourage development
Three-jaw chuck (wrist extended and ulnarly deviated); maturing release	52–56 weeks (1 year)		Toys requiring a strong radial finger hold and blocks and containers providing repeated motions will encourage strong grasp and release

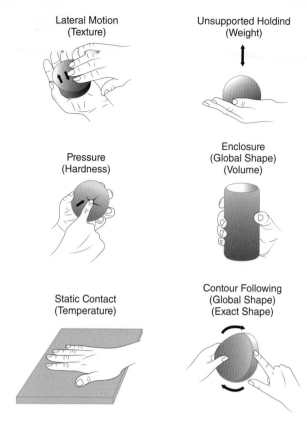

Lateral Motion
(Texture)

Unsupported Holding
(Weight)

Pressure
(Hardness)

Enclosure
(Global Shape)
(Volume)

Static Contact
(Temperature)

Contour Following
(Global Shape)
(Exact Shape)

Fig. 12.7 Haptic exploratory procedures. (Lederman SJ, Klatzky RL. Haptic perception: a tutorial. *Atten Percept Psychophys.* 2009;71:1439–1459.)

by 15 months.[97] Ball throwing is an example of release that improves in control and accuracy as the infant moves into childhood.

Bimanual Coordination

The development of bilateral arm and hand use combines the components of prehensile function. Initially, asymmetry predominates, as seen in the 2-month-old, and antigravity control is limited. The 3-month-old displays greater symmetry, as seen during bilateral hand play on the chest in midline. The 4-month-old often displays a bilateral, or two-handed, approach to reach objects visible in midline. After 5 months of age, object presentation and size determine whether the reach will be unilateral or bilateral. The 5-month-old crudely transfers objects from one hand to the other. Midline hand play away from the chest becomes more extensive as shoulder girdle strength improves. At this age,

the infant can hold a bottle with two hands and display more active object manipulation, such as banging and shaking toys. The 6- to 7-month-old displays a stronger unilateral reach and a mature hand-to-hand transfer. Despite the tendencies present in bilateral development, most infants seem to move easily between these two patterns throughout the first year.[72]

Differentiated bimanual movements begin at 8–10 months, when the two hands begin to have different roles or functions. For instance, one hand can hold the bottle while the other reaches to grasp a new toy. By 12–18 months of age, differentiated movements are advancing; each hand assumes either the active or stabilizing role. For example, the *active* hand may operate the dial of a toy with the index finger, and the *stabilizing* hand may hold the edge of the toy. After 2 years of age, the complexity of bimanual coordination/control or two-handed tasks increase significantly as does capability. Brakke and Pacheco studied drumming in toddlers from 15 to 27 months of age to better understand the development of bimanual coordination. The performance of a coordinated action such as an inverse, or antiphase, drumming results from interactions among the toddler, task requirements, and the environment. The toddlers became better at the task over the course of at least 3 months but more importantly, they were found to use different strategies to achieve antiphase coordination. These strategies involved varying oscillation frequency, amplitude ratio, and position of arm joints during drumming.

Gross Motor Development and Prehension

Advances in manual performance, visuomotor skill, and cognition coincide with exploration of objects and the environment made available through gross motor skill development. When making gross motor transitions from one position to another, the infant strengthens and stretches various muscle groups that are later used in numerous prehensile tasks. For instance, weight bearing on extended arms in a quadruped position activates shoulder and trunk muscles to contract for stability, and weight shifting alternates pressure from the ulnar to the radial side of the hand, stretching out the intrinsic muscles. Although strength and early prehensile skills naturally develop through activities executed in prone, supine, and quadruped, once postural control in sitting develops, prehensile ability improves dramatically. "Learning to sit sets up the necessary conditions for looking around and handling objects while stationary and moving—common situations in everyday life."[2] As trunk and upper limb strength and motor control expand, the infant reaches unilaterally and bilaterally with graded control. Studies examining the development of postural control in sitting reveal basic, direction-specific synergies, including APAs, adapted to task-specific conditions. Nine-month-old infants demonstrated anticipatory control by activating proximal trunk muscles before reaching for a toy in a study by Southgate and associates.[98] This finding suggests the beginning of anticipatory postural control in sitting. Visual-postural abilities may also undergo sensorimotor recalibration in newly sitting infants prior to learning to stand and walk.[99] Infants return to two-handed reaching when learning to walk. Corbetta and Bojczyk[100] and Claxton et al.[101] found that holding objects can help stabilize standing in infants.

Preschool Child

During the preschool years, prehensile patterns and eye-hand coordination skills are refined and practiced. Prehensile tasks are learned through trial and error and rehearsal from a model in collaboration with developing perceptual and cognitive processes. Often, a young child is unable to demonstrate a particular skill independently yet can do so in the presence of an adult or more capable peer. A 3-year-old child may be unable to cut paper with scissors independently yet may be successful in the presence of another capable 3-year-old by internalizing the perceptual and cognitive strategies provided. This phenomenon is known as the *Zone of Proximal Development*.[40,102] Skilled hand function and the use of implements develop rapidly during this period as preschool children expand their repertoire of play behaviors.

Reach and Grip Formation

Adultlike reaching patterns are assumed by 2 years of age yet continue to be refined through late childhood. Consistent temporal coordination across arm segments for multijoint reaching improves up until 3 years of age.[68] Kuhtz-Buschbeck and colleagues[79] compared reach and grip formation (hand preshaping) in children 4–12 years of age against adult behaviors. They found younger children opened their hand wider before object contact than did the older children or adults, suggesting that they grasp using a higher safety margin of error to prevent missing the target. They also reported that younger

children seemed to be more dependent on vision to scale their grip aperture to the target. With increasing age, the dependence on vision decreased and reaching trajectories became straighter. These studies suggest that anticipatory reach-to-grasp behaviors continue to develop through the preschool years and are refined into late childhood.

Intersegmental and interjoint coordination between the arm and trunk while reaching to grasp is known to continue to develop into late childhood.[103] Head, arm, and trunk coordination during reaching was studied in children from 2.8 to 11.8 years of age.[17] Five groups of children, divided by age, performed a reaching task. Young children reached and grasped a piece of food while older children reached for and grasped a cube. Six adults also reached and grasped a cube. The pattern of head and trunk coupling was different along different axes of rotation. Children used an HSS strategy and adults used a fixed head-trunk coordination pattern.

Grasp and Manipulation

Preschool children gradually become more socialized and begin to engage in activities that require grasp and manipulation of various implements. Implements commonly used at this age include utensils, such as eating devices and banging instruments; tools, such as scissors or writing devices; and self-care items, such as fasteners, shoelaces, and hairbrushes.

The use of implements requires the employment of one or all three forms of manipulation: sustained grip or pinch force, in-hand manipulation, and bimanual coordination. As strength of the intrinsic muscles develops, the child usually can demonstrate *sustained pinch force* on items such as a crayon when coloring. Young children improve in the ability to coordinate fingertip forces with practice but still demonstrate inefficient control. For example, they may crush fragile objects such as paper cups or potato chips or lift light objects too quickly. This lack of anticipatory control may be due in part to insufficient internal representations for the properties of the lifted objects.

As distal control improves, crayon and pencil grips are modified. A typical sequence of pencil grip development is outlined in Table 12.5. Before in-hand manipulation skill advances, the child often adjusts the crayon position in one hand with the contralateral hand. Once fingertip force coordination improves and in-hand manipulation develops, the crayon can be translated,

Pencil Grip	Age	Description	Illustration
TABLE 12.5 **Sequential Acquisition of Pencil Grip**			
Palmar supinate	1–2 years	Pencil or crayon is held by fisted hand; forearm slightly supinated; wrist slightly flexed; shoulder motion produces movement of pencil	
Digital pronate	2–3 years	Pencil or crayon is held by fingers and thumb; forearm pronated; wrist ulnarly deviated; pencil controlled by shoulder movement	
Static tripod	3+ years	Pencil held proximally between thumb and radial two fingers; minimal wrist mobility; pencil controlled by shoulder movement	
Dynamic tripod	4+ years	Pencil is held distally through thumb opposition to the index and long fingers, with the ring and small fingers stabilizing in flexion; small movements at the metacarpophalangeal and interphalangeal joints control the pencil; stabilization occurs at the shoulder, elbow, forearm, and wrist	

Data from Erhardt RP. *Developmental Hand Dysfunction: Theory, Assessment, and Treatment*. Laurel, MD: RAMSCO; 1982:9-3; Knobloch H, Stevens F, Malone AF. *Manual of Developmental Diagnosis: The Administration and Interpretation of the Revised Gesell and Amatruda's Developmental and Neurological Exam*. Houston, TX: Developmental Evaluation Materials; 1987:24-260; Rosenbloom L, Horton ME. The maturation of fine prehension in young children. *Dev Med Child Neurol*. 1971;13:3-8.

rotated, or shifted ipsilaterally without assistance from the opposite hand.

Bimanual coordination for symmetrical and asymmetrical tasks expands through the preschool years as children begin to incorporate anticipatory prehensile behaviors as needed for such tasks as catching a ball (Fig. 12.8). Many skills develop as each hand begins to refine coordinated, asymmetrical roles. Initially, the child may need to stabilize the paper she is coloring using both elbows, but eventually just the opposite hand is needed. Other examples of bimanual skills a typical preschooler engages in by 5 years of age are cutting paper with scissors, buttoning clothing, zipping zippers, and tying shoelaces. Motor planning, the ability to execute novel motor acts, and task-specific practice play significant roles in the acquisition of new fine-motor tasks such as those described earlier. Through trial and error, modeling, and practice, the preschooler expands and refines sustained pinch ability, in-hand manipulation, and bilateral hand use. By the end of this period,

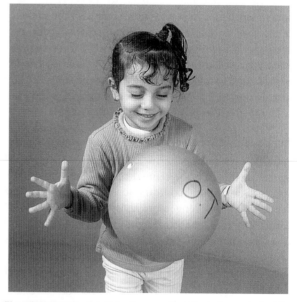

Fig. 12.8 Bimanual anticipatory reach and grip formation exhibited by a 4-year-old when catching a ball.

hand preference for specific tasks such as coloring and cutting with scissors may be demonstrated.

Hand Preference

Hand preference and hand dominance are often confused in definition. *Hand preference* refers to a *tendency* to use one hand for prehension instead of the other. *Hand dominance* is the *consistent use* of one hand over the other for tasks such as throwing a ball, writing with a pencil, and eating with a fork. Hand preference can be verified through interview and observation of performance during select tasks. The preschooler develops a hand preference as she practices skilled tasks, such as eating with utensils, coloring, and throwing a ball. By 4–6 years of age, hand preference is well established. Lateralization of the brain, the process by which the hemispheres become specialized for particular functions, is generally thought to be one factor affecting hand dominance.[104,105] Consistent use of one hand for skilled tasks promotes lateralization. Some children may not demonstrate a hand preference during the preschool years because the preferred hand is not yet sufficiently influenced by the contralateral motor cortex. However, by 6–7 years of age, hand dominance is demonstrated through the consistent and superior use of one hand to hold a pencil during writing tasks. Most agree that the dominant hand performs better than the nondominant during fine, dexterous activities. However, for some manual tasks, it is possible that by altering the context requirements such as speed and accuracy of the task, performance between hands may become more similar.[106]

The influence of hand preference on grip strength was studied in children and adolescents.[107] The researchers found a difference in grip strength between the preferred and nonpreferred hand. They further explored whether being left-preferrent (LP) or right-preferrent (RP) would result in different grip strength and whether the 10% rule[108] of the dominant hand having greater grip strength would hold true.[108] RP children and adolescents demonstrated the 10% rule while LP children did not. Handedness is a complex trait that occurs through the interaction of genetics, epigenetics, and the environment.[109]

School-Aged Child
Mastery

During this period, children often demonstrate mastery of many components of prehension. A child's knowledge and abilities for an activity are considered domain- or task-specific, which allows for rapid encoding and response to certain fine-motor situations. The degree to which a particular skill is mastered depends on the amount of time spent practicing specific tasks and the strength of the supporting systems.

Reach-to-grasp behaviors expand in the school-aged child. For instance, 6-year-olds display an exaggerated grip aperture during reaching, whereas 12-year-olds can scale the grip aperture more closely to object size.[79] Although some children between 6 and 8 years of age may demonstrate adultlike fingertip force coordination when grasping and lifting objects, some do not achieve this capacity until 11 years of age or later.[87] Reportedly by 6 years of age, most children can demonstrate adequate in-hand manipulation, which allows for the expansion of prehensile activities in which they can engage.

Bagesteiro and associates[110] studied interjoint coordination in 6-year-old children reaching for a target with either their dominant or nondominant arm. They also tested a group of young adults performing the same actions. Manual asymmetries were present in strongly right-handed children and young adults. The two groups used different strategies to perform the task. Young adults utilized the elbow joint to perform rapid aiming movements to the ipsilateral target, with minimal shoulder joint movement. A similar strategy was used by the children when aiming at the ipsilateral target but less elbow movement was used when aiming at the contralateral targe. Overall, the children were slower and less coordinated in reaching for the target and much more influenced by the target location. Researchers concluded that control of multiple body axes is not yet mature in children. Not all aspects of reaching develop at the same time.

Symmetrical bimanual coordination in typically developing (TD) 8-year-old children was assessed and performance of the same task compared with same-aged children with unilateral spastic cerebral palsy.[111] Children were seated in a quiet room and asked to lift a 10 cm × 10 cm cube, hold it for 1–2 seconds, and return it to the start position. Each face of the cube recorded the forces used by the subjects. They reported no differences in force coordination and timing in the preload phase. "TD children demonstrated consistent increases in grasp and load forces during both the load and unload phases, with only small variations in isometric force development between subsequent lifts."[111] Both TD children and children with unilateral CP showed a bias toward the preferred hand during lifting the cube. TD children demonstrated greater smoothness of movement. TD children at this age are able to use feedback from the friction of the finger-surface friction and object weight to safely lift and hold an object. Control of grasp force is dependent on intact sensorimotor integration of the objects' properties.[112]

Complex asymmetrical bimanual coordination progresses during the school-aged period. For example, building model airplanes is a complex task that requires one hand to stabilize the base and the other hand to glue small parts onto that stable base. Children of the same age demonstrate very different levels of skill at building models. As a child matures into adolescence, interest and experience further guide the refinement of prehensile skills.

School-aged children often spend a large amount of their time involved in task-specific practice. For example, the demands for written work increase by 8–9 years of age, necessitating skill in holding and sustaining a pencil grip while completing the complex task of handwriting. Writing requires selective attention and other cognitive processes and is affected by the state of arousal.

Handwriting

Many of the components of prehension play a role in handwriting. Visual regard of the paper and pencil and accurate perception of the workspace are needed. When copying from a chalkboard, we must shift visual gaze from the board to the paper without losing our place. The spatial relationships between the desk, the paper, and the blackboard need to be accurately perceived, as do the spatial relationships between the letters, words, and sentences on a page. Position in space and form constancy will guide recognition of letters and numbers. Grasp and manipulation, sustained grip and pinch, in-hand manipulation, and bimanual coordination contribute to handwriting and can be analyzed separately for clarity.

Pencil grip is an example of sustained pinch. Examples are shown by order of frequency in Fig. 12.9. The most frequently used pencil grip is the dynamic tripod, which is demonstrated when a pencil is held between the pads of the index and thumb while it rests against the long finger. This position is considered the most efficient in terms of speed and dexterity because pencil movement is controlled distally by the fingers and thumb. Alternative pencil grips are considered efficient if the thumb and index form a circle or open web space, allowing for skillful distal manipulation. Inefficient grips limit the range, speed, and

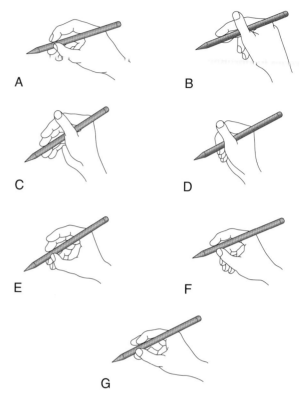

Fig. 12.9 Pencil grips. (**A**) Dynamic tripod. (**B**) Lateral tripod. (**C**) Transpalmar interdigital. (**D**) Cross-thumb. (**E**) Dynamic bipod. (**F**) Dynamic bipod with omitted third digit. (**G**) Static tripod. (Redrawn from Bergmann KP. Incidence of atypical pencil grasps among nondysfunctional adults. *Am J Occup Ther.* 1990;44:736–740.)

fluidity of distal movement and demand greater proximal movements of the wrist and elbow to control the pencil, reducing precision. The lateral tripod, considered a functional yet inefficient grip because the web space is closed, is used by up to 25% of nondysfunctional children and up to 10% of adults.[113] With adequate strength and somatosensory feedback, a child can sustain a hold on a pencil without the need for excess pressure. Endurance for sustained pinch, required during prolonged handwriting tasks, is gained with practice.

Grip and pinch strength increase throughout childhood and contribute to all prehensile abilities.[114-116] Fig. 12.10A depicts grip strength in 3- to 17-year-olds.[116] Pencil grip strength may be best inferred from palmar pinch and key pinch strength. Hager-Ross and Rosblad[114] studied grip strength in Swedish boys and girls from 4 to 16 years of age. The age-related increase in strength was approximately the same in boys and girls until 10 years of age, when boys became stronger than girls.[114] In the United States, Bohannon and colleagues[116] found that the dominant hand was stronger than nondominant; boys were stronger than girls and older children were stronger than younger children (Fig. 12.10A). Grip strength was associated with height, weight, sex, and age. Age explained the majority of the variance.

In-hand manipulation is frequently used for pencil writing. If a demand is made for quick writing and erasing, a child learns to adjust the pencil in one hand and rotate it longitudinally to use the eraser. The hand has to be stable enough to support the fingers when using a tool, in this example, a pencil.[117] Bimanual coordination is required for writing because one hand must stabilize the writing surface and the other hand must actively use the pencil.

Adolescence

During this phase of development, primary occupations include schoolwork, socialization, part-time employment, and prereadiness for later employment or career. The prehensile demands resemble those of the school-age child, except that the skill level required is often higher. Less time is spent in trial and error and more time is spent in perfecting skill. Skills performed with the dominant hand continue to advance beyond those of the nondominant hand. Bimanual skills, including the use of a computer keyboard, gaming platform, texting on a tablet/phone, or sports-related activities, do play a strong role at this stage of development. Adolescents often are cognitively aware of their strengths and weaknesses in terms of coordination and skill with manipulative tasks. Success heightens interest and helps boost self-esteem; thus, motivation for a task and practice are strongly correlated. Grip strength continues to increase in adolescence (see Fig. 12.10A). Young adults demonstrate a significant increase in grip and pinch strength, which may correlate with the functional gains seen in prehensile tasks.

By the time we reach adolescence, adultlike coordination of fingertip forces is demonstrated. Dayanidhi and colleagues[36] studied developmental improvements in dynamic control of fingertip forces. Finger dexterity measured by a novel paradigm of compressing springs continued to develop into late adolescence. Hand strength is highly correlated with measures of growth in adolescence.[118] In the study by Dayanidhi,[36] musculoskeletal strength and growth were poorly correlated with

improving dexterity. Success in the unstable manipulation task appeared dependent on improvements in sensorimotor processing. Manual dexterity allows an individual to fine-tune manual skills related to specific areas of interest.

Adulthood

Throughout adulthood, prehensile function is maintained and enhanced by occupational and recreational activities such as sports and hobbies.

Strength

The magnitude of grip and pinch strength needed to perform most activities of daily living tasks and job duties varies. Hand grip strength is a measure related to functional ability and health in adults and older adults.[119-123] Available grip and pinch strength may also influence our career choice. Conversely, grip and pinch strength increase if our occupational tasks require greater hand use.[119] For example, office workers have the weakest grips, and heavy manual workers have the strongest. Throughout the adult life span and across the globe, hand grip strength of men is greater than that of women.[119-121,124,125] Hand grip strength is also positively correlated with height, weight, and hand dominance.[119,121,125] Some studies have also found relationships between hand grip strength and cognition/level of education;[121] level of physical activity/cardiorespiratory fitness;[124] and nutritional status.[119] A negative correlation has been found between hand grip strength and waist circumference,[121] as well as hand grip strength and age.[119-121,124,125] Hand grip strength has also been found to be greater in developed countries as compared to developing countries.[119,126]

Hand dominance appears to impact grip strength. If the right hand is dominant, the strength of the right hand is approximately 10% greater than that of the left hand, and if the left hand is dominant, the strength of the two hands is usually equal.[107,108,127] However, other studies have found the grip strength of the dominant and nondominant hands to be relatively equal regardless of handedness.[128,129]

Hand grip strength peaks between 30 and 39 years of age.[119-121,124] Strength is maintained through middle adulthood, but then starts to decline in women at 50–59 years of age and at 60–69 years of age in men (see Fig. 12.10B).[119] Other studies confirm decline of hand grip strength accelerating after age 60 years for both men and women.[120,121,123-125]

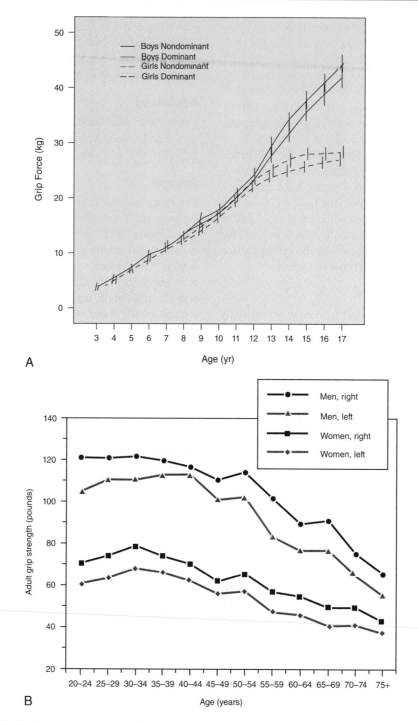

Fig. 12.10 (**A**) Hand grip strength for 3- to 17-year-olds. (**B**) Hand grip strength for individuals 18–85 years of age. (From (**A**) Bohannon RW, Wang YC, Bubela D, Gershon RC. Handgrip strength: a population-based study of norms and age trajectories for 3- to 17-year-olds. *Pediatr Phys Ther*. 2017;29:118–123. (**B**) Wang YC, Bohannon RW, Li X, et al. Hand-grip strength: normative reference values and equations for individuals 18 to 85 years of age residing in the United States. *J Orthop Sports Phys Ther*. 2018;48(9):685–693.)

Maintenance of Prehensile Skill and Function

In middle adulthood, most of the systems involved with prehension continue to function well, as long as they are maintained and not overextended. Performance in most activities of daily living is maintained easily because such activities are practiced repeatedly over the years and are generally nonstrenuous. When dysfunction does occur, it is commonly caused by congenital or traumatic limb loss, learned nonuse, peripheral neuropathy, or cumulative trauma disorders.

Maintenance of skill during the period of middle adulthood is differentiated from early adulthood in terms of performance, that is, the amount of domain-specific practice, motivation, and efficiency. When interest and motivation for activities drop, so does practice time. We may have been an expert at the piano at 25 years of age, but by age 50, we may spend too little time at the keyboard to maintain and preserve our former skill. Conversely, concert pianists, who continue to demonstrate fine technique well into their older adult years, may be able to maintain their skills because of continued practice. Sustained practice time promotes greater endurance, yet it is demanding. It requires us to maintain a high tolerance for aerobic work to avoid fatigue of associated structures.

Age differences in compensatory arm-trunk coordination during trunk-assisted reaching have been studied.[18] Young adults were gender matched to healthy adults over 60 years of age and asked to perform two tasks while seated. One task involved keeping a fixed hand position while flexing forward at the trunk (SHT). The other task involved reaching for a target while flexing forward at the trunk (RHT). The subjects completed the tasks with eyes closed using dominant and nondominant arms at slow and fast speeds under two conditions. The trunk was allowed to move versus blocking the trunk movement during the task. Researchers found that performance was similar regardless of which arm was used or the movement speed.[18] Older adults demonstrated efficient coordination of arm and trunk movements but exhibited more variability in movement times in RHT and in arm-trunk coordination in SHT than younger adults.

Older Adulthood

Manual performance and psychomotor behaviors decline as adults age.[130–132] Changes in prehension, manual dexterity, bimanual task performance, and overall hand function impact performance of activities of daily living (such as holding utensils, buttoning), work-related functions, and hobby-related activities for older adults.[48,132] These changes in manual skill reflect functional adaptation to changes in the visual, nervous, somatosensory, and musculoskeletal systems associated with aging. Metabolic disease, poor nutrition, and a sedentary lifestyle also contribute to the decline in hand function with aging.[132]

Older adults who regularly practice manual dexterity tasks, such as piano playing, are able to maintain hand function. It is recommended that older adults who regularly participate in an exercise program for hand strength and flexibility will slow the rate of functional decline.[132] Despite the system changes that occur with aging, overall eye-hand coordination and manipulative skills may be relatively maintained in older adults as long as task-specific practice is continued and the systems involved remain generally intact (Fig. 12.11). For example, although a reduction in sensibility typically affects fine-motor function, it may not reduce function in all tasks.[133]

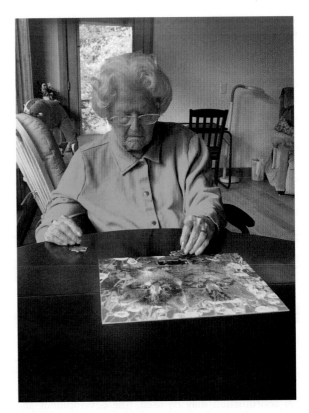

Fig. 12.11 Long-time hobbies contribute to maintained prehensile skills in 98-year-olds.

Structural and Functional Changes in the Hand With Aging

Changes in the central and peripheral nervous system influence hand function of older adults. Approximately, a 25%–40% decrease in motor axons can be seen in older adults, resulting in a decrease in motor units.[48,132] As described in Chapter 8, surviving motor units adapt and become larger and slower. These changes are especially noted in the thenar eminence. Fewer myelinated nerve fibers of smaller diameter from C7 to C8 also contribute to slower, less-effective hand use.[132] As nerve conduction velocity decreases, speed of grasp may also decrease Centrally, changes in the motor cortex, somatosensory cortex, subthalamic regions, and decreased gray matter are correlated with changes in bimanual activity.[48]

Musculoskeletal changes include changes to muscle, tendons, and intrinsic bones and joints. Although the decrease in muscle mass in the hand is not as great as in other skeletal muscles, after age 60 years, a 20%–25% decrease is seen in hand muscle fibers, especially in the thenar muscles.[132] Grip strength decreases beginning at approximately 50 years of age, with greatest declines after 80 years of age.[119,120,124,134] Increased stiffness of tendons is seen because of an increase in density of connective tissue with aging and circulatory changes. This contributes to diminished range of motion, decreased power in flexion, and less-effective joint control.[132] Bone loss with aging and degeneration of the articular cartilage can reduce the efficiency of joint movement, and reduced shock absorption also contributes to difficulties with grip and pinch abilities.

Sensory changes in the visual and somatosensory systems also impact hand function of older adults. Loss in sensibility through the arms and hands may be due to a decrease in sensory nerve conduction, alterations in mechanoreceptors, and a decline in spatial acuity of touch.[135] Furthermore, Cole and colleagues[133] reported that there is an increased threshold to touch pressure and a decreased sensitivity to vibration sense. Loss of cutaneous mechanoreceptors decreases tactile sensory perception and perception of temperature receptors and circulatory changes.[137] Visual acuity, imaging power of the retina, and the transparency of the lens are all reduced in older adulthood. In addition, there is a sharp decrease in depth perception from 60 to 75 years. Depth perception changes most influence distances reached and grip aperture during reach and grasp activities.[136] Visual perceptual changes do not appear to negatively impact accuracy of reach and grasp.[137–139]

Prehensile Skill and Function in Older Adulthood

Several functional changes are seen in older adult prehensile and hand skills. Decreased grip strength and grip stability are demonstrated in older adults, which affects prehension and reach-to-grasp activities.[134,138] Grip strength decline can also contribute to difficulties in performing housework and lifting objects.[122] When performing bimanual tasks, decreased accuracy, increased variability of grasp, and slower movement time are seen.[48] In reach and grasp activities, older adults demonstrate increased movement times, but accuracy is maintained.[138,139] Reach and grip stability during functional activities requires steady grip strength, perceptual feedback, arm coordination, and good attention span and working memory. Older adults have some difficulty with these functional activities because they need to hold an object with submaximal grip strength while the arm is moving.[134]

Decreased speed of muscle contraction will affect dexterity. This system change combined with reduced sensibility and greater time to plan precise distal movements may expand the time to task completion. For example, older adults may need more time to count out change at the checkout line.

In general, motivation and arousal for specific tasks do not decline with age. Therefore unless there are specific system deficits, prehensile skills can continue to be useful into older adulthood.

SUMMARY

During many everyday activities, the primary components of prehension are engaged: visual regard, reach, grasp, manipulation, and release. Depending on the task goal and constraints, postural control and bimanual coordination may be used. The development and maintenance of prehensile skill incorporate many interdependent systems. Indeed, strong relationships exist between prehension, postural control, cognition, and visuoperceptual skills. Flexible prehensile skills allow us to mold actions to constraints and environmental demands while meeting task goals. When prehension is viewed across the life span, we can only marvel at its highly developed features.

REFERENCES

1. Kahrs BA, Lockman JJ. Tool using. *Child Dev Perspect.* 2014;8:231–236. https://doi.org/10.1111/cdep.1287.

2. Rachwani J, Herzberg O, Golenia L, Adolph KE. Postural, visual, and manual coordination in the development of prehension. *Child Dev.* 2019;90:1559–1568. https://doi.org/10.1111/cdev.13282.

3. Kibler WB, Press J, Sciascia A. The role of core stability in athletic function. *Sports Med.* 2006;36(3):189–198.

4. Burnett R, Cornett N, Brahler CJ, et al. Investigating the association between core strength, postural control and fine motor performance in children. *Journal of Student Physical Therapy Research.* 2011;4(2):2..

5. Solanki DV, Soni N. Correlation between hand grip strength and core muscle activation in physical therapists of Gujarat. *Int Journal of Health Sciences and Research.* 2021;99(5). https://doi.org/10.52403/ijhsr.20210512.

6. Nuhami S. Correlation between core stability and upper extremity performance in male college athletes. *Medicina.* 2022;58:592.. https://doi.org/10.3390/medicina58080982.

7. Zemkova E, Zapletalová L. The role of neuromuscular control of posture and core stability in functional movement and athlete performance. *Front Physiol.* 2022;13:796097.. https://doi.org/10.3389/fphys2022.

8. Abd-Elfattah HM, Aly SM. Effect of core stability exercises on hand functions in children with hemiplegic cerebral pals. *Ann Rehab Med.* 2021;45:71–78. https://doi.org/10.5535/arm.20124.

9. Case-Smith J, Fisher AG, Bauer D. An analysis of the relationship between proximal and distal motor control. *Am J Occup Ther.* 1989;43:657–662.

10. Serrien B, Baeyens JP. The proximal-to-distal sequence in upper-limb motions on multiple levels and time scales. *Hum Mov Sci.* 2017;55:156–171. https://doi.org/10.1016/j.humov.2017.08.009.

11. Lumen Learning. Nervous system control of muscle tension. https://courses.lumenlearning.com/suny-ap1/chapter/nervous-system-control-of-muscle-tension/ Accessed December 31, 2022.

12. O'Driscoll SW, Horil E, Ness R, et al. The relationship between wrist position, grasp size, and grip strength. *J Hand Surg.* 1992;17:169–177.

13. Li ZM. The influence of wrist position on individual finger forces during forceful grip. *J Hand Surg Am.* 2002;27:886–896. https://doi.org/10.1053/jhsu.2002.35078.

14. Aoki T, Latash ML, Zatsiorsky VM. Adjustments to local friction in multifinger prehension. *J Mot Behv.* 2007;39:276–290. https://doi.org/10.3200/JMBR.39.4.276-290.

15. Hall LA, Karl JM, Thomas BL, Whishaw IQ. Reach and grasp reconfigurations reveal that proprioception assists reaching and hapsis assists grasping in peripheral vision. *Exp Brain Res.* 2014;232:2807–2819. https://doi.org/10.1007/s00221-014-3945-6.

16. Dale N, Sakkalou E, O'Reilly M, Springall C, De Haan M, Salt A. Functional vision and cognition in infants with congenital disorders of the peripheral visual system. *Dev Med Child Neurol.* 2017;59:725–731. https://doi.org/10.1111/dmcn.13429.

17. Sveistrup H, Schneiberg S, McKinley PA, McFadyen BJ, Levin MF. Head, arm and trunk coordination during reaching in children. *Exp Brain Res.* 2008;188(2):237–247. https://doi.org/10.1007/s00221-008-1357-1.

18. Khanafer S, Sveistrup H, Levin MF, Cressman EK. Age differences in arm-trunk coordination during trunk-assisted reaching. *Exp Brain Res.* 2019;237:223–236. https://doi.org/10.1007/s00221-018-5412-2.

19. Abend W, Bizzi E, Morasso P. Human arm trajectory formation. *Brain.* 1982;105:331–348. https://doi.org/10.1093/brain/105.2.331.

20. Paulignan Y, Jeannerod M. Visuomotor channels in prehension. In: Wing AM, Haggard P, Flanagan JR, eds.*Hand and Brain: The Neurophysiology and Psychology of Hand Movements.* New York: Academic Press; 1996:268..

21. Konczak J, Borutta M, Topka H, et al. The development of goal-directed reaching in infants: hand trajectory formation and joint torque control. *Exp Brain Res.* 1995;106(1):156–168.

22. Duff SV, Sainburg RL. Lateralization of motor adaptation reveals independence in trajectory and steady state position. *Exp Brain Res.* 2007;179(4):551–561.

23. Atkinson J, Braddick O. Visual development. *Handb Clin Neurol.* 2020;173:122–142. https://doi.org/10.1016/B978-0-444-64150-2.00013-7.

24. Karl JM, Slack BM, Wilson AM, Wilson CA, Bertoli ME. Increasing task precision demands reveals that the reach and grasp remain subject to different perception-action constraints in 12-month-old human infants. *Infant Behav Dev.* 2019;57:101382.. https://doi.org/10.1016/j.infbeh.2019.101382.

25. Jakobson LS, Goodale MA. Factors affecting higher-order movement planning: a kinematic analysis of human prehension. *Exp Brain Res.* 1991;86:199–208.

26. Ansuini C, Santello M, Massaccesi S, et al. Effects of end-goal on hand shaping. *J Neurophysiol.* 2005;95(4):2456–2465.

27. Pardhan S, Gonzalez-Alvarez C, Subramanian A. How does the presence and duration of central visual impairment affect reaching and grasping movements? *Ophthalmic Physiol Opt.* 2011;31:233–239. https://doi.org/10.1111/j.1475-1313.2010.00819.x.

28. Hou SW, Zhang Y, Christian L, Niechwiej-Szwedo E, Giaschi D. Evaluating visuomotor coordination in children with amblyopia. *Dev Psychobiol*. 2022;64: e22270.. https://doi.org/10.1002/dev.22270.

29. Niechwiej-Szwedo E, Colpa L, Wong A. The role of binocular vision in the control and development of visually guided upper limb movements. *Philos Trans R Soc Lond B Biol Sci*. 2023;378(1869): https://doi.org/10.1098/rstb.2021.0461. 20210461.

30. Napier JR. The prehensile movement of the human hand. *J Bone Joint Surg*. 1956;38:902–913.

31. Landsmeer JMF. Power grip and precision handling. *Ann Rheum Dis*. 1962;21:164–169.

32. Wong YJ, Whishaw IQ. Precision grasps of children and young and old adults: individual differences in digit contact strategy, purchase pattern, and digit posture. *Behav Brain Res*. 2004;154(1):113–123.

33. Casanova JS, Grunert BK. Adult prehension: patterns and nomenclature for pinches. *J Hand Ther*. 1989;2: 231–244.

34. Johansson RS, Cole KJ. Sensory-motor coordination during grasping and manipulative actions. *Curr Opin Neurobiol*. 1992;2:815–823.

35. Goodale MA, Cant JS. Coming to grips with vision and touch. Behavioral Brain. *Science*. 2007;30:209–210. https://doi.org/10.1017/S0140525X070011483.

36. Dayanidhi S, Hedberg A, Valero-Cuevas FJ, Forssberg H. Developmental improvements in dynamic control of fingertip forces last throughout childhood and into adolescence. *J Neurophysiol*. 2013;110:1583–1592. https://doi.org/10.1152/jn.00320.2013.

37. Chu-Santos CAR, Handog GB. Thumb opposition strength in healthy adults—a baseline study. *Acta Scientific Orthopaedics*. 2021;4:90–99. https://doi.org/10.31080/ASOR.2021.4323.

38. Raj R, Marquis C. Finger dominance. *J Hand Surg*. 1999;24:430..

39. Tubiana R. Architecture and functions of the hand. In: Tubiana R, Thomine JM, Mackin EJ, eds.*Examination of the Hand and Upper Limb*. Philadelphia: WB Saunders; 1984:1–98.

40. Exner C. The zone of proximal development in in-hand manipulation skills of nondysfunctional 3- and 4-year-old children. *Am J Occup Ther*. 1990;44:884–891.

41. Jarocka E, Pruszynski JA, Johansson RS. Human touch receptors are sensitive to spatial details on the scale of single fingerprint ridges. *J Neurosci*. 2021;41: 3622–3634. https://doi.org/10.1523/JNEUROSCI.1716-20.2021.

42. Liu M, Batista A, Bensmaia S, Weber DJ. Information about contact force and surface texture is mixed in the firing rates of cutaneous afferent neurons.

J Neurophysiol. 2021;125:496–508. https://doi.org/10.1152/jn.00725.2019.

43. Kazennikov O, Wiesendanger M. Bimanual coordination of bowing and fingering in violinists: effects of position changes and string changes. *Motor Control*. 2009;13(3):297–309.

44. Liao WW, Whitall J, Barton JE, McCombe Waller S. Neural motor control differs between bimanual common-goal vs. bimanual dual-goal tasks. *Exp Brain Res*. 2018;236:1789–1800. https://doi.org/10.1007/s00221-018-5261-z.

45. Sleimen-Malkoun R, Temprado JJ, Thefenne L, Berton E. Bimanual training in stroke: how do coupling and symmetry-breaking matter? *BMC Neurol*. 2011;11:11.. https://doi.org/10.1186/1471-2377-11-11.

46. Haken H, Kelso JA, Bunz H. A theoretical model of phase transitions in human hand movements. *Biol Cybern*. 1985;51:347–356. https://doi.org/10.1007/BF00336922.

47. Banerjee A, Jirsa VK. How do neural connectivity and time delays influence bimanual coordination? *Biol Cybern*. 2007;96(2):265–278. https://doi.org/10.1007/s00422-006-0114-4.

48. Krehbiel LM, Kang N, Cauraugh JH. Age-related differences in bimanual movements: A systematic review and meta-analysis. *Exp Gerontol*. 2017;98:199–206. https://doi.org/10.1016/j.exger.2017.09.001.

49. Lee MC, Hsu CC, Tsai YF, Chen CY, Lin CC, Wang CY. Criterion-referenced values of grip strength and usual gait speed using instrumental activities of daily living disability as the criterion. *J Geriatr Phys Ther*. 2018;41:14–19. https://doi.org/10.1519/JPT.0000000000000106.

50. Moore KL, Persaud TVN, Torchia MG.*The Developing Human*. 11th ed. Philadelphia: Elsevier; 2020.

51. Hepper PG. The developmental origins of laterality: fetal handedness. *Dev Psychobiol*. 2013;55:588–595. https://doi.org/10.1002/dev.21119.

52. de Vries JPP, Visser GHA, Prechtl HFR. The emergence of fetal behaviour. II. Quantitative aspects. *Early Hum Dev*. 1985;12:99–120.

53. Hepper PG, Shahidullah S, White R. Handedness in the human fetus. *Neuropsychologia*. 1991;29(11):1107–1111. https://doi.org/10.1016/0028-3932(91)90080-r.

54. McCartney G, Hepper P. Development of lateralized behaviour in the human fetus from 12 to 27 weeks' gestation. *Dev Med Child Neurol*. 1999;41:83–86.

55. Thelen E. Motor development: a new synthesis. *Am Psychol*. 1995;50:79–95.

56. Auer T, Pinter S, Kovacs N, et al. Does obstetric brachial plexus injury influence speech dominance? *Ann Neural*. 2009;65(1):57–66.

57. Adolph KE, Franchak JM. The development of motor behavior. *Wiley Interdiscip Rev Cogn Sci.* 2017;8 https://doi.org/10.1002/wcs.1430. 10.1002/wcs.1430.

58. Coren S, Ward LM, Enns JT, eds.*Sensation and Perception.* 5th ed. Orlando, FL: Harcourt Brace; 1999.

59. Rosander K, von Hofsten C. Visual-vestibular interaction in early infancy. *Exp Brain Res.* 2000;133:321–333.

60. Rosander K. Visual tracking and its relationship to cortical development. *Prog Brain Res.* 2007;164:105–122. https://doi.org/10.1016/S0079-6123(07)64006-0.

61. Liegeois F, Bentejec L, de Schonen S. When does inter-hemispheric integration of visual events emerge in infancy? A developmental study on 19- to 28-month-old infants. *Neuropsychologia.* 2000;38:1382–1389.

62. Kaul YF, Rosander K, von Hofsten C, et al. Visual tracking in very preterm infants at 4 mo predicts neurodevelopment at 3 y of age. *Pediatr Res.* 2016;80:35–42. https://doi.org/10.1038/pr.2016.37.

63. Kaul YF, Rosander K, Grönqvist H, Strand Brodd K, Hellström-Westas L, von Hofsten C. Reaching skills of infants born very preterm predict neurodevelopment at 2.5 years. *Infant Behav Dev.* 2019;57:101333.. https://doi.org/10.1016/j.infbeh.2019.101333.

64. Kaul YF, Rosander K, von Hofsten C, Strand Brodd K, Holmström G, Hellström-Westas L. Visual tracking at 4 months in preterm infants predicts 6.5-year cognition and attention. *Pediatr Res.* 2022;92:1082–1089. https://doi.org/10.1038/s41390-021-01895-8.

65. McBryde C, Zivani J. Proximal and distal upper limb motor development in 24-week-old infants. *Can J Occup Ther.* 1990;57:147–154. K.

66. Berthier NE, Keen R. Development of reaching in infancy. *Exp Brain Res.* 2006;169:507–518. https://doi.org/10.1007/s00221-005-0169-9.

67. Clifton RK, Muir DW, Ashmead DH, et al. Is visually guided reaching in early infancy a myth? *Child Dev.* 1993;64:1099–1110. K.

68. Konczak J, Dichgans J. The development toward stereotypic arm kinematics during reaching in the first 3 years of life. *Exp Brain Res.* 1997;117:346–354. K.

69. Rochat P. Self-sitting and reaching in 5- to 8-month-old infants: the impact of posture and its development on eye-hand coordination. *J Mot Behav.* 1992;24:210–220. K.

70. Out L, van Soest AJ, Savelsbergh GJP, Hopkins B. The effect of posture on early reaching movements. *J Motor Behav.* 1998;30:260–272. https://doi.org/10.1080/00222899809601341.

71. Soska KC, Adolph KE. Postural position constrains multimodal object exploration in infants. *Infancy.* 2014;19(2):138–161. https://doi.org/10.1111/infa.12039.

72. Corbetta D, Thelen E. The developmental origins of bimanual coordination: a dynamic perspective. *J Exp Psychol Hum Percept Perform.* 1996;22:502–522. K.

73. Courage ML, Frizzell LM, Walsh CS, Smith M. Toddlers using tablets: they engage, play, and learn. *Front Psychol.* 2021;12:564479.. https://doi.org/10.3389/fpsyg.2021.564479.

74. Rideout VJ.*The common sense census: media use by kids aged zero to eight.* San Francisco: Common Sense Media; 2017 https://www.commonsensemedia.org/research/the-common-sense-census-media-use-by-kids-age-zero-to-eight-2017. Accessed January 5, 2023.

75. Kirkorian HL. When and how do interactive digital media help children connect what they see on and off the screen. *Child Dev Perspect.* 2018;12:210–214. https://doi.org/10.1111/cdep.12290.

76. Dore RA, Shirilla M, Hopkins E, Collins M, Scott M, Schatz J, et al. Education in the app store: using a mobile game to support U.S. preschoolers' vocabulary learning. *J Child Media.* 2019;13:452–471. https://doi.org/10.1080/17482798.2019.1650788.

77. von Hofsten C, Fazel-Zandy S. Development of visually guided hand orientation in reaching. *J Exp Child Psychol.* 1984;38:208–219. K.

78. von Hofsten C, Ronnqvist L. Preparation for grasping an object: a developmental study. *J Exp Psychol Hum Percept Perform.* 1988;14:610–621. K.

79. Kuhtz-Buschbeck JP, Stolze H, Joehnk M, et al. Development of prehension movements in children. *Exp Brain Res.* 1998;122:424–432. K.

80. Jouen F, Molina M. Exploration of the newborn's manual activity: a window onto early cognitive processes. *Inf Behav Dev.* 2005;28:227–239. https://doi.org/10.1016/injbeh.2005.05.001.

81. Witherington DC. The development of prospective grasping control between 5 and 7 months: a longitudinal study. *Infancy.* 2005;7:143–161. https://doi.org/10.1207/s15327078in0702_2.

82. OT Tool Box. What is finger isolation? https://www.theottoolbox.com/what-is-finger-isolation-button-ring-craft/ Accessed December 28, 2022.

83. Monroy C, Gerson S, Hunnius S. Infants' motor proficiency and statistical learning for actions. *Front Psychol.* 2017;8:2174. https://doi.org/10.3389/fpsyg.2017.02174.

84. Zitelli BJ, McIntire SC, Nowalk AJ, eds.*Zitelli and Davis' Atlas of Pediatric Physical Diagnosis.* 8th ed. Philadelphia: Elsevier; 2023:76–79.

85. Lee MH, Liu YT, Newell KM. Longitudinal expressions of infant's prehension as a function of object properties. *Infant Behav Dev.* 2006;29:481–493. https://doi.org/10.1016/j.infbeh.2006.05.004.

86. Halverson HM. An experimental study of prehension in infants by means of systematic cinema recording. *Genet Psychol Monogr*. 1931;19:107–285. R.

87. Forssberg H, Eliasson AC, Kinoshita H, et al. Development of human precision grip. IV: tactile adaptation of isometric finger forces to the frictional condition. *Exp Brain Res*. 1995;104:323–330.

88. Barrett TM, Traupman E, Needham A. Infants' visual anticipation of object structure in grasp planning. *Infant Behav Dev*. 2008;31:1–9. https://doi.org/10.1016/j.infbeh.2007.05.004.

89. Steri A, Lhote M, Dutilleul S. Haptic perception in newborns. *Dev Sci*. 2000;3:319–327.

90. Rose SA. From hand to eye: findings and issues in infant cross-modal transfer. In: Lewkowicz DJ, Lickliter R, eds.*The Development of Intersensory Perception: Comparative Perspectives*. Hillsdale, NJ: Lawrence Erlbaum Associates; 1994:265–284. 265-284.

91. Jao RJ, James TWA, James KH. Crossmodal enhancement in the LOC for visuohaptic object recognition over development. *Neuropsychologia*. 2015;77:76–89. https://doi.org/10.1016/j.neuropsychologia.2015.08.008.

92. Kalagher H, Jones SS. Young children's haptic exploratory procedures. *J Exp Child Psychol*. 2011;110:592–602. https://doi.org/10.1016/j.jecp.2011.06.007.

93. Kalagher H, Jones SS. Developmental change in young children's use of haptic information in a visual task: the role of hand movements. *J Exp Child Psychol*. 2011;108:293–307. https://doi.org/10.1016/j.jecp.2010.09.004.

94. Bremner AJ, Spence C. The development of tactile perception. *Adv Child Dev Behav*. 2017;52:227–268. https://doi.org/10.1016/bs.acdb.2016.12.002.

95. Lederman SJ, Klatzky RL. Haptic perception: a tutorial. *Atten Percept Psychophys*. 2009;71:1439–1459. https://doi.org/10.3758/APP.71.7.1439.

96. Kahrimanovic M, Tiest WM, Kappers AM. Haptic perception of volume and surface area of 3-D objects. *Atten Percept Psychophys*. 2010;72:517–527. https://doi.org/10.3758/APP.72.2.517.

97. Hirschel A, Pehoski C, Coryell J. Environmental support and the development of grasp in infants. *Am J Occup Ther*. 1990;44:721–727.

98. Southgate V, Johnson MH, Osborne T, Caibra G. Predictive motor activation during action observation in human infants. *Biol Lett*. 2009;5:769–772. https://doi.org/10.1177/0956797612459766.

99. Chen L-C, Jeka J, Clark JE. Development of adaptive sensorimotor control in infant sitting posture. *Gait Posture*. 2016;45:157–163. https://doi.org/10.1016/j.gaitpost.2016.01.020.

100. Corbetta D, Bojczyk KE. Infants return to two-handed reaching when they are learning to walk. *J Mot Behav*. 2002;34:83–95. https://doi.org/10.1080/00222890209601933.

101. Claxton LJ, Haddad JM, Ponto K, Ryu JH, Newcomer SC. Newly standing infants increase postural stability when performing a supra-postural task. *PloS One*. 2013;8:e71288.. https://doi.org/10.1371/journal.pone.0071288.

102. Vygotsky L. Thought and Language. Cambridge, MA: MIT Press (Kozulin A, translator), 1986.

103. Schneiberg S, Sveistrup H, McFadyen B, McKinley P, Levin MF. The development of coordination for reach-to-grasp movements in children. *Exp Brain Res*. 2002;146:142–154. https://doi.org/10.1007/s00221-002-1156-z.

104. Sainburg RL. Handedness: differential specializations for control of trajectory and position. *Exerc Sport Sci Rev*. 2005;33(4):206–213.

105. Kovel CGF, Francks C. The molecular genetics of hand preference revisited. *Sci Rep*. 2019;9:5986.. https://doi.org/10.1038/s41598-019-42515-0.

106. Lewis SR, Duff SV, Gordon AM. Manual asymmetry during object release under varying task constraints. *Am J Occup Ther*. 2002;56(4):391–401.

107. Hepping AM, Ploegmakers JJ, Geertzen JH, Bulstra SK, Stevens M. The influence of hand preference on grip strength in children and adolescents; A cross-sectional study of 2284 children and adolescents. *PloS One*. 2015;10:e0143476.. https://doi.org/10.1371/journal.pone.0143476.

108. Peterson P, Petrick M, Connor H, et al. Grip strength and hand dominance: challenging the 10% rule. *Am J Occup Ther*. 1989;43:444–447.

109. Pfeifer LS, Heyers K, Berretz G, Metzen D, Packheiser J, Ocklenburg S. Broadening the scope: increasing phenotype diversity in laterality research. *Front Behav Neurosci*. 2022;16 https://doi.org/10.3389/fnbeh.2022.1048388.1048388.

110. Bagesteiro LB, Balthazar RB, Hughes CML. Movement kinematics and interjoint coordination are influenced by target location and arm in 6-year-old children. *Front Hum Neurosci*. 2020;14:554378.. https://doi.org/10.3389/fnhum.2020.554378.

111. Mutalib SA, Mace M, Burdet E. Bimanual coordination during a physically coupled task in unilateral spastic cerebral palsy children. *J Neuroeng Rehabil*. 2019;16:1.. https://doi.org/10.1186/s12984-018-0454-z.

112. Johansson RS. Sensory control of dexterous manipulation in humans. In: Wing AM, Haggard P, Flanagan JR, eds.*Hand and Brain: The Neurophysiology and Psycholo-*

gy of Hand Movements. San Diego, CA: Academic Press; 1996:381–414.

113. Schneck CM, Henderson A. Descriptive analysis of the developmental progression of grip position for pencil and crayon control in nondysfunctional children. *Am J Occup Ther*. 1990;44:893–900.

114. Häger-Ross C, Rösblad B. Norms for grip strength in children aged 4-16 years. *Acta Paediatr*. 2002;91:617–625. https://doi.org/10.1080/080352502760068990.

115. McQuiddy VA, Scheerer CR, Lavalley R, McGrath T, Lin L. Normative values for grip and pinch strength for 6- to 19-year-olds. *Arch Phys Med Rehabil*. 2015;96:1627–1633. https://doi.org/10.1016/j.apmr.2015.03.018.

116. Bohannon RW, Wang YC, Bubela D, Gershon RC. Handgrip strength: a population-based study of norms and age trajectories for 3- to 17-Year-Olds. *Pediatr Phys Ther*. 2017;29:118–123. https://doi.org/10.1097/PEP.0000000000000366.

117. Alaniz ML, Galit E, Necesito CI, Rosario ER. Hand Strength, handwriting, and functional skills in children with autism. *Am J Occup Ther*. 2015 https://doi.org/10.5014/ajot.2015.016022. 69:6904220030p1-9.

118. Häger-Ross C, Rösblad B. Norms for grip strength in children aged 4-16 years. *Acta Paediatr*. 2002;91:617–625.

119. Amaral CA, Amaral TLM, Monteiro GTR, Torres G, Vasconcellos MTL, Portela MC. Hand grip strength: reference values for adults and elderly people of Rio Branco, Acre, Brazil. *PLoS One*. 2019;14 https://doi.org/10.1371/journal.pone.0211452. e0211452.

120. Dodds RM, Syddall HE, Cooper R, Benzeval M, Deary IJ, Dennison EM, et al. Grip strength across the life course: normative data from twelve British studies. *PLoSOne*. 2014;9(12): https://doi.org/10.1371/journal.pone.0113637. e113637.

121. Lim SH, Kim YH, Lee JS. Normative data on grip strength in a population-based study with adjusting confounding factors: Sixth Korea National Health and Nutrition Examination Survey (2014-2015). *Int J Environ Res Public Health*. 2019;16:2235.. https://doi.org/10.3390/ijerph16.122235.

122. Roush JR, Gombold KL, Bay RC. Normative grip strength values in males and females, ages 50-89 years old. *The Internet Journal of Allied Health Sciences and Practice*. 2018;16(1): Article 7.

123. Pan PJ, Lin CH, Yang NP, Chen HC, Tsao HM, Chou P, Hsu NW. Normative data and associated factors of hand grip strength among elderly individuals: the Yilan Study. Taiwan. *Sci Rep*. 2020;10:6611.. https://doi.org/10.1038/s41598-020-63613-1.

124. Pratt J, DeVito G, Narici M, Segurado R, Dolan J, Conroy J, Boreham C. Grip strength performance from 9431 participants of the GenoFit study: normative data and associated factors. *GeoScience*. 2021;43:2533–2546. https://doi.org/10.1007/s11357-021-00410-5.

125. Wang YC, Bohannon RW, Li X, Sindhu B, Kapellusch J. Hand-Grip strength: normative reference values and equations for individuals 18 to 85 years of age residing in the United States. *J Orthop Sports Phys Ther*. 2018;48:685–693. https://doi.org/10.2519/jospt.2018.7851.

126. Dodds RM, Syddall SH, Cooper R, Kuh D, Cooper C, Sayer AA. Global variation in grip strength: a systematic review and meta-analysis of normative data. *Age Ageing*. 2016;45:209–216. https://doi.org/10.1093/ageing/afv192.

127. Incel NA, Ceceli E, Durukan B, Erdem HR, Yorgancioglu ZR. Grip strength: effect of hand dominance. *Singaport Med J*. 2002;43(5):234–237.

128. Armstrong CA, Oldman JA. A comparison of dominant and non-dominant hand strengths. *J Hand Surg*. 1999;24:421–425.

129. Mathiowetz V, Kashman N, Volland G, et al. Grip and pinch strength: normative data for adults. *Arch Phys Med Rehabil*. 1985;66:16–21.

130. Hughes S, Gibbs H, Dunlop D, et al. Predictors of decline in manual performance in older adults. *J Am Geriatr Soc*. 1997;45:905–910.

131. Weir PL, MacDonald JR, Mallat BJ, et al. Age-related differences in prehension: the influence of task goals. *J Mot Behav*. 1998;30:79–80.

132. Carmeli E, Patish H, Coleman R. The aging hand. *J Gerontol A Biol Sci Med Sci*. 2003; 58:146-152. 2003 https://doi.org/10.1093/gerona/58.2.m146.

133. Cole KJ, Rotella DL, Harper JG. Tactile impairments cannot explain the effect of age on a grasp and lift task. *Exp Brain Res*. 1998;121:263–269.

134. Lin BS, Kuo SF, Lee IJ, Lu LH, Chen PY, Wang PC, et al. The impact of aging and reaching movements on grip stability control during manual precision tasks. *BMC Geriatr*. 2021;21:703.. https://doi.org/10.1186/s12877-021-02663-3.

135. Stevens JC, Cruz LA. Spatial acuity of touch: ubiquitous decline with aging revealed by repeated threshold testing. *Somatosens Mot Res*. 1996;13:1–10.

136. Volcic R, Domini F. The endless visuomotor calibration of reach-to-grasp actions. *Sci Rep*. 2018;8:14803.. https://doi.org/10.1038/s41598-18-3309-6.

137. Couth S, Gower E, Poliakoff E. How does aging affect grasp, adaptation to a visual-haptic size conflict? *Ex Brain Res*. 2018;236:2173–2184. https://doi.org/10.1007/s00221-018-5288-1.

138. Runnarong N, Tretriluxana J, Walyasil W, Sittisupapong P, Tretriluxana S. Age-related changes in reach-to-grasp movements with partial visual occlusion. *PLoS One*. 2019;14:e022132.. https://doi.org/10.1371/journal.pone.0221320.

139. O'Rielly JL, Ma-Wyatt A. Changes to online control and eye-hand coordination with healthy aging. *Hum Mov Sci*. 2018;59:244–257. https://doi.org/10.1016/j.humov.2018.04.013.

Health and Fitness

OBJECTIVES

After studying this chapter, the reader will be able to:

1. Discuss the interrelationships between health, wellness, fitness, and physical activity.
2. Describe the contributions of health, fitness, and physical activity to the level of participation across the life span.
3. Understand the integrated role of all body systems in the development and maintenance of fitness and health.
4. Identify the effects of exercise and training on the body systems.
5. Identify age-related considerations in developing physical activity, exercise, training, and fitness programs.

Earlier units in this textbook discussed theories of development, motor control, and motor learning, as well as the roles of various body systems in relation to participation in meaningful functional physical activity. The International Classification of Functioning, Disability, and Health (ICF) model has been presented, reflecting the relationships between the person, their environment, and participation. The ability to function at our best in all activities throughout the life span is a goal shared by everyone. This chapter will focus on the importance of physical activity and physical fitness on health and participation. Healthy lifestyle habits such as physical activity contribute to the health of the individual, through epigenetic factors influencing overall health and maximizing efficient functioning of the body systems (Fig. 13.1). By supporting individuals to adopt a healthy lifestyle, health care providers assist the individual in optimizing the person's wellness and ability to function independently across the life span.

DEFINING HEALTH AND WELLNESS

Health

Since the 1940s, the World Health Organization has defined *health* as "a state of complete physical, mental, and social well-being, and not merely the absence of disease or infirmity."[1] In reality, health is a condition of the human body and mind. As a condition, health is represented on a continuum from good health to poor health. Good health reflects the ability to enjoy life and to withstand challenges, with the highest level of functional capability. Poor health reflects morbidity and ultimately mortality. Diseases such as arthritis, heart disease, and diabetes have the potential to diminish functional capacity. These limitations in physical function can also interfere with the ability to actively meet social demands and to participate in leisure-time activities. A person's health is measured at a specific point of time and may fall any place in the continuum from good to poor health. Individuals may strive to engage in a healthier lifestyle and improve their health, often making lifestyle changes in diet, exercise, and tobacco use. Making these types of lifestyle changes can have a positive epigenetic influence on a person's genetic template and has been shown to decrease risk for chronic disease.[2-4] As health is optimized in all three domains (physical, social, and mental), a person is best able to participate in life activities.[5] Additional components of health that have been identified include consideration of both emotional and intellectual components of the mental domain, and spirituality.[6]

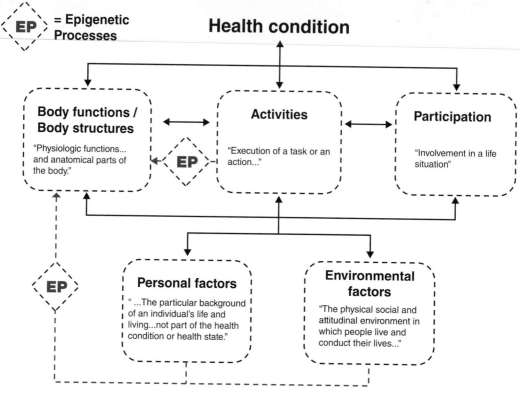

Fig. 13.1 Epigenetic processes *(EPs)* may biologically mediate the interrelationships among several International Classification of Functioning, Disability, and Health (ICF) domains. Activities (e.g., exercise), environmental factors (e.g., social determinants of health), and personal factors (e.g., smoking, alcohol abuse) may yield epigenetic adaptations of tissues that culminate in positive or negative outcomes in body functions or structures. (From Shields RK, Dudley-Javorski. Epigenetics, ICF model, and population health. *Phys Ther.* 2022;110:1–11.)

Wellness

The term *wellness*, which comprises biological and psychological well-being, is also used to denote a state of positive health.[7] This term reflects a holistic concept of health. A more comprehensive definition of wellness might incorporate promotion of physical, mental, and social health. Wellness is multidimensional and incorporates an understanding of the cognitive components of wellness and a commitment to a lifestyle, including wellness behaviors and practices.[8] Wellness also reflects a person´s enjoyment of a happy, fulfilled life, with decreased risk of illness.[6]

Other Definitions

Well-being is defined as the state of being comfortable, happy, and healthy. Health influences well-being and well-being influences health.[9] Well-being incorporates the life experiences and satisfaction with life of an individual. Well-being of an individual includes social, economic, psychological, medical, and spiritual components.[10] Health and well-being are reflected by a person's ability to successfully meet personal functional needs and those of society, as well as meet the challenges of daily life and experience satisfaction with life.[9]

Quality of life may also reflect a person's satisfaction with life. Within the ICF model, quality of life is thought to be reflected by the component of participation, which reflects a person´s involvement in meaningful activities across the life span. These meaningful activities may include going to a birthday party as a child, successfully working and supporting a family as an adult, or enjoying leisure activities such as golf or gardening. Health and quality of life are both influenced by functional, psychological, and social factors, as well presence or absence of disease or pain/discomfort.[10] Quality of life is a common measure of health status in health professions research.

Population health is the overall health of a defined population. It reflects the health outcomes/status of a group of individuals over their lifetime and is influenced by a variety of factors.[11] These factors include *social determinants of health*, which make up the social and physical environment in which people live. Economic stability (employment, safe housing, access to healthy food), access to education and healthcare, and environmental conditions are some of the social determinants of health and are reflected in the environment component of the ICF.[2] The World Health Organization (WHO) offers this definition of social determinants of health: "The conditions in which people are born, grow, live, work, and age."[12] Healthy People 2030[13] also uses this definition and focuses on the social determinants of health. As health care providers better understand the concept of population health, they can actively play a role in advocating for social policies aimed at preventing disease and development of programs that support health promotion and wellness within communities.[3]

Health promotion is the process of enabling people to increase control over and improve their health.[14] Health promotion practices and education can address the health behaviors of the individual, such as diet, exercise, maintaining a healthy body weight, and smoking cessation. Health promotion also includes addressing social and environmental factors that impact health, such as access to health care, clean air, water, and food. Environmental influences have been shown to have an epigenetic impact on health of individuals and the community. Factors such as childhood socioeconomic status can impact inflammatory processes which may influence later development of chronic diseases.[2,15] Personal factors such as inactivity and obesity may also epigenetically influence glucose regulation and development of diabetes.[2,16] Workplace safety and community-based programs supporting health are also a part of health promotion practice.

Summary: Health and Wellness

Each person, along with society, contributes to individual health and wellness (Fig. 13.2). Society contributes to the health of a community through policies such as laws mandating the use of seat belts, childhood immunization policies, and clean air regulations. Access to health care is also important, and social policies can assist in making health care available to all individuals.

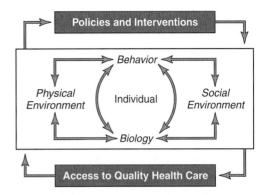

Fig. 13.2 Schematic model of determinants of health. (Redrawn from US Department of Health and Human Services. *Healthy People 2010: Understanding and Improving Health.* 2nd ed. Washington, DC: US Government Printing Office; 2000.)

Communities sponsor health promotion efforts aimed at the prevention of smoking or drug abuse, hoping to improve the health of their citizens. Communities can also develop and provide walking or bike paths to encourage physical activity among residents. Proximity to parks, public transportation, asnd grocery stores in the community are also important. Senior centers can be specifically designed to assist older adults to maintain fitness levels and provide additional nutrition. The social and physical environment in which we live contributes to the choices we make about following healthy lifestyles. Each individual has both genetic and medical profiles that may increase risk for specific diseases such as diabetes or heart disease. Each individual also makes choices about level of physical activity, smoking habits, and diet, which when paired with a person's health profile defines the individual's level of health and wellness. Health care providers contribute to the health and wellness of both individuals and the community through advocacy for federal, state, and local public policies that support health and enable individuals to make healthy choices about their lifestyle.

DEFINING PHYSICAL ACTIVITY AND FITNESS

Physical Activity

Physical activity is movement of the body to complete activities of daily living, occupational activities, sports, exercise, and leisure activities. The movement is produced by skeletal muscle and requires energy expenditure.[17] Physical activity is an important component of fitness and health. Participation in moderate and vigorous levels of physical activity contributes to levels of health.[18] Negative lifestyle changes, including decreasing amounts of time spent in physical activity and increased time spent in sedentary activity, are apparent across the globe.[19-27] Most recently, the COVID-19 outbreak has resulted in decreases in physical activity across the globe.[28] Decreases in physical activity seem to be related to a variety of negative health factors, such as obesity and cardiovascular disease, which remains as the number one cause of death in the United States.[4,5,19,20,26,29-33] It is important for health care providers to appreciate the interactions of physical activity and fitness in maintaining optimal levels of physical functioning and health throughout the life span. Health care providers, including physical and occupational therapists, are uniquely qualified to assist clients in reaching the goals of lifelong fitness, enhancing participation in meaningful life activity and maximizing overall quality of life.

Fitness

Some general definitions describe *fitness* as a state of optimal well-being and the capacity to successfully meet the present and potential physical challenges of life. To be fit is to be adapted, adjusted, qualified, or suited to some purpose, function, or aim. The term *fit* is also used to describe a person who is in good physical condition, someone who is healthy. *Physical fitness* is related to our ability to perform physical activity.[26,34] Fitness is defined by the World Health Organization as our ability to perform muscular work satisfactorily. Both genetic and environmental factors influence a person's level of physical fitness.[35] Physical fitness is best described as a collection of attributes that a person strives to achieve.[17]

Two major categories of physical fitness are health-related fitness and skill-related fitness (Table 13.1). *Health-related fitness*, reflected by cardiovascular and respiratory endurance, muscular strength and endurance, flexibility and body composition, reflects a person's level of health. Health-related fitness decreases the risk of developing chronic diseases and helps a person successfully perform activities of daily living. Power, an attribute generally considered a component of skill-related fitness, is also frequently considered a component of health-related fitness. *Skill-related fitness* reflects the level of skill and efficiency with which a person can

TABLE 13.1	**Physical Fitness**
Health-Related Fitness	**Skill-Related Fitness**
Cardiorespiratory endurance	Agility
Muscle strength	Balance
Muscle endurance	Coordination
Flexibility	Power[a]
Body composition	Speed
Power[a]	Reaction time

[a]Originally considered a component of skill-related fitness, power is now often considered a component of health-related fitness.

perform movement skills. Components of skill-related fitness include agility, balance, coordination, power, speed, and reaction time.[6] These components are very similar to the dimensions discussed in Chapter 1 that contributed to the quality of physical function. Motor competence, as introduced in Chapter 3, also contributes to and is related to physical fitness.[36] Within this model of physical fitness, it is evident that the components of health-related fitness contribute to skill-related fitness characteristics of agility, power, balance, coordination, and speed during physical activity. It is also important to consider that when components of skill-related fitness, such as balance, agility, and coordination, are optimized, they can decrease fall risk and associated injuries.[6]

The components of health-related fitness reflect the contribution of the different body systems to physical fitness and functional performance. *Cardiovascular* and *respiratory endurance* reflect the ability of the heart, vasculature, and lungs to provide oxygen to working muscle during physical activity. *Muscular strength* is the force that can be generated in a muscle, whereas *muscular endurance* reflects the ability of the muscle to complete many repetitions of muscle contraction before fatiguing. *Muscle power* refers to the ability of the muscle to exert force in a short period of time. Muscle strength and power are important to complete physical activities and functional tasks. *Flexibility*, the ability to move without restriction, depends on adequate muscle length and appropriate mobility within the joints of the body. Good flexibility improves efficiency of movement and decreases the potential for injury. *Body composition* refers to the amount of lean body mass (fat-free mass) and fat mass. Lean body mass includes muscle, bone, other nonfat substances (e.g., water, minerals), and a small amount of fat stored in the nervous system, bone marrow, and other body organs. During physical activity people must support and carry their body weight. Added non-lean body mass causes inefficiencies in movement function. Therefore lean body mass should exceed non-active fat mass.

FACTORS INFLUENCING HEALTH AND FITNESS

Individual factors such as heredity, age, sex, physical activity, lifestyle, and environment contribute to one's level of physical fitness. A model of the interactions between exercise, health, and fitness was developed by Bouchard and colleagues in 1990 (Fig. 13.3).[7] Personal attributes as defined for this diagram are age, sex, socio-economic status, personality, and motivation.

Physical Factors

Age, growth, and sex can influence fitness. The ability to perform physical activities with physiological efficiency improves through childhood, adolescence, and young adulthood. Performance is often maintained in adulthood but then declines in older adulthood. Some of this decline may be related to physical changes, such as loss of flexibility, strength, and muscle mass in older adults. Social and environmental factors also influence health and fitness. Functional losses in physical fitness may be due to decreased activity level in adulthood and older adulthood, rather than solely a result of aging.

Maintaining an active lifestyle appears to moderate physical changes related to aging within the various body systems and to contribute to overall fitness.[37-40] Physiological improvements through training occur at a similar rate and magnitude in all individuals, regardless of age.[34,41-43] Promoting an active lifestyle appears to play an important role in maintaining health and functioning in older age. Absence of physical activity leads to physiologic decline as people age.

Growth is most often recognized as the changes in height and weight measured through childhood. Loss of height in older adults also reflects a change. Individual organs such as the heart and lungs also change in size over the life span. In childhood, the developmental changes in aerobic capacity, muscular strength and endurance, and power are similar to the growth changes in height and weight.[44] Increase in stature gradually slows and ceases after adolescence, whereas weight increases into the mid-20s.[44] Bone growth continues through the life span, but peak bone mass is attained by the mid-20s. After age 35, body weight continues to slowly increase, reflecting an increase in adipose tissue. In older adulthood, both bone and muscle mass decrease, resulting in a decrease in lean body mass.[45] Loss in bone mass begins in the fifth decade in women and in the sixth decade in men,[46] with rate of loss accelerating immediately after menopause for women. Both trabecular and cortical bone are lost, with women losing more bone density than men.[42] Men appear to lose more muscle mass than women, with

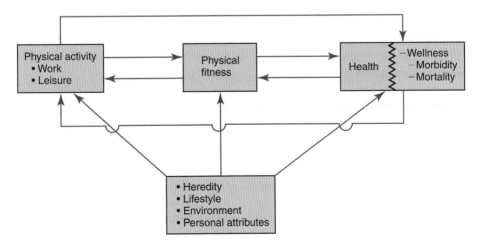

Fig. 13.3 Schematic model of the complex relationships between habitual physical activity, fitness, and health. (Redrawn from Bouchard C, Shepard RJ, Stephens T, et al. *Exercise, Fitness and Health: A Consensus of Current Knowledge.* Champaign, IL: Human Kinetics; 1990.)

1.0% loss in muscle mass per year in middle adulthood as they have more muscle mass to lose. In older adulthood, loss of muscle mass is more significant.[42,47,48]

Before puberty, gender does not appear to greatly affect fitness. Maximal aerobic capacity is slightly higher in boys than in girls through childhood.[49] After puberty, differences in maximal aerobic capacity between males and females become more dramatic. This change reflects the increased percentage of body fat seen in females, increased oxygen-carrying capacity of males compared with females because of increased levels of blood hemoglobin, and larger muscle fiber area in males compared with females.[49] Strength also increases more dramatically in males than females during puberty and young adulthood due to increased levels of testosterone.[42,50] In older adulthood, loss of muscle mass and muscle strength has been shown to be greater for men than women.[47]

Heredity

Heredity influences several factors that contribute to fitness, such as body size and muscle fiber composition. Whether we are tall or short is determined by heredity. The percentage of slow-twitch and fast-twitch muscle fibers found in skeletal muscle is determined genetically.[34,51,52] Heritability has been shown to influence strength, as well as flexibility.[35] Genetics is also a factor in determining maximal aerobic capacity, blood pressure, and heart rate.[53] Inherited factors may influence our selection of physical activities, such as choosing to be a sprinter rather than a marathon runner, or impose limits on the possible level of fitness we may achieve.

Environmental Factors

Environmental factors, as described earlier, can be considered as reflecting social determinants of health (Fig. 13.1). Physical environmental factors such as climate, oxygen pressure, and air quality can affect exercise performance. The epigenetic influences of the environment, such as air pollution, also impact an individual's ability to regulate their genetic template.[2] Extreme hot or cold climates stress the exercising individual trying to maintain internal body temperature. This is especially true for children and older adults. Children have a high ratio of surface area to body weight, allowing a greater rate of heat exchange with the environment. Children are also less able to sweat, making it more difficult to dissipate heat.[54] Some individuals may not live in a neighborhood that has safe and easy access including transportation to areas for exercise or physical activity. People who live and exercise in regions of high altitude must adjust to low oxygen pressures. Indoor air contaminants, such as cigarette smoke, radon, and wood smoke, may diminish air quality. Environmental air quality consists of by-products of industry and engine exhaust. Specific pollutants such as ozone and sulfur dioxide affect lung function.[55] Early life exposure to air pollution has been linked to increasing incidence of asthma and other conditions.[56,57]

Physical Activity

Participation in regular physical activity contributes positively to both health and fitness. Physical activity, which is defined as body movement that results in greater than resting levels of energy expenditure, can include leisure-time physical activity, housework, job-related physical tasks, exercise, and sport.[58] Physical activity has been demonstrated to improve muscle strength, cardiorespiratory endurance, bone mineral density, and physical function in older adults.[38,40,42,45,59,60] Across the life span, physical activity is a determinant of fat-free body mass.[61] Through adulthood, levels of fitness are influenced by exercise habits and body composition. Obesity, which has become a global concern, is often related to low levels of physical activity.[20,30,31,62] Regular physical activity and increased fitness diminish the risk for cardiovascular disease, type II diabetes mellitus, osteoporosis, cancer, and metabolic syndrome.[31,63–65]

Social Factors

Social factors play a role in determining an individual's involvement in physical activity and fitness, influencing health. Over the past decades, participation in sedentary activities such as television watching and computer use has increased, which seems to be related to increased incidence of obesity and development of health risk factors in children.[20,24,30,62] Children walk or ride their bikes less than they used to, more often being transported to activities by car.[23] As individuals of all ages spend more time in these sedentary activities, the amount of leisure time spent in physical activity is reduced. Social factors such as growing up in an environment of low socioeconomic status can epigenetically alter the inflammatory process and contribute to the development of cardiovascular disease and diabetes.[2,15]

Toddlers and preschoolers are very active. Their "job" is to learn new skills and to explore their environment through movement. Parents may influence this level of activity by guiding the child's choice of movement experiences and minimizing more sedentary activities such as television watching. By school age, children become more competitive, and achieving an adequate level of skill in sports and games is important for the child's social acceptance. Children who function well motorically are encouraged to continue with physical activities, whereas children who are less skilled may become frustrated and less active. Successful motor performance is a positive reinforcer for increasing levels of physical activity.[66] Functional motor skill competence (motor competence), as discussed in Chapter 3, has been related to levels of physical fitness, as well as cognitive function in children and adolescents across the globe.[67,68] Lower levels of motor competence in childhood and adolescence have also been related to decreased fitness levels, health, and well-being in adulthood.[36]

Physical activity decreases for both boys and girls in late adolescence. This reduction may be influenced by social models, peer pressure, and the need to enter the work force.[44] Adults report that job and family demands frequently do not allow time for exercise programs.[69] Socioeconomic status, safe access to recreational centers and parks, cultural norms, and social support are factors that may influence adult participation in physical activity.[70] Older adults' perceptions of their ability to participate in physical activity, as well as loneliness and lack of social support, contribute to low levels of physical activity in older adults.[71,72] The COVID-19 pandemic has further impacted levels of physical activity for individuals of all ages.[28,73-75] Society influences the awareness of and participation in fitness programs. With increased public awareness of the benefits of fitness, fitness centers and aerobic exercise programs have become more available in the United States. Community agencies sponsor fitness-related activities for individuals of all ages. Corporations also provide fitness programs for their employees, seeking to improve health and productivity. Many Medicare Advantage (Part C) programs cover the cost of gym membership. Globally, policy recommendations have focused on increasing participation in physical activity. As the communities we live and work in provide social and physical environments that foster increased levels of physical activity, individuals are encouraged to make positive choices regarding physical activity and fitness.

PERCEPTION: HOW FIT ARE WE?

Fitness has been associated with increased health and well-being. Improved quality of life and preventive health maintenance are valuable benefits of fitness. The US Department of Health and Human Services has promoted a public health agenda, Healthy People, focusing on health promotion and disease prevention for the past four decades. *Healthy People 2030* emphasizes health promotion and well-being for all and continues to include objectives that emphasize healthy behaviors such as weight status, physical activity, and fitness.[13] (Framework, HealthyPeople.gov) The vision of the Healthy People agendas has been to help members of society achieve their full potential for health and well-being across the life span.[9]

Over the past 40 years, positive changes have been seen in areas such as decreasing the rates of infant mortality; decreasing the number of deaths related to cancer and cardiac disease; and reducing risk factors such as cigarette smoking, hypertension, and elevated cholesterol.[13,76] On a less positive note, low levels of physical activity and increasing rates of overweight/obesity are global health concerns.

Childhood, adolescent, and adult levels of obesity are significant problems, which have been made worse by the COVID-19 pandemic.

(Spinelli et al., 2021,[77] WHO Fact Sheet overweight and obesity[78]) Just under 40% of the world's adult population and 20% of children are overweight, with almost 15% of adults and approximately 7% of children and adolescents being obese (WHO Fact Sheet overweight and obesity).[78] This global problem has grown significantly since the 1970s and is now a problem in low-, middle-, and high-income countries. Obesity of children is especially high in Asia (WHO Fact Sheet overweight and obesity).[78] In the United States, a steady increase in levels of obesity for youth (2–19 years of age) and adults has been seen (Fig. 13.4).[33,79]

Several organizations globally, including the World Health Organization (WHO Fact Sheet physical activity)[18], have published recommendations for daily physical activity and reduction of sedentary activity, such as television and computer time.[31,33,80-82] Even with these guidelines, minimal change has been seen in level of physical activity.[21,83,84] Sedentary lifestyle, increasing hours per day of screen time, diet, and obesity all contribute to decreasing levels of physical activity for individuals of all ages.

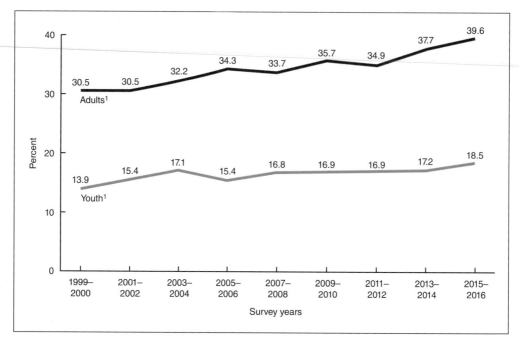

Fig. 13.4 Trends in obesity prevalence among adults ages 20 and over (age adjusted) and youth aged 2–19 years: United States, 1999–2000 through 2015–2016. (Hales, Craig M, Carroll, Margaret D, Fryar, Cheryl D, Ogden, Cynthia L. Prevalence of obesity among adults and youth: United States, 2015-2016. *NCHS Data Brief.* 2017;(288):1-8. URL: https://stacks.cdc.gov/view/cdc/49223. Accessed 4/3/2022.)

Significant numbers of individuals, of all ages, fail to meet the recommended levels of physical activity. A progressive and predictable decline in regular physical activity participation with age has been reported (Fig. 13.5).[34,69,85,86] Although levels of physical activity are high in children, activity rates decline from childhood to adolescence and then decline further through adulthood. A longitudinal study of children from 9–15 years of age showed that almost all children participated in physical activity for the recommended 60 minutes per day, but by 15 years of age, only 32% of children met the requirement on weekdays and 18% on weekends. In this study, the amount of time spent in moderately vigorous physical activity decreased by 35–40 minutes per year over the 6 years of the study.[87] Another cross-sectional study in the United States of 4- to 12-year-olds showed that 37% of children had low levels of activity play, 65% had high levels of sedentary activity ("screen time"), and 26% had both low levels of active play and high screen time. The children in this last category tended to be older, female, and had higher body mass index (BMI >95% for age-matched growth curves).[20] Globally, 80% of adolescents are reported to participate in insufficient levels of physical activity to meet current guidelines.[83] Adolescents demonstrate decreasing levels of cardiovascular endurance, strength, flexibility, agility, and speed.[26] Less than 50% of adults in the United States reported participating in the recommended 30 minutes of moderately vigorous physical activity at least 5 days a week, and of adults over the age of 65 years, less than 40% reported meeting the activity recommendations,[21] while almost 50% of European adults over the age of 18 years do not engage in physical activity or sports.[88] More than 25% of the world's adults fail to meet recommended physical activity levels.[18,84] Being physically active in midlife increases the odds of being active in old age. Promoting physical activity in later life might be best achieved by promoting sport participation earlier in the life course.[89] Participation in regular physical activity is influenced by other factors, and levels of participation decrease as education and income levels decrease.[21,33]

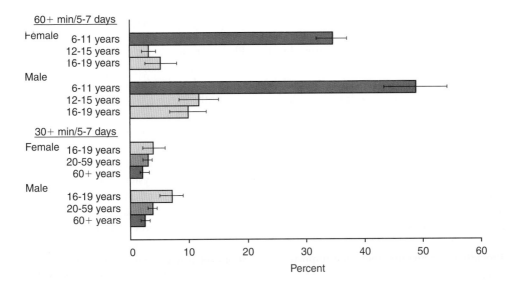

Fig. 13.5 Regular physical activity throughout life is important for maintaining a healthy body, enhancing psychological well-being, and preventing premature death. This graph shows the percentage of children, adolescents, and adults who achieved recommended levels of physical activity (as measured by accelerometer) in the United States in 2003–2004. Data from the National Health and Nutrition Examination Survey (NHANS, NCHS, CDC). (From Troiano RP, et al. Physical activity in the United States measured by accelerometer. *Med Sci Sports Exerc.* 2008;40(1):181-188.)

As obesity and low levels of physical activity increase health risks for individuals around the world, efforts by government agencies, public entities, and private groups are attempting to improve access and adherence to healthy lifestyle activities. According to the most recent published data (2016), obesity costs the US health care system $260.6 billion per year.[90] This is a substantial increase from 2009, when the estimated cost was $147 billion a year.[91] Public education programs have incorporated fitness programs into physical education and are increasing the time spent in promoting lifetime physical activities. Some schools, with local grants and support, are providing fitness equipment in their playgrounds (Fig. 13.6). To meet the needs of adults, increasing numbers of employers are providing workplace fitness programs. These programs benefit both the employee and the employer because there are fewer employee absences and less sick time. Community agencies also strive to provide physical activity programs for older adults. Older adults who are obese have much less participation in physical activity.[92] Older adults living in senior communities also take advantage of multiple opportunities for activities such as tennis, swimming, and offerings

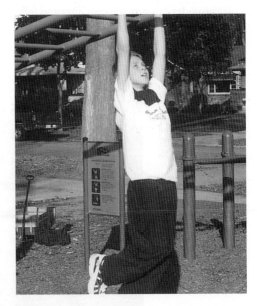

Fig. 13.6 Schools and communities work together to provide fitness equipment and programs for children. This fitness court was designed to be used with six individualized activity stations at an elementary school. A local community hospital donated the funds to build the court, which is enhanced by signs that describe the preferred regimens to be used for each activity.

at fitness club facilities, although these may be costly for many individuals (Fig. 13.7). Communities are also developing walking and bike paths and creating local playgrounds.

Individuals in any age group participate in leisure-time physical activity to varying degrees, with the most active tending to be the most fit. Significant efforts are being made to increase the public's awareness of the importance of physical activity and fitness. Public awareness of the importance of fitness may be increasing, but even though many individuals start exercise programs, often they will stop within a short period of time. Among the barriers to adhering to physical activity programs are time constraints and financial concerns. Making a behavioral change is challenging and complex. Providing information about the importance of physical activity for health promotion may help people be aware of a need for change but not the support to make health behavior changes. Health care providers can play an important role in supporting individuals as they strive to make changes. Health care providers can provide individualized education and evaluate an individual's motivation to make a change. As an individual feels confident and capable of making the change, the health care provider can provide coaching and follow-up to help sustain the individual's efforts.[93]

BODY SYSTEMS INVOLVED IN FITNESS

Physical fitness is achieved when several body systems—the cardiovascular, pulmonary, musculoskeletal, nervous, and endocrine systems—interact optimally and efficiently. In the course of development, changes in the body systems affect the way in which the body delivers fuel and produces energy for movement. Capacity for physical activity may vary throughout development as a result. In children, it is difficult to separate development of the body systems from development of physical fitness. Growth and maturation of the cardiovascular, pulmonary, musculoskeletal, and nervous systems contribute to the child's and adolescent's ability to move efficiently and effectively. Similarly, physical activity supports development of these systems.

Exercise and training have been found to improve body system function and levels of fitness. *Exercise* is defined as leisure-time physical activity[7] that is planned, repetitive, and purposeful.[34] Exercise includes participation in planned, structured physical activity for the purpose of improving fitness and health.[17,63] *Training* is regular and repeated exercise, carried out over several weeks or months, with the goal of developing physical or physiological fitness.[7] *Trainability* reflects the ability of different body systems to adapt to repeated exercise stimuli.[94]

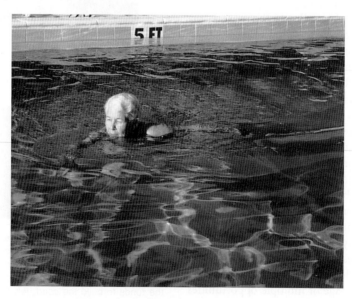

Fig. 13.7 Older adults can stay active by taking advantage of community facilities such as swimming pools.

Exercise and training affect an adult's body systems in different ways. Structural and functional changes are seen within each body system and will be discussed in more detail below. Exercise also appears to stimulate epigenetic modifications to the individual's genome. Some of the epigenetic changes are evident in the body's increased efficiency of glucose and lipid metabolism, insulin sensitivity, muscle regeneration, and mitochondrial function.[95,96] Exercise has also been related to telomere maintenance. This is important because the telomere is thought to be a marker of biologic aging.[97] The effects of exercise and training on the body systems are discussed in the following sections, with a focus on the response in adults. When available, information specific to children and adolescents is also provided. For additional information, the reader is referred to the specific system chapters in Unit II.

Effects of Exercise and Training on the Cardiovascular System

During exercise, the cardiovascular system must carry large amounts of oxygen to the muscle tissue and remove waste products associated with energy production.

Cardiovascular responses to exercise and training are summarized in Table 13.2.

Short-Term Adaptation

During aerobic exercise, skeletal muscle demand for oxygen increases, resulting in increased cardiac output and stroke volume. Heart rate and systolic blood pressure increases in proportion to the intensity of the exercise for 3–5 minutes. A steady state is then attained and maintained for short periods of exercise. Diastolic pressure should remain steady (within 10 mm Hg) during

TABLE 13.2   Body Systems' Response to Exercise and Training

Body System	Response to Acute Exercise	Response to Training
Cardiovascular	Increased heart rate Increased cardiac output Increased stroke volume Increased blood volume Decreased blood pressure following acute exercise session Decreased peripheral resistance	Increased heart weight Increased heart volume Increased blood volume Increased hemoglobin Decreased resting and submaximal heart rate Slightly decreased maximal heart rate Decreased blood pressure Increased arterial-to-venous oxygen difference Remodeling of arterial tree to more efficiently deliver oxygen to muscle tissue
Pulmonary	Increased minute ventilation Increased tidal volume Increased breathing frequency	Increased vital capacity Increased tidal volume Decreased respiratory rate at submaximal exercise Increased respiratory muscle strength and endurance
Musculoskeletal	Increased blood flow to working muscle	Increased bone mineral density Increased strength, flexibility of thickness of ligaments Increased thickness of articular cartilage Increased muscle strength Increased fat-free body mass Improved lipid profile (increase HDL, decrease LDL) Increased glucose tolerance Increased oxidative capacity Increased number of type I fibers Increased oxidative enzymes Increased mitochondria Onset of blood lactate accumulation at higher percent of maximum oxygen uptake

HDL, High-density lipoproteins; LDL, low-density lipoprotein.

exercise and should be halted if an increase or decrease more than 10^{93} mm Hg occurs. An increase in diastolic blood pressure of more than 10 mm Hg during or after exercise represents an unstable form of hypertension and may be associated with coronary artery disease.[98] A decrease in diastolic pressure could lead to cardiac ischemia. After 15–30 minutes, heart rate again begins to rise because of fatigue and increased body temperature. Blood volume increases, as hormones signal the kidney to retain fluids and plasma albumen increases. Following an acute exercise session, systolic and diastolic blood pressure decreases in response to input from the parasympathetic and sympathetic nervous system.[99–101] Moderate-intensity aerobic exercise has been shown to prevent hypertension and to help in the management of mild hypertension.[99] Additionally, resistance exercises, if done properly, contribute to lowering both systolic and diastolic blood pressures.[102] Vasodilation occurs, helping shunt blood flow to the working skeletal and heart muscles. Muscle contraction squeezes nearby veins, facilitating venous return. In general, dynamic, aerobic exercise results in increased cardiac contractility, decreased peripheral resistance, and increased venous return, all of which support efficient delivery of oxygen to the tissues.[34,100,103]

Long-Term Adaptation

Heart weight and volume, plasma volume, and hemoglobin levels increase with training.[34,104,105] Ventricular filling, stroke volume, and cardiac output also increase.[106] Therefore, more blood can be pumped per heartbeat, and necessary circulation is delivered to body tissues at a lower heart rate. Stroke volume increases because of greater end-diastolic volume of the left ventricle and more forceful contraction of strengthened cardiac muscle.[34,103] Increases in blood volume with training also contribute to increased stroke volume.[105] In prepubescent children, stroke volume increases, and an increase in cardiac size occurs in response to endurance training.[107]

Resting heart rate and heart rate during submaximal exercise decrease with long-term exercise, an effect that appears to be related to decreased sympathetic input. Maximum heart rate decreases slightly as left ventricular filling time and stroke volume increase, whereas maximum cardiac output and stroke volume increase.[100,105] Maximum heart rate remains stable for children after endurance training.[107]

Both systolic and diastolic blood pressures decrease with training.[34,101,105,108] In older adults, decreases in resting systolic blood pressure are seen, but minimal change is seen in diastolic blood pressure.[99] Decreases in blood pressure may be related to autonomic nervous system control, which decreases peripheral resistance to blood flow.[103] With training, changes are also seen in the arterial tree, with arterial wall thickness decreasing and diameter of the arteries increasing, further decreasing peripheral resistance.[100,105]

Exercise also appears to have a positive impact on the lipid levels circulating in the blood and the ability of the muscle to extract oxygen from the blood. With exercise, the levels of high-density lipoproteins (HDL) are increased and the levels of low-density lipoproteins (LDL) are decreased.[108,109] When our body is physiologically trained, we are better able to extract oxygen from the blood, as reflected by a widening of the arterial-to-venous oxygen difference (A-Vo$_2$ difference).[34,105] Increased capillary and mitochondrial capacities are seen in working muscle, improving the ability of the muscle to extract oxygen from the capillaries.[34,105] In children, no change in A-Vo$_2$ difference is seen.[107] In the older adult, even with exercise training, the ability to extract oxygen at the muscle cell level is diminished because of changes in both the muscle tissue and circulation; therefore dramatic changes are not seen in oxygen extraction. There is age-associated decline in the ability of older adults to increase O$_2$ delivery to active muscles due to decreased lung function, cardiac output, and muscle oxidative capacity.[110,111]

Effects of Exercise and Training on the Pulmonary System

During exercise, greater airflow is required to meet the oxygen demands of the body. Airflow is increased by taking deeper breaths and increasing the respiratory rate. Adaptations of the pulmonary system to exercise and training are summarized in Table 13.2.

Short-Term Adaptation

At the onset of exercise, ventilation increases rapidly and reaches a steady state.[34] The amount of air exchanged with the atmosphere per minute (*minute ventilation*) is increased as more air is moved in each breath (*tidal volume*) and as breathing frequency increases. At low-intensity exercise, changes in tidal volume are sufficient to maintain adequate minute ventilation. Greater tidal volume allows inspired air to perfuse more lung tissue, opening more alveoli and maximizing the ability for gas exchange between the capillaries and the alveoli. As exercise intensity becomes greater and tidal volume is 50%–60% of vital capacity, breathing rate increases.[37]

The breathing rate at rest is approximately 14 breaths per minute. During exercise, the respiratory rate may rise up to 40 breaths per minute. Even at these higher rates, there is enough time for alveolar gas exchange to occur because alveolar ventilation increases more than does pulmonary capillary blood flow. This process works until fatigue or cardiac function limits the exercise.

During light to moderate exercise, ventilation increases linearly with levels of oxygen consumption and carbon dioxide production. At higher exercise levels, ventilation increases in relation to increased carbon dioxide concentrations produced by anaerobic metabolism. For example, blood lactate levels increase during anaerobic metabolism and must be buffered to prevent acidosis. The end product of this buffering is carbon dioxide. As the carbon dioxide levels in the blood increase, chemoreceptors in the aortic and carotid bodies, as well as in the medulla, cue the system to increase ventilation.[34]

Long-Term Adaptation

After training, resting lung volumes show little change. Strength and endurance of respiratory muscles are improved.[112-114] People who exercise regularly develop an improved ability to consume oxygen during maximal exercise. This ability is measured using by VO_{2max}.[107] Regular exercise has the ability to increase the number of capillaries around the alveoli. Moreover, regular exercise can help capillaries dilate more, which in turn facilitates efficient exchange of gasses. The benefit comes mainly due because the lungs can now deliver oxygen to the cells of the body. Regular exercise also increases blood flow to the lungs, which in turn strengthens the lungs and ensures better exchange of gasses.[115] With training, increased mitochondria and capillarization of the respiratory muscles are seen, improving function of the respiratory muscles.[113] During submaximal exercise, the respiratory rate decreases and the tidal volume increases. Air stays in the lungs longer, allowing more oxygen to be extracted.[34] The amount of air that must be breathed in to deliver adequate oxygen to the tissues is decreased, requiring less work by the respiratory system.

Conclusive studies of the effects of training on the ventilatory system of children have not been done.[116]

Effects of Exercise and Training on the Musculoskeletal System

The muscular and skeletal systems form the mechanical basis for human movement. Muscle cells also contain energy stores necessary for movement. Within skeletal muscle, three types of muscle fibers (type I, type IIa, and type IIx) are found, and they are used differently to produce energy. Oxygen provided during respiration activates metabolic pathways that convert carbohydrates, fats, and proteins into stored energy sources in muscle. Type I and type IIa muscle fibers effectively work in these aerobic metabolic pathways. Type IIx muscle fibers assist in the production of energy via anaerobic pathways.

Adaptations of the musculoskeletal system to exercise and training are summarized in Table 13.2. Depending on the type of activity, type I, type IIa, and type IIx muscle fibers are affected differently.

Short-Term Adaptation

At the onset of exercise, blood flow to exercising muscle increases. Increased blood flow delivers more oxygen to the muscle and helps to dissipate heat, which results from muscular work. With exercise at less than 60%–70% of maximum aerobic power, first type I and then type IIa muscle fibers are recruited.

Long-Term Adaptation

Training affects all components of the musculoskeletal system. Both weight-bearing and the mechanical forces exerted by the muscles during activity contribute to musculoskeletal changes. Exercise increases the bone density[109,117-120] and strengthens the bone architecture. Ligaments become stronger, thicker, and more flexible. Articular cartilage also becomes thicker and more resistant to compression. Muscle tissue undergoes significant change, which varies with the type of exercise performed.

Resistance training increases muscle strength via hypertrophy of muscle fibers or neural recruitment of motor units. Children increase strength primarily via increased neural recruitment.[109,119,121] Neural recruitment also plays a major role in strength gains of older adults. In older adults, increases in strength also have been related to reversal of fast-twitch fiber atrophy. Muscle hypertrophy occurs after puberty, when increased levels of hormones such as testosterone, growth hormone, and other growth factors are present.[119] Muscle hypertrophy is seen in adults when high levels of resistance are used. Anaerobic metabolic pathways are used primarily in this type of exercise, resulting in increased anaerobic enzyme levels in type II muscle fibers.

With endurance training, oxidative capacity of the muscle is maximized, increasing the number of type I muscle fibers.[122] Levels of enzymes used by oxidative metabolic pathways increase, especially in oxidative type I and type IIa muscle fibers. The size and number of mitochondria increase with training, as does capillarization.[34,100,104,105] These changes all contribute to the efficient use of oxygen by muscle tissue, fueling the oxidative metabolic pathway. Aerobic exercise also improves the ability of the skeletal muscle to use glucose, improving glucose tolerance.[123] Muscle hypertrophy is seen and insulin sensitivity within the skeletal muscle is increased, improving muscle performance.[100]

High-intensity training increases the number of type II fibers active in anaerobic metabolism.[122] Anaerobic threshold increases during submaximal exercise as a result of increased mechanical efficiency and muscle strengthening. Blood lactate accumulation limits exercise during high-intensity training and begins at 50%–55% of maximal oxygen uptake in the untrained individual and at approximately 80%–90% of maximal oxygen uptake in the trained individual.[34] Both aerobic and anaerobic training have been shown to increase the lactate threshold (when lactate levels limit continued exercise), most likely related to the trained individuals' improved ability to clear lactate from their systems.[124,125] Prepubertal children are less able to use anaerobic metabolism because of lower muscle glycogen levels. Limited muscle mass in children also limits anaerobic metabolism.[34]

Metabolic, Endocrine, and Hormonal Contributions to Fitness and Training

The endocrine system (see Chapter 10) allows the body to adapt to vigorous physical activity and ensures that fuel is delivered to working muscles. Fuel can be supplied aerobically or anaerobically, through metabolism of carbohydrates or fats. Several endocrine organs are activated during exercise. The hormones they secrete play a role in the use of carbohydrates and fatty acids, maintenance of fluid volume, contractility of the heart, and distribution of blood within the vascular system (Table 13.3). Responses of children differ from adults

TABLE 13.3	Hormonal Activity Related to Physical Activity		
Hormone	**Response to Physical Activity**	**Secreted by**	**Action**
Growth Hormone	Increases	Anterior pituitary gland	Decreased carbohydrate use and increased fat use as energy source
Corticotropin	Increases	Anterior pituitary gland	Increased use of fat and protein for energy Stimulates secretion of cortisol
Antidiruetic hormone (ADH)	Increases	Posterior pituitary gland	Increased water retention by kidney
Norepinephrine/ epinephrine	Increases	Adrenal cortex	Increased cardiac activity; increased use of fatty acids and glucose for energy
Cortisol	Increases	Adrenal cortex	Transport protein and fatty acids into cells to use for energy
Aldosterone	Increases	Adrenal cortex	Increases sodium, potassium, and water retention
Insulin	Decreases	Pancreas	Allows transport of protein, fatty acids, and glucose into cells
Glucagon	Increases	Pancreas	Releases glucose from liver; increases fat metabolism

in that children metabolize fats during exercise, rather than carbohydrates.[126] Certain hormones make specific contributions to fitness and training.

Growth hormone, secreted by the anterior pituitary gland, decreases the use of carbohydrates and increases the use of fat metabolism for energy production. By maintaining glucose levels, growth hormone increases endurance. Growth hormone also promotes protein synthesis, cartilage formation, and skeletal growth. Intensity and duration of exercise affect the secretion of growth hormone. There does not appear to be a training effect that raises the levels of growth hormone in adults.[34] In prepubescent children, no change in growth hormone levels is noted during bouts of exercise.[126]

Corticotropin (ACTH), also secreted by the anterior pituitary gland, improves the mobilization of fat as an energy source, increases the rate of glucose formation, and stimulates the breakdown of proteins. ACTH also controls the secretion of hormones from the adrenal cortex, including cortisol, which is important during intense exercise. After training, ACTH levels are slightly elevated during exercise.[34]

Antidiuretic hormone secretion is controlled by the posterior pituitary gland. During exercise, this gland increases water retention by the kidneys, maintaining fluid volume.[34]

Norepinephrine and epinephrine secretion, by the adrenal medulla, is stimulated by exercise and increases as the intensity of the exercise increases. A greater response to exercise is seen in older rather than younger individuals and in men rather than in women. Also known as catecholamines, these hormones are related to activity of the sympathetic branch of the autonomic nervous system. They increase cardiac contractility, heart rate, distribution of blood within the vascular system, and so forth. They are also active in the breakdown of stored fat into free fatty acids and of glycogen into glucose.[34]

Cortisol is secreted by the adrenal cortex. It promotes the formation of glucose from proteins and fatty acids during intense exercise. ACTH stimulates the release of cortisol. After training, levels of cortisol are slightly increased with exercise.

Aldosterone, also secreted by the adrenal gland, regulates salt and water concentrations in the body. During exercise, aldosterone levels increase. Sodium, potassium, and water retention are activated by aldosterone, helping maintain increased plasma volume.

Insulin is secreted by the pancreas when blood glucose levels are too high. It inhibits the effects of epinephrine and glucagon on fat metabolism and facilitates glucose uptake by the muscle cells. Insulin secretion is usually decreased during exercise.[34,127] Insulin levels appear to increase during exercise in prepubertal children and remain stable in exercising pubescent children.[126] After training, levels of insulin are maintained at closer to resting levels during exercise.[34]

Glucagon also is secreted by the pancreas when blood glucose falls below a threshold. It stimulates the formation of glucose from liver glycogen stores and amino acids. It can also stimulate the breakdown of fat stores. Glucagon acts in opposition to insulin, functioning to raise blood glucose levels.[34] Similar to insulin, after training, glucagon levels remain closer to resting level during exercise.

Maximal Aerobic Capacity and Maximal Oxygen Uptake

All of the systems discussed here work together to allow our bodies to efficiently use their energy stores and to produce the mechanical work necessary for physical activity. A measure of how efficiently the body can perform this task is the maximal aerobic capacity, or maximal oxygen uptake (Vo_{2max}), which reflects the maximal rate at which oxygen can be used by the tissues during exercise. Both how well the cardiovascular and pulmonary systems deliver oxygen to the tissues and the ability of the tissues to use the oxygen contribute to Vo_{2max}. Maximal aerobic capacity measures the maximum level of work an individual can perform. It is a major determinant of overall functional ability and a good measure of aerobic fitness. Aerobic fitness has also been related to levels of health risk.

Maximal aerobic capacity appears to be closely related to our level of activity and body composition. This measure improves as our level of fitness improves and decreases with inactivity. Aerobic capacity decreases as the percent of body fat increases and is improved in individuals with lower percentages of body fat. Indeed, our habitual level of physical activity is thought to be more of a determinant of aerobic capacity than chronological age.

Age does affect maximal aerobic capacity. Maximal aerobic capacity appears to be lower in children than in adults, but it increases through childhood.[128] Through childhood, peak Vo_2 of boys is slightly greater than that of girls, with the difference increasing even more after puberty.[128] Cardiac size, cardiac output, and pulmonary capacity increase through childhood, but continue to be factors that limit the child's aerobic capacity. Other differences are seen in the cardiovascular system of children compared with adults. Blood volume and hemoglobin levels increase through childhood and are correlated with the peak Vo_2 that can be attained.[49] Because children have less hemoglobin than adults, they have less oxygen-carrying capacity than adults. Their ability to extract oxygen from the blood at the tissue level (A-Vo_2 difference) has been reported to increase slightly with age, especially after puberty, and reaches adult levels by late adolescence. This change may be related to the growing child's increased muscle mass, changes in muscle enzyme perfusion, and changes in the ratio of capillary to muscle fiber.[49,129]

The pulmonary system development also affects aerobic power in children. The growth of the lungs parallels the general growth of the child. Children's airways are small in diameter, resulting in higher resistance to airflow and increased work of breathing. Because children demonstrate poorer ventilatory efficiency than adults in both submaximal and maximal exercise, they must maintain a higher breathing frequency when performing similar tasks.

Training effects, specifically improvements in maximal aerobic power, in prepubescent children have been demonstrated, but the improvements in children are less than those seen in adults.[130-132] Increases in maximal aerobic power appear to be related to improvements in the child's stroke volume during maximal exercise.[107] High levels of habitual activity, mechanical inefficiency in performing physical activity, and body size limitations affect the maximal aerobic capacity of children.[133]

Aerobic capacity increases through adolescence in boys greater than in girls.[128,134] Studies of children and adolescents between 12 and 19 years of age in the United States have shown that Vo_{2max} increases with age in males, while Vo_{2max} of females decreases with age.[135] The increased muscle mass of boys compared with girls contributes to this difference.[49] Peak Vo_2 increases by 150% in boys and 80% in girls between the ages of 8 and 16 years. This increase also seems to be related to increased left ventricular size and stroke volume.[49] Adolescents' attainment of peak aerobic power appears to occur at the time of peak height velocity.[128] Higher levels of physical activity, less than 3 hours per day of

sedentary leisure activity, and normal weight were also related to higher levels of Vo_{2max} in 12- to 19-year-olds in the United States.[135] Aerobic power in adolescence also seems to predict performance in adulthood.[134]

Once adult levels of cardiovascular performance have been reached, some sex-related differences surface. The stroke volume of women is approximately 25% less than that of men. Men have 15–16 g Hb/100 mL blood, whereas women have 14 g Hb/100 mL blood; this gives men a greater oxygen-carrying capacity. Teenage and adult women have a 5%–10% higher cardiac output during submaximal exercise than do men, possibly to compensate for their decreased oxygen-carrying capacity.[34]

Longitudinal and cross-sectional studies of adults and older adults have demonstrated that aerobic capacity decreases through adulthood.[38,40,85,136,137] The decrease is most likely related to both age-related changes in the cardiovascular and musculoskeletal systems and to the level of physical activity. In middle age adults, decreases in cardiac output begin to limit aerobic capacity, while in older adults, skeletal muscle changes further limit aerobic capacity.[138] Longitudinal studies have indicated that the age-associated decrease in peak Vo_2 decreases 3%–6% per decade from ages 20–40 and accelerates greater than 20% per decade decline after the age of 70 years.[40,137-139]

Exercise capacity of older adults is also impacted by changes in the pulmonary system. For the older adult, structural pulmonary system changes, such as a stiffer bony thorax, increase the work of breathing. Decreased compliance of the lungs and airways increases resistance to airflow. As a result of structural and functional changes, the older adult's residual lung capacity is increased with age. Vital capacity, inspiratory reserve, and expiratory reserve volumes are decreased in both resting and dynamic states. Although changes in pulmonary function are seen with aging, older adults who remain physically active demonstrate less change than sedentary older adults.[34]

When considering the previously discussed cardiovascular, pulmonary, and musculoskeletal system changes with age, it is understandable that the ability to transport and oxygen at the tissue level would change with age. More specifically, the maximum heart rate does decrease with age regardless of training.[136] Muscle mass also decreases with age, affecting the amount of oxygen that can be used.

Not all of the changes in aerobic capacity of adults can be attributed to changes in the body systems. Lifestyle factors such as an increase in percent body fat and decreased levels of physical activity are major contributors to the diminishing aerobic capacity in adults. It has also been shown that individuals who have been physically active through childhood, adolescence, and young adulthood demonstrate higher levels of aerobic capacity in adulthood.[134] Older adults have also demonstrated increases in aerobic capacity after participating in exercise programs.[140]

EXERCISE AND TRAINING CONSIDERATIONS ACROSS THE LIFE SPAN

As body systems mature and develop across the life span and an individual's work and leisure habits are formed, regular participation in physical activity is important. Because of differences in the aerobic capacity and the ability of muscle tissue to respond to exercise, exercise programs must be designed for each individual based on his or her lifestyle and age. Especially with older adults, levels of physical functioning can vary significantly between senior athletes, community dwelling older adults, and frail elderly. Physical activity programs need to be individualized for each older adult, but even individuals who are frail can benefit from physical activity programs. Frailty is discussed in more depth in Box 13.1.

General recommendations regarding appropriate exercise for individuals of different ages are listed in Table 13.4, but it must be remembered that these are general recommendations and the health care provider must consider each individual's abilities and health when developing an exercise prescription.

Flexibility and Body Composition
Childhood and Adolescence

Especially after periods of skeletal growth, flexibility is an issue for children. Because bone growth precedes muscle growth, children should be reminded to stretch before exercising. Throughout childhood, girls are more flexible than boys.

CLINICAL IMPLICATIONS BOX 13.1
Frailty, a Geriatric Syndrome

Frailty is a multisystem geriatric syndrome characterized by a loss of physiological reserves and an inability to maintain homeostasis in the presence of stressors such as illness, surgery, or falls, which leads to disability. Homeostasis is unable to be maintained because of relentless physiological deterioration.[1] Fried et al.[2] define frailty as "a syndrome of decreased reserve and resistance to stressors, that result in cumulative declines across multiple physiologic systems, causing vulnerability to adverse outcomes."[3] The multiple system decline seen in frailty is different than the normal aging process and may include sarcopenia, osteoporosis, decreased cardiopulmonary function, and decreased immunological responses.[4] Frailty has a large public health impact, with 4%–60% prevalence in community dwelling older adults.[5,6]

Multiple components must be present to constitute frailty. Fried found that three of the following factors constitute frailty, and the presence of two factors may signal an increased risk for frailty within the next 3–4 years.[2] The factors include *loss of weight* (a decrease in 10 pounds or 5% body weight pounds lost unintentionally in past year), *self-reported exhaustion* using the Self-Report of Exhaustion on CES-D questions, *weakness* (specifically in grip strength and being in the lowest 20% adjusted for gender and BMI), *slow walking speed* (slowest 20% to walk 15 feet), and *low level of physical activity* (lowest quintile of weighted kilocalorie expended per week).[2] There is an inverse relationship between frailty and quality of life.[5]

Sarcopenia is considered a "biological substrate for physical frailty."[7] Sarcopenia predicts frailty, poor quality of life, and mortality.[8] Frailty and oxidative stress overlap in the older adult.[1] Fried's frailty phenotype is *primary* or *preclinical* and is associated with increased levels of reactive oxygen and nitrogen species (RONS). Primary frailty leads to *secondary* or *clinical frailty, clinical frailty*, which is associated with comorbidities or know disabilities (Fig. 13.9).

Clinical Implications: Working With the Frail Older Adult

Most studies suggest that therapists should recommend regular physical activity or exercise training for frail older adults. The evidence shows that regular physical activity or exercise is beneficial for older adults who are frail or at high risk of frailty.[6,9–12] Structured exercise training has a positive impact on the frail older adults and should be used for the management of frailty.[10] Exercise programs have been shown to improve strength, functional activity level, fat-free mass, and endurance of frail older adults. At the molecular level, exercise also decreases muscle inflammation and oxidative stress.[1,13]

Continued

CLINICAL IMPLICATIONS BOX 13.1
Frailty, a Geriatric Syndrome—cont'd

Exercise programs including physical activity, balance, and resistance training have been shown to decrease falls, improve functional performance, and improve frailty.[6,11] Aerobic exercise (such as walking) and flexibility are also important components to consider in an exercise program for a frail older adult.[6,13] It is also helpful if physical activities included in the program are similar to everyday tasks performed by the older adult.[6] All reviews demonstrated the superior nature of multicomponent exercise programs as opposed to single-component exercise programs.[9,11]

Barriers of different levels need to be taken into account and addressed prior to initiating exercise.[9] Older frail persons themselves may have self-efficacy and attitude issues. Health care personnel provide motivation and education at an appropriate level for the older adult. Although most trials studied resistance exercise training, frail older adults are encouraged to start with an aerobic activity, such as walking, as it is more accessible.[10] A longer-term multicomponent interventions with shorter-duration sessions (30–45 min) might be a better option for this population, especially for the prevention of adverse health consequences.[11,12] If possible, resistance exercise training should then be added. For individuals with severe frailty, evaluation by a rehabilitation professional is recommended.[10] Studies have shown that the number of adverse events is minimal and the gains of regular exercise clearly outweigh the risks.[10,13] Although there are still several areas related to the intervention that require further investigation, regular physical activity or exercise is highly recommended for older adults as a means to modify frailty and its adverse outcomes.[10] Rehabilitation of frail older adults can positively impact functional status and quality of life.

References

1. Liguori I, Russo G, Curcio F, Bulli G, Aran L, Della-Morte D, et al. Oxidative stress, aging, and disease. *Clin Interv Aging.* 2018;13:757–772.
2. Fried LP, Tangen CM, Walston J, Cardiovascular Health Study Collaborative Research Group. Frailty in older adults: evidence for a phenotype. *J Gerontol A Biol Sci Med Sci.* 2001;56(3):M146–M156.
3. Janz KF, Dawson JD, Mahoney LT. Tracking physical fitness and physical activity from childhood to adolescence: the Muscatine study. *Med Sci Sports Exerc.* 2000;32(7):1250–1257.
4. Bortz WM. A conceptual framework of frailty: a review. *J Gerontol A.* 2002;57(5):283–288.
5. Gustavson AM, Falvey JR, Jankowski CM, Stevens-Lapsley JE. Public Health Impact of frailty: role of physical therapists. *J Frailty Aging.* 2017;6:2–5.
6. Kidd T, Mold F, Jones C, Ream E, et al. What are the most effective interventions to improve physical performance in pre-frail and frail adults? A systematic review of randomized controlled trials. *BMC Geriatrics.* 2019;19:184.
7. Landi F, Calvani R, Cesari M, et al. Sarcopenia as the biological substrate of physical frailty. *Clin Geriatr Med.* 2015;31(3):367–374.
8. Gomes MJ, Martinez PF, Pagan LU, et al. Skeletal muscle aging: influence of oxidative stress and physical exercise. *Oncotarget.* 2017;8(12):20428–20440.
9. Freiberger E, Kemmler W, Siegrist M, et al. Frailty and exercise interventions. *Z Gerontol Geriat.* 2016;49:606–611.
10. Liu CK, Fielding RA. Exercise as an intervention for frailty. *Clin Geriatr Med.* 2011;27(1):101–110.
11. Stookey AD, Katzel LI. Home exercise interventions in frail older adults. *Curr Geriatr Rep.* 2020;9:163–175.
12. Stathokostas L, Roland KP, Jakobi JM, et al. The effectiveness of exercise interventions for the management of frailty: a systematic review. *J Aging Res.* 2011;2011:569194.
13. Aguirre LE, Villareal DT,. Physical Exercise as therapy for frailty. *Nestle Nutr Inst Workshop Ser.* 2015;83:83–92.

Through infancy, the amount of fat mass increases, but then it decreases once children start increasing muscle mass. Girls' fat mass is slightly higher than that of boys in early childhood, and the difference increases with puberty. Exercise and diet are important to control increased fat mass, and with strength training, increased bone density and muscle mass contribute to an increase in fat-free body mass.

Adulthood and Older Adulthood

Flexibility and body composition change through adulthood. Body fat increases 2%–2.5% per decade even in individuals who participate regularly in moderate- to high-intensity exercise.[136] Activities to increase muscle strength and mass, and to sustain or improve bone density, assist in the maintenance of fat-free body mass. Flexibility continues to decrease in older adults and is likely related to decreased compliance of connective tissue.[141,142]

Flexibility training is frequently not included in the general recommendations for older adults. Even though it has been found to increase flexibility and joint range of motion for older adults, flexibility training does not seem to improve functional outcomes.[143] Some sources recommend 2–3 days per week of flexibility or stretching exercise to maintain range of motion (ROM). Disease or specific disability may require more flexibility exercise to maintain function.[144]

TABLE 13.4	Physical Activity Recommendations Across the Life Span	
Age Group	**Activity Recommendations**	**Other Recommendations**
Infants less than 1 year	Floor-based active play many times across the day At least 30 min of tummy time (spread across day)	Not restrained more than 1 hr at a time (car seat, high chair, infant seats, etc.)
1–2 year olds	180 min of physical activity throughout day	Not restrained more than 1 hr at a time 1-year-old—no sedentary screen time 2-year-old—no more than 1 hr sedentary screen time/day
Preschooler	180 min of physical activity a day (variety of activities)	Not restrained more than 1 hr at a time Screen time no more than 1 hr a day
School-age children 5–17 years	60 min of moderate to vigorous physical activity/day Mainly aerobic, but also muscle strengthening 2–3 days a week	Limit sedentary activity and screen time
Adult	150–300 min of moderately vigorous aerobic activity/week, or 75–150 min of vigorous aerobic activity/week Muscle strengthening 2 days/week	Limit sedentary activity
Older adults	150 min of moderately vigorous physical activity per week Include balance training, aerobics, muscle strengthening	

From World Health Organization (WHO). *Fact Sheet: Physical Activity.* 2020 https://www.who.int/news-room/fact-sheets/detail/physical-activity; Office of Disease Prevention and Health Promotion. *Healthy People 2030.* US Department of Health and Human Services, 2021. https://health.gov/healthypeople/objectives-and-data/social-determinants-health; and National Center for Health Statistics, Center for Disease Control and Prevention. *Healthy People 2020: An end of a decade snapshot.* https://www.cec.gov/nchs/healthy_people/index.htm.

Exercise Considerations and Recommendations Across the Life Span

Participation in physical activity and high motor competence levels in childhood affect health and well-being in adults.[36] Individuals who are active in midlife have significantly better function in later life.[145,146] This supports the theory that exercise in middle years can delay aerobic capacity impairment and the occurrence of clinically manifest sarcopenia at old age. Participation in regular exercise or physical activity programs through childhood, adolescence, and adulthood can lead to higher levels of functional capabilities, maintenance of functional independence, postponed disability, and improved quality of life for older adults. Regular exercise and/or physical activity are important components for optimal aging and should even be encouraged/ prescribed for improved chronic disease management. Exercise prescriptions for older adults should account for each individual's health status and functional capacity. For most individuals, more benefits occur when the physical activity is performed at higher intensity, greater frequency, or longer duration.

Childhood

It is difficult to define optimal intensity, duration, and frequency of endurance training for children. Regular physical activity should be encouraged to promote optimal physiological fitness and to establish health behavior patterns for the child to carry into adulthood. Children are learning and perfecting motor skills that promote agility, balance, coordination, speed, and power. Fitness evaluations and programs for children should include a motor skills component.[44] Endurance activities that require anaerobic metabolism should be thoroughly evaluated for appropriateness. Children may have difficulty participating in strenuous activity that lasts more than 15–30 seconds because of immaturity of the glycolytic metabolism and decreased sympathetic nervous system activation.[126] Participation in events such as middle- or long-distance running should be monitored very closely with prepubescent children.

Older Adulthood

Normal aging is associated with reduced functional capacity and strength, and degenerative musculoskeletal conditions. Older adults are generally happy with their level of fitness but underestimate their ability to exercise.[69] As maximal exercise capacity decreases with age, it begins to affect the intensity of exercise that can be considered submaximal work. Older adults at any submaximal exercise load tend to exert a higher percentage of their maximal capacity and effort than younger persons. For example, activities of daily living are considered submaximal work. The energy required to perform these activities remains constant, but the percentage of maximal capacity they require increases as the maximal exercise capacity decreases. In older adults, activities such as walking or housework may be considered high-intensity exercise; in younger adults, these same activities offer a low-intensity exercise. For the older adult, these activities may become more stressful. If the individual can no longer complete activities of daily living because of the level of physiological stress, functional independence is decreased. Therefore, it is very important for older adults to maintain aerobic capacity and to maximize their functional independence.

Studies have shown that regular exercise, even in older adults, can increase maximal aerobic capacity and submaximal work capacity (Fig. 13.8).[38,41,60,147,148] It has been found that even older adults who exercise at less than 50% aerobic capacity show an improvement in submaximal exercise response.[149] To increase Vo_{2max}, exercise intensity should be at 50%–85% of Vo_{2max}.

Exercise programming for the older adult should emphasize the functional needs of the individual. A person's level of fitness and interests must be kept in mind. Aerobic exercise, resistance training flexibility, and balance exercises should be included in the older adult physical activity program to improve cardiovascular endurance, improve or maintain muscle strength, control

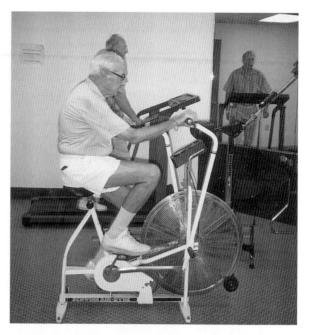

Fig. 13.8 Maintaining an active exercise program through older adulthood improves physical function.

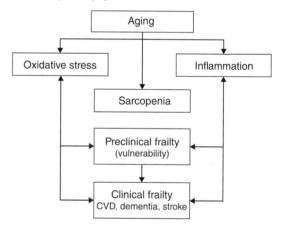

Fig. 13.9 Relationship among oxi-inflamm-aging, preclinical, and clinical frailty. (Clinical Interventions in Aging 2018:13 757–772′ – Originally published by and used with permission from Dove Medical Press Ltd).

weight and loss of bone mineral, and improve flexibility. Older adults will gain distinct benefits from aerobic exercise, strength or resistance training, flexibility or stretching exercises, and balance training to maintain or improve function.[144,150,151] Even individuals into their 8th to 10th decade can improve function with exercise. Exercise has also been shown to minimize and even reverse frailty.[152]

SUMMARY

We continue to emphasize a premise that is discussed throughout this book: exercise and training programs can improve our health, fitness, quality of life, and level of participation. Quality of life is improved when we feel better, do more, and develop a positive self-image. Exercise helps us attain and maintain body efficiency, allowing us to function optimally within the environment. This is why health promotion and maintenance of appropriate levels of physical activity are increasingly important in today's health care arena.

Our level of health and physical fitness is related to our level of physical activity. Many body systems work together to produce efficient, effective physical activity. Each of these systems develops uniquely, and this development can be enhanced by participation in physical fitness programs.

Because optimal health and fitness reflect our ability to maintain a physically active and independent lifestyle, fitness programming is an important focus of health care. Exercise planning and programming form a complex process. Detailed assessment of a person's ability to participate in an exercise program is necessary. Exercise programs differ according to age, health, level of fitness, and interests. As health care providers, we should become familiar with the age-related aspects of exercise and training programs to help our clients attain lifelong fitness, as well as to maintain a healthy lifestyle for ourselves.

REFERENCES

1. World Health Organization. *The First Ten Years of the World Health Organization*. Geneva: World Health Organization; 1958.
2. Shields RK, Dudley-Javorski S. Epigenetics and the International Classification of Functioning, Disability and Health model: bridging nature, nurture and patient-centered population health. *Phys Ther*. 2022;102:1–11. https://doi.org/10.1093/ptj/pzab247.
3. Magnusson DM, Rethorn ZD. Strengthening population health perspectives in physical therapist practice using epigenetics. *Phys Ther*. 2022;102:1–8. https://doi.org/10.1093/ptj/pzab244.
4. Severin R, Sabbahi A, Arena R, Phillips SA. Precision medicine and physical therapy: a healthy living medicine approach for the next century. *Phys Ther*. 2022;102(1):9. https://doi.org/10.1093/ptj/pzab253.
5. Dean E. Physical therapy in the 21st century (part I): toward practice informed by epidemiology and the crisis of lifestyle conditions. *Physiother Theory Pract*. 2009;25(5):330–353.
6. Corbin CB, LaMasurier GC, McConnell KE.*Fitness for Life*. 6th ed. Champaign, IL: Human Kinetics; 2014:17–23.
7. Bouchard C, Shepard RJ, Stephens T, et al. *Exercise Fitness and Health: A Consensus of Current Knowledge*. Champaign, IL: Human Kinetics; 1990.
8. Fair SE.*Wellness and Physical Therapy*. Boston: Jones and Bartlett; 2011.
9. Pronk N, Kleinman DV, Goekler SF, et al. Promoting health and well-being in Healthy People 2030. *J Public Health ManagPract*. 2021;27(Suppl 6):S242–S248. https://doi.org/10.1097/PHH0000000000001254.
10. Sfeatcu R, Scernusca-Mitariu M, Ionescu C, et al. The concept of wellbeing in relation to health and quality of life. *European Journal of Science and Theology*. 2014;10(4):123–128.
11. Kindig D, Stoddart g. What is population health? *J Public Health*. 2003;93:380–383.
12. World Health Organization (WHO). Social Determinants of Health. https://www.who.int/health-topics/social-determinants-of-health#tab=tab_1. Accessed 3/30/2022.
13. Office of Disease Prevention and Health Promotion. (2021). *Healthy People 2030*. U.S. Department of Health and Human Services.https://health.gov/healthypeople/objectives-and-data/social-determinants-health.
14. World Health Organization (WHO), 1986. *Ottawa Charter for Health Promotion*. http://www.who.int/healthpromotion/conferences/previous/ottawa/en/. Accessed 2/13/2022.
15. McDade TW, Ryan C, Jones MR, et al. Social and physical environments early in development predict DNA methylation of inflammatory genes in young adulthood. *Proc Natl Acad Sci USA*. 2018;114:7611–7616. https://doi.org/10.1073/pnas.1620661114.
16. Fernandez-Sanles A, Sayols-Baixeras S, Castro De Maura M, et al. Physical activity and genome-wide DNA methylation: the REGICOR Study. *Med Sci Sports Exerc*. 2020;52:589–597. https://doi.org/10.1249/MSS.0000000000001274.
17. Caspersen CJ, Powell KE, Christenson GM. Physical activity, exercise and physical fitness: Definitions and

distinctions for health-related research. *Public Health Reports.* 1985;100(2):126–131.

18. World Health Organization (WHO), 2020. *Fact Sheet: Physical Activity.* https://www.who.int/news-room/fact-sheets/detail/physical-activity.

19. Aires L, Silva P, Silva G, et al. Intensity of physical activity, cardiorespiratory fitness, and body mass index in youth. *J Phys Act Health.* 2010;7:54–59.

20. Anderson SE, Economos CD, Must A. Active play and screen time in US children aged 4 to 11 years in relation to sociodemographic and weight status characteristics: a nationally representative cross-sectional analysis. *BMC Public Health.* 2008;8:355. https://doi.org/10.1186/1471-2458/8/366.

21. CDC Prevalence of self-reported physically active adults – United States, 2007. *MMWR Morb Mortal Wkly Rep.* 2008;57(48):1297–1300.

22. Janz KF, Dawson JD, Mahoney LT. Tracking physical fitness and physical activity from childhood to adolescence: the Muscatine study. *Med Sci Sports Exerc.* 2000;32(7):1250–1257.

23. Mackett RL, Paskins J. Children's physical activity: the contribution of playing and walking. *Child Soc.* 2008;22:345–357.

24. Nelson MC, Neumark-Stzainer Hannan PJ, Sirary JR, et al. Longitudinal and secular trends in physical activity and sedentary behavior during adolescence. *Pediatrics.* 2006;118 e1627e1634.

25. Scholes S. 2017. *Health Survey for England 2016: Physical Activity in Adults.* Health and Social Care Information Centre. www.digital.NHS.UK@nhs.digital ISBN 978-1-78734-099-2.

26. Masonovic B, Gardasevic J, Marques A, et al. Trends in physical fitness among school aged children and adolescents: a systematic review. *Front. Pediatr.* 2020;8:627529. https://doi.org/10.3389/fped.2020.627529.

27. Mengesha MM, Roba HS, Ayele BH, Beyene AS. Levels of physical activity among urban adults and the socio-demographic correlates: a population-based cross-sectional study using the global physical activity questionnaire. *BMC Public Health.* 2019;19:1160. https://doi.org/10.1186/s12889-019-7465-y.

28. Ammar A, Trabelsi K, Branch M, et al. Effects of home confinement on mental health and lifestyle behaviours during the COVID-19 outbreak: Insights from ECLB-COVID19 multicentre study. *Biol Sport.* 2021;38(1):9–21. https://doi.org/10.5114/biolsport.2020.96857.

29. Hallal PC, Victora CG, Azevedo MR, et al. Adolescent physical activity and health: a systematic review. *Sports Med.* 2006;36(12):1019–1030.

30. Mitchell JA, Mattocks C, Ness AR, et al. Sedentary behavior and obesity in a large cohort of children. *Obesity.* 2009;17(8):1596–1602.

31. Strong WB, Malina RM, Blimkie CJR, et al. Evidence based physical activity for school-age youth. *J Pediatr.* 2005;146:732–737.

32. Whitaker RC, Orzol SM. Obesity among US urban preschool children: relationships to race, ethnicity, and socioeconomic status. *Arch Pediatr Adolesc Med.* 2006;160:578–584.

33. Singh R, Pattisapu A, Emery M. US physical activity guidelines: current state, impact and future directions. *Trends in Cardiovascular Medicine.* 2020;30(7):407–412. https://doi.org/10.1016/j.tcm.2019.10.002.

34. McArdle WD, Katch FI, Katch VL. *Exercise Physiology: Energy, Nutrition and Human Performance.* 7th ed. Philadelphia: Wolter Kluwer/Lippincott, Williams & Wilkins; 2010.

35. Okuda E, Horii D, Kano T. Genetic and environmental effects on physical fitness and motor performance. *International Journal of Sport and Health Science.* 2005;3:1–9.

36. Weedon BD, Liu F, Mahmoud W, et al. The relationship of gross upper and lower limb motor competence to measures of health and fitness in adolescents aged 13–14 years. *BMJ Open Sport & Exercise Medicine.* 2018;4:e000288. https://doi.org/10.1136/bmjsem-2017-000288.

37. Frontera WR, Evans WJ. Exercise performance and endurance training in the elderly. *Top Geriatr Rehabil.* 1986;2:17–32.

38. Lemura LM, VonDuvillard SO, Mookerjee S. The effects of physical training of functional capacity in adults ages 46-90: a meta-analysis. *J Sports Med Phys Fitness.* 2000;40:1–10.

39. Sarkisian CA, Liu H, Gutierrez PR, et al. Modifiable risk factors predict functional decline among older women: a prospectively validated clinical prediction tool. *J Am Geriatr Soc.* 2000;48:170–176.

40. Jackson AS, Sui X, Hebert JR, et al. Role of lifestyle and aging on the longitudinal change in cardiorespiratory fitness. *Arch Intern Med.* 2009;169(19):1781–1787.

41. Green JS, Crouse SF. The effects of endurance training on functional capacity in the elderly: a meta-analysis. *Med Sci Sports Exerc.* 1995;27:920–926.

42. Suominen H. Physical activity and health: musculoskeletal issues. *Adv Physiother.* 2007;9:65–75.

43. Moreno-Agostino D, Daskalopoulou C, Wu YT, et al. The impact of physical activity on healthy ageing trajectories: evidence from eight cohort studies. *Int J Behav Nutr Phys Act.* 2020;17:92. https://doi.org/10.1186/s12966-020-00995.

44. Malina RM. Growth, exercise fitness and later outcomes. In: Bouchard C, Shepard RJ, Stephens T, eds. *Exercise, Fitness and Health: A Consensus of Current Knowledge.* Champaign, IL: Human Kinetics; 1990:637–653.

45. Sattelmair JR, Pertman JH, Forman DE. Effects of physical activity on cardiovascular and noncardiovascular

outcomes in older adults. *Clin Geriatr Med.* 2009;25:677–702.

46. Alswat KA. Gender disparaties in osteoporosis. *J Clin Med Res.* 2017;9(5):382–387.

47. Goodpaster BH, Park SW, Harris TB, et al. The loss of skeletal muscle strength, mass, and quality in older adults: the health, aging and body composition study. *J Gerontol A Biol Sci Med Sci.* 2006;61A(10):1059–1064.

48. Azzolino D, Spolidoro GC, Saporiti D, Luchetti C, Agostoni C, Cesari M. Musculoskeletal changes across the lifespan: nutrition and the life-course approach to prevention. *Front Med.* 2021;8:697954. https://doi.org/10.3389/fmed2021.697954.

49. Armstrong N, Welsman JR. Development of aerobic fitness during childhood and adolescence. *Pediatr Exerc Sci.* 2000;12:128–149.

50. Vingren JL, Kraemer WJ, Ratamess NA, Anderson JM, Volek JS, Maresh CM. Testosterone physiology in resistance exercise and training: the up-stream regulatory elements. *Sports Med.* 2010;40(12):1037–1053. https://doi.org/10.2165/11536910-000000000-00000. PMID: 21058750.

51. Faulkner JA, White TP. Adaptation of skeletal muscle to physical activity. In: Bouchard C, Shepard RJ, Stephens T, eds. *Exercise, Fitness and Health: A Consensus of Current Knowledge.* Champaign, IL: Human Kinetics; 1990:256–279.

52. Mustafina LJ, Naumov VA, Cieszczyk P, et al. AGTR2 gene polymorphism is associated with muscle fiber composition, athletic status, and aerobic performance. *Exp Physiol.* 2014;99(8):1042–1052. https://doi.org/10.1113/expphysiol.2014.079335.

53. Bouchard C, Perusse L. Heredity, activity level, fitness and health. In: Bouchard C, Shephard RJ, Stephens T, eds. *Physical Activity, Fitness and Health: International Proceedings and Consensus Statement.* Champaign, IL: Human Kinetics; 1994:106–118.

54. Bar-Or O. The growth and development of children's physiologic and perceptional responses to exercise. In: Ilmannen J, Valimaki I, eds. *Children and Sport-Pediatric Work Physiology.* New York: Springer Verlag; 1984:3–17.

55. Folinsbee LJ. Discussion: exercise and environment. In: Bouchard C, Shepard RJ, Stephens T, eds. *Exercise, Fitness and Health: A Consensus of Current Knowledge.* Champaign, IL: Human Kinetics; 1990:179–183. editiors.

56. To T, Zhu J, Stieb D, et al. Early life exposure to air pollution and incidence of childhood asthma, allergic rhinitis and eczema. *Eur Respir J.* 2020;55:1900913. https://doi.org/10.1183/13993003.00913-2019.

57. Holst GJ, Pederson CB, Thygesen M, et al. Air pollution and family determinants of asthma onset and persistent wheezing in children: nationwide case-control study. *Bmj2020: 370.* 2020:m2791. https://doi.org/10.1136/bmj.m2791.

58. Bouchard C, Shephard RJ. Physical activity, fitness, and health: the model and key concepts. In: Bouchard C, Shephard RJ, Stephens T, eds. *Physical Activity, Fitness and Health: International Proceedings and Consensus Statement.* Champaign, IL: Human Kinetics; 1994:77–88.

59. Lovell DI, Cuneo R, Gass GC. Can aerobic training improve muscle strength and power in older men? *J Aging Phys Act.* 2010;18:14–26.

60. Cress ME, Buchner DM, Quiestad KA, et al. Exercise effects on physical functional performance in older adults. *J Gerontol.* 1999;54A M242M238.

61. Westerterp KR, Yamada Y, Sagayama H, et al. Physical activity and fat free mass during growth and in later life. *Am J Clin Nutr;.* 2021;114:1583–1589. https://doi.org/10.1093/ajcn/nqab260.

62. Aires L, Andersen LB, Mendonca D, et al. A 3-year longitudinal analysis of changes in fitness, physical activity, fatness and screen time. *Acta Paediatr.* 2010;99:140–144.

63. Vuori I. Physical activity and health: metabolic and cardiovascular issues. *Adv Physiother.* 2007;9:50–64.

64. Perpera G, Hadjiandrea S, Iliadis I, et al. Associations between cardiorespiratory fitness, fatness, hemodynamic characteristics and sedentary behavior in primary school-aged children. *BMC Sports Science, Medicine and Rehabilitation.* 2022;14:16. https://doi.org/10.1186/S13102-022-00411-7.

65. Feinberg AP. The key role of epigenetics in human disease prevention and mitigation. *N Engl J Med.* 2018;378:1323–1324. https://doi.org/10.1056/NEJMra1402513.

66. King-Dowling S, Proudfoot NA, Cairney J, Timmons BW. Motor Competence, physical activity and fitness across early childhood. *Med.Sci.Sports Exerc.* 2020;52(11):2342–2348. https://doi.org/10.1249/MSS.0000000000002388.

67. Bolger LA, Bolger LA, O'Neill C, et al. Global levels of fundamental motor skills in children: a systematic review. *Journal of Sports Sciences.* 2020. https://doi.org/10.1080/02640414.2020.1841405.

68. Schmutz EA, Leegor-Aschmann CS, Kakabeeke TH, et al. Motor competetence and physical activity in early childhood: Stability and relationship. *Front Public Health.* 2020;8(39). https://doi.org/10.3389/fpubh.2020.00039.

69. Buskirk ER. Exercise, fitness and aging. In: Bouchard C, Shepard RJ, Stephens T, eds. *Exercise, Fitness and*

Health: A Consensus of Current Knowledge. Champaign, IL: Human Kinetics; 1990:687–697.

70. Mansfield ED, Ducharme N, Koski KG. Individual, social and environmental factors influencing physical activity levels and behaviors of multi-ethnic, socio-economically disadvantaged urban mothers in Canada: a mixed methods approach. *International Journal of Behavioral Nutrition and Physical Activity.* 2012;9:42.

71. Lindsay Smith G, Banting L, Eime R, et al. The association between social support and physical activity in older adults: a systematic review. *International Journal of Behavioral Nutrition and Physical Activity.* 2017;14:6. https://doi.org/10.1186/s12966-017-0509-8.

72. Park CH, Elavsky S, Koo KM. Factors influencing physical activity in older adults. *Journal of Exercise Rehabilitation.* 2014;10(1):45–52.

73. Statistics Canada, 2021. Youth—but not adults—reported less physical activity during COVID-19 pandemic. Catalogue no. 45-28-0001. https://www150.statcan.gc.ca/n1/pub/45-28-0001/2021001/article/00032-eng.htm. Accessed 3/4/2022

74. Kaur H, Singh T, Arya YK, Mittal S. Physical fitness and exercise during the COVID-19 pandemic: a qualitative enquiry. *Front Psychol.* 2020;11:590172. https://doi.org/10.3389/fpsyg.2020.590172.

75. Goo Y, Liao M, Cai W, et al. Physical activity, screen exposure and sleep among students during the pandemic of COVID-19. *Nature.* 2021;11:8529. https://doi.org/10.1038/s41598-021-88071-4.

76. National Center for Health Statistics, Center for Disease Control and Prevention. Healthy People 2020: *An end of a decade snapshot.* https://www.cdc.gov/nchs/healthy_people/index.htm. Accessed March 2, 2022 (cdc.gov)

77. Spinelli A, Buoncristiano M, Nardone P, et al. Thinness, overweight, and obesity in 6- to 9-year-old children from 36 countries: The World Health Organization European Childhood Obesity Surveillance Initiative-COSI 2015-2017. *Obesity Reviews.* 2021;22(Suppl 6):e13214. https://doi.org/10.1111/0br.13214.

78. World Health Organization (WHO) Fact Sheet - Obesity and overweight. https://www.who.int/news-room/fact-sheets/detail/obesity and overweight. published 6/9/2021.

79. Hales, Craig M., Carroll, Margaret D., Fryar, Cheryl D., Ogden, Cynthia L. Prevalence of obesity among adults and youth: United States, 2015-2016. Corporate Authors(s): National Center for Health Statistics (U.S.), 2017, Series: NCHS data brief; no. 288; DHHS publication; no. (PHS) 2018–1209; URL: https://stacks.cdc.gov/view/cdc/49223.

80. Nelson ME, Rejeski WJ, Blair SN, et al. Physical activity and public health in older adults: recommen-dation from the American College of Sports Medicine and the American Heart Association. *Circulation.* 2007;116:1094–1105.

81. Haskell WL, Lee IM, Pate RR, et al. Physical activity and public health: updated recommendations for adults from the American College of Sports Medicine and the American Heart Association. *Med Sci Sports Exerc.* 2007;39:1423–1434.

82. Bull FC, Al-Ansar SS, Biddle S, et al. World Health Organization 2020 guidelines on physical activity and sedentary behavior. *Br J Sports Med;.* 2020;54:1451–1462.

83. Guthold R, Stevens GA, Riley LM, Bull FC. Global trends in insufficient physical activity among adolescents: a pooled analysis of 298 population-based surveys with 1.6 million participants. *Lancet Child Adolesc Health.* 2020;4:23–35. https://doi.org/10.1016/S2352-4642(19)30323-2.

84. Guthold R, Stevens GA, Riley LM, Bull FC. Worldwide trends in insufficient physical activity from 2001-2015: a pooled analysis of 358 population-based surveys with 1.9 million participants. *Lancet Glob Health;.* 2018;6:e1077–e1086.

85. Talbot LA, Metter EJ, Fleg JL. Leisure time physical activities and their relationship to cardiorespiratory fitness in healthy men and women, 18-95 years old. *Med Sci Sports Exerc.* 2000;32:417–425.

86. Jenkin CR, Eime RM, Westerbeek H, et al. Sport and ageing: a systematic review of the determinants and trends of participation in sport for older adults. *BMC Public Health.* 2017;17:976. https://doi.org/10.1186/s12889-017-4970-8.

87. Nader PR, Bradley RH, Houts RM, et al. Moderate-to-vigorous physical activity from ages 9 to 15 years. *JAMA.* 2008;300(3):295–305.

88. Klemm K, Krell-Roesch J, DeClerck IL, Brehm W, Boes K. Health related fitness in adults from 8 European countries—an analysis based on data from the European Fitness Badge. *Frontiers in Physiology.* 2021;11:615237. https://doi.org/10.3389/fphys.2020.615237.

89. Aggio D, Papacosta O, Lennon L, et al. Association between physical activity levels in mid-life with physical activity in old age: a 20-year tracking study in a prospective cohort. *BMJ Open.* 2017;7:e017378. https://doi.org/10.1136/bmjopen-2017-017378.

90. Cawley J, Biener A, Meyerhoefer C, Ding Y, Zvenyach T, Smolarz BG, Ramasamy A. Direct medical costs of obesity in the United States and the most populous states. *J Manag Care Spec Pharm.* 2021 Mar;27(3):354–366. https://doi.org/10.18553/jmcp.2021.20410. Epub 2021 Jan 20. PMID: 33470881.

91. Finkelstein EA, Trogdon JG, Cohen JW, Dietz W. Annual medical spending attributable to obesity: payer- and

service-specific estimates. *Health Aff.* 2009;28(5): w822–w883.

92. Suryadinata RV, Wirjatmadi B, Adriani M, Lorensia A. Effect of age and weight on physical activity. *J Public Health Res.* 2020;9(2):1840. https://doi.org/10.4081/jphr.2020.1840. Published July 3, 2020.

93. Dean E. Physical therapy in the 21st century (part II): evidence-based practice within the context of evidence-informed practice. *Physiother Theory Pract.* 2008;25(5–6):354–368.

94. Bar-Or O. The prepubescent female. In: Shangold MM, Mirken G, eds.*Women and Exercise: Physiology and Sports Medicine.* Philadelphia: FA Davis; 1988:109–119.

95. Barron-Cabrera E, Ramos-Lopez O, Gonzalez-Becerra K, et al. Epigenetic modifications as outcomes of exercise interventions related to specific metabolic alterations: a systematic review. *Lifestyle Genom.* 2019;12:25–44. https://doi.org/10.1159/000503289.

96. Plaza-Diaz J, Izquierdo D, Torres-Martos A, et al. Impact of physical activity and exercise on the epigenome in skeletal muscle and effects on systemic metabolism. *Biomedicines.* 2022;10:126. https://doi.org/10.3390/biomedicines.10010126.

97. Sellami M, Bragazzi N, Prince MS, Denham J, Elrayess M. Regular intense exercise training as a healthy aging lifestyle strategy: preventing DNA damage, telomere shortening, and adverse DNA methylation changes over a lifetime. *Front.Genet.* 2021;12:652297. https://doi.org/10.3389/fgene.2021.652497.

98. Kelley GA, Kelley KS. Progressive resistance exercise and resting blood pressure: a meta-analysis of randomized controlled trials. *Hypertension.* 2000;3:838–843.

99. Kelley GA, Kelley KS. Aerobic exercise and resting blood pressure in older adults: a meta-analytic review of randomized controlled trials. *J Gerontol A Biol Sci Med Sci.* 2001;56(5):M298M303.

100. Farrell C., Turgeon D., 2021. Normal versus chronic adaptation to aerobic exercise. [updated July 15, 2021]. In: STATPearls [Internet] Treasure Island (FL): STATPearls Publishing; Jan. 2022 – Available from: https://www.ncbi.nlm.nih.gov/books/NBK572066/. Accessed 3/8/2022.

101. Carpio-Rivera E, Moncada-Jimenez J, Salazai-Rojas W, Solera-Herra A. Acute effects of exercise on blood pressure: a meta-analytic investigation. *Arq Bras Cardiol.* 2016;106(5):422–433. https://doi.org/10.5935/abc.20160064.

102. Ghadieh AS, Saab B. Evidence for exercise training in the management of hypertension in adults. *Can Fam Physician.* 2015;61(3):233–239.

103. Mitchell JH, Raven PB. Cardiovascular adaptation to physical activity. In: Bouchard C, Shephard RJ, Stephens T, eds. *Physical Activity, Fitness and Health: International-*

104. Green HJ. Discussion: adaptation of skeletal muscle to physical activity. In: Bouchard C, Shepard RJ, Stephens T, eds. *Exercise, Fitness and Health: a Consensus of Current Knowledge.* Champaign, IL: Human Kinetics; 1990:281–291.

105. Hallsten Y, Nyberg M. Cardiovascular adaptations to exercise training. *Comprehensive Physiology.* 2016;6(1):1–32. https://doi.org/10.1002/cphys.c140080.

106. Saltin B. Cardiovascular and pulmonary adaptation to physical activity. In: Bouchard C, Shepard RJ, Stephens T, eds. *Exercise, Fitness and Health: A Consensus of Current Knowledge.* Champaign, IL: Human Kinetics; 1990:187–203.

107. Obert P, Mandigouts S, Nottin S, et al. Cardiovascular responses to endurance training in children: effect of gender. *Eur J Clin Invest.* 2003;33(3):199–208.

108. Nystoriak MA, Bhatnagar A. Cardiovascular effects and benefits of exercise. *Front. Cardiovasc. Med.* 2018;5:135. https://doi.org/10.3389/fcvm.2018.00135.

109. Faigenbaum AD. State of the art reviews: resistance training for children and adolescents: are there health outcomes? *Am J Lifestyle Med.* 2007;1:190–200.

110. DeLorey DS, Paterson DH, Kowalchuk JM. Effects of ageing on muscle O2 utilization and muscle oxygenation during the transition to moderate-intensity exercise. *Appl Physiol Nutr Metab.* 2007;32(6): 1251–1262. https://doi.org/10.1139/H07-121.

111. Burtscher M. Exercise limitations by the oxygen delivery and utilization systems in aging and disease: coordinated adaptation and deadaptation of the lung-heart muscle axis—a mini-review. *Gerontol.* 2013;59:289–296. https://doi.org/10.1159/000343990.

112. Babcock MA, Dempsey JA. Pulmonary system adaptations: limitations to exercise. In: Bouchard C, Shephard RJ, Stephens T, eds. *Physical Activity, Fitness and Health: International Proceedings and Consensus Statement.* Champaign, IL: Human Kinetics; 1994:320–330.

113. Chlif M, Chaouachi A, Ahmaida S. Effect of aerobic exercise training on ventilatory efficiancy and respiratory drive in obese subjects. *Respir Care.* 2017;67(7):936–946. https://doi.org/10.4187/respcare.04923.

114. Hackett DA. Lung function and respiratory muscle adaptations of endurance- and stength-trained males. *Sports.* 2020;8(12):160. https://doi.org/10.3390/Sports8120160.

115. Amann M. Pulmonary system limitations to endurance exercise performance in humans. *Exp Physiol.* 2012;97(3):311–318. https://doi.org/10.1113/expphysiol.2011.058800.

al Proceedings and Consensus Statement. Champaign, IL. Human Kinetics; 1994:286–301.

116. Mahon AD, Vaccaro T. Ventilatory threshold and VO_{2max} changes in children following endurance training. *Med Sci Sports Exerc.* 1989;21:425–431.

117. Kemper HC. Skeletal development during childhood and adolescence and the effects of physical activity. *Pediatr Exerc Sci.* 2000;12:198–216.

118. Hass CJ, Feigenbaum S, Franklin BA. Prescription of resistance training for healthy populations. *Sports Med.* 2001;31(14):953–964.

119. Faigenbaum AD, Kraemer WJ, Blimkie CJR, et al. Youth resistance training: updated position statement paper from the National Strength and Conditioning Association. *J Strength Cond Res.* 2009;23(5): s60s79.

120. Behm DG, Faigenbaum AD, Falk B, et al. Canadian Society for Exercise Physiology position paper: resistance training in children and adolescents. *Appl Physiol Nutr Metab.* 2008;33:547–561.

121. Van Praagh E, Dore E. Short-term muscle power during growth and maturation. *Sports Med.* 2002;32(11):701–728.

122. Van Praagh E. Development of anaerobic function during childhood and adolescence. *Pediatr Exerc Sci.* 2000;12:150–173.

123. Thompson L. Physiologic changes associated with ag-ing. In: Guccione K, ed. *Geriatric Physical Therapy.* 2nd ed,. St Louis: Mosby; 2000.

124. Messonnier LA, Emhoff CA, Fattor JA, et al. Lactate kinetics at the lactate threshold in trained and untrained men. *J Appl. Physiol.* 2013;114:1593–1602. https://doi.org/10.1152/japplphysiol.00043.2013.

125. Green JM, Hornsby JH, Pritchett RC, Pritchett K. Lactate threshold comparison in anaerobic versus aerobic athletes and untrained participants. *International Journal of Exercise Science.* 2014;7(4):329–338.

126. Boisseau N, Delamarche P. Metabolic and hormonal responses to exercise in children and adolescents. *Sports Med.* 2000;30(6):405–422.

127. Sutton JR, Farrell PA, Harber VJ. Hormonal adaptation to physical activity. In: Bouchard C, Shepard RJ, Stephens T, eds. *Exercise, Fitness and Health: a Consensus of Current Knowledge.* Champaign, IL: Human Kinetics; 1990:217–257.

128. Geithner CA, Thomis MA, Eynde BV, et al. Growth in peak aerobic power during adolescence. *Med.Sci.Sports. Exerc.* 2004;36(9):1616–1624.

129. Cunningham DA, Paterson DH, Blimke CJR. The development of the cardiorespiratory system with growth and physical activity. In: Bouleau RA, ed. *Advances in Pediatric Sport Science. Biological Issues.* 1. Champaign, IL: Human Kinetics; 1984:85–116.

130. Mandigout S, Lecoq AM, Courteix D, et al. Effect of gender in response to an aerobic training programme in prepubertal children. *Acta Paediatr.* 2001;90:9–15.

131. Mandigout S, Melin A, Lecoq AM, et al. Effect of two aerobic training regimens on the cardiorespiratory response of prepubertal boys and girls. *Acta Paediatr.* 2002;91:403–408.

132. Baquet G, Van Praagh E, Berthoin S. Endurance training and aerobic fitness in young people. *Sports Med.* 2003;33(15):1127–1143.

133. Bar-Or O. *Pediatric Sports Medicine for the Practitioner.* New York: Springer Verlag; 1983.

134. Westerstahl M, Jansonn E, Barnekow-Bergkvist M, Aasa U. 2018. Longitudinal changes in physical capacity from adolescence to middle age in men and women. www.nature.com/Scientific. *Reports.* 2018;8:14767. https://doi.org/10.1038/s41598-018-33141-3.

135. Pate RR, Wang CY, Dowada M, et al. Cardiorespiratory fitness levels among US youth 12 to 19 years of age: findings from the 1999-2002 National Health and Nutrition Examination Survey. *Arch Pediatr Adolesc Med.* 2006;160:1005–1012.

136. Pollock ML, Mengelkoch LJ, Graves JE, et al. Twenty-year follow-up of aerobic power and body composition of older track athletes. *J Appl Physiol.* 1997;82:1508–1516.

137. Fleg AJ, Morrell CH, Bos AG, et al. Accelerated longitudinal decline of aerobic capacity in healthy older adults. *Circulation.* 2005;112:674–682.

138. Betik AC, Wepple RT. Determinates of VO2Max decline with aging: an integrated perspective. *Applied Physiology, Nutrition, Metabolism.* 2008;33(1). https://doi.org/10.1139/H07-174.

139. Alul LAU, Gomez-Campos R, Almonacid-Fierro A, et al. Aerobic capacity of Chilean adults and elderly: proposal of classification by regional percentiles. *Rev Bras Med E Sporte.* 2019;25(5):390. https://doi.org/10.1590/1517-869220192505185893.

140. Woo JS, Derleth C, Stratton JR, Levy WC. The influence of age, gender and training on exercise efficiency. *Journal of the American College of Cardiology.* 2006;45(5):1049–1057. https://doi.org/10.1016/j.jacc.2005.09.066.

141. Stathokostas L, McDonald Mw, Little RMD, Paterson DH. 2013. Flexibility of older adults aged 55-86 years and the influence of physical activity. *J Aging Res.* 2013:743843. https://doi.org/10.1155/2013/7433843.

142. Wilke J, Macchi V, DeCaro R, Stecco C. Fascia thickness, aging and flexibility: is there an association. *Journal of Anatomy.* 2019;234:43–49. https://doi.org/10.1111/joa12902.

143. Stathokostas L, Little RMD, Vandervoort AA, Patersen DH. 2012. Flexibility training and functional ability in older adults: a systematic review. *J Aging Res.* 2012:306818. https://doi.org/10.1155/2012/306818.

144. Lee PG, Jackson EA, Richardson CR. Exercise prescriptions in older adults. *Am Fam Physician*. 2017;95(7):425–432.

145. Chang M, Saczynski JS, Snaedal J. Midlife physical activity preserves lower extremity function in older adults: age gene/environment susceptibility-Reykjavik study. *J Am Geriatr Soc*. 2013;61(2):237–242. https://doi.org/10.1111/jgs.12077.

146. Edholm P, Veen J, Kadi F, Nilsson A. Muscle mass and aerobic capacity in older women: impact of regular exercise at middle age. *Experimental Gerontology*. 2021;147.

147. Cunningham DA, Paterson DH. Discussion: exercise, fitness and aging. In: Bouchard C, Shepard RJ, Stephens T, eds. *Exercise, Fitness and Health: A Consensus of Current Knowledge*. Champaign, IL: Human Kinetics; 1990:699–704.

148. Villareal DT, Smith GI, Sinacore DA, Shah K, Mittendorfer B. Regular multi-component exercise increases physical fitness and muscle protein anabolism in frail, obese, older adults. *Obesity*. 2011;19(2):312–318. https://doi.org/10.1038/oby.2010.110.

149. DeVito G, Hernandez R, Gonzalez V, et al. Low intensity physical training in older subjects. *J Sports Med Phys Fitness*. 1997;37:72–77.

150. Pugard Larsen JB, et al. Maximal oxygen uptake, muscle strength and walking speed in 85-year-old women: effects of increased physical activity. *Aging*. 2000;12(3):180–189.

151. Hruda KV, Hicks AL, et al. Training for muscle power in older adults: effects on functional abilities. *Can J Appl Physiol*. 2003;28(2):178–189.

152. Brown MB, Sinacore DR, Binder EF, et al. Physical and performance measures for the identification of mild to moderate frailty. *J Gerentol Med Sci*. 2000;6: M350–M355.

INDEX

Note: Page numbers followed by *b* indicates boxes, *f* indicates figures, and *t* indicates tables.